Progress in
Cancer Research and Therapy
Volume 14

HORMONES AND CANCER

Progress in Cancer Research and Therapy

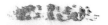

Progress in
Cancer Research and Therapy
Volume 14

Hormones and Cancer

Editors

Stefano Iacobelli

Laboratory of Molecular Endocrinology
S. Cuore Catholic University
Rome, Italy

R. J. B. King

Hormone Biochemistry Department
Imperial Cancer Research Fund
London, England

Hans R. Lindner

Department of Hormone Research
The Weizmann Institute of Science
Rehovot, Israel

Marc E. Lippman

Medicine Branch
National Cancer Institute
National Institutes of Health
Bethesda, Maryland, U.S.A.

Raven Press ■ New York

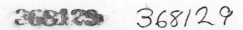

Raven Press, 1140 Avenue of the Americas, New York, New York 10036

Great care has been taken to maintain the accuracy of the information contained in the volume. However, Raven Press cannot be held responsible for errors or for any consequences arising from the use of the information contained herein.

Library of Congress Cataloging in Publication Data

Main entry under title:

Hormones and cancer.

    (Progress in cancer research and therapy; v. 14)
    Includes bibliographical references and index.
    1. Cancer—Congresses. 2. Hormones—Congresses.
3. Hormone receptors—Congresses. I. Iacobelli,
Stefano. II. Series. [DNLM: 1. Hormones—
Pharmacodynamics—Congresses. 2. Neoplasms—
Physiopathology—Congresses. W1 PR667M v. 14/QZ200
H812 1979]
RC261.A2H67   616.99′4   79-5292
ISBN 0-89004-486-4

Preface

Those individuals charged with the responsibility for the primary care of the cancer patient and those searching for new clues to the essential nature of the disease must keep abreast of developments in a wide range of scientific disciplines. Conversely, the phenomenon of malignancy, i.e., the escape from the controls normally governing cell proliferation and differentiation, has become the legitimate concern of students of almost every branch of regulatory biology. This overlap of interests is particularly evident in the fields of oncology and endocrinology, with respect to both the clinical and the basic aspects of the disciplines, as hormones do have striking effects on both the rate of proliferation and the degree of differentiation of many cell types. Also, some of the classic "target organs" of hormones, such as the breast, the prostate, or the lymphatic system, seem particularly prone to malignant change in man.

Information on the mode of action of hormones at the level of the cell membrane and at the level of the genome has been accumulating at a staggering rate. Some of this information has had significant, although thus far limited, impact on the management of malignant disease. Hormone receptor assays are now considered indispensable for the choice of treatment for those cancers that are potentially amenable to restraint by manipulation of the endocrine milieu, be it by hormone supplementation or hormone deprivation. For the latter purpose, more sophisticated techniques, such as use of the aromatase inhibitors or antagonistic hormone analogs discussed in this volume, may in time supplant mutilating ablative surgery. Beyond their use as prognostic markers, receptors for hormones or for peptide growth factors (in at least some of the more common tumors) may serve to provide a homing signal for cytotoxic drugs linked to the appropriate hormone, so as to ensure selective uptake of the drug by the cancer cell.

The frequent occurrence of ectopic hormone production by tumor cells provides a further topic of common interest to oncologists and endocrinologists. Given the close cooperation of workers in both specialties, this feature can be made into a powerful diagnostic tool, as shown in this volume for the case of lung cancer. The question as to whether hormonal means of fertility control or endocrine replacement therapy for the postmenopausal syndrome may entail increased risk of cancer again properly comes under the joint purview of experts in both fields, as do other epidemiological aspects of hormone-related tumors. Finally, to the pure biologist the cancer cell represents an experiment of nature from which we may learn something about normal control mechanisms, including the mode of hormone action. Hence tumor cell lines find ever-increasing use in endocrine research laboratories.

Clearly, then, increased opportunity for dialogue between oncologists and scientists engaged in hormone research is desirable. This volume recognizes this need and will be of interest to all concerned with treatment of and research on malignancy.

Hans R. Lindner

Acknowledgments

The editors thank the members of the International Scientific Committee and Advisory Board and the Local Organizing Committee for their counsel and devoted work in helping to make the meeting on which this volume is based an exciting event.

Contents

Steroid Antagonists

Clinical Use of Receptor Assay

Predisposing Factors

New Therapeutic Approaches

Contributors

Susan C. Aitken
Medicine Branch
National Cancer Institute
National Institutes of Health
Bethesda, Maryland 20205

A. Amar-Costesec
International Institute of Cellular and
   Molecular Pathology
B-1200 Brussels, Belgium

A. Amsterdam
Department of Hormone Research
The Weizmann Institute of Science
Rehovot, Israel

Péter Arányi
Department of Cell Growth and Regula-
tion
Sidney Farber Cancer Institute
Charles A. Dana Cancer Center
Boston, Massachusetts 02115

Emilio Bajetta
National Tumor Institute
Milan, Italy

Emanuela Bartoccioni
Laboratory of Molecular Endocrinology
S. Cuore Catholic University
00168 Rome, Italy

E. E. Baulieu
Hormone Laboratory
I.N.S.E.R.M. Unit 33
94270 Bicêtre, France

P. A. Bell
Tenovus Institute for Cancer Research
Welsh National School of Medicine
Cardiff CF4 4XX, Wales

Alan Bennett
Department of Surgery
King's College Hospital Medical School
London SE5 8RX, England

D. C. Bennett
The Salk Institute
San Diego, California 92138

Frederick J. Bex
Section of Endocrinology
Wyeth Laboratories, Inc.
Philadelphia, Pennsylvania 19101

Clara D. Bloomfield
Section of Medical Oncology
Department of Medicine
University of Minnesota Health Sciences
   Center
Minneapolis, Minnesota 55455

Gianni Bonadonna
National Tumor Institute
Milan, Italy

J. Bonte
Gynecology Clinics
Saint Rafaël Academic Hospital
University of Louvain
B-3000 Louvain, Belgium

N. M. Borthwick
Tenovus Institute for Cancer Research
Welsh National School of Medicine
Cardiff CF4 4XX, Wales

Suzanne Bourgeois
Regulatory Biology Laboratory
The Salk Institute
San Diego, California 92138

Angela M. H. Brodie
Department of Pharmacology and Experimental Therapeutics
University of Maryland School of Medicine
Baltimore, Maryland 21201

Nicholas Bruchovsky
Department of Cancer Endocrinology
Cancer Control Agency of British Columbia
Vancouver, B.C. V5Z 3J3, Canada

F. Celotti
Department of Endocrinology
University of Milan
20129 Milan, Italy

J. H. Clark
Department of Cell Biology
Baylor College of Medicine
Houston, Texas 77030

Ericque Coezy
Unit of Cellular and Molecular Endocrinology
I.N.S.E.R.M. Unit 148
34100 Montpellier, France

Philip Coffino
Departments of Medicine and Microbiology and Immunology
University of California
San Francisco, California 94143

G. Concolino
Institute of General Clinical Medicine and Medical Therapy V
University of Rome
00100 Rome, Italy

C. Conti
Institute of General Clinical Medicine and Medical Therapy V
University of Rome
00100 Rome, Italy

Alan Corbin
Section of Endocrinology
Wyeth Laboratories, Inc.
Philadelphia, Pennsylvania 19101

J. R. Couchman
Unilever Research
Colworth Laboratory
Sharnbrook, Bedfordshire MK44 1LQ, England

Gerald R. Crabtree
National Cancer Institute
National Institutes of Health
Bethesda, Maryland 20205

Lionel Cusan
MRC Group in Molecular Endocrinology
Le Centre Hospitalier
Laval University
Quebec G1V 4G2, Canada

Erik Dahlberg
Departments of Chemistry and Medical Nutrition
Karolinska Institutet
S-104 01 Stockholm, Sweden

T. C. Dembinski
Tenovus Institute for Cancer Research
Welsh National School of Medicine
Cardiff CF4 4XX, Wales

N. Devleeschouwer
Department of Medicine
Henri Tagnon Laboratory of Clinical Investigation
Jules Bordet Institute
1000 Brussels, Belgium

Giovanni di Fronzo
National Tumor Institute
Milan, Italy

F. Di Silverio
Institute of Clinical Urology
University of Chieti
Chieti, Italy

Jean Djiane
Laboratory of the Physiology of Lactation
National Institute of Agronomy Research
78350 Jouey-en-Josas, France

D. Duval
Department of Physiology and Pharmacology
I.N.S.E.R.M. Unit 7
Necker Hospital
75015 Paris, France

Richard L. Eckert
Departments of Physiology and Biophysics
University of Illinois College of Medicine
Urbana, Illinois 61801

P. M. Edwards
International Institute of Cellular and
Molecular Pathology
B-1200 Brussels, Belgium

Peter Ekman
Department of Urology
Karolinska Hospital
Karolinska Institutet
S-104 01 Stockholm, Sweden

M. El Etr
Hormone Laboratory
I.N.S.E.R.M. Unit 33
94270 Bicêtre, France

M. F. El Etreby
Department of Endocrine Pharmacology
Schering AG
D-1000 Berlin 65, West Germany

Guidalberto Fabris
Institute of Pathology
University of Ferrara
44100 Ferrara, Italy

Alex Ferenczy
Department of Pathology
Sir Mortimer B. Davis Jewish General
Hospital
Montreal, Quebec, Canada

P. Ferraboschi
Department of Endocrinology
University of Milan
20129 Milan, Italy

Glauco Frizzera
Department of Laboratory Medicine and
Pathology
University of Minnesota Health Sciences
Center
Minneapolis, Minnesota 55455

Kazimiera J. Gajl-Peczalska
Department of Laboratory Medicine and
Pathology
University of Minnesota Health Sciences
Center
Minneapolis, Minnesota 55455

Ulrich Gehring
Institute for Biological Chemistry
University of Heidelberg
69 Heidelberg, West Germany

C. Gelly
C.N.R.S. Steroid Hormone Research Unit
Foundation for Hormone Research
75014 Paris, France

Steven Gillis
Hematology Research Laboratory
Department of Medicine
Dartmouth Medical School
Hanover, New Hampshire 03755

D. K. Granner
Departments of Internal Medicine and
Biochemistry
University of Iowa College of Medicine
and
Veterans Administration Hospital
Iowa City, Iowa 52242

K. Griffiths
Tenovus Institute for Cancer Research
Welsh National School of Medicine
Cardiff, CF4 4XX, Wales

G. V. Groom
Tenovus Institute for Cancer Research
Welsh National School of Medicine
Cardiff CF4 4XX, Wales

A. Gulino
C.N.R.S. Steroid Hormone Research Unit
Foundation for Hormone Research
75014 Paris, France

Pietro M. Gullino
Laboratory of Pathophysiology
National Cancer Institute
National Institutes of Health
Bethesda, Maryland 20205

Jan-Åke Gustafsson
Departments of Chemistry and Medical
  Nutrition
Karolinska Institutet
S-104 01 Stockholm, Sweden

Paul Guyre
Departments of Physiology and Medicine
Dartmouth Medical School
Hanover, New Hampshire 03755

G. L. Hammond
Reproductive Endocrinology Center
University of California
San Francisco, California 94143

J. W. Hardin
Department of Cell Biology
Baylor College of Medicine
Houston, Texas 77030

J. M. Harmon
Laboratory of Biochemistry
National Cancer Institute
National Institutes of Health
Bethesda, Maryland 20205

J. L. Harousseau
Hematology Service
Saint Louis Hospital
75475 Paris Cedex 10, France

M. E. Harper
Tenovus Institute for Cancer Research
Welsh National School of Medicine
Cardiff CF4 4XX, Wales

James R. Hayes
Department of Physiology and Biophysics
University of Illinois College of Medicine
Urbana, Illinois 61801

J. C. Heuson
Department of Medicine
Henri Tagnon Laboratory of Clinical In-
  vestigation
Jules Bordet Institute
1000 Brussels, Belgium

Laurie Hildebrandt
Department of Medicine
Dartmouth Medical School
Hanover, New Hampshire 03755

D. Hodges
Department of Cell Biology
Baylor College of Medicine
Houston, Texas 77030

Bertil Högberg
Department of Pharmacology
Karolinska Institutet
S-104 01 Stockholm, Sweden

F. Homo
Department of Physiology and Pharmacol-
  ogy
I.N.S.E.R.M. Unit 7
Necker Hospital
75015 Paris, France

Stefano Iacobelli
Laboratory of Molecular Endocrinology
S. Cuore Catholic University
00168 Rome, Italy

V. H. T. James
Department of Chemical Pathology
St. Mary's Hospital Medical School
London W2 1PG, England

Ethel Joly
Unit of Cellular and Molecular Endocri-
    nology
I.N.S.E.R.M. Unit 148
34100 Montpellier, France

Benita S. Katzenellenbogen
Department of Physiology and Biophysics
University of Illinois
Urbana, Illinois 61801

John A. Katzenellenbogen
Department of Chemistry
University of Illinois College of Medicine
Urbana, Illinois 61801

Alvin M. Kaye
Department of Hormone Research
The Weizmann Institute of Science
Rehovot, Israel

Paul A. Kelly
MRC Group in Molecular Endocrinology
Le Centre Hospitalier
Laval University
Quebec G1V 4G2, Canada

John H. Kersey
Department of Laboratory Medicine and
    Pathology
University of Minnesota Health Sciences
    Center
Minneapolis, Minnesota 55455

W. R. Kidwell
Laboratory of Pathophysiology
National Cancer Institute
National Institutes of Health
Bethesda, Maryland 20205

R. J. B. King
Hormone Biochemistry Department
Imperial Cancer Research Fund
London WC2A 3PX, England

R. Kling
Department of Cell Biology
Baylor College of Medicine
Houston, Texas 77030

F. Kohen
Department of Hormone Research
The Weizmann Institute of Science
Rehovot, Israel

P. H. Kohn
Medicine Branch
National Cancer Institute
National Institutes of Health
Bethesda, Maryland 20205

Fernand Labrie
MRC Group in Molecular Endocrinology
Le Centre Hospitalier
Laval University
Quebec G1V 4G2, Canada

G. Leclercq
Department of Medicine
Henri Tagnon Laboratory of Clinical In-
    vestigation
Jules Bordet Institute
1000 Brussels, Belgium

N. Legros
Department of Medicine
Henri Tagnon Laboratory of Clinical In-
    vestigation
Jules Bordet Institute
1000 Brussels, Belgium

M. Liberti
Institute of Clinical Urology
University of Rome
00100 Rome, Italy

H. R. Lindner
Department of Hormone Research
The Weizmann Institute of Science
Rehovot, Israel

Marc E. Lippman
Medicine Branch
National Cancer Institute
National Institutes of Health
Bethesda, Maryland 20205

Ivan S. Login
Department of Neurology
University of Virginia School of Medicine
Charlottesville, Virginia 22908

Paola Longo
Laboratory of Molecular Endocrinology
S. Cuore Catholic University
00168 Rome, Italy

Robert T. Lyons
The E. Henry Keutman Laboratories
Division of Endocrinology and Metabolism
Department of Medicine
University of Rochester School of Medicine
   and Dentistry
Rochester, New York 14642

Robert M. MacLeod
Department of Medicine
University of Virginia School of Medicine
Charlottesville, Virginia 22908

Raffaella Malandrino
Institute of Clinical Pediatrics
S. Cuore Catholic University
00168 Rome, Italy

Elisabetta Marchetti
Institute of Pathology
University of Ferrara
44100 Ferrara, Italy

Paolo Marchetti
Laboratory of Molecular Endocrinology
S. Cuore Catholic University
00168 Rome, Italy

A. Marocchi
Institute of General Clinical Medicine and
   Medical Therapy V
University of Rome
00100 Rome, Italy

Luciano Martini
Department of Endocrinology
University of Milan
20129 Milan, Italy

Andrea Marzola
Institute of Pathology
University of Ferrara
44100 Ferrara, Italy

Renato Mastrangelo
Institute of Clinical Pediatrics
S. Cuore Catholic University
00168 Rome, Italy

S. A. McCormack
Department of Cell Biology
Baylor College of Medicine
Houston, Texas 77030

William L. McGuire
Department of Medicine/Oncology
University of Texas Health Science Center
San Antonio, Texas 78284

M. E. Monaco
Department of Physiology and Biophysics
New York University School of Medicine
New York, New York 10016

R. Enzio Müller
Department of Biochemistry
Boston University School of Medicine
Boston, Massachusetts 02188

Allan Munck
Department of Physiology
Dartmouth Medical School
Hanover, New Hampshire 03755

Ivan Nagy
Department of Medicine
University of Virginia School of Medicine
Charlottesville, Virginia 22908

P. Negri-Cesi
Department of Endocrinology
University of Milan
20129 Milan, Italy

Italo Nenci
Institute of Pathology
University of Ferrara
44100 Ferrara, Italy

F. Neumann
Research Laboratories
Schering AG
D-1000 Berlin 65, West Germany

Ronald F. Newby
Regulatory Biology Laboratory
The Salk Institute
San Diego, California 92138

B. L. Nguyen
C.N.R.S. Steroid Hormone Research Unit
Foundation for Hormone Research
75014 Paris, France

Mary L. Nicholson
The E. Henry Keutman Laboratories
Division of Endocrinology and Metabolism
Department of Medicine
University of Rochester School of Medicine
and Dentistry
Rochester, New York 14642

J. A. Nisker
Reproductive Endocrinology Center
University of California
San Francisco, California 94143

M. R. Norman
Department of Chemical Pathology
King's College Hospital Medical School
London, England

J. R. Pasqualini
C.N.R.S. Steroid Hormone Research Unit
Foundation for Hormone Research
75014 Paris, France

W. B. Peeling
Department of Urology
St. Woolos Hospital
Newport, Gwent, Wales

Bruce A. Peterson
Section of Medical Oncology
Department of Medicine
University of Minnesota Health Sciences
Center
Minneapolis, Minnesota 55455

Åke Pousette
Departments of Chemistry and Medical
Nutrition
Karolinska Institutet
S-104 01 Stockholm, Sweden

Franco O. Ranelletti
Institute of Histology and Embryology
S. Cuore Catholic University
00168 Rome, Italy

M. J. Reed
Department of Chemical Pathology
St. Mary's Hospital Medical School
London W2 1PG, England

Nachum Reiss
Department of Hormone Research
The Weizmann Institute of Science
Rehovot, Israel

Paul S. Rennie
Department of Cancer Endocrinology
Cancer Control Agency of British Colum-
bia
Vancouver, B.C. V5Z 3J3, Canada

David W. Robertson
Department of Chemistry
University of Illinois
Urbana, Illinois 61801

Henri Rochefort
Unit of Cellular and Molecular Endocrinology
I.N.S.E.R.M. Unit 148
34100 Montpellier, France

Eugene Rosanoff
Section of Virology
Wyeth Laboratories, Inc.
Philadelphia, Pennsylvania 19101

G. G. Rousseau
International Institute of Cellular and
Molecular Pathology
B-1200 Brussels, Belgium

P. S. Rudland
The Ludwig Institute for Cancer Research
Royal Marsden Hospital
Sutton, Surrey, England

Gordon H. Sato
Biology Department
University of California, San Diego
La Jolla, California 92093

T. J. Schmidt
Fels Research Institute
Temple University Medical School
Philadelphia, Pennsylvania 19140

S. Schorderet Slatkine
Department of Obstetrics and Gynecology
University of Geneva
Geneva, Switzerland

Carl Séguin
MRC Group in Molecular Endocrinology
Le Centre Hospitalier
Laval University
Quebec G1V 4G2, Canada

Theodor K. Shnitka
Department of Pathology
University of Alberta
Edmonton, Alberta T6G 2G3, Canada

P. E. C. Sibley
Tenovus Institute for Cancer Research
Welsh National School of Medicine
Cardiff CF4 4XX, Wales

P. K. Siiteri
Reproductive Endocrinology Center
University of California
San Francisco, California 94143

Kendall A. Smith
Hematology Research Laboratory
Department of Medicine
Dartmouth Medical School
Hanover, New Hampshire 03755

Marek Snochowski
Polish Academy of Sciences
Warsaw, Poland

Frank A. Snyder
Department of Medicine
University of Virginia School of Medicine
Charlottesville, Virginia 22908

J. S. Strobl
Medicine Branch
National Cancer Institute
National Institutes of Health
Bethesda, Maryland 20205

C. Sumida
C.N.R.S. Steroid Hormone Research Unit
Foundation for Hormone Research
75014 Paris, France

Gabriele Tancini
National Tumor Institute
Milan, Italy

J. Tardy
C.N.R.S. Steroid Hormone Research Unit
Foundation for Hormone Research
75014 Paris, France

Tochiro Tatee
Department of Chemistry
University of Illinois
Urbana, Illinois 61801

R. Tenaglia
Institute of Clinical Urology
University of Rome
00100 Rome, Italy

C. Thierry
Department of Immunopharmacology of
*   Tumors*
Paul Lamarque Center
St. Eloi Hospital
34059 Montpellier, France

E. Brad Thompson
Laboratory of Biochemistry
National Cancer Institute
National Institutes of Health
Bethesda, Maryland 20205

Abdulmaged Traish
Department of Biochemistry
Boston University School of Medicine
Boston, Massachusetts 02188

Lucile Turcot-Lemay
MRC Group in Molecular Endocrinology
Le Centre Hospitalier
Laval University
Quebec G1V 4G2, Canada

Ten-lin S. Tsai
Department of Physiology and Biophysics
University of Illinois
Urbana, Illinois 61801

Carlos A. Valdenegro
Department of Medicine
University of Virginia School of Medicine
Charlottesville, Virginia 22908

M. Verhaegen
International Institute of Cellular and
 Molecular Pathology
B-1200 Brussels, Belgium

Françoise Vignon
I.N.S.E.R.M. Unit 148
34100 Montpellier, France

Bruce P. Voris
The E. Henry Keutman Laboratories
Division of Endocrinology and Metabolism
Department of Medicine
University of Rochester School of Medicine
 and Dentistry
Rochester, New York 14642

M. J. Warburton
The Ludwig Institute for Cancer Research
Royal Marsden Hospital
Sutton, Surrey, England

Bruce Westley
Unit of Cellular and Molecular Endocri-
 nology
I.N.S.E.R.M. Unit 148
34100 Montpellier, France

H. Herbert Wotiz
Department of Biochemistry
Boston University School of Medicine
Boston, Massachusetts 02188

Jean Yates
Hormone Biochemistry Department
Imperial Cancer Research Fund
London WC2A 3PX, England

Donald A. Young
The E. Henry Keutman Laboratories
Division of Endocrinology and Metabolism
Department of Medicine
University of Rochester School of Medicine
 and Dentistry
Rochester, New York 14642

JoAnn Zaleskas
Section of Medical Oncology
Department of Medicine
University of Minnesota Health Sciences
 Center
Minneapolis, Minnesota 55455

Hormone Action in Normal and Neoplastic Tissues: Sex Steroids

Hormones and Cancer, edited by S. Iacobelli et al.
Raven Press, New York © 1980.

Estrogen and Antiestrogen Effects on Thymidine Utilization by MCF-7 Human Breast Cancer Cells in Tissue Culture

Marc E. Lippman and Susan C. Aitken

Medicine Branch, National Cancer Institute, National Institutes of Health, Bethesda, Maryland 20205

While incorporation of radioactive thymidine into acid-insoluble material is probably the most common method employed to estimate DNA synthesis, it may lead to erroneous conclusions. Conflicting data on the effects of estrogen on proliferation in MCF-7 cells made us wonder whether a more detailed analysis of precursor incorporation might elucidate some of the problems. A number of serious difficulties complicate the interpretation of incorporation data using this high specific activity trace.

First, the accurate determination of the true specific activity of labeled precursor in every experimental situation is critical.

Second, feedback (both positive and negative) by thymidine on a variety of key enzymatic steps in pyrimidine synthesis which affect its own utilization can occur. This is further complicated by the fact that intracellular-thymidine pools are relatively small. Consequently, addition of even small amounts of trace may seriously perturb the experimental system.

Third, deoxynucleotide pools may be compartmentalized intracellularly and differential incorporation of salvage and *de novo* derived thymidine may prevent legitimate projections to net DNA synthetic rates.

Fourth, and finally it is possible that metabolism of labeled precursor to products capable of eventual incorporation into material which is not DNA may occur.

The experiments summarized here are directed toward an accurate assessment of the role of the salvage pathway of pyrimidine synthesis and utilization in the response of the MCF-7 cell line to administration of estrogens and antiestrogens.

MATERIALS AND METHODS

MCF-7 cells, maintained in continuous tissue culture, were repeatedly shown to be free of mycoplasma contamination during this study. Conditions of culture have been previously described (1). Cells underwent two passages in IMEM supplemented with 2.5% charcoal-treated calf serum and 10^{-7} moles/liter insulin prior to replicate plating in four or six well tissue culture dishes. When cells became subconfluent medium was replaced with IMEM containing 10^{-5} moles/ liter phosphate and lacking asparagine. This reduction in phosphate content is necessary to obtain substantial incorporation of $[^{32}P]P_i$ into DNA. These experimental conditions do not affect growth curves or incorporation of radioactive precursors into macromolecular components of MCF-7 cells during the limited duration of these experiments (1). Four to twelve hr later medium was replaced with IMEM (10^{-5} moles/liter P_i), estradiol (5×10^{-9} moles/liter), or tamoxifen (2×10^{-6} moles/liter).

Before harvest, cells were incubated for 6 or 8 hr with $[^{32}P]P_i$ (1 μCi/ml) and/or $[^3H]dThd$ (1–10 μCi/ml, 42–46 μCi/mmole) for a 2-hr period. The necessity for such a labeling procedure lies in the relatively long equilibration period required for $[^{32}P]P_i$ in this experimental system and the known perturbation of the system produced by radioactive thymidine. The details of any given experiment are described in Results.

An outline for the fractionation procedure for cell pellets following harvest can be found in Fig. 1. Detailed validation of fractionation and isolation methodologies will be found elsewhere (1).

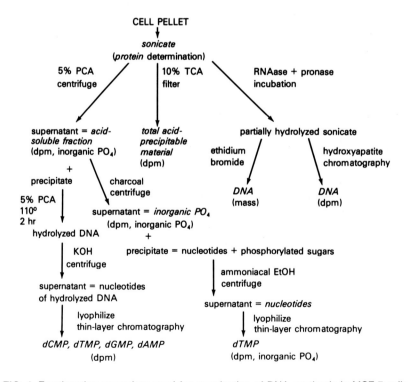

FIG. 1. Fractionation procedure used for examination of DNA synthesis in MCF-7 cells.

PARAMETERS

M	Size of intracellular pool
a	rate of entry of label into intracellular pool
b	rate of exit of label from intracellular pool

VARIABLES

L	dependent variable - amount of label in intracellular pool at any time t
t	independent variable - time after addition of label

EQUATIONS

$L(t) = M + (a-b)t -M(1+((a-b)/M)t)^{(-b/(a-b))}$ condition $a \neq b$

$L(t) = M(1-exp(-at/M))$ condition $a = b$

$S(t) = L(t)/(M + (a-b)t)$ $S = \%$ of pool saturation

FIG. 2. Terms and equations related to kinetic analyses (MLAB) of incorporation data.

Kinetic analyses were based on the determination of radioactivity incorporated into acid-soluble fractions and DNA versus time. The coupling of such experiments with a modified isotope dilution technique (7) and subsequent analysis utilizing the NIH DEC-10 computer system and programming package MLAB (4) as previously described (1) permitted accurate measurement of thymidine pool size and analysis of thymidine kinetics. The parameters employed in the MLAB analysis are shown in Fig. 2. The precise details of such experiments will be presented in Results.

RESULTS

Three conditions are essential to the accurate use of thymidine in monitoring DNA synthetic rates: (a) exogenous dThd must be in equilibrium with intracellular precursor pools; (b) the true specific activity of thymidine in the system must be available; and (c) the perturbation of the system due to addition of trace must be appropriately controlled. A series of experiments relating to each of these conditions will be presented employing MCF-7 human breast cancer cells.

To establish the time required for equilibration of exogenous [³H]dThd with precursor thymidine pools, the time course of incorporation of label into acid-soluble pools (Fig. 3A) and DNA (Fig. 3B) under varying experimental conditions was first examined. At time 0 [³H]dThd was added to all wells and cells harvested at varying times thereafter. The time course of uptake of label into the acid-soluble pool of MCF-7 cells was between 1 and 60 min and is seen

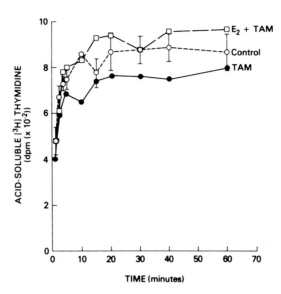

FIG. 3. A: Incorporation of ³H dThd into the acid-soluble pool of MCF-7 cells. Cells were transferred to 10^{-5} moles/liter phosphate medium hormones (10^{-8} moles/liter estradiol, 10^{-8} moles/liter estradiol + 2×10^{-6} moles/liter tamoxifen) 32 hr prior to addition of [³H]dThd (2 μCi/ml). Cells were harvested at the times indicated following addition of label. Values are the mean of two determinations and are normalized per unit protein. Standard deviations are presented only for control cells but did not exceed 10% for any group of samples.

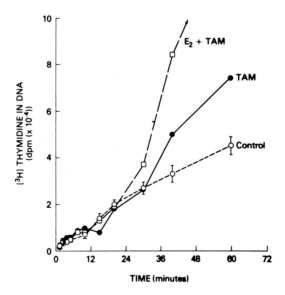

FIG. 3. B: Incorporation of [³H]dThd into DNA of MCF-7 cells. Incorporation into DNA was determined by acid-precipitation on millipore filters. Values were normalized per unit protein and are presented as the mean of two determinations. Standard deviations are shown only for controls but were similar in all experimental groups.

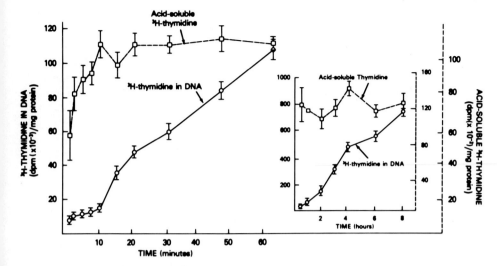

FIG. 3. C: Incorporation of [³H]dThd into DNA and acid-soluble pool of MCF-7 cells. Cells were treated as previously described but were placed in 10^{-5} moles/liter phosphate medium 24 hr prior to addition of [³H]dThd at time 0. Two separate experiments representing a short period of study (1–60 min and a longer time period (0.5–8 hr) are depicted. The latter is shown as an *inset*. In both experiments values are normalized per unit protein and are the average of three determinations ± 1 SD. DNA *(circles)* and acid-soluble *(squares)* fractions were isolated as previously described.

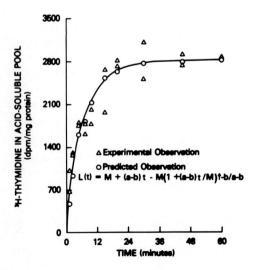

FIG. 3. D: Saturation curve for incorporation of [³H]dThd into acid-soluble pool of MCF-7 cells. Data obtained as described in Fig. 3A (dpm/mg protein) were fitted to the function $L(t) = M + (a - b)t - M(1 + (a - b)t/M)^{(-b/(a-b))}$ employing the computer programming package MLAB as previously described.

in Fig. 3A. Constant radioactivity was observed with 20 min of exposure to radioactive trace. No significant differences in the amount of label accumulating at equilibrium as a consequence of hormone treatment were detected. The incorporation of [³H]dThd into partially purified DNA is presented in Fig. 3B. Incorporation became linear within 20 min, again suggesting that equilibration of the thymidine precursor pool for DNA synthesis had been attained. Figure 3B shows that both estrogen-treated and tamoxifen-treated cells displayed a higher rate of incorporation of dThd into DNA than did control cells. An explanation for this paradoxical observation following tamoxifen treatment—a condition long known to produce inhibition of thymidine incorporation (5,9)—is presented below.

The kinetics of incorporation of thymidine over a more extended time period are shown in Fig. 3C. Equilibrium conditions were maintained for the 8 hr of exposure to trace. Only the results observed in control cells are presented; however, a similar stability was evident in estrogen- and tamoxifen-treated MCF-7 cells. Figures 3A–C show that the 2-hr labeling period (which will be employed in subsequent experiments) satisfies the first condition of this study: equilibration of thymidine precursor pools within the time frame of a given experiment.

The next series of experiments to be discussed involve detailed kinetic analysis of thymidine pools employing three distinct analytic techniques: (a) MLAB (4); (b) linear regression analysis of incorporation into acid-soluble pools and DNA; and (c) a modified isotope dilution procedure (7). The MLAB computer programming package for graphic display and modeling of kinetic data and the equations developed by Cooper for two compartment systems (2) constitute the first approach to the complex issue of thymidine pools. MCF-7 cells are experimentally treated as previously described. The incorporation of label into the acid-soluble pool of control cells versus time (1–60 min) is fit to a function representing a two compartment system in which rate of entry and exit of label are approximately equal. Such a fit is shown in Fig. 3D for untreated MCF-7 cells. The excellent fit of data and function suggest that this program can yield significant information on the utilization of exogenous thymidine through the salvage pathway in MCF-7 cells. The parameters that can be defined by such computer assisted analysis (Fig. 2) include pool size (M) and rate of entry (a) and exit (b) of thymidine from the total acid-soluble pool.

Linear regression analysis can also be applied to incorporation data for label in acid-soluble pools and DNA versus time (Fig. 3A and 3B). The slopes of these lines (dpm/min) indicate the rate of incorporation of label. In the case of the acid-soluble pool, the initial velocity of the incorporation is of interest and only the earliest time points can be employed. In the case of incorporation into DNA, only the period of linearity at later time points is of interest.

However, neither MLAB analysis nor the linear regression analysis of incorporation data can establish pool parameters in terms of actual mass of thymidine in the absence of information on the effective specific activity of [³H]dThd in (a) the extracellular environment and (b) the intracellular pool. In order to investigate this question a modified isotope dilution technique (7) can be applied to the MCF-7 cell system. The basis of such an analysis is the ability of preexisting thymidine pools to compete with added labeled thymidine with respect to incorporation into a given end-product. Generally, three to four concentrations of thymidine are utilized in any given experiment. Cells are harvested after exogenous thymidine has equilibrated with intracellular precursor pools for DNA and the radioactivity in the acid-soluble pool and DNA is determined. Application of the equation presented in the legend of Table 1 to the acid-soluble pool provides an index of the extracellular competitive pool for thymidine incorporation. Applying this analysis to incorporation into DNA provides estimates of actual intracellular pool size. Table 1 demonstrates results obtained in control MCF-7 cells. These results suggest that substantial amounts of thymidine are available both extra- and intracellularly and that there is considerable variation in pool size over time in serum-free medium. The fact that addition of labeled thymidine in the range of 1 to 2 μCi (2–5×10^{-8} moles/liter) constitutes only 5 to 10% of total thymidine incorporated into intracellular pools and DNA suggests that [³H]dThd incorporation is likely to provide highly inaccurate estimates of actual rates of DNA synthesis in the absence of information on the condition of said pools. It should be pointed out that IMEM contains no thymidine and that the charcoal-treated calf serum has negligible residual nucleoside.

Hormonal influences on thymidine pool kinetics were studied at 24, 36, and 48 hr after estrogen or tamoxifen treatment. These studies represent separate

TABLE 1. *Effective intracellular and extracellular pools of dThd*

Time (hr)	Extracellular pool (moles/liter)	Intracellular pool (moles/liter)	Protein (mg)
0	2.38×10^{-6}	6.30×10^{-8}	0.783
12	2.30×10^{-6}	1.67×10^{-7}	0.804
24	3.59×10^{-6}	6.38×10^{-7}	0.998
36	8.36×10^{-7}	7.12×10^{-7}	1.299
48	7.18×10^{-7}	5.67×10^{-7}	1.089

MCF-7 cells were replicately plated as previously described. Eight hours before time 0 cells were transferred to 10^{-5} moles/liter phosphate medium. Medium was again replaced 1 hr before time 0. [³H]dThd (10 μCi/ml, 1 hr) was added with varying amounts of unlabeled dThd to achieve estimated extracellular molarities of 2×10^{-7}, 5×10^{-7}, or 10^{-6} moles/liter 1 hr before harvest. Cells were harvested at the times indicated (column 1) and aliquots were taken for determination of acid-soluble radioactivity (column 2), acid-precipitable radioactivity (column 3), and protein (column 4). Values for incorporation were normalized per unit protein. The effective pool size was determined according to Scudiero et al. (7) as follows:

T_1 = lower concentration of dThd
T_2 = Higher concentration of dThd
Q = ratio of label incorporated at concentration T_1 and T_2 (cpm 1/cpm 2)

Then P (effective pool size) $+ (T_2 - (T_1 \times Q))/(Q - 1)$

experiments in which the incorporation of [³H]dThd into the acid-soluble pool and DNA of MCF-7 cells were determined as a function of time of exposure to trace (1–60 min) and in which cells were additionally exposed to varying concentrations of dThd (2×10^{-8}, 5×10^{-8}, 10^{-6}, and 2×10^{-6} moles/liter) for a constant period of time (60 min). Coupling of experimental results employing MLAB, linear regression, and isotope dilution (described above) allows a rigorous analysis of thymidine pools and permits determination of whether extracellular salvage or intracellular dThd is primarily utilized in DNA synthesis. The parameters that can be estimated by this methodology are presented in Table 2. The contributions of extracellular salvage-derived thymidine to net DNA synthesis (b(s)/b) and to intracellular pools (a(s)/a) are of particular interest. These methods do not allow a breakdown of intracellular dThd into (thymidine derived from internal breakdown of DNA) or from the reduction and methylation of uridine derived from turnover of RNA. The term "salvage"

TABLE 2. *Significance and derivation of parameters utilized in analysis of thymidine pools in MCF-7 cells*

Parameter	Significance	Method of determination
1. M	Intracellular pool size (pmoles)	MLAB kinetic analysis [dpm/(spec. act. × ECDF × IDCF)]
2. L	[³H]dThd component of intracellular pool (pmoles)	MLAB kinetic analysis [dpm/spec. act.]
3. a	Rate of entrance of dThd into intracellular pool (pmoles/min)	MLAB kinetic analysis [dpm/(spec. act. × ECDF × ICDF)]
4. a(s)	Rate of entrance of extracellular dThd into intracellular pool (pmoles/min)	Slope of line for incorporation of [³H]dThd into acid-soluble pool [dpm/(spec. act. × ECDF)]
5. a(s)/a	Percent of dThd entering the intracellular pool from extracellular sources	Ratio of parameters 3 and 4
6. ECDF	Factor by which [³H]dThd is diluted by extracellular dThd in medium	Method of Scudiero et al. (7) (isotope dilution)
7. b	Rate of exit of dThd from extracellular pool (pmoles/min)	MLAB kinetic analysis [dpm/(spec. act. × ECDF × ICDF)]
8. b(d)	Rate of incorporation of dThd into DNA (pmoles/min)	Slope of line for incorporation of ³H dThd into DNA [(spec. act. × ECDF × IDCF)]
9. b(m)	Rate of loss of dThd from intracellular pool due to metabolism (pmoles/min)	b − b(d) (parameters 7 and 8)
10. b(s)	Rate of incorporation of extracellular dThd into DNA (pmoles/min)	Slope of line for incorporation of [³H]dThd into DNA [dpm/(spec. act. × ECDF)]
11. b(s)/b(d)	Percent of dThd in DNA derived from extracellular sources	Ratio of parameters 10 and 8
12. ICDF	Factor by which [³H]dThd is diluted by intracellular sources of dThd	Method of Scudiero et al. (7) (isotope dilution)

refers to the capacity of MCF-7 cells to respond to the availability of pyrimidine during a 1- to 2-hr period and does not suggest that the ultimate source of thymidine is other than *de novo* synthesis prior to this labeling period.

The results of the study are presented in Table 3. Parameters are shown in column 1. Values are shown for control, tamoxifen-treated, and estrogen-treated cells at 24, 36, and 48 hr. Units are picomoles and picomoles per minute per unit protein. M (pool size) size is presented in row 1. At all times after tamoxifen treatment, pool size was reduced to 20 to 25% of control levels. In contrast, estrogen + tamoxifen administration increased thymidine pool size two- to threefold over controls. L (accumulation of added trace in the intracellular pool) was only slightly (30%) increased by estrogen treatment at 24, 36, and 48-hr time points. Tamoxifen had little effect on the accumulation of label at either time. These data suggest that the ability to accumulate exogenous thymidine in intracellular pools is not significantly affected by tamoxifen treatment.

The rates of entry of total thymidine (a, row 3) and of extracellular thymidine [a(s), row 4] were dramatically affected by hormonal manipulation. Estrogen increased total thymidine synthesis two- to threefold whereas tamoxifen produced a 15 to 30% decrease below control rates, indicating that some fundamental process in thymidine synthesis is sensitive to hormonal manipulation. The rate of extracellular salvage uptake of dThd was increased 24 hr after estrogen administration, unaltered at 36 hr and decreased at 48 hr. Tamoxifen decreased the rate of thymidine uptake at 24- and 48-hr time points. On examining the ratio of the extracellular contribution to total thymidine synthesis [a(s)/a, row 5] it is apparent that the salvage component decreases with incubation time and estrogen treatment to as little as 5% of the total pool. However, in tamoxifen-treated cells salvage dThd represents 60 to 70% of thymidine synthesis, suggesting that the essential lesion in thymidine synthesis may lie in the *de novo* pathway.

The extracellular dilution factor (ECDF, row 6) is the ratio of total thymidine available in the medium to the mass of trace added and is a correction factor in conversion of radioactivity (dpm) to mass units. The intracellular dilution factor (ICDF, row 12) is the ratio of total intracellular dThd to total extracellular dThd and is utilized in a similar fashion. Comparing experimental groups with respect to these factors provides immediate information on relative extra- and intracellular pool sizes. The extracellular pools (row 6) do not appear to vary greatly with hormonal treatment. However, intracellular pools (row 12) are uniformly increased by estrogen treatment and decreased by exposure to tamoxifen. The method of establishing these ratios is based on the ability of existing pools to compete with the incorporation of [^{3}H]dThd at the rate-limiting step in incorporation. Thus, the ECDF may be an overestimate, particularly if deoxycytidine and deoxyuridine compete for a rate-limiting step in incorporation into the acid-soluble pool.

Examination of the rate of exit of total thymidine from the intracellular pool, (b, row 7) reveals a substantial estrogen-produced stimulation (two- to threefold) and a tamoxifen inhibition of approximately 60%. The amount of thymidine

TABLE 3. Hormonal influence on dThd pools and kinetics in MCF-7 cells

Parameters	24 hr			36 hr			48 hr		
	C	TAM	E_2 + TAM	C	TAM	E_2 + TAM	C	TAM	E_2 + TAM
1. M	20.60	4.64	52.30	18.70	6.76	32.40	26.30	6.76	65.90
2. L	3.59	2.69	4.55	3.40	3.90	4.60	4.68	5.09	5.10
3. a	3.85	1.05	11.73	1.40	0.72	3.72	8.68	1.11	15.40
4. a(s)	1.41	0.76	4.50	0.34	0.37	0.28	1.22	0.67	0.05
5. a(s)/a	0.37	0.72	0.34	0.25	0.51	0.08	0.14	0.61	0.05
6. ECDF	2.30	2.30	3.10	4.08	3.27	3.56	1.81	1.82	2.45
7. b	3.68	1.00	11.16	1.36	1.24	7.21	8.69	2.04	17.49
8. b(d)	3.40	0.84	5.86	0.42	0.41	2.29	1.22	0.50	7.29
9. b(m)	0.28	0.16	5.30	0.95	0.84	4.92	7.47	1.54	10.20
10. b(s)	0.60	0.67	2.22	0.18	0.27	0.61	0.39	0.68	1.36
11. b(s)/b(d)	0.18	0.80	0.42	0.43	0.66	0.22	0.32	1.00	0.19
12. ICDF	2.50	0.75	3.71	2.32	1.52	3.75	3.12	0.73	5.37

Cells were transferred to 10^{-5} moles/liter phosphate medium 8 hr before time 0. At time 0 medium was again replaced and estradiol (10^{-8} moles/liter) and tamoxifen (TAM) (2×10^{-6} moles/liter) were added as indicated. Thirty and sixty minutes prior to harvest, (24, 36, and 48 hr after hormonal treatment as indicated above), a minimum of three different concentrations of [^{3}H]dThd between 2×10^{-6} and 2×10^{-7} moles/liter were added to incubation wells. Concomitantly, a time course of incorporation (1–60 min) was conducted employing a single concentration of [^{3}H]dThd. The computer programming package MLAB (4) was utilized as previously described to obtain estimates for M, L, a, and b. The rates of incorporation of label into acid-soluble pools, a(s), and into DNA, b(d), were obtained by least squares regression analysis as the slopes of the lines for incorporation versus time. The method of Scudiero et al. (7) was employed to obtain factors for the dilution of the initial specific activity of [^{3}H]dThd by extracellular pools (ECDF) and intracellular pools (ICDF). Conversion of all data from dpm to mass units was based on the initial known specific activity of [^{3}H]dThd (46 Ci/mmole = 110 dpm/fmole) and application of appropriate dilution factors. All values were normalized per unit protein. In all cases multiple determinations were performed and the standard deviations of the reported values were within 15%. The 24-, 36-, and 48-hr studies represent independent experiments. C, control.

lost via incorporation of DNA [b(d), row 8] is similarly affected by hormonal administration. This parameter is one of key interest, providing the actual values for rate of net DNA synthesis and the standard against which breakdown into extracellular salvage and intracellular components must be conducted. It provides the most accurate estimate of DNA synthesis. Tamoxifen inhibition is clearly seen here as is a clear-cut estrogen stimulation. The portion of thymidine derived from extracellular sources and incorporated into DNA [b(s)] is seen in row 10. Both estrogen and tamoxifen increase this parameter. However, this salvage component comprised almost all dThd incorporated into DNA in tamoxifen-treated samples [b(s)/b(d), row 11]. Estrogen increased relative salvage utilization at 24 hr but decreased this ratio after 48 hr.

The second major route by which thymidine may exit the total acid-soluble pool is via metabolism (dephosphorylation, or catabolism to β-aminoisobutyric acid). It appears that a substantial proportion of the thymidine pool is lost through this mechanism [b(m), row 9].

In summary it appears that the pattern of thymidine synthesis and utilization varies considerably with both hormonal treatment and time. Tamoxifen treatment sharply decreases whereas estrogen increases the size of intracellular dThd pools. Apparent increases in incorporation of [³H]dThd (dpm) into DNA following tamoxifen administration reflect an effective increase in specific activity relative to controls rather than a true increase in DNA synthesis as would be falsely concluded from a cursory inspection of raw incorporation data (dpm in DNA). Indeed, tamoxifen profoundly decreases the actual mass of dThd incorporated into DNA. Careful analysis suggests that the paradoxical stimulation of [³H]dThd incorporation into DNA observed here after tamoxifen administration is a result of depletion of intracellular pools following a cessation of intracellular *(de novo)* thymidine synthesis. On the other hand, the stimulatory effects of estrogen are greatly augmented when appropriate corrections for dilution of exogenous label by preexisting pools are applied. It should also be noted that the percentage of extracellular dThd in the acid-soluble pool (row 5) is significantly lower than the percentage in DNA (row 11), suggesting that salvage-derived dThd may be preferentially used in DNA synthesis and that intracellular compartmentalization of *de novo* and salvage thymidine is possible.

Concentrations of dThd in the range of anticipated pool sizes were used in order to obtain accurate isotope dilution estimates. These concentrations of thymidine are considerably higher (5–10 μCi/ml) than those generally used in thymidine incorporation studies and may have contributed to the disparity between the tamoxifen stimulation of [³H]dThd incorporation observed here and previous reports (5,9). Thus, we asked whether hormonal treatment and available dThd concentration constituted independent experimental variables (Table 4). Values observed in control samples were taken as 1.00 and other experimental groups were adjusted accordingly. The observed stimulation of [³H]dThd incorporation into DNA by tamoxifen is dependent on thymidine concentration. Inhibition was seen at low levels of added label. After correction

TABLE 4. Effects of varying thymidine concentration on rates of thymidine incorporation into DNA in control and hormone-treated cells

Time (hr)	Group	dThd pool (moles/liter)	[³H]dThd incorporation into DNA			
			1 µCi/ml	2 µCi/ml	5 µCi/ml	10 µCi/ml
24	Control	0.256	1.00 ± 0.02	1.00 ± 0.10	1.00 ± 0.04	1.00 ± 0.10
	TAM	0.066	0.67 ± 0.08	0.69 ± 0.01	1.27 ± 0.33	1.44 ± 0.11
			0.17 ± 0.03	*0.18 ± 0.01*	*0.33 ± 0.08*	*0.37 ± 0.03*
	E₂ + TAM	0.980	0.94 ± 0.06	1.63 ± 0.05	2.25 ± 0.71	1.79 ± 0.39
			3.59 ± 0.23	*6.24 ± 0.39*	*8.61 ± 2.72*	*6.85 ± 1.49*
32	Control	0.111	1.00 ± 0.02	1.00 ± 0.06	1.00 ± 0.03	1.00 ± 0.02
	TAM	0.044	0.67 ± 0.08	1.22 ± 0.08	1.65 ± 0.44	1.35 ± 0.16
			0.27 ± 0.03	*0.48 ± 0.03*	*0.65 ± 0.17*	*0.53 ± 0.06*
	E₂ + TAM	0.448	1.38 ± 0.07	2.24 ± 0.09	2.22 ± 0.09	2.51 ± 0.57
			5.57 ± 0.49	*9.18 ± 0.37*	*9.09 ± 0.37*	*10.28 ± 0.33*

MCF-7 cells were transferred to 10^{-5} moles/liter phosphate medium 8 hr before time 0. At time 0 medium was again replaced and hormonal additions performed. [³H]dThd was added as indicated 2 hr before harvest. Total acid-precipitable radioactivity was determined as previously described. All values represent the mean of three independent determinations ± 1 SD and were normalized per unit protein. The time after hormone treatment at which cells were harvested is presented in column 1. Column 2 represents the experimental treatments. Column 3 displays the pool size of dThd as estimated according to Scudiero et al. (7). Columns 4–7 present the ratios of incorporated label [dpm[³H]dThd] to label in control cells at varying added concentrations of labeled [³H]dThd. The ratios of incorporated label (mass) following correction for variation in dilution of specific activity due to endogenous pools of dThd (column 3) are presented in italic.

for specific activity, tamoxifen was inhibitory (values in italics) regardless of thymidine concentration. Estrogen stimulation was greater when concentrations of [³H]dThd in excess of 2×10^{-8} moles/liter of thymidine were employed, suggesting that stimulation at these time points is at least partially dependent on the amount of available exogenous dThd. Following correction for actual specific activity, estrogen stimulation was greatly enhanced.

In order to more firmly establish the actual relationship of salvage and net DNA synthesis and to further illustrate the difficulties associated with the interpretation of [³H]dThd incorporation, an experiment employing [³²P]P$_i$ as an index of net DNA synthesis was conducted. The experimental conditions under which ³²P incorporation truly reflects net DNA synthesis are not reviewed at this time (1).

Figure 4A shows the pattern of estrogen stimulation of net DNA synthesis (phosphate) and the salvage pathway ([³H]dThd) in MCF-7 cells versus incubation time. Distinct peaks of DNA synthesis occur (24 and 48 hr), only the first of which is detectable by measuring [³H]dThd incorporation. The ability of estrogen to increase incorporation of extracellular salvage thymidine is limited to early incubation times and is associated with the general entrance of cells into DNA synthesis (S phase). The pattern of change of extra- and intracellular thymidine pools (data not shown) is clearly associated with the time of entrance of cells into S.

Figure 4B illustrates the relationship between salvage utilization of [³H]dThd and net DNA synthesis (phosphate incorporation) following administration of tamoxifen. The tremendous increase in incorporation of labeled thymidine is

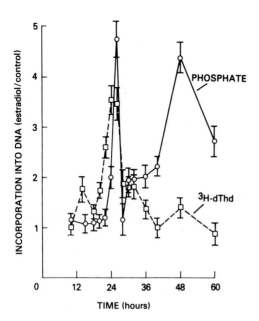

FIG. 4. A: Effect of estradiol on net and salvage DNA synthesis in MCF-7 cells. Cells were transferred to 10^{-5} moles/liter phosphate medium 8 hr before time 0. At time 0 medium $\pm$ 17β-estradiol (5×10^{-9} moles/liter) was again exchanged. Cells were harvested at the times indicated, 6 or 8 hr prior to harvest. [³²P]P$_i$ (1 μCi/ml) was added to samples which were concomitantly labeled with ³²P for 8 hr. DNA and acid-soluble fractions were isolated as previously described. Values for incorporation of ³²P into DNA were corrected to mass units of phosphate incorporated as previously described (1). All data were normalized per unit DNA content. Results are the average of three determinations $\pm$ 1 SD and are presented as the ratio of estrogen-treated to control values.

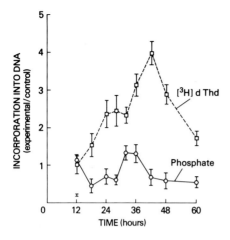

FIG. 4. B: Effect of tamoxifen on net and salvage DNA synthesis in MCF-7 cells.

not correlated with the pattern of net DNA synthesis, which is inhibited to approximately 50% of controls. Increases in incorporation of [³H]dThd vary due to relative increases in intracellular specific activity of [³H]dThd in tamoxifen-treated cells, not an increase in salvage activity.

In summary it can be seen that estradiol and the antiestrogen tamoxifen exert powerful regulatory effects on thymidine synthesis and DNA synthesis in the MCF-7 cell line. Cells preferentially utilize extracellular sources of thymidine during the early stages of incubation in serum-free medium, but the dependency of DNA synthesis on exogenous sources of dThd is greatly diminished at later times. Administration of estradiol decreases the proportion of thymidine incorporated into DNA via the salvage pathway while increasing intracellular pool size. Absolute amounts of exogenous dThd incorporated are increased by estrogen. In contrast, tamoxifen administration results in drastic drops in intracellular thymidine pools and virtual complete dependence on extracellular sources of thymidine for DNA synthesis. However, the capacity of tamoxifen-treated cells to utilize the salvage pathway of thymidine synthesis is only slightly impaired and can be stimulated over controls thymidine in excess of 10^{-7} moles/liter.

DISCUSSION

The use of thymidine to estimate rates of DNA synthesis involves a number of complex problems. Comparison of the data obtained here with the data from other tissue culture systems suggests that these issues may be equally applicable to the MCF-7 cell line. Exogenous thymidine label added to animal cells in culture has consistently been observed to equilibrate with intracellular pools within 5 to 10 min of addition (6). MCF-7 cells appear to require a somewhat longer period of 15 min for equilibration with the DNA precursor pools. Further, the projections made from isotope dilution studies in MCF-7 cells indicate that the effective pool size of intracellular dThd is in the range of 10^{-6} moles/liter.

Salvage and *de novo* pathways of pyrimidine production have been suggested to have distinct roles in the induction of growth and differentiation processes in a variety of different systems (3,8). At any given time the intracellular pool of thymidine is comprised of thymidine triphosphate (dTTP) derived *de novo* and a supply of precursor available from intracellular RNA metabolism or from extracellular sources such as dead or dying cells or a population of feeder cells. The ability to utilize preformed pyrimidines is a reflection of salvage activity and represents a variable element both *in vitro* and *in vivo*. Even in the absence of exogenous dThd in tissue culture systems, it cannot be assumed that the salvage pathway is nonfunctional and the extent of its contribution cannot be readily assessed. In MCF-7 cells under serum-free conditions a substantial pool (molar) of thymidine appears available for transport and DNA synthesis (Table 3). The method of estimation of this pool is, however, kinetic rather than direct and is consequently dependent on the nucleoside specificity of the rate-limiting step in incorporation into intracellular pools. It also appears that the rate-limiting step in thymidine uptake is significantly modulated by hormonal treatment. Twenty-four hours of estrogen treatment results in two- to threefold increases in rates of uptake of exogenous dThd (Table 3). However, stimulation was not evident at later incubation times and the salvage component of intracellular pools was proportionally less significant. Tamoxifen treatment did not appreciably affect the ability of MCF-7 cells to incorporate exogenous label into acid-soluble pools [Table 3: L, a(s)]. However, it has been previously noted that at very low concentrations of dThd, inhibitory effects of tamoxifen on salvage routes of incorporation are seen.

Comparing the amount of thymidine incorporated into DNA in MCF-7 cells to the amount lost through metabolism [Table 3: b(m)] reveals that the latter is an extremely significant component (40–50%) of the total loss of thymidine from intracellular pools. Potential routes for such loss include dephosphorylation, demethylation to other pyrimidine derivatives, and complete catabolism to β-aminoisobutyric acid. We have no data on the relative importance of these processes in MCF-7 cells. The dephosphorylation mechanism which is known to function in a highly regulatory fashion in other cell systems is of most interest. MCF-7 cells, as previously noted, release large quantities of competitors for thymidine transport into culture medium (Table 1) and by far the most likely route of such release is dephosphorylation (thymidine phosphorylase) to nucleoside derivatives. Estrogen increases both thymidine extracellular pool sizes and thymidine metabolism. Conversely, tamoxifen decreases both pool size and metabolism. It is possible that dephosphorylation of dTTP synthesized *de novo* to extracellular thymidine results in a reservoir which becomes available to cells via the salvage pathway on induction of DNA synthesis but which becomes progressively depleted during the course of DNA synthesis. The capacity of tamoxifen-treated cells to replenish extracellular pools is impaired.

This variation in extracellular dThd concentration in MCF-7 cells may itself constitute a significant regulatory factor in salvage and *de novo* thymidine synthesis. There is abundant evidence that the availability of exogenous dThd affects the relative activity of salvage, *de novo,* and intermediary pathways of pyrimidine synthesis as well as the relative utilization of pyrimidines derived from these respective sources.

The intracellular dThd pool in MCF-7 cells is composed of salvage and *de novo* derived nucleotides. Since repair is less than 1% of replicative DNA synthesis in these cells (1), extracellular scavenger activity constitutes the major portion of the salvage component. Since turnover of uridine from RNA metabolism is very small compared with the enormous background pool of uridine in other cell systems, the capacity of MCF-7 cells to utilize exogenous thymidine may be considered to represent total salvage activity.

Our data suggest that the intracellular thymidine pool in MCF-7 cells may be compartmentalized. The proportion of salvage thymidine incorporated into DNA is up to fourfold greater than the proportion of salvage thymidine incorporated into acid-soluble pools, suggesting that the salvage pathway constitutes a preferential route of DNA synthesis.

Hormonal administration has distinct effects on *de novo* and salvage pool compartments. Estrogen increases total intracellular pool size, net rate of thymidine synthesis, and net rate of DNA synthesis while decreasing the relative contribution of the salvage pathway to all parameters. Moreover, the salvage component becomes less important with incubation time. Estrogen-induced increases in ability to incorporate exogenous dThd is limited to early incubation stages (24–32 hr). Also the increase in extracellular thymidine pools over controls is associated with the early wave of DNA synthesis.

In contrast, tamoxifen administration reduces the size of intra- and extracellular pools, rate of thymidine synthesis, and net rate of DNA synthesis. Cells are entirely dependent on salvage sources of dThd to carry on DNA synthesis. *De novo* synthesis of thymidine is essentially curtailed. These effects are reversible with concomitant administration of estrogen, indicating that nonspecific toxicity is not involved. It is also possible that feedback effects, as discussed above for estrogen, are involved in the maintenance of high levels of salvage activity in tamoxifen-treated cells. Increased incorporation of label versus controls is evident only when exogenous dThd concentrations are relatively high. This implies a decrease in the activity of some rate-limiting protein in the salvage pathway as a consequence of antiestrogen administration.

The significance of information on the status of thymidine pools in any given experimental situation is evident on examining the disparity between the incorporation of [³H]dThd into DNA and net DNA synthesis (phosphate incorporation) in Fig. 4A and B. The correspondence between the discrete period of [³H]dThd incorporation into DNA and net DNA synthesis (24 hr) indicates that the ability of MCF-7 cells to initiate salvage utilization of thymidine is tightly coupled to net DNA synthesis. The ability of MCF-7 cells to increase net DNA synthesis within a 2-hr period of exposure to nucleoside but only at specific incubation times suggests that the cell system is highly synchronized. Apparently, cells are primed to enter S but thymidine availability is limiting. The permissive action of dThd in initiating DNA synthesis in MCF-7 cells suggests that a specific rate-limiting and estrogen-sensitive lesion relating to *de novo* thymidine synthesis is involved in regulation of growth in this cell system.

We conclude that estrogenic effects on growth and DNA synthesis in MCF-7 cells are linked to the *de novo* pathway of thymidine synthesis. The rate-limiting step in estrogen induction of thymidine synthesis is unclear but may be related to activity of intermediary enzymes such as ribonucleotide reductase, deoxycytidine deaminase, or thymidylate synthetase. The capacity to precisely measure net DNA synthesis in this synchronized cell system coupled with ability to identify salvage and *de novo* routes of pyrimidine synthesis may yield significant information mechanisms of growth regulation.

REFERENCES

1. Aitken, S. C., and Lippman, M. E.: *Cancer Res. (submitted).*
2. Cooper, H. L. (1973): *Anal. Biochem.,* 53:49–63.
3. DiBattista, W. J., Nishikawara, M. T., and Leung, Y. F., (1978): *J. Reprod. Fertil.,* 54:249–253.
4. Knott, G. D., and Reese, D. (1972): MLAB: An on-line modeling laboratory. Reference Manual, 7th edition, Division of Computer Research and Technology, National Institutes of Health, Bethesda, Maryland.
5. Lippman, M. E., Bolan, G., and Huff, K. (1976): *Cancer Res.,* 36:4595–4601.
6. Plageman, P. G., and Erbe, J. (1972): *J. Cell Biol.,* 33:757–775.
7. Scudiero, D., Henderson, E., Norin, A., and Strauss, B. (1975): *Mutation Res.,* 29:473–488.
8. Taylor, A. T., Stafford, M. A., and Jones, O. W. (1972): *J. Biol. Chem.,* 247:1930–35.
9. Zava, D. T., Chamness, G. C., Horwitz, K. B., and McGuire, W. L. (1977): *Science,* 196:663–664.

Hormones and Cancer, edited by S. Iacobelli et al.
Raven Press, New York © 1980.

Hormonal Control of Breast Cancer in Cell Culture

Henri Rochefort, Ericque Coezy, Ethel Joly, Bruce Westley, and Françoise Vignon

Unité d'Endocrinologie Cellulaire et Moléculaire, I.N.S.E.R.M., 34100 Montpellier, France

Previous *in vivo* studies on experimental mammary cancer in animals have given information concerning the regulation by hormones of steroid receptor sites, gene products, and tumor growth (6,13,16). The growth of hormone-dependent mammary cancer is thought to be stimulated mainly by two classes of hormones, estrogen and prolactin. Conversely, high doses of androgens, progesterone, glucocorticoids, and synthetic antiestrogens have been reported to reduce tumor growth by unknown mechanisms. However, *in vivo,* it is difficult to define which hormone is responsible for the observed effect. For example, the effect of estrogen on the growth of mammary tumors in rats appears to be mostly due to an indirect effect of prolactin released from the pituitary and not to a direct interaction of estrogen with the estrogen receptor (R_E) located in the tumor (19).

During the last 3 years we have studied the mechanism of action of steroid hormones in breast cancer using cell culture in addition to *in vivo* experiments. The ultimate aim of these studies was to reach a better understanding of the mechanism by which hormones regulate the growth of breast cancer cells. Practically, these studies might be of considerable help in the therapy of breast cancer by finding new selective therapeutical approaches and better markers of hormone responsiveness for growth. Presented below are the results of our studies, which were guided by three major questions concerning the mechanism of regulation of tumor growth by a steroid hormone:

1. Which hormones, or metabolites, directly control cell proliferation and/or gene expression?
2. Which receptors mediate the effects of these hormones, since one hormone might interact with different types of receptors (21)?
3. How do hormones regulate cell growth and, more precisely, do hormone receptor complexes act directly in the nucleus or indirectly via endogenous growth factors?

These questions are considered in the Discussion in relation to the results of our studies performed in the nitrosomethylurea (NMU) rat mammary adenocarcinoma cell line, which we have found to be stimulated mainly by glucocorti-coids (25), and in the human MCF-7 breast cancer cell line (24), which is known to be mainly responsive to estrogens and antiestrogens (15). The detailed protocol for each experiment can be found in the quoted references.

HORMONE REGULATION OF THE GROWTH OF NMU RAT MAMMARY CANCER CELLS

Mammary tumors induced in the rat by the carcinogens dimethylbenz [a] anthracene (DMBA) and NMU generally regress after ovariectomy (8,10), and estrogen and prolactin appear to be the major hormones stimulating their growth. Two continuous cell lines, RBA and NMU, have been established from these two tumors (5) and we have studied the receptor content and the effect of hormones in these cell lines (25). These cells are epithelial and tumorigenic; they have a chromosome number of 51–77 (RBA) and 66–70 (NMU) and a doubling time of 36 hr. To define the steroid hormones modulating the growth of these cells, we have screened the cells for their steroid receptor content. We found (25) that the two cell lines RBA and NMU contained negligible amounts of R_E and no progesterone receptor (R_P). Conversely, they had high concentrations of androgen (R_A) and glucocorticoid receptors (R_G) ($\approx$100 and 500 fmoles/mg protein, respectively). Both receptors could be translocated into the nucleus and, while dexamethasone stimulated cell growth and incorporation of [^{3}H]thymidine into DNA, dihydrotestosterone (DHT) was only able to stimu-late [^{3}H]thymidine incorporation (14). Progesterone also stimulated thymidine incorporation by itself and prevented the growth of the cells cultured with glucocorticoid. This model system, which is markedly different from the original tumor that it was derived from, was of interest in determining the possible role of R_G and R_A in the growth of mammary cancer and the mechanism of action of progesterone which is currently used to treat some breast cancers. The most popular hypothesis for the mechanism of progesterone action is that

TABLE 1. *Steroid hormone regulation in the NMU rat mammary adenocarcinoma cell line*

Hormones	Receptors[a]		Responses[b]		
	Cytosol	nt	^{3}HT	Cell no.	SIP
Glucocorticoid	+	+	++	+	+
Androgen	+	+	+	0	0
Estrogen	0	nd	0	nd	0
Progesterone	0	nd	+	0	nd

[a] Receptor results are detailed in ref. 25. nt, hormone-dependent nuclear translocation.
[b] [^{3}H]thymidine incorporation (^{3}HT) into DNA was performed according to ref. 3. Cell number (cell no.) was counted directly using a Coulter counter. Secreted induced proteins (SIP) were shown as in ref. 28. nd, not determined.
Data from E. Joly and B. Westley *(unpublished)*.

it prevents cell growth by antagonizing estrogen action. This is unlikely here, since these cells have no R_E and their growth is not stimulated by estrogen. As there is no R_P, it is also unlikely that progesterone could act *via* its own receptor. However, the effect of progesterone could be mediated by interacting with R_G, R_A, or both, since progestins are known to be a glucocorticoid (22) and androgen antagonist (4).

At present, it seems most likely that progesterone acts as a partial agonist–antagonist on the R_G rather than on the R_A. We have found (14), using SDS polyacrylamide gel electrophoresis of [^{35}S]methionine-labeled proteins, that secreted proteins are induced specifically by glucocorticoid but not by androgen or estrogen. Thus, for both cell growth and effects on protein synthesis, these cells are mostly responsive to glucocorticoids.

These results, summarized in Table 1, show that, by assaying steroid receptors, it is easy to eliminate the hormone that cannot stimulate growth at physiological concentrations via its own receptor. It is more difficult to specify which receptor is responsible for a given hormone effect when this hormone is able to bind to different receptors. We have also found that glucocorticoids in rats can stimulate the growth of mammary tumor cells both *in vitro* and *in vivo* in nude mice (Vignon, *unpublished experiments*). The mechanism of this stimulation, which could be either direct or indirect via other growth factors or hormones present in the serum, or via the secretion of endogenous growth factors, is presently unknown.

EFFECT OF ESTROGEN ON THE BIOSYNTHESIS OF SPECIFIC SECRETED PROTEINS IN THE MCF-7 HUMAN BREAST CANCER CELLS

As estrogens are probably the most important steroids which stimulate the growth of human breast cancer, we have focused our efforts on human breast cancer cell lines containing high concentrations of R_E and responding to estrogens. The growth of these cells is slightly stimulated by estrogen and markedly prevented by antiestrogens (9,15). The effect of antiestrogen is totally overcome by estradiol, and is absent in R_E (−) cell lines, strongly suggesting that it is specific and mediated by R_E.

The only available specific marker of response to estrogen in these cells is the R_P (9). Since the R_P is a minor protein and since it does not appear to be a perfect marker for the response to estrogens and antiestrogens for tumor cell proliferation, we looked for other estrogen-induced proteins that might be more closely related to tumor growth using [^{35}S]methionine-labeled proteins analyzed by SDS polyacrylamide gel electrophoresis (1). The MCF-7 cells were first withdrawn in a medium containing 10% charcoal-treated serum; they were then cultured in the same medium containing different hormones or antihormones and were finally labeled with [^{35}S]methionine. The labeled proteins of a cell lysate and of the medium were then analyzed by SDS polyacrylamide gel electrophoresis. The fluorograms of these gels revealed different bands whose intensity could be quantified in a gel scanner. We found no clear effect of estradiol on the labeling of intracellular proteins by this technique. Using the 2D O'Farrell technique (17), we found three spots constantly stimulated by estradiol (28). However, the most dramatic effect of estradiol was seen for the secreted proteins (28). We found that starting from 12 hr of treatment, a protein of 46,000 dalton molecular weight (46 K) was induced by estradiol. Near optimal induction was obtained with 0.1 nM estradiol (29). In addition to this 46-K protein, some other proteins were also stimulated. The induction was found to be specific for R_E ligands, since estrone and estriol were $\simeq$10-fold less efficient than E_2 and progesterone and dexamethasone were inactive. DHT was only active from 5 μM concentration (29), which is consistent with its action being mediated by the R_E (20,21). An interesting property was that tamoxifen did not induce the 46-K protein but prevented its induction by estradiol at a molar ratio of 10^4. Monohydroxytamoxifen (a metabolite of tamoxifen which binds R_E with high affinity) was found in our laboratory to be accumulated *in vivo* in nuclei of target cells (rat uterus, chick liver) (2). It is shown here (Fig. 1) that hydroxy-tamoxifen is 10-fold more potent than tamoxifen for blocking the induction of the secreted protein by estradiol. We also found that these two antiestrogens inhibited the induction of the 46-K protein by DHT in a ratio corresponding roughly to the relative affinities of these three ligands for the R_E.

Finally, estrogen-3-sulfates but not the 17-sulfates induced the 46-K protein in MCF-7 cells (Fig. 2). This finding was surprising since estrogen sulfates have a very low affinity for the R_E. However, using [^{3}H]estrone sulfate we found that MCF-7 cells were able to hydrolyze the sulfate ester bond, thus liberating [^{3}H]estrogens which were recovered bound to the nuclear R_E (26). These results demonstrate that MCF-7 cells have an aryl-sulfatase activity, but not a 17-sulfatase activity. Moreover, the estrogen sulfates are not completely removed by charcoal treatment and the serum treated by charcoal (to deplete steroids for cell cluture experiments) in fact contained up to 30 nM estrogen sulfate (26). These results lead us to propose that the culture medium contains estrogen sulfate which can be used as biologically active estrogens by the cell. It is possible that the estrogen sulfates remaining in the charcoal-treated serum stimulate cell growth in the control "estrogen-free" medium.

The secreted 46-K protein is now being characterized using 2D gel electrophoresis; it is resolved into five different spots of decreasing pI and increasing MW (29). We have found by [^{3}H]fucose incorporation and neuraminidase digestion that this secreted protein is probably a glycoprotein. The identity and function of this 46-K protein is presently unknown. However, we can exclude the major milk proteins which have very different MW. Finally, a protein of the same MW and sensitivity to estrogens has been found in the ZR_{75-1} line which also contains R_E. It was stimulated by estrogen and present only in low amounts in two other hormone cell lines not containing R_E (29).

In conclusion, we have found a protein with a molecular weight of 46 K which is secreted by hormone responsive breast cancer cells and which is specifi-

MW

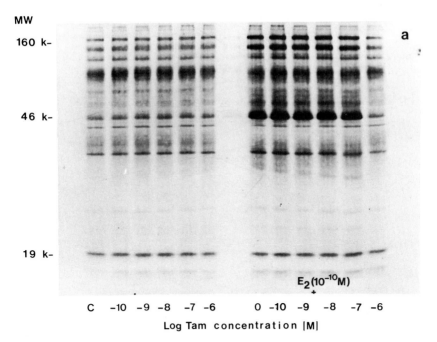

160 k-

46 k-

19 k-

$E_2(10^{-10}M)$
+

C   -10 -9 -8 -7 -6   0 -10 -9 -8 -7 -6

Log Tam concentration [M]

MW

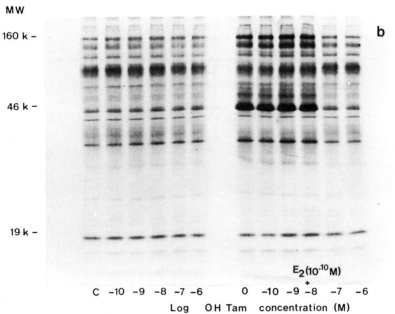

160 k -

46 k -

19 k -

$E_2(10^{-10}M)$
+

C -10 -9 -8 -7 -6   0   -10 -9 -8 -7 -6

Log   OH Tam   concentration (M)

FIG. 1. Effect of antiestrogens on secreted proteins in MCF-7 cells. Tamoxifen (Tam: *trans*-1-(*p*-dimethylaminoethoxyphenyl)-1,2-diphenylbut-1-ene) **(a)** and the monohydroxytamox-ifen (OH Tam) **(b)** were incubated with MCF-7 cells for 2 days either with or without estradiol (0.1 nM). The secreted proteins, labeled by [35S]methionine, were then analyzed by SDS polya-crylamide gel electrophoresis. The major estrogen-induced proteins are seen at MW of 46 and 160 K.

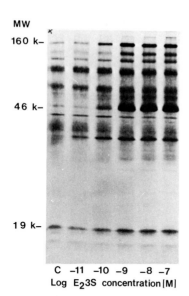

MW

160 k–

46 k–

19 k–

C –11 –10 –9 –8 –7
Log E₂3S concentration|M|

FIG. 2. Induction of the 46-K MW secreted induced protein by estradiol-3-sulfate. Same protocol as in Fig. 1.

cally induced by estrogen. This protein represents 40% of the total secreted proteins and appears to be a good marker for studying the mechanism of action of estrogen and antiestrogen in these cells.

We propose that the 46-K protein, if present in primary breast cancers, would also be an excellent marker to predict hormone responsiveness of breast cancer growth. At present, the R_P is the only marker for responsiveness to estrogen currently available in human breast cancer, though there are now several arguments which suggest that it is not ideal. First, although the simultaneous assay of R_E and R_P improves the prediction of hormone responsiveness in breast cancer (18), the prediction is not 100%, as there are approximately 20% of R_P (−) patients who respond to endocrine therapy and 20% of R_P (+) who do not respond (18). Second, R_P is present in MCF-7 cells in the absence of estrogens. Third, tamoxifen which prevents growth of MCF-7 cells induces R_P (9,18). Finally, estrogen induces R_P but does not stimulate growth in the transplantable MTW-9B hormone independent rat mammary tumor (12) or in some primary tumors induced by DMBA (12). The estrogen induced 46-K protein, however, might be a better marker for cell growth than the R_P since in MCF-7 cells it is not induced by tamoxifen. Our current goal is now to determine its identity and function.

GENERAL DISCUSSION

The Nature of the Steroid Hormone–Receptor Complexes Active in Regulating Specific Gene Expression in Experimental and Human Breast Cancer

The hormones that cannot be acting through their own receptor at physiological concentration can be eliminated by determining the steroid receptors present, since there is no evidence that a hormone can act without its classical receptor in somatic cells. This was found to be the case for progesterone and estrogen in the NMU cell line which does not contain receptors for these hormones. However, a hormone can act at pharmacological concentrations through another receptor. For instance, we found that high concentrations of progesterone stimulate the incorporation of thymidine into DNA in an R_P negative cell line (NMU) and we therefore suggest that the effect of progesterone is mediated by another class of steroid receptors (for glucocorticoid or androgen). Another example of this is the effect of the androgen DHT which is mediated by the estrogen receptor (7,20). These results strongly suggest that the final response observed is specific to the type of receptor that has been activated rather than to the nature of the hormone activating it. It is thus possible to define the receptor responsible for an observed effect by using two types of experiment:

1. A quantitative comparison of the dose response and the saturation curves for the different receptors able to bind one given hormone. In the case of androgen action on R_E, this is easy, since quite different concentrations of androgen are required to saturate the R_A and the R_E, respectively (7,20).

2. A qualitative comparison of the specific responses stimulated by physiological concentrations of various hormones. Thus, for example, if a particular response is obtained by physiological concentrations of a hormone A and by high concentrations of another hormone B, it strongly suggests that hormone B acts through the receptor for hormone A. This is the case for high doses of androgen which act on the R_E and can give several estrogen-specific responses (21). We have found that analysis of [^{35}S]methionine-labeled secreted proteins by SDS polyacrylamide gel electrophoresis (28) is an excellent method of screening for hormone-induced proteins in breast cancer cell lines. This method (17) also appears to be highly suitable for screening a wide variety of cells and tissues for hormone-induced proteins.

The Mechanism of Stimulation of Cell Proliferation by Steroid Hormones

First, we observed that the effect of a hormone on the incorporation of thymidine into DNA can be dissociated from its effect on cell growth, for example, the effect of DHT on NMU cells, which under our conditions stimulates thymidine incorporation without increasing the cell number. The direct measure of cell number or DNA content therefore appears to be more valid than thymidine incorporation as a measure of cell proliferation. Second, we have found that *in vivo* it is difficult to specify whether a given steroid hormone regulates cell proliferation directly or indirectly. This problem should be easier to solve using cell culture, though this approach will ultimately require that cell lines are grown in chemically defined medium (11). In addition to a direct effect of the R-h complex on the chromosomes to stimulate DNA replication and mitosis, the R-h complex might also be acting indirectly by facilitating the action of exogenous growth factors present in the serum (Fig. 3) (23). It could also be

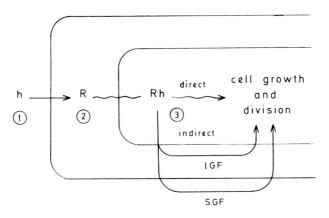

FIG. 3. Schematic representation of a steroid hormone (h), the receptor mediating its effect (R), and three possible pathways by which the R-h complex might influence cell growth and division in a target cell. IGF, intracellular endogenous growth factor; SGF, secreted endogenous growth factor.

acting indirectly by inducing some endogenous growth factor which would then be acting in the cell (internal growth factor) or on the cell membrane (external growth factor) after secretion into the medium. We are currently investigating the possibility that the protein specifically induced by estrogen that we have found secreted by the R_E (+) breast cancer cell lines might be such an endogenous external growth factor.

Our results support the idea that breast cancer cells in culture are good model systems to study the mechanism of hormone action in cancer cells. In some cases, such as the NMU cell line, the cell lines have a different hormone responsiveness to the tumor from which they were derived. However, the human breast cancer lines which have maintained high concentrations of R_E have kept their ability to respond to estrogen for some gene products such as the R_P and the secreted induced proteins that we have described (29) and to respond to antiestrogen for cell growth. They therefore constitute very good model systems to study the mechanism of action of estrogens and antiestrogens and might be useful in the understanding of the regulation of tumor growth by hormones.

ACKNOWLEDGMENTS

This study was supported by INSERM, the NCI-INSERM cooperation on Hormone and Cancer, the "Fondation pour la Recherche Médicale Française," and INSERM Grant 49.77.81. B.W. was a recipient of an MRC-INSERM exchange fellowship. We thank Mrs. D. Derocq and J. Vanbiervliet for their excellent technical assistance and Miss E. Barrié for the preparation of the manuscript. We are grateful to Drs. P. C. Chan, M. Lippman, and M. Rich for kindly providing us with mammary cell lines.

REFERENCES

1. Bonner, W. M., and Laskey, R. A. (1974): *Eur. J. Biochem.,* 46:83–88.
2. Borgna, J. L., and Rochefort, H. (1979): *C.R. Acad. Sci. (Paris),* 289:1141–1144.
3. Brooks, R. F. (1977): *Cell,* 12:311–317.
4. Bullock, L., Bardin, C. W., and Sherman, M. R. (1978): *Endocrinology,* 103:1768.
5. Cohen, L. A., Tsuang, J., and Chan, P. C. (1974): *In Vitro,* 10:51–62.
6. Dao, T. L., editor (1972): *Estrogen Target Tissues and Neoplasia.* University of Chicago Press, Chicago.
7. Garcia, M., and Rochefort, H. (1977): *Steroids,* 29:111–124.
8. Gullino, P. M., Pettigrew, H. M., and Grantham, F. Y. (1975): *J. Natl. Cancer Inst.,* 54:401–414.
9. Horwitz, K. B., and McGuire, W. L. (1978): *J. Biol. Chem.,* 253:2223–2228.
10. Huggins, C., Briziarelli, G., and Sutton, H., Jr. (1959): *J. Exp. Med.,* 109:25.
11. Hutchings, S. E., and Sato, G. (1978): *Proc. Natl. Acad. Sci. USA,* 75:901–904.
12. Ip, M., Milholland, R. J., Rosen, F., and Kim, U. (1979): *Science,* 203:361–363.
13. Jensen, E. V., and De Sombre, E. R. (1972): *Annu. Rev. Biochem.,* 41:203–230.
14. Joly, E. et al. (1980): *In preparation.*
15. Lippman, M., Bolan, G., and Huff, K. (1976): *Cancer Res.,* 36:4595–4601.
16. McGuire, W. L., Chamness, G., Costlow, M. E., and Horwitz, K. B. (1976): In: *Modern Pharmacology,* edited by G. S. Levey, pp. 265–299. Dekker, New York.
17. O'Farrell, P. H. (1975): *J. Biol. Chem.,* 250:4007–4025.
18. Osborne, C. K., and McGuire, W. L. (1979): *Bull. Cancer,* 66:203–210.
19. Pearson, O. H., Llerena, O., Llerena, L., Molina, A., and Butler, T. (1963): *Trans. Assoc. Am. Physicians,* 82:481–484.
20. Rochefort, H., and Garcia, M. (1976): *Steroids,* 28:549–560.
21. Rochefort, H., and Garcia, M. (1979): In: *Proceedings of the Satellite Symposium of the VII International Congress of Pharmacology* (Turine, Italy, July 23–25, 1978). Raven Press, New York.
22. Samuels, H. H., and Tomkins, G. M. (1970): *J. Mol. Biol.,* 52:57–74.
23. Sirbasku, D. A. (1978): *Proc. Natl. Acad. Sci. USA,* 75:3786–3790.
24. Soule, H. D., Vazquez, J., Long, A., Albert, S., and Brennan, M. (1973): *J. Natl. Cancer Inst.,* 51:1409–1416.
25. Vignon, F., Chan, P. C., and Rochefort, H. (1979): *Mol. Cell. Endocrinol.,* 13:191–202.
26. Vignon, F., Terqui, M., Westley, B., and Rochefort, H. (1980): *Endocrinology,* 106:1079–1086.
27. Vignon, F. (1979): Etapes initiales de l'action des hormones stéroides dans les tumeurs mammaires. Ph.D. Thesis, Université des Sciences et Techniques de Montpellier.
28. Westley, B., and Rochefort, H. (1979): *Biochem. Biophys. Res. Commun.,* 90:410–416.
29. Westley, B., and Rochefort, H. (1980): *Cell,* 20:352–362.

Hormones and Cancer, edited by S. Iacobelli et al.
Raven Press, New York © 1980.

Androgen Effects on Growth, Morphology, and Sensitivity of S115 Mouse Mammary Tumor Cells in Culture

Jean Yates, *J. R. Couchman, and R. J. B. King

*Hormone Biochemistry Department, Imperial Cancer Research Fund, London WC2A 3PX; and *Unilever Research, Colworth Laboratory, Sharnbrook, Bedfordshire MK44 1LQ, United Kingdom*

Two statements appear, in one form or another, in virtually every article on steroid-mediated growth of mammary tumors: (a) Steroids affect the proliferation of mammary tumor cells but the biochemical mechanisms are not clear. (b) Objective remissions are achieved by steroid therapy in about a third of women with breast cancer but the remissions so induced are of a temporary nature. This chapter describes experiments with mammary tumor cells in culture that give clues as to postreceptor events involved in the regulation of cell proliferation and that may provide an explanation for the temporary nature of endocrine-induced remissions in some human breast cancer.

We have been studying the growth of Shionogi mouse mammary tumor cells (S115 cells) in cell culture and their responsiveness to androgens such as dihydrotestosterone (DHT) and testosterone. The publications by ourselves and others have established that androgen receptors are involved in the growth regulation, that growth in culture is responsive to, but not dependent on, androgens (18, 31,36), and that unresponsive variants can be generated by growth in the absence of androgen (5,18,41). The androgen receptor machinery in S115 cells has been studied in some detail (6,11,16,18,19) whereas only fragmentary data are available on postreceptor events. Protein synthesis is increased in the presence of testosterone (29) as is ribosomal but not messenger RNA (15,18,35). Amino acid but not sugar transport across the cell membrane is increased by androgen (27,28) whereas there is no change in cyclic adenosine monophosphate (cyclic AMP) content of the cells (30).

It is difficult to fit these data into a cohesive model and further markers of androgen action are required. We have exploited two features of S115 cell growth to this aim. First, androgen withdrawal leads to a change from fibroblastic to epithelial morphology (11,30) and secondly, 2 to 3 weeks growth in the absence of androgen results in loss of androgen sensitivity with minimal detectable change in the receptor machinery (18,19). It is thus possible to compare responsive cells with unresponsive counterparts derived from them.

The morphological change seen on androgen withdrawal raises the possibility that androgens modulate cell proliferation by affecting membrane sensitivity to other agents (40,41). This hypothesis was, in part, engendered by the growing body of evidence indicating that the sensitivity of cultured cells to various stimuli is markedly influenced by morphology (12,13,24). Cell morphology in culture is largely determined by cytoskeletal elements (26,38) and we therefore decided to study the effects of androgen withdrawal on microfilament and microtubule organization using immunofluorescent techniques (10). These experiments clearly indicate that testosterone withdrawal leads to the formation of microfilament bundles (Fig. 1) without changing the arrangement of microtubules (Fig. 2). The increased organization of the actin-containing microfilaments was correlated with the change from fibroblastic to epithelial morphology (Fig. 3). Interference reflection microscopy further indicated that the adoption of an epithelial shape was associated with the formation of specific focal adhesions between the underside of the cell and the culture dish (Fig. 4). Focal adhesions are zones of membrane specialization which form the termini of microfilament bundles at the cell membrane (1). These structures have been correlated with cell stability for growth, rather than with locomotion, which can proceed in their absence (8,9). Time-lapse cinematography of S115 cells indicates little directional movement in either the presence or absence of testosterone. The cell surface-associated fibronectin, which was present in amorphous patches in the fibroblastic cells, assumed a more fibrillar arrangement following androgen withdrawal.

The kinetics of these changes are ill-defined. The results described thus far certainly occur within 3 weeks of testosterone withdrawal and some changes are evident within 1 week (10). Scanning electron microscopy suggests that

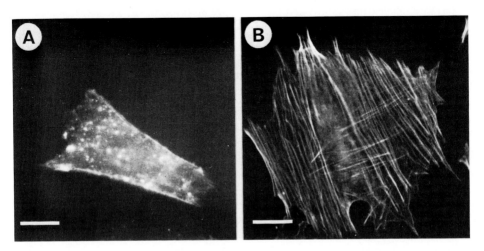

FIG. 1. Arrangement of microfilament bundles in the presence **(A)** and absence **(B)** of testosterone. Bar is 20 μm.

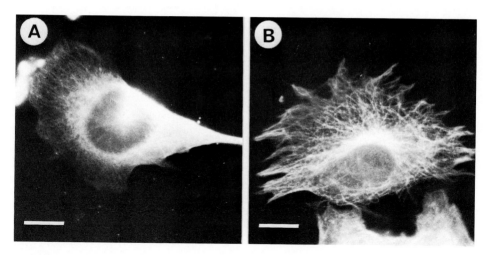

FIG. 2. Microtubule distribution in the presence **(A)** and absence **(B)** of testosterone. Bar is 20 μm.

signs of morphological change are evident within 1 day of testosterone withdrawal (41). Our present observations indicate that androgens can modify cell morphology by a mechanism that may involve microfilament organization; the question, as yet unanswered, concerns the molecular nature of that organization. Since actin is a major component of microfilament bundles (26), logical candidates for the testosterone-induced changes could be alterations in synthesis of actin or the machinery involved in the polymerization reaction. These are currently under investigation.

The next question to be addressed is the physiological effects of morphological change. It is reasonable to suppose that changes in membrane sensitivity to proliferative stimuli would accompany the epithelial transition. We therefore compared several parameters of membrane sensitivity in fibroblastic and epithelial S115 cells; parameters studied were androgen responsiveness, serum sensitivity, density regulation, and anchorage dependence (Fig. 5) (40,41). Loss of androgen response was accompanied by increased sensitivity to serum, increased density regulation (lower saturation density), and much greater dependence on attachment to the substrate for proliferation. When the timecourse of these androgen-associated effects was studied they all appeared to change concomitantly (40) (Fig. 6). However, the 7-day time interval between data points leaves open the possibility of sequential changes. Evidently, when testosterone is removed a number of membrane-associated activities change, which would certainly be compatible with the alterations in microfilament bundles noted earlier.

It is interesting to relate our results to cell transformation. The behavior of testosterone-treated cells resembles that of many transformed cells in culture whereas the testosterone-deprived S115 cells are similar to untransformed cells

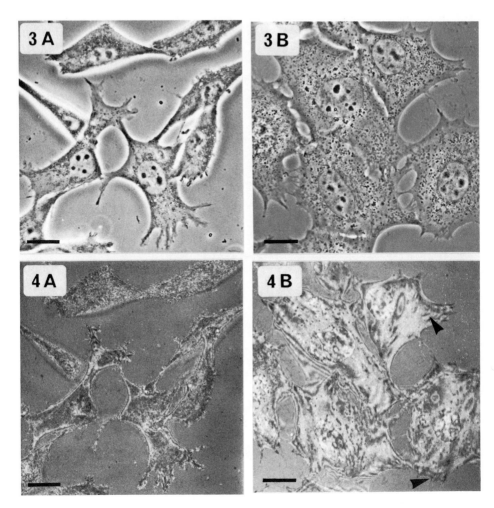

FIG. 3. Phase contrast micrographs of S115 cells in the presence **(A)** and absence **(B)** of testosterone. Bar is 20 μm.

FIG. 4. Interference reflection micrographs of the same cells as Fig. 3 showing the development of focal adhesions *(arrowheads)*. Bar is 20 μm.

(25,39). Of particular importance is the change in anchorage dependence, an effect noted earlier by Stanley et al. (36). This particular property is currently thought to be the one most closely correlated with tumorigenicity (4). It could thus be suggested that in S115 cells, androgens are changing the cells from normal to transformed phenotype, perhaps in an analogous manner to transformation by temperature-sensitive mutant viruses. In the presence of androgen they grow as though at the permissive temperature, whereas steroid withdrawal

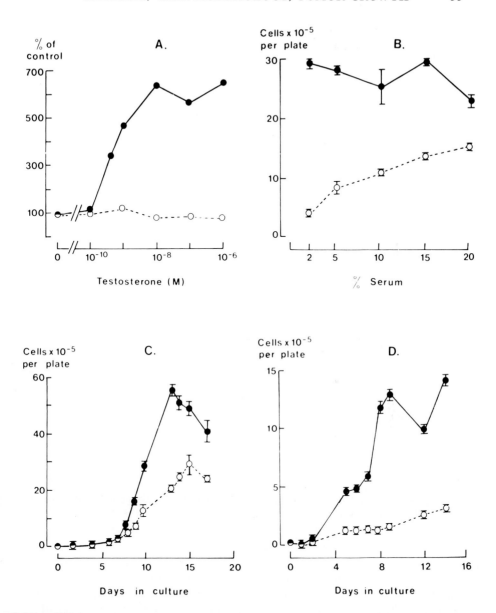

FIG. 5. Proliferation rates of androgen-maintained S115 cells *(closed circles)* and of cells deprived of testosterone for 6 weeks *(open circles)*. **A:** Response to administration for 4 days of varying concentrations of testosterone in the presence of 2% fetal calf serum. **B:** Effect of varying concentrations of fetal calf serum in the presence of 3.5×10^{-8} M testosterone. **C:** Growth in monolayer culture in 2% serum and 3.5×10^{-8} M testosterone showing the lower growth rate and increased density regulation of androgen-deprived cells. **D:** Growth in suspension culture in 2% serum and 3.5×10^{-8} M testosterone showing the increased anchorage dependence of androgen-deprived cells.

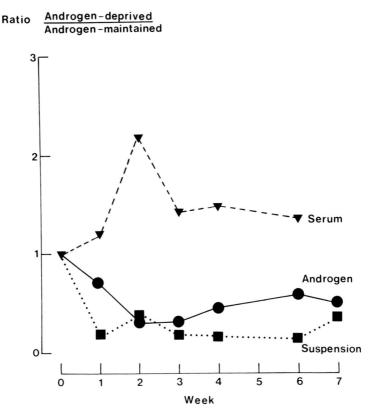

FIG. 6. Time course of proliferative changes in androgen and serum sensitivity and the ability to grow in suspension culture following androgen deprivation.

is analogous to a shift to the nonpermissive mode. This idea has interesting molecular implications which are discussed below, but the comparison does have a major limitation. The S115 cells were derived from an androgen-responsive mammary tumor growing in male mice (23). Technically, therefore, they are transformed cells. Furthermore, transplantation into castrated male nude mice of androgen-insensitive S115 cells exhibiting "normal" behavior in culture gave rise to tumors (42). With the S115 cells it is clear that equating transformation as applied to cell culture characteristics with tumorigenicity is not justified.

The androgen-induced transformation in culture might be exploited to determine molecular events in androgen action. Given the features of cell transformation, the main possibility to consider is that androgens are switching on the production of a transforming virus. The original S115 tumor arose in a mouse derived from the DD strain (23) which are known to contain mouse mammary tumor virus (MMTV) (14). However, several data indicate that virus production is unlikely to explain our results. No virus particles can be seen in electron micrographs and negligible RNA-dependent DNA synthesis is associated with the S115 cells cultured in either the presence or absence of testosterone (Yates et al., *unpublished observations*). MMTV synthesis is greatly enhanced by glucocorticoids (37), yet in S115 cells glucocorticoids inhibit rather than stimulate growth and do not transform the epithelial morphology (34). Nevertheless, despite these evidences against involvement of complete MMTV, it remains a possibility that a residual viral component such as the oncogene or some analogue thereof might be activated by androgens. The exciting data showing that the protein product of the oncogene of sarcoma virus is involved in protein phosphorylation (7,21) and may be related to actin depolymerization (22,33) deserves application to the S115 system.

The working model that we have adopted from these experiments is shown in Fig. 7. Androgens work via the intracellular receptor machinery to alter microfilament structure, which in turn modulates membrane sensitivity to external agents. Such a model has important clinical implications that are discussed below, but some other points should first be made about this model: (a) It only allocates a permissive role to the steroids, a point that has been fully discussed elsewhere (17,18). (b) Data are accumulating that glucocorticoids may affect cell proliferation in culture by an analogous mechanism (2,3,32). (c) The location within the model of androgen-mediated effects on DNA synthesis is uncertain. Changes in DNA synthesis occur within 10 hr of testosterone addition to S115 cells (35) as compared with approximately 1 day for the earliest detectable changes in morphology. The time discrepancy may simply reflect differing methodological sensitivities, but it could be that androgens affect proliferation both directly as well as indirectly via the cell membrane. An intriguing possibility that would link cytoskeletal elements to both mechanisms comes from the suggestion that the cytoskeleton can regulate RNA metabolism (20).

Provided that results obtained with S115 cells can be related to the behavior of human breast cancer cells, the clinical implications of the present results relate to the second statement made at the beginning of this article—Why are endocrine-induced remissions of a temporary nature? The common answer is that outgrowth of unresponsive cells occurs from within the mass of responsive cells. While this undoubtedly occurs, an additional mechanism would be that, because of their changed sensitivity to other agents (cell contacts, blood supply, other hormones), regrowth is of phenotypically but not genotypically changed responsive cells (17).

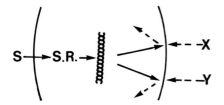

FIG. 7. Diagrammatic representation of a model by which steroid (S) can influence cell sensitivity to external agents (X and Y). R, receptor.

ACKNOWLEDGMENTS

We should like to thank Miss S. Ord and Miss C. B. Evans for assistance with cell culture and photography, respectively, and Dr. R. A. Badley for the provision of antisera and advice on immunofluorescent techniques.

REFERENCES

1. Badley, R. A., Lloyd, C. W., Woods, A., Carruthers, L., Allcock, C., and Rees, D. A. (1978): *Exp. Cell Res.,* 117:231–244.
2. Baker, J. B., Barsh, G. S., Carney, D. H., and Cunningham, D. D. (1978): *Proc. Natl. Acad. Sci. USA,* 75:1882–1886.
3. Baker, J. B., Simmer, R. L., Glenn, K. C., and Cunningham, D. D. (1979): *J. Cell. Physiol.,* 98:561–570.
4. Barret, J. C., Crawford, B. D., Mixter, L. O., Schechtman, L. M., Ts'o, P. O. P., and Pollack, R. (1979): *Cancer Res.,* 39:1504–1510.
5. Bruchovsky, N., and Meakin, J. W. (1973): *Cancer Res.,* 33:1689–1695.
6. Bruchovsky, N., Sutherland, D. J. A., Meakin, J. W., and Minesita, T. (1975): *Biochim. Biophys. Acta,* 381:61–71.
7. Collett, M. S., and Erikson, R. L. (1978): *Proc. Natl. Acad. Sci. USA,* 75:2021–2024.
8. Couchman, J. R., and Rees, D. A. (1979): *Cell Biol. Int. Rep.,* 3:431–439.
9. Couchman, J. R., and Rees, D. A. (1979): *J. Cell Sci.,* 39:149–165.
10. Couchman, J. R., Yates, J., King, R. J. B., and Badley, R. A. (1980): *Submitted.*
11. Desmond, W. J., Jr., Wolbers, S. J., and Sato, G. (1976): *Cell,* 8:79–86.
12. Folkman, J., and Moscona, A. (1978): *Nature,* 273:345–349.
13. Gospodarowicz, D., Greenburg, G., and Birdwell, C. R. (1978): *Cancer Res.,* 38:4155–4171.
14. Heston, W. E., and Vlahakis, G. (1971): *Int. J. Cancer,* 7:141–148.
15. Jagus, R. (1979): *Exp. Cell Res.,* 118:115–125.
16. Jung-Testas, I., Desmond, W., and Baulieu, E.-E. (1976): *Exp. Cell Res.,* 97:219–232.
17. King, R. J. B. (1979): In: *Biochemical Actions of Hormones, Vol. 6,* edited by G. Litwack, pp. 247–264. Academic, New York.
18. King, R. J. B., Cambray, G. J., Jagus-Smith, R., Robinson, J. H., and Smith, J. A. (1976): In: *Receptors and Mechanisms of Steroid Hormones,* edited by J. R. Pasqualini, pp. 215–261. Dekker, New York.
19. King, R. J. B., Cambray, G. J., and Robinson, J. H. (1976): *J. Steroid Biochem.,* 7:869–783.
20. Lenk, R., and Penman, S. (1979): *Cell,* 16:289–301.
21. Levinson, A. D., Oppermann, H., Levintow, L., Varmus, H. E., and Bishop, J. M. (1978): *Cell,* 15:561–572.
22. McClain, D. A., Maness, P. F., and Edelman, G. M. (1978): *Proc. Natl. Acad. Sci. USA,* 75:2750–2754.
23. Minesita, T., and Yamaguchi, K. (1965): *Cancer Res.,* 25:1168–1175.
24. O'Neill, C. H., Riddle, P. N., and Jordan, P. W. (1979): *Cell,* 16:909–918.
25. Pastan, I., and Willingham, M. (1978): *Nature,* 274:645–650.
26. Pollack, R., and Rifkin, D. B. (1976): In: *Cell Motility, Book A,* edited by R. Goldman, T. Pollard, and J. Rosenbaum, pp. 389–401. Cold Spring Harbor Laboratory, Cold Spring Harbor.
27. Robinson, J. H. (1976): *J. Cell. Physiol.,* 89:101–109.
28. Robinson, J. H., and Smith, J. A. (1976): *J. Cell. Physiol.,* 89:111–122.
29. Robinson, J. H., Smith, J. A., and Dee, L. A. (1976): *Exp. Cell Res.,* 102:117–126.
30. Robinson, J. H., Smith, J. A., and King, R. J. B. (1974): *Cell,* 3:361–365.
31. Robinson, J. H., Smith, J. A., Totty, N. F., and Riddle, P. N. (1976): *Nature,* 262:298–300.
32. Rudland, P. S., and Jimenez de Asua, L. (1979): *Biochim. Biophys. Acta,* 560:91–133.
33. Sen, A., and Todaro, G. J. (1979): *Cell,* 17:347–356.
34. Sica, G., Yates, J., and King, R. J. B. (1979): *Cancer Treatment Reports,* 63:1175.
35. Smith, J. A., Robinson, J. H., Jagus-Smith, R., and King, R. J. B. (1975): In: *Regulation of Growth and Differentiated Function in Eukaryote Cells,* edited by G. P. Talwar, pp. 355–367. Raven Press, New York.
36. Stanley, E. R., Palmer, R. E., and Sohn, U. (1977): *Cell,* 10:35–44.

37. Varmus, H. E., Ringold, G., and Yamamoto, K. R. (1979): In: *Glucocorticoid Hormone Action,* edited by J. D. Baxter and G. C. Rousseau, pp. 254–271. Springer-Verlag, Berlin.
38. Vasiliev, J. M., and Gelfand, I. M. (1977): *Int. Rev. Cytol.,* 50:159–274.
39. Watt, F. M., Harris, H., Weber, K., and Osborn, M. (1978): *J. Cell Sci.,* 32:419–432.
40. Yates, J., and King, R. J. B. (1978): *Cancer Res.,* 38:4135–4137.
41. Yates, J., and King, R. J. B. (1980): *Submitted.*
42. Yates, J., and King, R. J. B.: *In preparation.*

Hormones and Cancer, edited by S. Iacobelli et al.
Raven Press, New York © 1980.

The "Estrogen-Induced Protein" in Normal and Neoplastic Cells

Alvin M. Kaye, Nachum Reiss, *Stefano Iacobelli, *Emanuela Bartoccioni, and *Paolo Marchetti

*Department of Hormone Research, The Weizmann Institute of Science, Rehovot, Israel; and *Laboratorio Endocrinologia Molecolare, Università Cattolica S. Cuore, 00168 Roma, Italia*

The "estrogen-induced protein" in the rat uterus (IP), first described by Notides and Gorski (30), has proven to be a very useful marker for estrogen action in normal cells and promises to be equally useful in the analysis of the estrogen responsiveness of tumor cells. The two characteristics of IP that combine to make it so suitable are the rapidity with which it is induced and the fact that it can be reproducibly induced *in vitro.* Within 15 min after injection of estradiol-17β into immature rats, increased synthesis of mRNA for IP can be detected (12). By 40 min after estrogen treatment, an increased rate of synthesis of IP is measurable (1). This increase in IP synthetic rate can be induced, although to a lower extent than *in vivo,* by incubating surviving uterus in the presence of physiological concentrations of estradiol (17). Thus, induction of IP could prove to be a valuable system for testing the responsiveness of tumors (e.g., biopsy samples) to estrogen, as a necessary adjunct to measurement of estrogen and progesterone receptors, for prediction of a tumor's response to hormonal therapy.

IP has been characterized in several laboratories (11,16,18,23,32) as a cytoplasmic protein with an isoelectric point between 4.5 and 4.7 and a molecular weight between 39,000 and 50,000. The rapid response of uterus to estradiol by increased IP synthesis led to the suggestion that IP might be a "key intermediary protein" which is necessary to enable expression of later processes in the response to estradiol (2). However, until recently (19) no function could be attributed to IP (14).

Iacobelli et al. (15) have shown by radioimmunoassay (RIA) that the concentration of IP is doubled 12 hr after estradiol injection. The increase in IP concentration, 12 or 24 hr after estradiol injection, could also be demonstrated by electrophoresis of uterine extracts on sodium dodecyl sulfate (SDS) polyacrylamide gels and staining with Coomassie brilliant blue (N. Reiss, *unpublished data*).

The constitutive presence of IP in untreated uteri has been demonstrated

41

(34) by the use of SDS polyacrylamide gel electrophoresis (24) and fluorography (7). Using this technique, the constitutive presence of IP in organs other than uterus was demonstrated (35); it was found to be a major constitutive protein in the pituitary, hypothalamus, and cerebral cortex of immature rats. The identity between uterine and nonuterine IP was shown by comparison of limited protease digestion (10) patterns. Total rat brain soluble protein was found to be rich in IP; it is one of the most prominent cytosol proteins (after tubulin and actin) at 25 to 30 days of life.

PURIFICATION OF IP FROM IMMATURE RAT BRAIN

The rat brain was chosen as the most convenient source of material for IP purification (19,21). In brief, brains from 25-day-old rats were excised and immediately frozen in liquid nitrogen. A small quantity of [^{35}S]methionine-labeled uterine protein was taken from animals injected 1 hr earlier with estradiol-17β and prepared as previously described (33); it was then added to the brain homogenate to permit fluorographic visualization and comparison of brain and uterine IP at each step of the purification. IP-containing fractions were detected on analytical SDS polyacrylamide gel slabs. A brain homogenate was prepared, using an Ultraturrax homogenizer, and centrifuged for 30 min at 40,000 $\times$ g. The supernatant was fractionated by ammonium sulfate precipitation. The fraction precipitating at 40 to 63% saturation was applied to a DEAE cellulose column (Whatman DE52) and developed with a linear salt gradient from 100 to 165 mM NaCl, 100 mM Tris-HCl, pH 7.5. The fractions from DEAE chromatography, which contained IP as the major protein, were pooled for preparative slab gel electrophoresis (25) as modified in our laboratory (21). IP was collected by precipitation in 20% TCA. This procedure resulted in approximately 70-fold purification (we estimate that this preparation is approximately 85% pure) with a yield of 26%, based on planimetric evaluation of densitometric scans of Coomassie brilliant blue stained gels.

IMMUNOCHEMICAL STUDIES

For injections into rabbits, the IP precipitate was washed twice with diethyl ether and dissolved by boiling in a small volume of 0.5% SDS, 10% glycerol. Two doses of 200 μg of rat brain IP in 50% saline and 50% complete Freund's adjuvant were injected intradermally at 14-day intervals into each of 2 male rabbits and 2 female rabbits (2 month old), followed by an additional 30-μg dose 14 days later. Blood was collected from the ear vein of the rabbits 24 and 38 days after the first injection.

Cytosol from estradiol-treated uterus, which was labeled *in vitro* with [^{35}S]methionine, was treated with normal and anti-IP serum for 3 hr at 4°C. The immune complex was prepared for analytical polyacrylamide SDS gel electrophoresis by precipitation with formalin-inactivated *Staphylococcus aureus* (22) and elution by boiling for 5 min in electrophoresis sample buffer (24). The results of gel fluorography confirmed the previous report (35) of the close similarity or identity between the uterine protein and the brain protein, since uterine IP was preferentially precipitated by antiserum raised in response to brain IP. The reaction of antiserum against the denatured brain IP with uterine cytosol was approximately equal to the reaction with antiserum prepared against uterine IP (15; see below).

We labeled organs *in vitro* with [^{35}S]methionine as described previously for the rat uterus (33) and prepared cytosol extracts of uteri from control and estrogen-treated rats, and pituitary and vagina of control rats. By immune precipitation (Fig. 1), we demonstrated the increased synthesis of IP in the rat uterus induced by estradiol (lanes c and d). The presence of IP was shown in vagina and pituitary (Fig. 1, lanes f and h), and in rat mammary tumor induced by dimethylbenzanthracene (DMBA) (Fig. 1, lanes j and k).

For the quantitation of IP by RIA, IP was prepared from rat uteri using

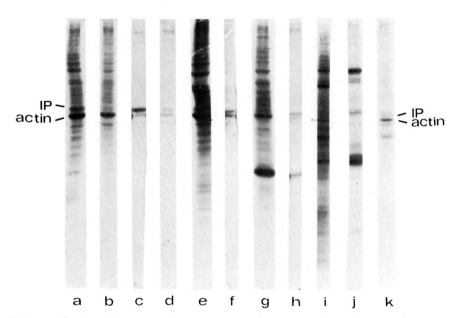

FIG. 1. Demonstration of the presence of IP in extracts of rat organs, and DMBA-induced rat mammary tumors, and their precipitates with anti-IP. Samples were subjected to SDS polyacrylamide gel electrophoresis followed by fluorography. The lanes are uterine 100,000 × *g* supernatant fractions (S$_{100}$) of estradiol-treated **(a)** and control **(b)** rats and their immune precipitates (**c** and **d,** respectively); S$_{100}$ from vagina **(e)** and pituitary of untreated rats **(g)** with their corresponding immune precipitates (**f** and **h,** respectively); S$_{100}$ fraction from DMBA-induced rat mammary tumor **(i)** and its corresponding immune precipitate **(k).** Lane **j:** IP fraction (~10% faster migration than bovine serum albumin) from Cellogel electrophoresis of the S$_{100}$ from DMBA-induced mammary tumor. (Tumor samples were obtained in collaboration with Avraham Geier, Institute of Endocrinology, Tel Hashomer, Israel.)

described procedures (16) and preparative electrophoresis on Cellogel (33). SDS polyacrylamide gel electrophoresis of the IP preparation showed a major component migrating in the range of 45,000 to 48,000 M_r and two minor components migrating in the range of M_r ~90,000 and ~25,000. As judged by the staining intensity, the 45,000 to 48,000 component represented more than 85% of the total protein visualized on the gel. Antibodies to IP were raised in rabbits as previously described (15). The sera were tested for the presence of IP antibody by immunodiffusion in agarose gel. After 4 weeks, antisera against IP were detected in all rabbits; one of the sera was found to be suitable for RIA. IP was iodinated by the chloramine-T method.

Assay of serial dilutions of rat uterus cytosol gave a dose–response curve parallel to the standard curve for the IP preparation used for immunization, whereas serum or cytosol from skeletal muscle did not show a significant inhibition (Fig. 2). The results from different tissues examined by RIA are presented in Table 1. In female rats, IP was found in high concentration in the brain (about 0.13% of the total cytosol protein from rats 12 to 16 weeks old), oviduct, uterus, and vagina, and in lower concentrations in cytosols from hypophysis, skin, kidney, and spleen. Male rat brains also contained high concentrations of IP.

Two weeks after ovariectomy, the concentrations of IP decreased by approximately 70% in the uterus (Table 2) whereas a significant increase (45%) was seen in the brain. No modifications of IP content were observed in the kidney.

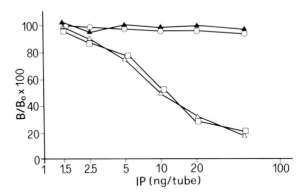

FIG. 2. RIA standard inhibition curve. The incubation mixture consisted of 100 μl of [^{125}I]-IP (15,000 cpm) (15), 100 μl standard IP preparation or appropriately diluted sample, and 100 μl antiserum [diluted 1:10,000 in phosphate-buffered saline (PBS) containing 2.5% of preimmune rabbit serum]. After incubation for 3 hr at 37°C, 100 μl of sheep antirabbit gamma globulin (DASP, Organon N.V., Oss, Holland), which had been diluted 1:10 in PBS containing 5% bovine serum albumin (BSA), was added to each tube. Tubes were incubated for 2 hr at 37°C followed by 15 min at 0–4°C and centrifuged at 10,000 × g for 5 min. Precipitates were washed with 2 ml PBS containing 2% BSA for counting in an automated gamma counter. Points represent serial dilutions of IP *(open triangles)* or cytosols from uterus *(squares)* skeletal muscle *(closed triangles)*, or serum *(circles)*. Each point represents the mean of triplicate determinations.

TABLE 1. *Concentration of IP in cytosol from rat organs*

Organ	IP (μg/mg cytosol protein)	
	Female	Male
Brain	1.28 ± 0.11	1.21 ± 0.08
Oviduct	1.19 ± 0.09	
Uterus	0.66 ± 0.02	
Vagina	0.61 ± 0.07	
Hypophysis	0.48 ± 0.05	0.29 ± 0.05
Skin	0.28 ± 0.03	0.23 ± 0.03
Kidney	0.25 ± 0.03	0.26 ± 0.04
Spleen	0.25 ± 0.04	<
Liver		<
(Serum)		<

Values shown are means of four determinations ± SD. Values below 1.5 ng/tube are indicated by <.

IP responded to estradiol administration (50 μg/kg body weight) in both the brain and the uterus, although in opposite directions. Thus, while the concentration of IP in the brain was reduced to about 45% of the original value within 12 hr, the level of IP in the uterus increased by about 70% in the same period of time. The concentrations of IP in the kidney were not significantly changed.

RIA of IP in Dimethylbenzanthracene (DMBA)-Induced Mammary Tumors

The availability of a sensitive RIA for IP permitted investigation of IP estrogen-inducibility in DMBA-induced mammary tumors. Mammary tumors were induced in 50-day-old female Sprague-Dawley rats by oral administration of 20 mg DMBA in sesame oil. Under ether anesthesia, approximately one-half of each tumor was resected and analyzed for IP content by RIA; the residual

TABLE 2. *Effects of ovariectomy and estradiol administration on IP content of female rat tissues*

Organ	IP (μg/mg cytosol protein)	
	Ovx	Ovx + estradiol
Uterus	0.20 ± 0.05	0.34 ± 0.05
Brain	1.86 ± 0.07	0.81 ± 0.07
Kidney	0.27 ± 0.06	0.23 ± 0.04

Values shown are means of four determinations ± SD. Ovx, ovariectomized 2 weeks previously. Ovx + estradiol, 50 μg estradiol-17β/kg body wt was injected into ovariectomized rats 12 hr before killing.

TABLE 3. *Concentration of IP in cytosol from DMBA-induced mammary tumors*

	IP (μg/mg cytosol protein)	
Tumor	Control	Estradiol-treated
1	0.61	0.85
2	0.21	0.23
3	0.23	0.33
4	0.33	0.41
5	0.39	n.d.
6	0.45	0.52
7	0.22	n.d.
8	0.49	0.68
9	0.15	0.26
10	0.59	0.61
Total	0.36 ± 0.16	0.48 ± 0.22

Rats were injected with 50 μg estradiol-17β/kg body wt 4 hr before extirpation of the tumor.
n.d., not detectable.

part of each tumor was left *in situ* and examined for IP after the animals were injected with estradiol (50 μg/kg body weight).

As shown in Table 3, cytosols from all ten tumors examined contained IP (mean 0.36 ± 0.16 μg/mg total cytosol protein). Moreover, the dilution curve obtained with these cytosols was parallel to the standard curve, indicating that the IP of DMBA-induced mammary tumor and that of the uterus were immunologically identical. Four hours after treatment with estradiol, the IP concentrations were increased in six of eight tumors examined and, in the two other cases, were not significantly different from pretreatment values. Preliminary results from our laboratories indicate that a protein with physicochemical properties similar to those of IP can be induced in the human uterus after estrogen stimulation (20). This finding calls for further studies on the occurrence of IP in normal and neoplastic human breast tissue.

COMPARISON OF IP WITH THE ACIDIC (γ) ISOZYME OF ENOLASE

Since IP was found to be one of the major soluble proteins of the brain, we were convinced that it must have been described by neurobiologists under some other name. Therefore we searched the literature for descriptions of brain proteins with physicochemical characteristics similar to those of IP.

In 1968, two groups described the isolation of acidic proteins from rat (4) and bovine (29) brain which were designated antigen α and 14-3-2, respectively. These proteins have very similar amino acid compositions (26) and electrophoretic mobilities (3) and exhibit high immunological cross-reactivity (3). Thus, antigen α and 14-3-2 are thought to be the same protein (3,26). Antigen 14-3-

2 was reported to be brain specific (4,9) but not species specific (3). The presence of 14-3-2 in the brain of cat (27), chicken (8), and other species has been reported. The concentration of 14-3-2 in nonnervous tissues was found to be negligible, but uterus was not studied.

It was recently reported (5,28) that 14-3-2 preparations show enolase (2-phospho-D-glycerate hydrolase, EC 4.2.1.11) activity. There were no detectable contaminants (28) in these preparations that could account for the enolase activity. Analysis of enolase isozyme patterns of rat brain revealed the presence of three enolase isozymes of which the acidic isozyme (γ dimer) was reported to be brain specific (6,28) but has recently been found in the neuroendocrine amine-precursor uptake and decarboxylation (APUD) cells of pancreas and adrenal gland (31). The other isozymes are a neutral form (α dimer) which is not neuron specific and an intermediate form which shows immunologic cross-reactivity with both subunits.

The isoelectric point of 14-3-2 is 4.7 (26) and its molecular weight is 48,000 to 50,000 (26,29). The concentration of 14-3-2 in rat brain was found to be approximately 1% of the soluble brain proteins (3,27). The close similarity in isoelectric point, molecular weight, and concentration which was found for IP and 14-3-2 in brain prompted us to examine the relationship between IP, 14-3-2, and the acidic isozyme of enolase.

Enolase Isozymes in Uterus and Brain

Cytosol of uterus and brain were prepared in 5 mM $MgSO_4$, 0.4 mM EDTA, and 50 mM Tris-HCl (pH 6.8) at a concentration of 4 volumes buffer per gram tissue. The cytosol was further diluted five times in the same buffer, but at pH 7.9, and aggregates were removed by centrifugation. The supernatant solution was applied to a DEAE cellulose column which was eluted with a linear salt gradient of 10 to 250 mM NaCl in 100 mM Tris-HCl (pH 7.5), 5 mM $MgSO_4$, and 0.4 mM EDTA. Enolase activity was assayed (28) in a reaction volume of 0.5 ml using a Gilford recording spectrophotometer.

The uterine enolase isozyme pattern (Fig. 3A) as revealed by DEAE cellulose chromatography is analogous to the pattern from brain (Fig. 3B). The ratios among the isozymes in these tissues differ, but the presence of a small but significant acidic enolase activity in uterus is reproducibly detectable (Fig. 3A, insert). The peak of acidic enolase activity in uterine fractions correlates well with the peak fraction of IP as visualized by SDS polyacrylamide gel electrophoresis (Fig. 4, bottom) of the appropriate fractions from DEAE cellulose column chromatography.

To test for estradiol-induced increases in γ enolase activity in uterus and brain, these organs were collected from 30-day-old rats at various times after estradiol injection. Tissues (0.5–2.0 g) were homogenized at pH 6.4 and the cytosol fractions applied to a small DEAE cellulose column (1 ml) at pH 7.9.

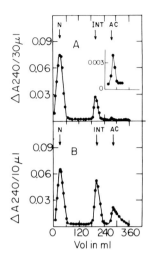

FIG. 3. Pattern of enolase isozymes, of uterine **(A)** and brain **(B)** S_{100} fractions, separated by DEAE cellulose chromatography. Forms of enolase: N, neutral; INT, intermediate; AC, acidic. **Insert** shows the acidic isozyme peak using the same abscissa and a 10-fold expanded ordinate.

The neutral isozyme was not absorbed to the column. The intermediate isozyme was eluted with 40 mM NaCl, 100 mM Tris-HCl (pH 6.4), 5 mM $MgSO_4$, and 0.4 mM EDTA. The acidic isozyme was eluted with 250 mM NaCl in the same buffer. No significant changes were observed in neutral and intermediate enolase isozyme activities in uterus (Fig. 5a and b) in response to estradiol. However, the acidic isozyme (Fig. 5c) showed a 40% increase at 2 hr, 150% at 12 hr, and 170% at 24 hr after estradiol injection.

In brain, both the intermediate (Fig. 5e) and acidic enolase isozymes (Fig. 5f) responded to estradiol injection by a decrease in activity. The percentage of the intermediate isozyme decreased rapidly to about 25% of its original value (Fig. 5e) between 8 and 24 hr after injection. The acidic enolase was reduced to 45% of its original value within 8 hr; but returned to 63% of its original value at 24 hr. The ratio of intermediate to acidic isozyme was approximately 2:1 before estradiol injection and reached a value of 0.8:1 within 12 to 24 hr after injection. SDS polyacrylamide electrophoresis revealed a decrease in IP concentration within 8 hr of estradiol injection (N. Reiss, *unpublished data*). RIA data (see above) have shown that IP decreased to about 50% of its original value in the brain of the ovariectomized rat, after estradiol injection. As a result of the decrease in the intermediate and acidic forms of enolase in brain (Fig. 5e and f) the relative percentage of the neutral enolase appears to increase (from approximately half to over three-quarters of the total enolase activity).

Partial purification of IP from brain under conditions closely similar to those reported for 14-3-2, using DEAE cellulose column chromatography as a final step, yielded an IP preparation which contained negligible contamination in the region of 40,000 to 60,000 molecular weight (N. Reiss, *unpublished data*). At this stage, the specific activity of acidic enolase was 15 units/mg which is a purification of approximately 80-fold. Using the same procedure, we obtained

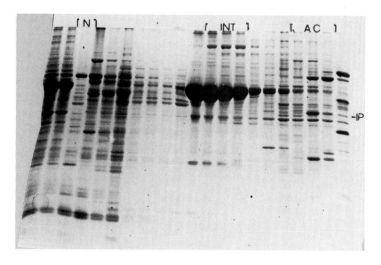

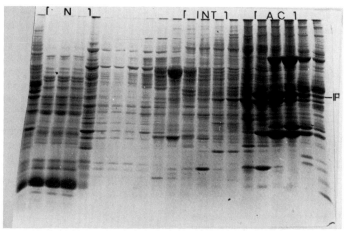

FIG. 4. Protein patterns (Coomassie brilliant blue staining) of 100,000 × *g* supernatant fractions (S$_{100}$) separated by DEAE cellulose chromatography and then subjected to SDS polyacrylamide gel electrophoresis. *Upper panel,* uterus; *lower panel,* brain. Enolase positions: N, neutral; INT, intermediate; AC, acid. Note IP band appearing in the position of the acidic enolase isozyme.

a uterine IP preparation which showed acidic enolase activity of 2 units/mg (approximately 600-fold purification). Although IP was the major protein in the preparation (N. Reiss, *unpublished data*), further purification is necessary to obtain pure IP. IP appearance in the eluate from the DEAE cellulose column, as visualized by SDS polyacrylamide gel electrophoresis, coincided exactly with the appearance of the acidic enolase activity measured by the enzyme assay (N. Reiss, *unpublished data*).

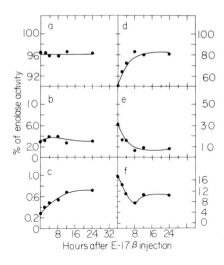

FIG. 5. Percentage of uterine neutral **(a)**, intermediate **(b)**, and acidic **(c)** enolase isozymes; and brain neutral **(d)**, intermediate **(e)**, and acidic **(f)** enolase isozymes, following injection of estradiol-17β. There was no significant change in the overall specific activity of enolase in uterus or brain after estradiol treatment.

DISCUSSION AND FUTURE PROSPECTS

Since the acidic enolase isozyme constitutes only 0.3 and 16% of enolase activity in uterus and brain, respectively, its importance in the energy generating system of these tissues remains to be clarified. IP may interact, either directly or indirectly, in a totally different metabolic process. Precedents exist for an intermediate in one pathway regulating another metabolic pathway; for example, the recent report that a glycolytic intermediate, glucose-6-phosphate, regulates initiation of protein synthesis in reticulocyte lysates (13). The present finding of the association of enolase activity with IP provides an additional characteristic in the search for the precise biological role of IP.

For investigating the mechanism of IP induction, we require a specific hybridization probe for sensitive measurement of mRNA for IP. For this purpose, poly A-rich RNA was prepared from rat brain and uterus; its capacity for directing the translation of IP was demonstrated by specific immunoprecipitation of the products of a rabbit reticulocyte lysate protein synthesizing system, and two-dimensional polyacrylamide gel analysis, i.e., isoelectric focusing in the first dimension followed by electrophoresis in the presence of SDS in the second dimension (M. Walker, *unpublished data*).

In collaboration with colleagues in the Department of Neurobiology of our Institute, a sucrose gradient fraction of brain mRNA enriched for IP message was obtained. This was subsequently transcribed into a cDNA copy, the complementary strand synthesized, and the resulting double-stranded DNA inserted into the pBR 322 plasmid using standard techniques. This plasmid was used to transform *Escherichia coli*. Probing for IP clones is presently underway.

SUMMARY

The estrogen-induced protein of uterus is a preferred marker for estrogen action because of its rapid induction both *in vivo* and *in vitro*. Its usefulness for determining the steroid responsiveness of tumors is now increased due to the availability of RIA for IP and the finding of an enzymic activity in IP preparations.

Our finding of IP in brain led us to compare IP with a specific brain protein called antigen 14-3-2 which shows enolase activity. We have shown in this report that the acidic enolase isozyme is also present in the uterus: The uterus and brain contain a similar complement of enolase isozymes, though the ratio of the isozymes is different in these two organs. The acidic (γ) enolase isozyme was also shown to be estradiol responsive in both uterus and brain, increasing in uterus and decreasing in brain after estradiol injection.

In addition to these data, the physicochemical characteristics reported for IP and 14-3-2 as well as their abundance in brain are closely similar. Therefore, there is a high probability that IP is identical to the brain protein 14-3-2 and that IP has intrinsic enolase activity.

ACKNOWLEDGMENTS

This work was supported in part by research grants from the Ford Foundation and Population Council to Prof. H. R. Lindner, and by C. N. R. Progetto Finalizzato "Biologia della Riprodozione." We thank Prof. H. R. Lindner for his help and encouragement, Michael Walker for his helpful suggestions, and Dr. Avraham Geir for DMBA-induced rat mammary tumor.

REFERENCES

1. Barnea, A., and Gorski, J. (1970): *Biochemistry,* 9:1899–1904.
2. Baulieu, E. E., Wira, C. R., Milgrom, E., and Reynaud-Jammet, C. (1972): In: *Karolinska Symposia on Research Methods in Reproductive Endocrinology, 5th Symposium,* pp. 396–419.
3. Bennet, G. S. (1974): *Brain Res.,* 68:365–369.
4. Bennett, G. S., and Edelman, G. M. (1968): *J. Biol. Chem.,* 243:6234–6241.
5. Bock, E., and Dissing, J. (1975): *Scand. J. Immunol.,* 4(suppl. 2):31–36.
6. Bock, E., Fletcher, L., Rider, C. C., and Taylor, C. B. (1978): *J. Neurochem.,* 30:181–185.
7. Bonner, W. M., and Laskey, R. A. (1974): *Eur. J. Biochem.,* 46:83–88.
8. Cicero, T. J., Cowan, W. N., and Moore, B. W. (1970): *Brain Res.,* 24:1–10.
9. Cicero, T. J., Cowan, W. M., Moore, B. W., and Suntzeff, V. (1970): *Brain Res.,* 18:25–34.
10. Cleveland, D. W., Fischer, S. G., Kirschner, M. W., and Laemmli, U. K. (1977): *J. Biol. Chem.,* 252:1102–1106.
11. Cohen, M. E., and Hamilton, T. H. (1975): *Biochem. Biophys. Res. Commun.,* 64:633–639.
12. DeAngelo, A. B., and Gorski, J. (1970): *Proc. Natl. Acad. Sci. USA,* 66:693–700.
13. Ernst, V., Levin, D. H., and London, I. M. (1978): *J. Biol. Chem.,* 253:7163–7172.
14. Galand, P., Flandroy, L., and Mairesse, N. (1978): *Life Sci.,* 22:217–238.
15. Iacobelli, S., King, R. J. B., and Vokaer, A. (1977): *Biochem. Biophys. Res. Commun.,* 76:1230–1237.

16. Iacobelli, S., Paparatti, L., and Bompiani, A. (1973): *FEBS Lett.,* 32:199–203.
17. Katzenellenbogen, B. S., and Gorski, J. (1972): *J. Biol. Chem.,* 247:1299–1305.
18. Katzenellenbogen, B. S., and Williams, L. B. (1974): *Proc. Natl. Acad. Sci. USA,* 71:1281–1285.
19. Kaye, A. M., and Reiss, N. (1980): In: *Steroid Induced Uterine Proteins,* edited by M. Beato, pp. 3–19. Elsevier/North Holland, Amsterdam.
20. Kaye, A. M. et al. (1980): *In preparation.*
21. Kaye, A. M., Reiss, N., and Walker, M. D. (1980): In: *Development of Responsiveness to Steroid Hormones,* edited by A. M. Kaye and M. Kaye, pp. 1–20. Pergamon, Oxford.
22. Kessler, S. W. (1975): *J. Immunol.,* 115:1617–1624.
23. King, R. J. B., Sömjen, D., Kaye, A. M., and Lindner, H. R. (1974): *Mol. Cell. Endocrinol.,* 1:21–36.
24. Laemmli, U. K. (1971): *Nature,* 227:680–685.
25. LeStourgon, W. M., and Beyer, A. L. (1977): *Methods Cell Biol.,* 16:387–406.
26. Marangos, P. J., Zomzely-Neurath, C., Luk, D. C. M., and York, C. (1975): *J. Biol. Chem.,* 250:1884–1891.
27. Marangos, P. J., Zomzely-Neurath, C., and York, C. (1975): *Arch. Biochem. Biophys.,* 170:289–293.
28. Marangos, P. J., Zomzely-Neurath, C., and York, C. (1976): *Biochem. Biophys. Res. Commun.,* 68:1309–1316.
29. Moore, B. W., and Perez, V. J. (1968): In: *Physiological and Biochemical Aspects of Nervous Integration,* edited by F. D. Carlson, pp. 343–360. Prentice–Hall, Engelwood Cliffs, New Jersey.
30. Notides, A., and Gorski, J. (1966): *Proc. Natl. Acad. Sci. USA,* 56:230–235.
31. Schmechel, D., Marangos, P. J., and Brightman, M. (1978): *Nature,* 276:834–836.
32. Sömjen, D., King, R. J. B., Kaye, A. M., and Lindner, H. R. (1973): *Isr. J. Med. Sci.,* 9:546–547.
33. Sömjen, D., Sömjen, G., King, R. J. B., Kaye, A. M., and Lindner, H. R. (1973): *Biochem. J.,* 136:25–33.
34. Walker, M. D., Gozes, I., Kaye, A. M., Reiss, N., and Littauer, U. Z. (1976): *J. Steroid Biochem.,* 7:1083–1085.
35. Walker, M. D., Negreanu, V., Gozes, I., and Kaye, A. M. (1979): *FEBS Lett.,* 98:187–191.

Hormones and Cancer, edited by S. Iacobelli et al.
Raven Press, New York © 1980.

Recent Data on Receptors and Biological Action of Estrogens and Antiestrogens in the Fetal Uterus of Guinea Pig

J. R. Pasqualini, C. Sumida, A. Gulino, B. L. Nguyen, J. Tardy, and C. Gelly

C.N.R.S. Steroid Hormone Research Unit, Foundation for Hormone Research, 75014 Paris, France

It is well established that estrogens and progesterone are steroid hormones which are essential for conception and gestation and that the biological action of progesterone is significantly increased by the influence of estrogens. Furthermore, the production rates and plasma concentrations of these hormones increase very significantly during pregnancy in the human and in some other mammalian species.

At present, only limited information is available on the biological role of these hormones and their effect on the maturation of the different fetal tissues. In 1971, steroid hormone receptors were found to be present in the fetal compartment: aldosterone was found in the fetal kidney of guinea pig (14), and estradiol in the fetal brain (13); later, estrogen receptors were also found in the fetal uterus, lung, kidney, and testes of the same animal species (15). In subsequent years, cortisol receptors were detected in the fetal lung of rabbit (7), and androgen receptors in reproductive tracts of fetal rat (8). This chapter summarizes different aspects of the biological action of estrogens and antiestrogens, which include their effect on the synthesis of the progesterone receptor protein in the fetal uterus of guinea pig as well as their uterotrophic effect.

SELECTIVE UPTAKE OF ESTRADIOL BY THE FETAL UTERUS OF GUINEA PIG

Figure 1 indicates the concentration of radioactivity in various fetal tissues of guinea pig at different periods after subcutaneous injection *in vivo* and *in situ* of [³H]estradiol to the fetus. In the fetal uterus, lung, and kidney, the maximal concentration of radioactivity is found 1 hr after the injection and the concentration (dpm/g tissue) is 13 to 16 times higher in the fetal uterus. It is interesting to note that a similar relationship of the concentration of estradiol-specific binding sites is found in these fetal tissues (19).

Table 1 indicates the distribution of the radioactivity, characterized by chroma-

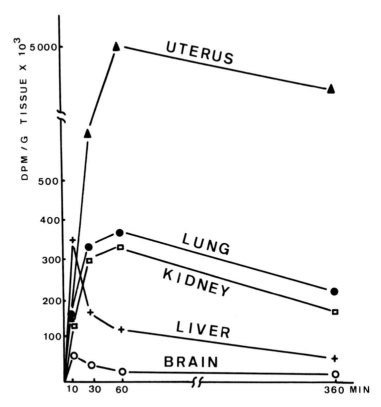

FIG. 1. Time curve of [³H]estradiol in the different fetal tissues after s.c. injection of 30 μCi [³H]estradiol to the fetus of guinea pig. Each point represents the quantitative value of the unmetabolized [³H]estradiol and is the average of two determinations.

tographic analysis as [³H]estradiol and [³H]estrone, in the cytosol and nucleus of the fetal uterus after injection of [³H]estradiol. It can be observed that the maximal values are obtained 1 hr after the injection, at which time 70% of the [³H]estradiol is present in the nucleus. Moreover, significant quantities of [³H]estrone are present in the two subcellular fractions.

PRESENCE OF ESTRADIOL AND PROGESTERONE RECEPTORS IN THE FETAL UTERUS OF GUINEA PIG

The physicochemical properties of the specific binding of both estradiol and progesterone are indicated in Table 2. These studies were carried out with the fetal uterus of guinea pig at the end of gestation. It is observed that these properties are the same as those found in the uterus during extrauterine life in different animal species. It is to be remarked that the concentration of the estradiol receptor is 8 to 10 times greater than that of the progesterone receptor.

TABLE 1. *Time curve of [³H]estradiol and [³H]estrone in the cytosol and nuclei of the fetal uterus of guinea pig after S.C. administration of [³H]estradiol to the fetus*

Time after injection (min)	Cytosol		Nuclei	
	[³H]estradiol	[³H]estrone	[³H]estradiol	[³H]estrone
10	8,000	4,400	3,600	400
30	45,000	45,000	152,000	24,000
60	200,000	61,000	350,000	29,000
360	70,000	2,300	186,000	1,500

[³H]estradiol (30 μCi) was injected *in situ* to each fetus (51–61 days of gestation), and at different periods (10, 30, 60 min and 6 hr) the fetuses were removed, decapitated, and the uteri separated and homogenized in 0.25 M sucrose, 0.01 M Tris-HCl, 0.003 M CaCl₂ buffer. After centrifugation at 900 × g, the 900 × g supernatant was centrifuged at 200,000 × g to separate the soluble cytosol. The 900 × g pellet was washed with 0.4 M sucrose, 0.01 M Tris-HCl, and 0.003 M CaCl₂, centrifuged again at 2,000–3,000 × g, homogenized in 2 M sucrose and 0.01 M Tris, and centrifuged at 200,000 × g to obtain the purified nuclei. The radioactive material of the cytosol and nuclei was extracted with ethanol and [³H]estradiol and [³H]estrone, identified, and evaluated. The values are expressed in dpm/100 mg tissue and represent the average of two to three determinations.

SUBCELLULAR DISTRIBUTION OF ESTRADIOL RECEPTOR SITES IN THE UTERUS OF GUINEA PIG FETUSES

The effect of endogenous estradiol on the subcellular distribution of estradiol receptor sites between the cytosol and nuclear fractions and the proportion of available and occupied binding sites in fetal uterus of guinea pig was determined by an exchange assay in protamine sulfate precipitates of cytosol and nuclear extracts (2,20,21). The total concentration of estradiol receptor was 11 to 15

TABLE 2. *Physicochemical characteristics of estradiol, progesterone, and R-5020-R receptors in the fetal uterus of guinea pig (end of gestation)*

Characteristics	E₂-R	P-R	R-5020-R[a]
Dissociation constant	2–5 × 10⁻¹⁰ M	3.3 ± 1.7 × 10⁻⁹ M	0.7 ± 0.3 × 10⁻⁹ M
Sedimentation coefficient	8;4	6–7;4	—
Isoelectric point	6.2	5–5.5	—
Specific binding sites (pmoles/mg DNA)[b]			
Cytosol	12.60 ± 2.47	1.34 ± 0.62	3.29 ± 1.15
Nuclei	0.65 ± 0.66	0.07 ± 0.07	0.38 ± 0.15

[a]R-5020: 17α,21-Dimethyl-19-nor-pregna-4,9-diene-3,20-dione.
[b]Occupied and unoccupied.
The dissociation constants were determined by application of the Scatchard method. The fetal uterine cytosol was incubated with 1 × 10⁻¹⁰ M to 3.5 × 10⁻⁹ M of the radioactive steroid with or without 5 × 10⁻⁷ M of the unlabeled steroids at 4°C for 18 hr. The sedimentation coefficient was determined in low salt 5–20% wt/vol sucrose density gradients. The isoelectric points were measured by electrofocusing on polyacrylamide plates as described previously (11).

pmoles/mg DNA which is two to three times higher than the values found in the uterus of immature or castrated rats (3,21). Eighty-seven percent of these binding sites are not occupied by endogenous estrogen and practically all are in the cytosol fraction. The remaining 13% which are the occupied sites (1.7 pmoles/mg DNA or 9 pmoles/g tissue) are in the range of the endogenous estradiol plus estrone concentration (7 pmoles/g tissue) found in the uterus by radioimmunoassay (19). This concentration of occupied estradiol receptor is comparable to the values of total estradiol receptor in immature or adult rat uterus which have been found to be the concentrations required to account for the biological response to estrogens in this target tissue (1,4).

EVOLUTION OF ESTRADIOL AND PROGESTERONE RECEPTOR IN THE UTERUS OF GUINEA PIG FETUSES DURING DEVELOPMENT

A study on the evolution of the estradiol and progesterone receptors in the fetal uterus during the course of fetal development revealed that the estradiol receptor can be measured at least from 34 to 35 days of gestation while the progesterone receptor remains undetectable until 50 days of gestation (Table 3). This observation suggested a causal relationship between the estradiol receptor and the stimulation of the progesterone receptor proteins under normal, physiological conditions.

EFFECT OF ESTRADIOL TREATMENT ON PROGESTERONE RECEPTORS IN THE UTERUS OF FETAL AND NEWBORN GUINEA PIGS

Since the appearance of progesterone receptors seemed to follow the rise in estradiol receptors during development, it was interesting to see if exogenously

TABLE 3. *Evolution of estradiol and progesterone receptors in fetal uterine cytosol*

Days of gestation	E-R	P-R
34–35	85–95	nd
36–37	140–200	nd
44–45	300–490	nd
50–54	550–680	30–45
55–65	580–880	70–140

Cytosol fractions of uteri of guinea pig fetuses were incubated with 4×10^{-9} M [^{3}H]estradiol (E-R) or [^{3}H]progesterone (P-R) (with or without a 100-fold molar excess of unlabeled steroid) for 4 hr at 4°C. Dextran-coated charcoal was used to separate bound and unbound steroids. The values are expressed in fmoles/mg protein and represent the extremes of four to five determinations. nd, not detectable.
Data from Pasqualini et al., ref. 17.

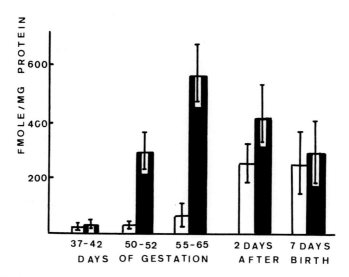

FIG. 2. Effect of estradiol treatment on specific binding of [³H]progesterone in uterine cytosol during development. Pregnant guinea pigs were injected s.c. with 1 mg/kg/day of estradiol (E₂-treated animals) or 40% ethanol-saline vehicle (control animals) for 3 days. On day 4, the animals were anesthetized, the fetuses separated, and the fetal uterus removed and cytosol fraction prepared. The newborn animals were injected s.c. for 1 day with 1–100 μg estradiol in 5% ethanol-saline. Animals were sacrificed on day 2 and uterine cytosol isolated. Cytosols were incubated with $3-4 \times 10^{-9}$ M [³H]progesterone with or without a 100-fold molar excess of unlabeled progesterone for 4–18 hr at 4°C.

administered estradiol could induce or stimulate the progesterone receptor. Figure 2 shows that progesterone receptors could be induced at a gestational age when they were normally at the limit of detection and could be increased 7 to 10 times at the end of gestation by estradiol-priming of the guinea pig mothers. After birth, there is a smaller stimulatory effect above the control values which are higher in newborn animals than in fetuses.

EFFECT OF ESTRADIOL ON THE UPTAKE OF [³H]PROGESTERONE IN THE FETAL UTERUS OF GUINEA PIG

The uptake and subcellular localization of the radioactivity after injection of [³H]progesterone to the fetus were studied by autoradiography in nontreated animals and in estradiol-primed animals. [³H]progesterone was injected to the fetus *in situ* and *in vivo* in the control animal and in animals treated with estradiol (1 mg/kg/day) for 3 days. After 30 min, the animals were anesthetized, the fetuses separated from the mother, and the fetal uterus removed and processed for autoradiography as described by Stumpf and Roth (18) with the modification indicated in a previous publication (17). As indicated in Fig. 3, the uterine accumulation of radioactivity in the estradiol-treated animals is many times

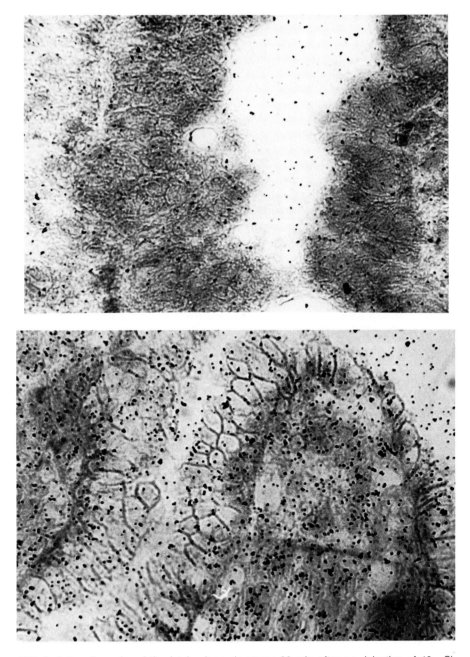

FIG. 3. Autoradiography of the fetal guinea pig uterus 30 min after s.c. injection of 40 μCi [³H]progesterone to the fetus. **Top:** Fetal uterus of nontreated animals. **Bottom:** Fetal uterus of estradiol-primed animals (1 mg estradiol/kg/day during 3 days). Magnification 520×. Exposure time, 94 days. (From Pasqualini et al., ref. 17, with permission.)

higher than in nontreated animals, which agrees with other results obtained on the stimulation of progesterone-specific binding sites by the action of estradiol.

TIME COURSE OF THE EFFECT OF ESTRADIOL ON PROGESTERONE RECEPTORS IN THE UTERUS OF FETAL GUINEA PIGS

Pregnant guinea pigs were injected with 1 mg of estradiol for increasing lengths of time up to 24 hr and with daily injections up to 3 days at which time the treatment was stopped. As indicated in Fig. 4, the progesterone receptor already begins to increase at 6 hr after estradiol administration and reaches maximal values by 15 hr. Repeated injections do not increase this effect and cessation of treatment does not lead to a loss of progesterone receptors even up to 4 days after the last injection. On the other hand, uterine wet weight only increased after 3 daily injections of estradiol, showing that the uterotrophic response and the progesterone receptor stimulation are two parameters of estrogen action which are widely separated in time in the uterus of the fetus.

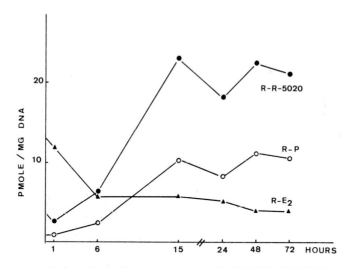

FIG. 4. Time curve of effect of estradiol on progesterone (R-P), R-5020 (R-R-5020), and estradiol (R-E₂) receptors in the fetal uterus of guinea pig (total specific binding: cytosol + nucleus). Pregnant guinea pigs (55–60 days of gestation) were injected with 1 mg estradiol/kg body weight in 50% ethanol saline and animals were sacrificed after 1, 6, and 24 hr. Another group of animals was injected for 2 (48 hr) or 3 (72 hr) consecutive days before sacrifice 24 hr after the last injection. Specific binding of [³H]progesterone and ³H-R-5020 were measured in the cytosol fraction and 0.6 M KCl nuclear extract of fetal uterus by incubations at 4°C for 18 hr with 4 × 10⁻⁹ M radioactive steroid (with and without a 100-fold molar excess of unlabeled steroid). Bound steroid was separated by charcoal-dextran adsorption. Specific binding of [³H]estradiol was assayed in protamine sulfate precipitates of cytosol and 0.6 M KCl nuclear extract by incubation with 1 × 10⁻⁸ M [³H]estradiol (with and without a 100-fold molar excess of unlabeled estradiol) under exchange conditions which measure total binding.

COMPARATIVE EFFECT OF DIFFERENT ESTROGENS (ESTRONE, ESTRADIOL, ESTRIOL) ON UTERINE GROWTH AND ON THE STIMULATION OF THE PROGESTERONE RECEPTOR IN THE FETAL UTERUS OF GUINEA PIG

Uterotrophic Effect

The action of these estrogens on fetal uterine growth was studied in the fetal uterus of guinea pig at the end of gestation and compared in the newborn animals. As indicated in Table 4, the uterotrophic effect is similar for these three estrogens in the fetal uterus, but the action in the uterus of newborns is three to five times higher with estradiol or estrone than with estriol.

Effect on the Uterine Progesterone Receptors

It was demonstrated that, after injection of [³H]estradiol to the fetus of guinea pig, a significant percentage of this hormone is converted to estrone (16). Furthermore, important quantities of this steroid circulate in the fetal plasma, and the concentration in the fetal uterus is evaluated to be six to eight times higher than in the plasma. In addition, the data indicated in Table 2 show that significant quantities of this estrogen are localized in the nuclei. Consequently, it was interesting to compare the action of estrone on the concentration of progesterone receptors in the fetal uterus of guinea pig. Table 5 indicates that the three estrogens studied have a similar effect in increasing the progesterone receptor. Particularly interesting is the data obtained with estriol, because it is well known that this is quantitatively the most important estrogen circulating during human pregnancy.

TABLE 4. *Uterotrophic response to estradiol, estriol, and estrone in the fetal and newborn guinea pig*

	Uterine wet wt (mg)			
	Control (nontreated animals)	+ Estradiol	+ Estriol	+ Estrone
Fetal uterus	50–110	95–140	92–120	106–126
Newborn uterus	80–107	355–509	150–178	280–435

Pregnant guinea pigs (57–65 days of gestation) were injected s.c. with 1 mg estrone, estradiol, or estriol (1 mg/kg/day) for 3 days and sacrificed on day 4. Three-day-old guinea pigs were treated s.c. with 0.5 μg of estrone, estradiol, or estriol (dissolved in saline solution) for 6 days and sacrificed on day 7. Uteri were excised, stripped of adhering fat, and weighed. The values represent the extremes of four to five determinations.

TABLE 5. *Comparative effect of estradiol, estriol, and estrone on the progesterone and R-5020-R receptors in the fetal uterus of guinea pig*

Treatment	P-R		R-5020-R[a]	
	Cytosol	Nuclei	Cytosol	Nuclei
Control (nontreated)	70–140	4–50	100–250	23–70
+ Estradiol	500–920	101–203	1150–1680	279–480
+ Estriol	710–1030	43–200	890–1920	150–350
+ Estrone	440–580	31–75	1050–1220	—

[a] R-5020: 17α-21-Dimethyl-19-nor-pregna-4,9-diene-3,20-dione.

Pregnant guinea pigs (57–62 days of gestation) were injected with 1 mg estradiol, estriol, or estrone/kg/day for 3 consecutive days (controls received vehicle alone). On day 4, the fetuses were removed, fetal uteri were excised, and cytosol fraction (C) and 0.6 M KCl nuclear extract (N) of fetal uterus were prepared. Specific binding of [^{3}H]progesterone (P-R) and ^{3}H-R-5020 was determined by incubations with 4×10^{-9} M radioactive steroid (with and without a 100-fold excess of unlabeled steroid) at 4°C overnight. The values are expressed in fmoles/mg protein and represent the extremes of two to six determinations. —: not carried out.

ACTION OF ANTIESTROGENS (TAMOXIFEN AND NAFOXIDINE) ON UTERINE GROWTH AND PROGESTERONE RECEPTORS IN THE FETAL UTERUS OF GUINEA PIG

In order to study the effect of these antiestrogens in the fetal uterus of guinea pig, 1 mg of nafoxidine or tamoxifen was injected to the pregnant guinea pig (58–62 days of gestation) for 3 days and the weight of the fetal uterus and the concentration of specific binding sites for progesterone were evaluated on day 4.

Uterotrophic Effect

Table 6 shows the action of nafoxidine and tamoxifen on the weight of the fetal uterus. An 80 to 100% increase is observed in relation to nontreated animals. This effect is similar to that obtained with estradiol.

TABLE 6. *Effect of nafoxidine, tamoxifen, and estradiol on the weight of fetal uterus of guinea pig*

Treatment	Uterine wet wt (mg)
Control (nontreated)	50–110
Nafoxidine	120–150
Tamoxifen	100–190

Pregnant guinea pigs (57–64 days of gestation) were injected s.c. with 1 mg/kg/day for 3 consecutive days with nafoxidine, tamoxifen, or estradiol. Animals were sacrificed on day 4 and the fetal uteri weighed. Values represent the extremes of 8–15 determinations.

TABLE 7. *Action of nafoxidine and tamoxifen on the progesterone receptor in the fetal uterus of guinea pig*

Treatment	Progesterone receptors (pmoles/mg DNA)	
	Cytosol	Nuclei
Control	0.9	0.03
Tamoxifen	2.0	0.26
Nafoxidine	2.6	0.18
Estradiol	9.0	0.40

Pregnant guinea pigs (57–64 days of gestation) were injected s.c. with 1 mg/kg/day of tamoxifen, nafoxidine, or estradiol during 3 consecutive days. On day 4, the fetuses were removed and the progesterone receptors in the cytosol and nuclei of the fetal uteri were determined as indicated in the legend to Table 5.

Effect on Fetal Uterine Progesterone Receptors

As indicated in Table 7, the action of these antiestrogens on the biosynthesis of the progesterone receptor protein is limited and represents only one-third of the effect of the different estrogens (see Table 5).

DISCUSSION AND CONCLUSIONS

The study of different aspects of receptors and the biological action of estrogens in the fetal uterus of guinea pig gives a series of results which lead us to the conclusion that the uterus responds to hormone action during intrauterine life.

The data in Fig. 1 and Table 1 show the very selective uptake of circulating estradiol by the fetal uterus and after 1 hr of [³H]estradiol administration, the ratio of radioactivity/gram uterine tissue to radioactivity/milliliter of fetal plasma is 30 to 50; this relationship is of the same order as that found for concentrations of endogenous estrogens (19).

The analysis of the occupied specific binding sites of estradiol in the fetal uterine tissue shows values which are relatively high (2–3 pmoles/mg DNA) (20), and the fact that estrogen receptors appear in the fetal uterus at an early period of fetal development, but that progesterone receptors are only present at the end of gestation (19), suggests the possibility of an action of estradiol on the biosynthesis of progesterone receptor protein which is proved by the administration of estradiol to the mother (see Fig. 2).

The most interesting aspect of this stimulation is that the effect of estradiol is many times higher in the fetal uterus than in the uterus of newborn animals. Furthermore, as is indicated in Fig. 4, there is a significant disappearance of the total (occupied and unoccupied) specific binding sites of estradiol in the fetal uterine tissue after injection of estradiol. These data are contrary to those observed in immature rat uterus (10), but a similar effect was recently observed in human breast cancer (MCF-7 cell line) (9). This decrease in the concentration of estradiol binding sites could be related to recent data in which a prolonged effect of estradiol on the stimulation of the progesterone receptor in the fetal uterus was observed. These results indicate that 5 days after the administration of the last dose of estradiol the concentration of progesterone receptors is the same as that evaluated only 24 hr after the last injection (17). This effect is also different from that of estradiol on progesterone receptor in adult castrated guinea pigs treated with diethylstilbestrol, in which most of the stimulated progesterone receptor disappears 48 hr after the treatment (6). Consequently, it could be suggested that, in the fetal uterus, estradiol can have a negative control of its own receptor.

An interesting aspect of this finding is the similar effect, in fetal uterus, of the three estrogens, estrone, estradiol, and estriol, on both actions: increase in uterine weight and stimulation of the progesterone receptors. The effect of estriol can be of particular interest, as it is well known that this steroid is quantitatively the most important estrogen circulating throughout human pregnancy. As indicated in Table 5, the action of estriol can be very different in the fetal compartment and in extrauterine life; the uterotrophic effect of estriol is many times less intense in the uterus of the newborns than in the fetal uterus. Clark et al. (5) explained this difference by a shorter nuclear retention of estriol than of estradiol.

Studies with the antiestrogens nafoxidine and tamoxifen show that these drugs, which are generally used as antiestrogens, can have a potent estrogenic effect, at least with regard to the uterotrophic action. Complementary studies on the histological effect of these drugs, as well as the effect on the nuclear translocation of the estrogen receptors, are needed to clarify this action.

It is concluded that some aspects of the estrogen receptor and estrogen action are different in the fetal and in the extrauterine life and the fetal uterus of guinea pig is a useful model for studying the different biochemical events of the action of estrogens and anti-estrogens.

ACKNOWLEDGMENTS

Part of the expense of this work was defrayed by a grant from the "Centre National de la Recherche Scientifique" (C.N.R.S.), France ("Equipe de Recherche CNRS No. 187"). This chapter is dedicated to Elwood V. Jensen on the occasion of his sixtieth birthday.

REFERENCES

1. Anderson, J. N., Peck, E. J., Jr., and Clark, J. H. (1973): *Endocrinology,* 92:1488–1495.
2. Chamness, G. C., Huff, K., and McGuire, W. L. (1975): *Steroids,* 25:627–635.

3. Clark, J. H., Anderson, J., and Peck, E. J. Jr., (1972): *Science,* 176:528–530.
4. Clark, J. H., Eriksson, H. A., and Hardin, J. W. (1976): *J. Steroid Biochem.,* 7:1039–1044
5. Clark, J. H., Paszko, Z., and Peck, E. J. (1977): *Endocrinology,* 100:91–96.
6. Freifeld, M. L., Feil, P. D., and Bardin, C. W. (1974): *Steroids,* 23:93–103.
7. Giannopoulus, G., Mulay, S., and Solomon, S. (1972): *Biochem. Biophys., Res. Commun.,* 47:411–418.
8. Gupta, C., and Bloch, E. (1976): *Endocrinology,* 99:389–399.
9. Horwitz, K. B., and McGuire, W. L. (1978): *J. Biol. Chem.,* 253:2223–2228.
10. Katzenellenbogen, B. S., and Ferguson, E. R. (1975): *Endocrinology,* 97:1–12.
11. Pasqualini, J. R., and Cosquer-Clavreul, C. (1978): *Experientia,* 34:268–269.
12. Pasqualini, J. R., and Nguyen, B. L. (1980): *Endocrinology,* 106:1160–1165.
13. Pasqualini, J. R., and Palmada, M. (1971): *Endocrinology (Suppl.),* 88:A242.
14. Pasqualini, J. R., and Sumida, C. (1971): *C. R. Acad. Sci. Ser. D.,* 273:1061–1063.
15. Pasqualini, J. R., Sumida, C., and Gelly, C. (1976): *J. Steroid Biochem.,* 7:1031–1038.
16. Pasqualini, J. R., Sumida, C., and Gelly, C. (1976): *Acta Endocrinol.,* 83:811–828.
17. Pasqualini, J. R., Sumida, C., Nguyen, B. L., Tardy, J., and Gelly, C. (1980): *J. Steroid Biochem.,* 12:65–72.
18. Stumpf, W. E., and Roth, L. J. (1966): *J. Histochem. Cytochem.,* 14:274–287.
19. Sumida, C., and Pasqualin, J. R. (1979): *J. Steroid Biochem.,* 11:267–272.
20. Sumida, C., and Pasqualini, J. R. (1979): *Endocrinology,* 105:406–413.
21. Zava, D. T., Harrington, N. Y., and McGuire, W. L. (1976): *Biochemistry,* 15:4292–4297.

Hormone Action in Normal and Neoplastic Tissues: Glucocorticoids

Hormones and Cancer, edited by S. Iacobelli et al.
Raven Press, New York © 1980.

Genetic Analysis of Glucocorticoid Action on Lymphoid Cell Lines

Suzanne Bourgeois and Ronald F. Newby

The Salk Institute, Regulatory Biology Laboratory, San Diego, California 92138

The somatic cell genetic approach to hormone action requires the use of a genetically uniform population of responsive cells in which rare unresponsive variants can easily be recognized, selected, and cloned for further genetic and biochemical characterization of their defect. This approach can be used to study the mode of action of glucocorticoids because of the availability of a number of neoplastic lymphoid cell lines which have been established in tissue culture, and which retain many of the differentiated properties of normal thymocytes or lymphocytes. In particular, mouse thymomas and thymus-derived lymphoma lines that undergo cytolysis in response to glucocorticoids have been cloned. Unresponsive variants can be selected by their resistance to the killing effect of the steroid, and cloned. Cell fusion can be used to perform dominance and complementation analysis of the defects involved, and the glucocorticoid receptor of resistant variants can be measured and characterized.

The murine lymphoma line S49, adapted to tissue culture and cloned by Horibata and Harris (12), has been used extensively for such studies. However, some properties of the S49 line raised questions about the validity of using that line for a genetic analysis of the mechanism of lymphocytolysis. In particular, the frequency of appearance of glucocorticoid-resistant S49 variants, of the order of 10^{-6} to 10^{-5} is surprisingly high for a genetic event in a pseudodiploid somatic cell (1,10,20,21). Moreover, this high frequency appeared to be independent of cell ploidy, in that it was observed in a pseudotetraploid S49 line as well as in pseudodiploids (10,20,21). This behavior suggested the possibility that the appearance of resistance involved a stable phenotypic variation in the expression of the genome, rather than a change in the primary structure of DNA, i.e., an "epigenetic" rather than a genetic event.

Because of this and other problems encountered with the S49 line, we have turned to another glucocorticoid-sensitive lymphoid line, the murine thymoma WEHI-7 (W7). Our studies with the W7 line (1,3,16–18) confirm the genetic nature of the acquisition of resistance to glucocorticoids, and clarify some of the earlier observations made with the S49 line. W7 variants and hybrids have also been useful in investigating the correlation between the glucocorticoid receptor content of lymphoid cells and their cytolytic response (2).

HEMIZYGOSITY OF THE GLUCOCORTICOID RECEPTOR GENE

The W7 line was established in tissue culture and cloned by Harris et al. (9) from a thymoma that arose in a female BALB/c mouse after X-ray irradiation. We have derived from this line (1) a variant, W7TB, resistant to thymidine and to 5-bromo-2′-deoxyuridine (BUdR) and another variant, W7TG, resistant to 6-thioguanine (TG). The introduction of these markers does not affect the response of these lines to glucocorticoids, but allows the selection of hybrids between BUdR-resistant and TG-resistant lines in a medium containing hypoxanthine, aminopterin, and thymidine (15). All glucocorticoid-resistant variants were derived from the glucocorticoid-sensitive W7TB or W7TG line, and Fig. 1 shows the origin of the different lines used in this study.

Both the W7TB and W7TG lines are highly sensitive to the synthetic glucocorticoid dexamethasone, like their W7 parent. Figure 2a illustrates the effect of 10^{-5} M dexamethasone on the growth of these lines. In the absence of glucocorticoid, the doubling time of the W7 lines is approximately 15 hr. In the presence of 10^{-5} M dexamethasone, the number of living cells decreases; pyknotic cells and cells unable to exclude trypan blue appear in the culture which will eventually lyse. Figure 3a shows a Scatchard plot analysis of the data obtained for the specific binding of [³H]dexamethasone to whole cells, using the assay described elsewhere (18). The W7TB and W7TG lines both contain approximately 30,000 dexamethasone receptor sites per cell, and bind this steroid with an affinity, $K_D = 1.3 \pm 0.3 \times 10^{-8}$ M. In the conditions of the assay (18) used to measure the extent of transfer of these bound receptors to the nucleus, approximately 70% of the receptors of the W7TB and W7TG lines are found in the nuclear fraction (data not shown).

Our interest in the W7 line was prompted by the observation of A. Harris *(personal communication)* that no dexamethasone-resistant variant could ever be spontaneously derived from this line, in contrast to the high frequency of such variants mentioned earlier for the S49 line. Table 1 shows that no resistant variant was found when populations of approximately 3×10^8 W7TG or W7TB cells were exposed to 10^{-6} M dexamethasone, confirming that the frequency

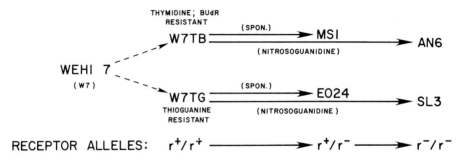

FIG. 1. Lineages of the cell lines described in the text.

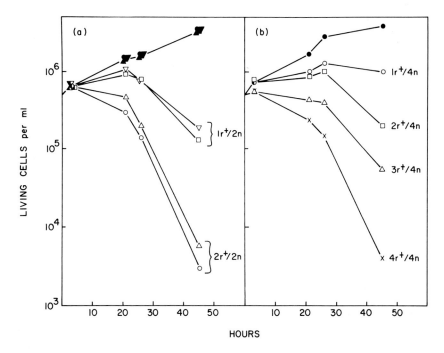

FIG. 2. Growth curves of parental and hybrid lines in the presence of dexamethasone. *Open symbols:* Cultures in the presence of 10^{-5} M dexamethasone. *Closed symbols:* Control cultures without dexamethasone. Conditions used for growth have been described elsewhere (1). "Living" cells are defined as those cells which exclude trypan blue. All cultures were inoculated with 5×10^5 cells/ml. **a:** Parental lines: W7TB *(open circles);* W7TG *(upward open triangles);* MS1 *(open squares);* EO24 *(downward open triangles);* same four cell lines without dexamethasone *(closed symbols).* **b:** Hybrid clones: W7TB $\times$ W7TG *(cross);* MS1 $\times$ W7TG *(triangles);* W7TB $\times$ SL3 *(squares);* MS1 $\times$ SL3 *(open circles);* control culture of MS1 $\times$ SL3 hybrid in the absence of dexamethasone *(closed circles).* The growths without dexamethasone of the other hybrid lines (not shown) were very similar to that of the MS1 $\times$ SL3 control. $Xr^+ = X$ gene doses for dexamethasone receptor; n value = ploidy.

of this event is very low, $< 3 \times 10^{-9}$. This frequency can be increased to values of 10^{-7} to 10^{-6} (see Table 1) by mutagenic treatment with N-methyl-N'-nitro-N-nitrosoguanidine, as was shown to be the case also for the S49 line (20). However, when exposed to lower concentrations of dexamethasone (5×10^{-9} M) the W7TG and W7TB lines gave rise spontaneously, and with a frequency of approximately 2×10^{-6}, to variants resistant to this concentration of the steroid (see Table 1).

Two such variants, MS1 derived from W7TB and EO24 derived from W7TG (see Fig. 1), were cloned and further characterized. Figure 2a shows that these variants, which formed clones in 5×10^{-9} M dexamethasone, are also less sensitive than their parental lines to 10^{-5} M dexamethasone: the number of living cells in these cultures increased from 5×10^5 cells/ml to approximately 10^6

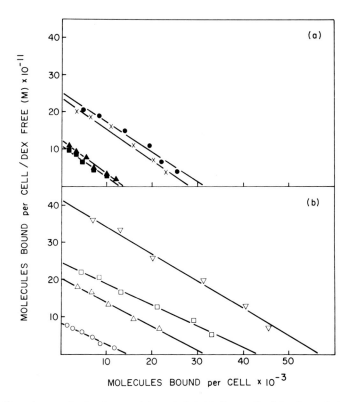

FIG. 3. Receptor content of parental and hybrid lines. Scatchard analysis of [1,2-^{3}H]dexamethasone specific binding data obtained in the whole-cell assay described elsewhere (18). **a:** Parental lines: W7TG *(circles)*; W7TB *(crosses)*; MS1 *(triangles)*; EO24 *(squares)*. **b:** Hybrid clones: The data shown represent averaged values obtained, at identical dexamethasone concentrations, for several clones containing one *(circles)*, two *(upward triangles)*, three *(squares)*, or four *(downward triangles)* copies of the r[+] receptor allele. *Circles:* average of four clones resulting from an MS1 (r[+]/r[−]) × SL3 (r[−]/r[−]) fusion. *Upward triangles:* average of one clone from a W7TB (r[+]/r[+]) × SL3 (r[−]/r[−]) fusion, one clone from a MS1 (r[+]/r[−]) × EO24 (r[+]/r[−]) fusion, and one clone from a AN6 (r[−]/r[−]) × W7TG (r[+]/r[+]) fusion. *Squares:* average of one clone from an MS1 (r[+]/r[−]) × W7TG (r[+]/r[+]) fusion and of one clone from a W7TB (r[+]/r[+]) × EO24 (r[+]/r[−]) fusion. *Downward triangles:* average of two clones from a W7TB (r[+]/r[+]) × W7TG (r[+]/r[+]) fusion.

cells/ml during the first 20 hr of exposure before a decline in the living cell population and lysis were observed. The receptor content of the MS1 and EO24 lines is shown in Fig. 3a: both lines contain approximately 15,000 receptor sites per cell, which bind dexamethasone with the same affinity as their parental lines. The extent of transfer of these steroid–receptor complexes to the nucleus in the conditions of our assay is 70%, also identical to that of their parental lines (17).

The MS1 and EO24 lines, which have a reduced sensitivity to dexamethasone, have half the parental amount of receptor which appears, however, to be normal.

TABLE 1. *Frequencies of dexamethasone-resistant variants*

Cell line	Receptor alleles	No. r^+ alleles/cell	Dex. conc. (M)	Mutagen (μg/ml)	No. cells in sample	No. variants in sample	Frequency[a]
W7TG	r^+/r^+	2	10^{-6}	None	2.8×10^8	0	$<3.6 \times 10^{-9}$ [b]
W7TB	r^+/r^+	2	10^{-6}	None	3.5×10^8	0	$<2.9 \times 10^{-9}$ [b]
W7TG	r^+/r^+	2	10^{-6}	NG^d (1.25)	1.8×10^8	26	1.4×10^{-7} [b]
W7TB	r^+/r^+	2	10^{-6}	NG^d (1.25)	5.9×10^7	76	1.3×10^{-6} [b]
W7TG	r^+/r^+	2	5×10^{-9}	None	2.9×10^6	7	2.4×10^{-6} [b]
W7TB	r^+/r^+	2	5×10^{-9}	None	8.6×10^6	17	2.0×10^{-6} [b]
E024	r^+/r^-	1	10^{-5}	None	2.4×10^6	36	1.5×10^{-5} [b]
MS1	r^+/r^-	1	10^{-6}	None	2.4×10^6	10	4.2×10^{-6} [b]
MS1 × SL3	$r^+/r^- \times r^-/r^-$	1	10^{-5}	None	3.0×10^5	348	1.6×10^{-3} [c]
AN6 × W7TG	$r^-/r^- \times r^+/r^+$	2	10^{-5}	None	9.0×10^7	218	7.6×10^{-6} [c]
W7TB × E024	$r^+/r^+ \times r^+/r^-$	3	10^{-5}	None	1.4×10^8	0	$<7.1 \times 10^{-9}$
W7TB × W7TG	$r^+/r^+ \times r^+/r^+$	4	10^{-5}	None	4.0×10^7	0	$<2.5 \times 10^{-8}$

[a] The number of cells in the sample is the total number of cells present in the culture at the time of addition of dexamethasone. Since the number of living cells increases for a period of time after addition of the steroid, the actual number of cells giving rise to resistant variants cannot be accurately known. Thus, the calculated frequencies may be overestimated to a degree depending on the amount of growth of each line in the presence of dexamethasone, which could be considerable especially at low dexamethasone concentration and in the case of the hybrid MS1 × SL3 partially resistant to 10^{-5} M dexamethasone.

[b] Data published elsewhere by Bourgeois and Newby (1).

[c] Values corrected for cloning efficiencies of 73% in the case of MS1 × SL3 and of 32% in the case of AN6 × W7TG.

[d] NG: *N*-methyl-*N'*-nitro-*N*-nitrosoguanidine.

The dexamethasone-resistant variants were selected as clones growing in liquid medium in the presence of the indicated concentration of the steroid, as described elsewhere (1).

The phenotype of these lines seems, therefore, to be the result of a reduction in the quantity of receptor rather than of a change in its properties. Another important characteristic of the MS1 and EO24 lines is shown in Table 1: they give rise with a high frequency (10^{-6}–10^{-5}) to variants that are fully resistant to high concentrations of dexamethasone. As described elsewhere (17), the vast majority of the fully resistant variants derived from MS1 and EO24 are "receptorless," i.e., lack any detectable dexamethasone receptor, while a few of them are "nuclear transfer defective," i.e., have receptors altered in their capacity to be transferred to the nucleus.

These results can be explained most simply by the following model: while two copies of a gene, r^+, coding for the glucocorticoid receptor would be present in the W7 parental line (r^+/r^+), as expected for a pseudodiploid somatic cell, the MS1 and EO24 derivatives would be functionally hemizygous at that locus (r^+/r^-). The presence of half the amount of receptor in these lines would reflect an r^+ gene dosage effect, while the high frequency of appearance of variants resistant to high dexamethasone concentrations would be due to the fact that a single genetic event is required to inactivate the only r^+ allele present in the hemizygous (r^+/r^-) MS1 and EO24 lines, while two events would be necessary to inactivate both copies of the r^+ gene in the W7 (r^+/r^+) parental lines.

In the W7 system, then, the frequency of appearance of glucocorticoid-resistant variants appears to be strictly dependent on the ploidy of the r^+ allele, as expected for a *bona fide* genetic phenomenon. How can these results be reconciled with the observations made with the S49 line? It is striking that the MS1 and EO24 lines described above behave like S49 in that they give rise, with high frequency, to fully resistant variants which are of the same types, "receptorless" and "nuclear transfer defective," and which are obtained in the same proportion in both systems (17,20). Moreover, we have shown elsewhere that the S49 line also contains 15,000 dexamethasone binding sites per cell, and displays the same level of sensitivity as MS1 and EO24 to the cytolytic effect of the steroid (1). These similarities strongly suggest that, like the MS1 and EO24 lines, the S49 line is functionally hemizygous at the r locus (r^+/r^-). As far as the high frequency of resistant variants observed in a S49 pseudotetraploid line is concerned (10,20,21), we will show later that this phenomenon can be accounted for by chromosome segregation in tetraploid cells.

CORRELATION BETWEEN GLUCOCORTICOID RECEPTOR CONTENT AND SENSITIVITY OF CELL HYBRIDS

The question of the correlation between glucocorticoid receptor content and cytolytic response of lymphoid cells is of great interest, because such a correlation would support the idea that glucocorticoid receptor measurements in human leukemic lymphocytes and in lymphomas would be useful in predicting the outcome of glucocorticoid therapy. The W7 thymoma line and its derivatives offer the possibility of investigating this controversial issue in a murine model system.

Three types of cells differing in their glucocorticoid receptor content are available: the homozygous r^+/r^+ W7 parental lines, the hemizygous r^+/r^- lines selected for resistance at 5×10^{-9} M dexamethasone, and the homozygous r^-/r^- lines induced by mutagenic treatment and resistant to 10^{-6} M dexamethasone (see Table 1). The AN6 (r^-/r^-) line was derived from the W7TB parent, and the SL3 (r^-/r^-) line from the W7TG parent, as shown in Fig. 1. Because of the presence of the TG resistance or TB resistance marker in these lines, hybrids can be selected after cell fusion which contain one ($r^+/r^- \times r^-/r^-$), two ($r^+/r^+ \times r^-/r^-$ or $r^+/r^- \times r^+/r^-$), three ($r^+/r^+ \times r^+/r^-$), or four ($r^+/r^+ \times r^+/r^+$) copies of the r^+ allele. By selection for hybrids in hypoxanthine–aminopterin–thymidine medium, no selective pressure is imposed for any level of resistance to glucocorticoids. In fact, the hybrid clones described below had never been exposed to glucocorticoids before the receptor assays and the tests of sensitivity to dexamethasone were performed.

Cell fusions were induced by polyethylene glycol (6), and hybrids were observed at frequencies of 1×10^{-7}–2×10^{-6}. Figure 3b shows that hybrids were obtained in which the receptor content reflects the number of copies of the r^+ allele: the number of dexamethasone binding sites per cell was approximately 15,000, 32,000, 43,000, and 57,000 for hybrids containing one, two, three, or four r^+ alleles, respectively. The effect of 10^{-5} M dexamethasone on the growth of these hybrids is illustrated in Fig. 2b. The rate of the cytolytic response is tightly correlated with the receptor content, and their sensitivity increases with the number of receptor sites per cell. The hybrid containing a single dose of receptor per tetraploid cell ($1r^+/4n$) is the most resistant, the number of living cells increasing for 30 hr, although slow lysis will eventually occur at later times. At the concentration of dexamethasone used, 10^{-5} M, all the cellular receptors are saturated and the response is limited by the receptor concentration. Studies carried out at dexamethasone concentrations in the range of 10^{-9}–10^{-8} M have shown that, in these hybrids, the response can be further limited by the degree of occupancy of the receptors (2): the number of receptor–steroid complexes limits the cytolytic response.

CHROMOSOME SEGREGATION IN CELL HYBRIDS

The hybrids described above can also be used to examine the correlation between the number of copies of the r^+ allele and the frequencies of variants resistant to 10^{-5} M dexamethasone. We have seen earlier (see Table 1) that, in diploid cells, these frequencies are dependent on the homo- or hemizygous state of the r locus, the r^+/r^+ cells giving rise to variants at very low frequencies of $< 3 \times 10^{-9}$, while values of 10^{-6}–10^{-5} were observed for r^+/r^- cells. The frequencies of resistant variants derived from hybrids containing one, two, three, or four copies of the r^+ allele are also listed in Table 1. In the case of the hybrid (MS1 × SL3) containing a single copy of the r^+ allele, a frequency of approximately 10^{-3} was observed, three orders of magnitude higher than in the case of the diploid cell, r^+/r^-, containing a single r^+ allele. Similarly, the frequency obtained in the case of the hybrid (AN6 × W7TG) containing two r^+ alleles is $7.5 × 10^{-6}$, at least three orders of magnitude higher than the value of $< 3 × 10^{-9}$ observed for r^+/r^+ diploid cells. Hybrids containing three or four r^+ alleles, however, did not give rise to variants at a frequency high enough to be precisely estimated in these experiments: these values are $< 10^{-8}$ or $< 10^{-9}$.

These results suggest that, in the case of tetraploid cells, resistance can be acquired not only by mutations but also by segregation of chromosomes, involving loss or rearrangements of the chromosome(s) carrying the r^+ allele(s). Figure 4 shows that chromosome losses do, indeed, occur in these hybrids. The karyotype of a AN6 (r^-/r^-) × W7TG (r^+/r^+) hybrid clone (Fig. 4a) reveals that the majority of these cells contain 80 chromosomes. A variant resistant to 10^{-5} M dexamethasone was selected from this hybrid and karyotyped. Figure 4b illustrates that the majority of the cells of this variant population contain 78 chromosomes. In the course of the growth of the AN6 × W7TG hybrid and

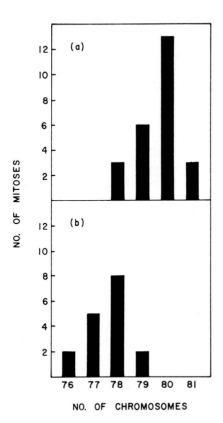

FIG. 4. Karyotypes of a hybrid and its dexamethasone-resistant variant. The procedure used for chromosome analysis has been described elsewhere (1). **a:** AN6 (r^-/r^-) × W7TG (r^+/r^+) hybrid clone. **b:** Clone resistant to 10^{-5} M dexamethasone derived from the same AN6 × W7TG hybrid.

of the selection of its dexamethasone-resistant variant, approximately two chromosomes have been lost.

Segregation-like events have been observed in the case of other intraspecific hybrids (4,8) and, recently, in W7 $\times$ S49 hybrids (16). Such events result in apparent frequencies of variants which are abnormally high because they are not only due to mutations but, in addition, to chromosome losses and to translocations leading to the inactivation of some alleles. This behavior of hybrids most likely is responsible for the early observation that the frequency of dexamethasone-resistant variants of S49 was the same in diploid or pseudotetraploid S49 cells (10,20,21). The case of the pseudotetraploid hybrid AN6 $\times$ W7TG, containing two r^+ alleles, is very similar to the situations of pseudotetraploid S49 cells; as shown in Table 1, the frequency observed for that hybrid is 7.5×10^{-6}, of the same order of magnitude as the values of 10^{-5} to 10^{-6} obtained for the hemizygous (r^+/r^-) cells, EO24 and MS1. Because of segregation-like events, the frequency of variations to dexamethasone resistance behaves as if it were independent of ploidy when diploid cells containing a single r^+ allele are compared with tetraploid cells containing two r^+ alleles.

DISCUSSION AND CONCLUSIONS

Our results have been interpreted in terms of a single genetic locus, r, coding for the glucocorticoid receptor or a receptor subunit, and which could be present in the homozygous active state (r^+/r^+), the hemizygous state (r^+/r^-), or the homozygous inactive state (r^-/r^-). Two alternative models should, however, be considered. One is the existence of two distinct loci, coding for nonidentical subunits of the receptor, and which could each be inactivated independently. Another possibility is that the receptor could be inactivated by defects in a locus coding for a receptor "activation" protein such as a receptor-specific kinase (19). Both these models involve at least two different genes which would be necessary for receptor activity and, therefore, predict that complementation should occur in hybrids between different receptor defective variants. Hybrids between a series of variants of the "receptorless" or "nuclear transfer defective" phenotype have been examined, and no evidence of complementation was found (16). This result, without ruling out the existence of two different genes necessary for active receptor, does not support such models.

Our study points to some potential problems to be aware of when using a somatic cell genetic approach to hormone action. In particular, one cannot take for granted that somatic cell lines established in culture are functionally diploid at every locus. Partial hemizygosity can be expected and has been observed (8) in some aneuploid cell lines, which do not contain the normal diploid number of chromosomes and show, upon karyotyping, many chromosomal rearrangements and translocations. Our data indicate, however, that functional hemizygosity can also occur in a pseudodiploid line, like S49, which appears to have a normal and stable diploid complement of 40 chromosomes. No chromosome banding studies have been done in this cell line to examine possible chromosome rearrangements. It is probable that, in the case of the S49 line, the inactivation of one of the two copies of the r^+ gene is the result of a mutation rather than of a chromosome rearrangement. Whatever the mechanism of r^+ inactivation, the S49 hemizygote must have been selected because of its resistance to low concentrations of glucocorticoids. This selection could have occurred in the animal, or in tissue culture, in the course of numerous transfers of the S49 in media with serum containing low levels of glucocorticoids. In general, the possibility of unwanted selection of variants with an altered sensitivity to one of the hormones present in the serum of tissue culture media should be kept in mind. In addition, selection for variants independent of a hormone for growth could occur upon transfers in medium with a serum deficient in that hormone.

The segregation-like events which seem to occur in cell hybrids introduce another complication in the genetic analysis of variants. These events, by increasing the frequencies of variants arising from hybrids, may obscure the results of complementation or dominance tests. Although the hybrids described here contain approximately the sum of the receptor present in each parent, it has been shown elsewhere (16) that this is not necessarily the case and that, in some hybrids, the expression of the genes is also complex.

Altogether, our studies with W7 cells have clarified some of the problems encountered with the S49 cell line. One can hope that the W7 system will allow further analysis of glucocorticoid action and, in particular, yield variants blocked at a step beyond the receptor. Such variants, which should complement receptor defective variants in hybrids, have been called "deathless" by Sibley and Tomkins (21) but have, in fact, never been demonstrated. One can now understand that, in S49 cells, the isolation of such a variant would be extremely unlikely because the hemizygosity of the r gene, whatever the product this gene encodes, strongly favors the isolation of resistant variants resulting from a defect at that locus. The use of the W7 (r^+/r^+) line should allow the selection for defect in other genes, if a function(s) other than the receptor is involved in the response. However, over 100 dexamethasone-resistant variants of W7 induced by various mutagens have been examined so far, and all result from defects in the receptor (3).

W7 cell hybrids have provided a simple animal cell system to show a tight correlation between glucocorticoid receptor content and cytolytic response. In the case of human leukemias, recent studies find little correlation between receptor levels and clinical response or glucocorticoid sensitivity of cells *in vitro* (5,11), although early studies (13,14) indicated such a correlation. The model system we are using, which consists of a homogeneous population of cloned and exponentially growing cells, is likely to be more favorable than clinical samples of lymphocytes to demonstrate such a correlation. Although the lymphocytolytic response in mice, a glucocorticoid sensitive species, may not be directly comparable to the inhibitory effects of glucocorticoids in humans, our results are certainly encouraging.

ACKNOWLEDGMENTS

This work was supported by Grant 5-RO1-GM20868 from the National Institute of General Medical Sciences, and by a grant from the Whitehall Foundation.

REFERENCES

1. Bourgeois, S., and Newby, R. (1977): *Cell,* 11:423–430.
2. Bourgeois, S., and Newby, R. F. (1979): *Cancer Res.,* 39:4749–4751.
3. Bourgeois, S., Newby, R. F., and Huet, M. (1978): *Cancer Res.,* 38:4279–4284.
4. Chasin, L. A., and Urlaub, G. (1975): *Science,* 187:1091–1093.
5. Crabtree, G. R., Smith, K. A., and Munck, A. (1978): *Cancer Res.,* 38:4268–4272.
6. Davidson, R. L., and Gerald, P. S. (1976): *Somatic Cell Genetics,* 2:165–176.
7. Farrell, S. A., and Worton, R. G. (1977): *Somatic Cell Genetics,* 3:539–551.
8. Gupta, R. S., and Siminovitch, L. (1978): *Somatic Cell Genetics,* 4:715–735.
9. Harris, A. W., Bankhurst, A. D., Mason, S., and Warner, N. L. (1973): *J. Immunol.,* 110:431–438.
10. Harris, A. W., and Cohn, M. (1970): In: *Development Aspects of Antibody Formation and Structure,* edited by J. Sterzl and I. Riha, pp. 275–279. Academia Publishing House of the Czechoslovak Academy of Sciences, Prague.
11. Homo, F., Duval, D., and Meyer, P. (1975): *C.R. Acad. Sci. Paris,* 280:1923–1926.
12. Horibata, K., and Harris, A. W. (1970): *Exp. Cell Res.,* 60:61–77.
13. Lippman, M., Halterman, R., Perry, S., Leventhal, B., and Thompson, E. B. (1973): *Nature (New Biol.),* 242:157–158.
14. Lippman, M. E., Perry, S., and Thompson, E. B. (1975): *Am. J. Med.,* 59:224–227.
15. Littlefield, J. W. (1966): *Exp. Cell Res.,* 41:190–196.
16. Pfahl, M., and Bourgeois, S. (1980): *Somatic Cell Genet.,* 6:63–74.
17. Pfahl, M., Kelleher, R. J., and Bourgeois, S. (1978): *Mol. Cell. Endocrinol.,* 10:193–207.
18. Pfahl, M., Sandros, T., and Bourgeois, S. (1978): *Mol. Cell. Endocrinol.,* 10:175–191.
19. Sando, J. J., Hammond, N. D., Stratford, C. A., and Pratt, W. B. (1979): *J. Biol. Chem.,* 254:4779–4789.
20. Sibley, C. H., and Tomkins, G. M. (1974): *Cell,* 2:213–220.
21. Sibley, C. H., and Tomkins, G. M. (1974): *Cell,* 2:221–227.

Hormones and Cancer, edited by S. Iacobelli et al.
Raven Press, New York © 1980.

Genetic and Biochemical Studies on Glucocorticoid Receptors

Ulrich Gehring

Institute for Biological Chemistry, University of Heidelberg, 69 Heidelberg, West Germany

Glucocorticoids exert striking inhibitory effects on certain types of lymphoid cells, both normal and neoplastic. The latter cells offer the advantage that they can be adapted to grow in continous culture. By cloning of such cells it is possible to obtain genetically homogenous cell populations suitable for investigating the glucocorticoid-specific cell response. Moreover, the cell-inhibitory hormone effects allow one to select for cell clones which are fully or partially resistant to glucocorticoids. Based on these considerations, a cell genetic approach to steroid hormone action was begun several years ago (18) using murine lymphoma cells of line S49.1 as a model system. As will be described, these investigations in effect turned out to be a study of the genetics of glucocorticoid receptors. Several other lymphoid cell lines of higher glucocorticoid sensitivity than S49.1 have also been investigated in recent years (1,2,11,12). While the present report concentrates on S49.1 cells, two of these high-sensitivity cell lines have been used in a comparative study which will be described at the end of this chapter.

GLUCOCORTICOID RESPONSE IN SENSITIVE LYMPHOMA CELLS

Upon addition of glucocorticoids to the culture medium of S49.1 mouse lymphoma cells, the rate of transport of nutrients from the medium into the cells decreases (7) and cell replication comes to a halt (6,10), causing the cells to preferentially accumulate in the G_1 phase of the cell cycle (6). Upon prolonged exposure to the steroid, cell viability is affected with cell survival declining exponentially (10). Using some of these effects, glucocorticoid sensitivity can be measured in sensitive cells either by quantitating growth inhibition (10), by counting the number of dead cells in a suspension culture exposed to glucocorticoid (7), or by measuring the relative efficiency of cell cloning in the presence of steroid (Fig. 1). If, for example, the synthetic glucocorticoid dexamethasone is added at increasing concentrations to the cloning medium, the cloning efficiency decreases drastically (14) and approaches 0% at 100 nM dexamethasone (Fig. 1). The few colonies which grow up at such high concentrations turn out to be permanently resistant (14) and reclone in the presence of dexamethasone

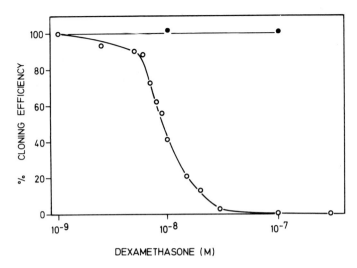

FIG. 1. Cloning in the presence of dexamethasone. Wild-type S49.1 cells *(open circles)* were cloned in soft agar over a feeder layer of mouse embryo fibroblasts (14). One clone which grew in 100 nM dexamethasone *(closed circles)* was recloned in the presence of dexamethasone. (Data from ref. 4.)

with high efficiency (Fig. 1). In experiments like this a large number of fully resistant subclones of S49.1 have been isolated using dexamethasone at 0.5 to 10 μM concentrations (13,15,18).

RECEPTORS IN GLUCOCORTICOID-RESISTANT LYMPHOMA CELLS

Three major phenotypes of glucocorticoid resistance have been observed upon analysis of a large number of resistant S49.1 subclones (13,18). Most abundant are resistant variants with negligible or greatly reduced levels of specific receptor as detected either by diminished retention of radiolabeled steroid in whole cell incubations or by decreased binding in cytosol preparations (13,15,18). These variants have been termed "receptorless" (r^-) (15). Lack of specific steroid binding could result either from a defect in the steroid binding site of the receptor protein or from the absence of the receptor molecule altogether. Distinction between these alternative possibilities will depend on the use of specific antisera raised against the glucocorticoid receptors of these lymphoma cells.

About 10 to 20% of resistant S49.1 clones contain receptors at roughly normal levels (13,18). The majority of these clones show abnormalities in receptor distribution between cytoplasmic and nuclear fractions as compared with wild-type cells. Variants with decreased nuclear binding of the receptor–steroid complex have been designated "nuclear transfer deficient" (nt^-) (15,19) and those with increased nuclear accumulation have been termed "increased nuclear trans-

TABLE 1. *Binding of receptor–dexamethasone complexes to nuclei from wild-type and nt⁻ cells*

Cytosol receptor from:	Nuclei from:	Specifically bound dexamethasone (molecules/nucleus)
wt	wt	4,170
nt⁻	nt⁻	310
wt	nt⁻	4,680
nt⁻	wt	370

Cytosols were pretreated at 0°C with 50 nм [³H]dexamethasone and incubated at 20°C with 10⁸ nuclei. The incubation contained 3.8 mg cytosol protein of wt and nt⁻ S49.1 cells, corresponding to 0.87 and 0.63 pmoles specifically bound steroid per mg protein, respectively (data from ref. 7).

fer" (nt^i) (19). In both situations the defect has been localized in the cytoplasmic rather than in the nuclear compartments of these cells. Cell-free nuclear transfer experiments with nuclei and cytosol preparations from wild-type and nt⁻ cells (Table 1) clearly show that the defect in nt⁻ cells lies in the cytoplasmic receptor system rather than in the nucleus. The same result was found for nt^i cells in similar transfer experiments (Table 2). These conclusions have been substantiated in a series of experiments in which binding to DNA was used as a model for nuclear binding (7,18,19). While the receptor–steroid complex from wild-type cells readily binds to isolated DNA, the complex from nt⁻ cells is not retained by DNA to any appreciable extent. In contrast, the complex from nt^i cells

TABLE 2. *Binding of receptor–dexamethasone complexes to nuclei from wt and nt^i cells*

	Cytosol receptor from:	Nuclei from:	Specifically bound dexamethasone (molecules/nucleus)
Exp. A	wt	wt	2,900
	nt^i	nt^i	10,880
	wt	nt^i	2,830
	nt^i	wt	9,880
Exp. B	wt	wt	2,580
	nt^i	nt^i	6,070
	wt	nt^i	3,330
	nt^i	wt	6,710

Cytosols were pretreated at 0°C with 50 nм [³H]dexamethasone and incubated at 20°C with 10⁸ nuclei. In experiment A the incubations contained 3.6 mg cytosol protein of wt and nt^i S49.1 cells, corresponding to 0.60 and 1.6 pmoles specifically bound steroid per mg protein, respectively. In experiment B the incubations contained equal amounts of specifically bound dexamethasone (50,000 cpm), corresponding to 4.1 and 1.8 mg cytosol protein of wt and nt^i cells, respectively (Gehring, *unpublished experiments*).

exhibits greatly increased affinity to DNA as compared with the wild-type complex (18). These observations as well as some differences in physicochemical properties (18) point to the fact that lymphoma cells of nt^- and nt^i phenotypes carry defects in their glucocorticoid-specific receptors.

GLUCOCORTICOID SENSITIVITY AND RECEPTORS OF HYBRID LYMPHOMA CELLS

The defects in the above-mentioned phenotypes of resistant lymphoma cells were studied under *in vivo* conditions by use of somatic cell hybridization which allows one to test for dominance or recessiveness of glucocorticoid resistance. This approach appeared suitable for distinguishing between alternative explanations for the nt^- and nt^i phenotypes. For example, the receptors of both types of variants might be defective in such a way that nuclear binding is affected. Alternatively, modulators of the nuclear binding reaction might be associated with the receptors and their relative levels could determine nt^- and nt^i resistance. Inhibitors of nuclear receptor binding might operate in wild-type cells in a limiting fashion and could be more active in nt^- cells or absent from nt^i cells, thereby causing decreased or increased nuclear binding, respectively. Conversely, activators of nuclear interaction could be overproduced in nt^i cells but missing from nt^- cells. Excess of an inhibitor in nt^- cells would result in steroid resistance in $nt^- \times$ wt hybrids. Likewise, overproduction of an activator in nt^i cells should result in steroid resistance in $nt^i \times$ wt hybrids. In contrast, lack of an activator in nt^- or of an inhibitor in nt^i cells should allow complementation to steroid sensitivity in $nt^- \times nt^i$ hybrids and in $r^- \times nt^-$ and $r^- \times nt^i$ hybrids provided that the r^- variants continue to produce these putative modulators. If, however, the nuclear interaction site of the receptor molecule were affected in nt^- and nt^i variants and if no modulators of the postulated types were involved in the normal response, one would expect to find dominance of wild-type responsiveness over r^-, nt^-, and nt^i resistance, and complementation between r^-, nt^-, and nt^i would probably not occur.

With these considerations in mind, two major series of cell hybridizations were carried out. In the experiments shown in Table 3, two subclones of S49.1 were hybridized with EL4 mouse lymphoma cells. EL4 cells were glucocorticoid resistant when first tested and had an nt^- phenotype (3). As a partner in cell fusion with S49.1 they offer several advantages: they are more fusogenic than S49.1; they originated from a mouse strain of distinguishable histocompatibility antigens (facilitating the identification of hybrid cells), and possess marker chromosomes; EL4 also contains glucocorticoid receptors which can be distinguished from those of S49.1 (3,4). As shown in Table 3, S49.1 (wt) $\times$ EL4 (nt^-) hybrids are glucocorticoid sensitive. This result clearly establishes dominance of the wild-type response over nt^- resistance and thus rules out the hypothesis of a diffusible inhibitor of nuclear receptor binding as the cause for the nt^- phenotype. S49.1 (r^-) $\times$ EL4 (nt^-) hybrids are steroid resistant (Table 3), suggesting that

TABLE 3. Characteristics of S49.1, EL4, and hybrid cells

Cell line	Chromosome no.: mode (range)	Response to steroid: relative cloning efficiency in 1 μM dexamethasone
S49.1 (wt)	40 (38–41)	2.5×10^{-4}
S49.1 (r⁻)	40 (38–43)	0.98
EL4 (nt⁻)	39 (36–42)	1,10
S49.1 (wt) × EL4 (nt⁻)	77 (72–80)	2.4×10^{-2}
S49.1 (r⁻) × EL4 (nt⁻)	78 (73–79)	0,98

Data from refs. 3 and 4.

the nt⁻ phenotype does not result from the lack of an activator of nuclear binding.

These studies were extended to cell hybridizations within the S49.1 cell system in which a series of resistant sublines was available (4,18). The S49.1 × S49.1 hybrids were examined for dominance relationships and for complementation (Table 4). Hybrids between wild-type cells and resistant variants of different phenotypes again showed dominance of the wild-type response over resistance, while hybrids between resistant variants either of the same or of different phenotypes failed to complement to wild-type sensitivity. It was also found that all hybrid cell clones investigated contained the types of receptors of the respective parental cells (Table 4). This proves that more than one receptor type can be expressed in the same cell but that the presence of the wild-type receptor determines cellular responsiveness. These hybridization studies rule out the possibility of activators or inhibitors of nuclear receptor interaction as the cause for nt⁻ and ntⁱ resistance. The altered nuclear binding properties of receptors in these phenotypes appear to be caused by defects in the nuclear interaction sites of

TABLE 4. Characteristics of S49.1 × S49.1 hybrid cells

Type of hybrid	Response to dexamethasone	Relative cloning efficiency in 1 μM dexamethasone	Type of receptor present
wt × wt	Sensitive	3×10^{-6}–2×10^{-5}	wt
wt × r⁻	Sensitive	2.3×10^{-2}	wt
wt × nt⁻	Sensitive	2.5×10^{-2}	wt and nt⁻
wt × ntⁱ	Sensitive	1.3×10^{-2}	wt and ntⁱ
r⁻ × r⁻	Resistant	1.03	—
r⁻ × nt⁻	Resistant	1.00	nt⁻
r⁻ × ntⁱ	Resistant	1.01	ntⁱ
nt⁻ × nt⁻	Resistant	0.96	nt⁻
nt⁻ × ntⁱ	Resistant	1.02	nt⁻ and ntⁱ

Data from ref. 4.

the receptor molecules themselves. Lack of complementation between r⁻ and nt⁻ or nt^i resistance suggests that the two active domains of the wild-type receptor for steroid binding and for nuclear interaction, respectively, reside within the same molecular unit, possibly the same polypeptide chain. This view is also supported by recent biochemical observations with purified glucocorticoid receptors from rat liver (9) which are in favor of a homodimer rather than a heterodimer subunit structure. Moreover, limited proteolysis of the crude rat liver glucocorticoid receptor yields a receptor form of lower molecular size which has lost the ability to bind to isolated nuclei and DNA (17). With both steroid and nuclear interaction sites on the same molecular structure it would not be surprising if alterations of the nuclear interaction site in nt⁻ and nt^i receptors also cause some subtle change in steroid binding properties (7).

CHROMOSOME SEGREGATION AND INCREASED RATE OF RESISTANCE IN HYBRID LYMPHOMA CELLS

Even though glucocorticoid sensitivity was found to be dominant over resistance, lymphoma cell hybrids of the types S49.1 (wt) × EL4 (nt⁻) and S49.1 (wt) × S49.1 (resistant) always contained 1 to 3% fully resistant cells (Tables 3 and 4). This frequency is about 100-fold higher than that seen in the sensitive parental S49.1 cell line (Table 3). In fact, resistance appeared to arise at a high rate in these hybrid cells as was particularly obvious when a hybrid cell clone was propagated for several months (Fig. 2). During that time the modal

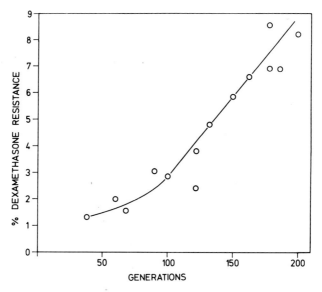

FIG. 2. Development of resistance in S49.1 (wt) × EL4 hybrids. One randomly picked hybrid cell clone was propagated for several months; the fraction of resistant cells was determined by cloning in the presence of 1 μM dexamethasone. (Data from ref. 4.)

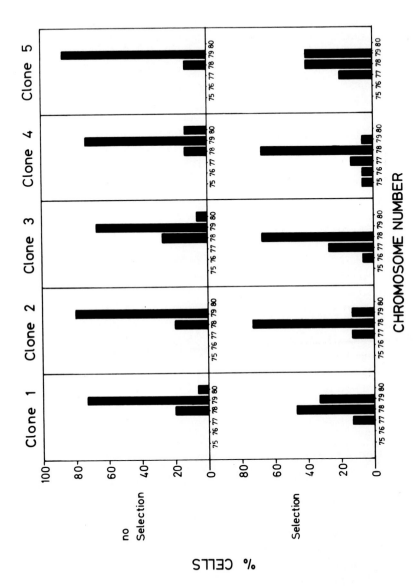

FIG. 3. Chromosome segregation in hybrid cell clones. Five separate clones of S49.1 (wt) × EL4 were treated with (selection) or without (no selection) 1 μM dexamethasone; chromosome numbers were determined in treated and untreated cultures. (Data from refs. 4 and 5.)

chromosome number decreased, suggesting a link between chromosome loss and glucocorticoid resistance. In order to investigate this hypothesis, several sensitive clones of S49.1 (wt) × EL4 were subjected to dexamethasone early after isolation and the chromosome numbers were determined in both treated and untreated cultures. The data of Fig. 3 clearly show that chromosome segregation is the major cause for resistance in these hybrid cells and that, in the majority of cells, resistance is accompanied by the loss of *one* chromosome. When the receptors of some of these clones were investigated it was found that, following selection, the hybrid cells had lost the S49.1-specific receptor (5). This proves that S49.1 lymphoma cells contain only one functional allele of the glucocorticoid receptor gene as had previously been suggested using a different experimental approach (1,2). Moreover, these experiments show that S49.1 × EL4 hybrids are a suitable cell system for assigning the glucocorticoid receptor gene to a specific chromosome.

LYMPHOMA CELLS WITH DECREASED GLUCOCORTICOID SENSITIVITY

In order to isolate S49.1 subclones of intermediate glucocorticoid sensitivity, a cloning experiment similar to that described in Fig. 1 was carried out and cell colonies growing up at 10 nM dexamethasone were isolated. Figure 4 compares the growth properties of one such cell clone in the presence of dexamethasone with a fully sensitive S49.1 clone. While the fully sensitive clone clearly responds to 30 nM dexamethasone, a 10-fold higher steroid concentration is required to achieve about the same effect in the variant cells. While sensitive S49.1 cells contain 13,000 to 20,000 glucocorticoid receptor sites per cell (16), the low sensitivity variant has only about 20 to 25% of that number of cellular receptors (8). This clearly characterizes a situation in which the cellular receptor content plays an important role in determining responsiveness.

GLUCOCORTICOID SENSITIVITY AND CELLULAR RECEPTOR CONTENT

Previous experiments by Bourgeois et al. (1,2) compared the glucocorticoid sensitivity of S49.1 cells with that of the more sensitive thymic lymphoma line WEHI-7 and found about twice the number of glucocorticoid receptors in the latter cells. This has led to the proposal of a gene dose effect in these cells with S49.1 being haploid and WEHI-7 diploid for the receptor gene (1,2). Very careful sensitivity measurements and receptor determinations were recently carried out by us (16) using several S49.1 clones and the thymic lymphoma lines WEHI-7 and WEHI-22. As shown in Fig. 5 there is in fact a direct relationship between glucocorticoid sensitivity and cellular receptor content in the lines studied. Moreover, in these cells the same number of receptors has to be occupied by the hormone in order to elicit a defined biological response. However, the

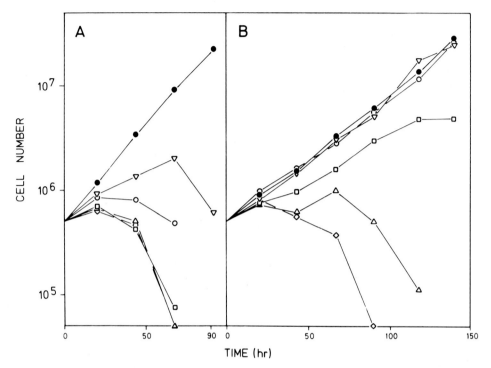

FIG. 4. Growth of suspension cultures in the presence of dexamethasone. Cells of a wild-type S49.1 clone **(A)** and of a clone with decreased glucocorticoid sensitivity **(B)** were grown in the absence *(closed circles)* or presence of dexamethasone at 30 nM *(downward triangles)*, 100 nM *(open circles)*, 300 nM *(squares)* 1 μM *(upward triangles)*, or 10 μM *(diamonds)* concentrations. (Data from refs. 4 and 6.)

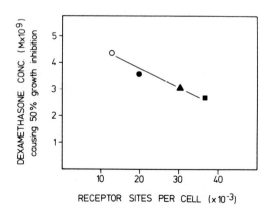

FIG. 5. Glucocorticoid sensitivity and cellular receptor levels. Sensitivity was determined by measuring growth inhibition after a time period sufficient for control cultures to grow through 6–7 cell generations (10). The number of cellular receptor sites was determined in whole cell binding experiments (16). Lines S49.1TB.4 *(open circle)*, S49.1G.3.5 *(closed circle)*, WEHI-22 *(triangle)*, and WEHI 7 *(square)*, were used. (Data from ref. 16.)

two clones of S49.1 included in Fig. 5 are quite different with respect to both sensitivity and receptor content. Thus a simple gene dose hypothesis is not sufficient to explain the results. Other cellular factors besides the dose of receptor gene per cell control the receptor level and hence determine glucocorticoid sensitivity of lymphoma cells.

ACKNOWLEDGMENTS

This work was supported by a grant from the Deutsche Forschungsgemeinschaft. I am grateful to Dr. A. W. Harris for supplying the cell lines WEHI-7 and WEHI-22 and to B. Segnitz and M. Behringer for skillful technical assistance.

REFERENCES

1. Bourgeois, S., and Newby, R. F. (1977): *Cell,* 11:423–430.
2. Bourgeois, S., Newby, R. F., and Huet, M. (1978): *Cancer Res.,* 38:4279–4284.
3. Gehring, U. (1977): In: *Endocrinology, Proceedings of the Fifth International Congress of Endocrinology, Vol. 1,* edited by V. H. T. James, pp. 536–541. Excerpta Medica, Amsterdam.
4. Gehring, U. (1979): In: *Advances in Enzyme Regulation, Vol. 17,* edited by G. Weber, pp. 343–361. Pergamon, Oxford.
5. Gehring, U. (1980): *In preparation.*
6. Gehring, U., Gray, J. W., and Tomkins, G. M. (1976): In: *Pulse-Cytophotometry,* edited by T. Büchner, W. Göhde, and J. Schumann, pp. 284–289. European Press, Gent.
7. Gehring, U., and Tomkins, G. M. (1974): *Cell,* 3:301–306.
8. Gehring, U., and Ulrich, J. (1980): *In preparation.*
9. Govindan, M. V. (1979): *J. Steroid Biochem.,* 11:323–332.
10. Harris, A. W. (1970): *Exp. Cell Res.,* 60:341–353.
11. Harris, A. W. (1978): In: *Protides of the Biological Fluids, 25th Colloquium,* edited by H. Peeters, pp. 601–604. Pergamon, Oxford.
12. Harris, A. W., and Baxter, J. D. (1979): In: *Glucocorticoid Hormone Action,* edited by J. D. Baxter and G. G. Rousseau, pp. 423–448. Springer-Verlag, Berlin.
13. Pfahl, M., Kelleher, R. J., and Bourgeois, S. (1978): *Mol. Cell. Endocrinol.,* 10:193–207.
14. Sibley, C. H., and Tomkins, G. M. (1974): *Cell,* 2:213–220.
15. Sibley, C. H., and Tomkins, G. M. (1974): *Cell,* 2:221–227.
16. Ulrich, J., and Gehring, U. (1979): *Hoppe Seylers Z. Physiol. Chem.,* 360:1201.
17. Wrange, Ö., and Gustafsson, J.-Å. (1978): *J. Biol. Chem.,* 253:856–865.
18. Yamamoto, K. R., Gehring, U., Stampfer, M. R., and Sibley, C. H. (1976): *Recent Prog. Horm. Res.,* 32:3–32.
19. Yamamoto, K. R., Stampfer, M. R., and Tomkins, G. M. (1974): *Proc. Natl. Acad. Sci. USA,* 71:3901–3905.

Hormones and Cancer, edited by S. Iacobelli et al.
Raven Press, New York 1980.

Glucocorticoid Actions in a Human Acute Lymphoblastic Leukemia, T-Cell Line: A Model System for Understanding Steroid Therapy

E. Brad Thompson, J. M. Harmon, *M. R. Norman, and
**T. J. Schmidt

Laboratory of Biochemistry, National Cancer Institute, National Institutes of Health, Bethesda, Maryland 20205

The advantages of cultured cells for studying hormone action are now generally recognized. To provide a model for glucocorticoid hormone actions in human acute lymphoblastic leukemia (ALL), we have characterized in some detail the effects of that class of steroids on an established line of ALL cells. Called CEM cells, this line has given rise to a number of steroid-sensitive clones of cells. The glucocorticoid receptors of these cells have been quantified and characterized with respect to steroid affinity and specificity, and the cellular effects of glucocorticoids have been correlated with occupancy of these receptors. Furthermore, we have established the spontaneous rate at which resistant cells arise from a sensitive clone and have partially characterized the glucocorticoid receptor phenotype of a number of both spontaneous and mutagenized resistant clones.

In this chapter, rather than reviewing all the above in detail, we will discuss certain aspects of our work which may have relevance to the use of corticosteroids in the therapy of ALL. We will also try to stress the danger of uncritically generalizing the results from any model system such as this one to all clinical situations.

It was recognized quite early after their discovery that glucocorticoids exerted lympholytic and immunosuppressive activity (11,13,35,47,49,53). Experiments on rodent thymocytes showed that such steroids were capable of directly lysing these cells (8,34). This activity was soon tested clinically, as glucocorticoids were administered for the treatment of many leukemias (14,16–18,27,43,48). In these circumstances, these steroids were often found to produce remissions, especially in ALL of children; but as with many single-drug therapies, relapses were frequent (5,42,54). Nevertheless, the value of steroids is still recognized, and they are a cornerstone in today's more successful multidrug regimens (16,17).

---

* Present address: Department of Chemical Pathology, King's College Hospital Medical School, London, England.
** Present address: Fels Research Institute, Temple University Medical School, Philadelphia, Pennsylvania 19140.

Despite the increased successfulness of combination chemotherapy in ALL, relapses still occur; permanent remissions are not achieved in 100% of patients. Among the many factors involved in this problem, such as sequestered sites of cells, leukemic cell type, and the narrow therapeutic index of the drugs used, we have been concerned with the question of the mechanism by which the leukemic blast cells acquire resistance to steroids.

GLUCOCORTICOID RECEPTORS IN ALL BLAST CELLS

In the initial study of glucocorticoid receptors in human ALL cells, we found that 100% of the patients who had received no previous treatment yielded cells that contained receptors, as did about half the patients in relapse after one or more rounds of chemotherapy. These receptors showed steroid affinities such that they would be killed by therapeutic levels of hormone. All these receptor-positive patients (studied in retrospect) responded to initial or further steroid-containing chemotherapy. The other group of patients in relapse all had received several courses of combination chemotherapy. These few patients' leukemic blast cells were found to have little or no cytoplasmic receptors (30,31). These data fit well with the large body of results in rodent model systems. There, receptor occupancy by glucocorticoids correlated well with various cell-inhibitory effects of the steroids, and quite telling was the finding that virtually all steroid-resistant mouse lymphoid cells had receptor defects. Most lacked receptors altogether, and the rest seemed to contain altered receptors (3,6,37, 38,55).

However, hopes for a simple test of glucocorticoid sensitivity, based on the mere presence of receptors have not been met. Although it is generally agreed that the absence of receptors ensures lack of response to all but heroic concentrations of steroids, i.e., $\sim 10^{-3}$ M, the simple presence of receptors does not guarantee response. We first predicted this likelihood on the basis of studies on mouse and human leukemic tissue culture cells (32); in fact, even earlier studies on steroid-*inducible* rat hepatoma cells had presaged the same conclusion (28). Now, many lines of evidence lead to the same conclusion.

Resistance to the lethal effects of steroids has been found in receptor-containing transplantable rodent lymphomas (22,39), in normal rodent and human lymphocytes (12,21,29,50), and in the cells from a variety of human leukemias (4,52). *In vitro* tests of leukemic cell sensitivity to steroids, such as inhibition of thymidine or glucose uptake, haven't always been found to correlate quantitatively with steroid receptor concentration; and these biochemical alterations sometimes fail to correlate with cell lysis and/or clinical response to therapy (9).

In light of these complications, a tissue culture system might be useful in revealing the common phenotype of steroid-resistant ALL cells and in showing how such cells become resistant. Does resistance correlate with receptor changes at all? The above-cited data on clinical material, for example, often does not enable one to tell whether the observed receptors are functioning normally.

The tissue–culture system permits clear tests of the functional nature of the receptors.

PROPERTIES OF CEM CELLS

The CEM line of cells was derived from a female patient with childhood ALL (15). They possess T-cell surface antigen and form E rosettes (23,51). Uncloned cultures of CEM cells show partial (41) to no (32) steroid sensitivity, but unselected clones derived from the mass cultures often are fully sensitive (41). These cells contain about 2×10^4 receptor sites/cell, and these receptors specifically bind glucocorticoids and their antagonists (41). The relative affinities of a series of steroids correspond to their potency as glucocorticoids. Direct microscopic examination shows that the cells are lysed by the steroid treatment (41; A. Truitt and E. B. Thompson, *unpublished observations*). Dose–response studies show that as receptor occupancy approaches 100%, so does maximum cell kill, inhibition of growth, and inhibition of cloning. Thus these sensitive clones of CEM cells would appear to be good models for the high-receptor content type of T-cell (and probably null-cell) ALL. They reinforce the conclusion that in clinical situations, the efficacy of the usual pharmacologic doses of glucocorticosteroids is related to their ability to occupy receptor sites in the leukemic blast cell, which is eventually lysed by some direct action of the steroid.

KINETICS OF KILL AND CELL CYCLE EFFECTS

When one observes the time course of cell kill by following growth curves or the ability to form colonies, or by electron microscopy of cells, it is apparent that a considerable time must elapse before CEM cells begin to die (19,41). For approximately 24 hr after adding steroid to the culture, there is no reduction in growth, no loss of cloning efficiency, and no obvious change in cell ultrastructure. During this time, cells can be washed free from steroid and then grown without loss of viability. This is in marked contrast to the relatively rapid effects of glucocorticoids on rodent thymocytes or lymphoid lines, in which killing occurs within 10 to 12 hr or less after addition of the steroid. Figure 1 shows the results of an experiment in which this delay can be seen. The curve in the lower half of the figure displays the loss of cloning efficiency after addition of dexamethasone. Also shown, in the upper half of the figure, is the time course of accumulation of cells in the G_1 phase of the cell cycle. As can be seen, a delay very similar to that of the lower curve occurs before cells begin to accumulate in G_1.

We have in fact analyzed the effects of steroids on the cell cycle of logarithmically growing CEM cells in some detail, utilizing flow microfluorometry to distinguish cell growth compartments (19). The results of these studies indicated that effective steroids irretrievably blocked CEM cells in the G_1 phase of the

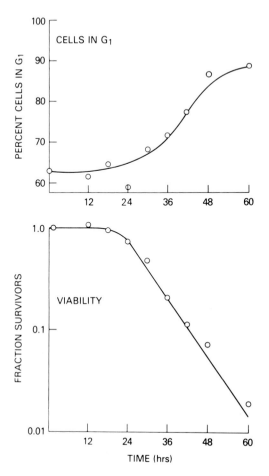

FIG. 1. Time course of loss of viability and G_1 accumulation. Cells were grown in 10^{-6} M dexamethasone for various lengths of time and then assayed for cell cycle distribution *(upper panel)* and viability *(lower panel)*. (Reprinted from Harmon et al., ref. 19, with permission.)

cycle. In timing, steroid specificity, and dose response, this block correlated closely with effects on cell viability. We concluded from those studies that the primary result of treating CEM cells with potent glucocorticoids is to fix them in the G_1 phase of the cell cycle, where they eventually lyse.

The above results have several messages of possible clinical relevance. They suggest that not only must doses of steroids be administered adequate to saturate the glucocorticoid receptors of sensitive leukemic cells, but also that these doses must be maintained for several days to achieve maximum kill. The failure of many steroidal treatment regimens might be explained, in retrospect, by the failure to meet this requirement, as might the success of more recent high-dose, several-day regimens (17). It has long been of concern that if steroids blocked cells in G_1, simultaneous administration of steroids with cycle-active drugs might protect some of the leukemic cell population against the cycle-active agents (25,26,33). Our studies with CEM cells suggest that this is not the case; that the irreversibility of the G_1 block caused by steroids should result in their acting independently of (other) cycle-active agents, unless of course the other agents protected against steroid killing by temporarily blocking cells in compartments other than G_1.

CEM CELLS USED TO ANALYZE MULTIDRUG INTERACTIONS

Extensive studies have not as yet been carried out utilizing CEM cells to study the effects of drug combinations. Our single pilot study in this area, however, suggests that they may have considerable usefulness in such studies (40). In that study we found that CEM cells were sensitive to reasonable pharmacologic concentrations of methotrexate, 6-mercaptopurine, and vincristine. Each of these compounds was tested for its ability to inhibit cloning when added singly, or in combination with a receptor-saturating concentration of prednisolone. The results were analyzed for drug interactions by comparing the inhibitory effects of each drug given alone with those obtained when given together with the steroid. Table 1 shows that methotrexate and vincristine acted essentially independently of the steroid, but that 6-mercaptopurine and prednisolone were antagonists. Flow microfluorometric analysis of cell cycle populations suggested that this may have been due to 6-mercaptopurine holding cells up in S phase and thereby protecting them from the steroid. In any case, these preliminary studies suggest that methotrexate or vincristine and prednisolone act indepen-

TABLE 1. *Interactions of prednisolone with other antileukemic drugs*

| | Fractional survivors | | | | |
| | Experimental | | | Predicted | |
Drug B	S_A	S_B	S_{AB}	$(S_A \times S_B)$	Interaction
Vincristine (5×10^{-9} M)	0.289	0.161	0.027	0.046	Weak synergists?
Methotrexate (5×10^{-6} M)	0.289	0.183	0.030	0.053	Weak synergists?
6-Mercaptopurine (10^{-4} M)	0.289	0.199	0.155	0.058	Antagonists

The lethal effects of vincristine (5×10^{-9} M), methotrexate (5×10^{-6} M), and 6-mercaptopurine (10^{-4} M) when added to CEM-C7 cells are listed. Drugs were added during the last 24 hr to cells that were treated for a total of 48 hr with prednisolone (10^{-6} M), or to cells which were not treated with steroid (control). Antagonism was inferred if $S_{AB} > S_A \times S_B$, independence was inferred if $S_{AB} = S_A \times S_B$, and synergism was inferred if $S_{AB} < S_A \times S_B$, where S_A equals fractional survival in 10^{-6} M prednisolone and S_B equals fractional survival in second drug.
Reprinted from Norman et al., ref. 40, with permission.

dently (or possibly as very weak synergists), while 6-mercaptopurine and predniso-lone given simultaneously may be partially antagonistic.

THE GENETICS OF STEROID RESISTANCE IN CEM CELLS

Luria-Delbruck fluctuation analysis experiments have been carried out which show that CEM-cell resistance to killing by glucocorticoids occurs through spon-taneous, independent events and not by general adaptation of the entire popula-tion at risk (J. Harmon and E. B. Thompson, *unpublished results*). These events occur at the order of 1 per 10^5 cells per generation. Thus, a simple calculation will show that from 10^5 growing, wild-type leukemic cells, approximately 1,800 steroid-resistant cells emerge in only 10 generations in a total population of $\sim 10^8$ cells. If these rates were to apply to a patient, an untreated individual who had just achieved a total burden of 10^8 leukemic blast cells might be expected to have a few thousand steroid-resistant cells already. While it would be very unwise to push such calculations too far, they readily give one a feeling for understanding some mechanisms behind the difficulty in achieving lasting remissions with single-drug steroid therapy of ALL, and for the often seen correlation between treatment failure and increasing tumor cell burden at the time of initiating therapy.

The resistant CEM cells show a remarkably constant phenotype. Some sixty independent, spontaneously resistant clones have been screened, and all contain reduced, but measurable quantities of receptors, with reduced capacity to un-dergo nuclear translocation. Several, in fact, showed no translocation at all. Steroid binding studies on these residual receptors revealed that their affinity for steroids was the same or only slightly less than that of receptors from sensitive cells. More detailed studies show that the receptors from the resistant cells are markedly more labile than are those from sensitive cells (44).

The potential clinical relevance of these results is clear. All the spontaneous clones so far obtained showed measureable (but less than wild type) levels of glucocorticoid receptor by the whole-cell assay technique employed. These results seem to correspond with the frequently observed presence of receptors in steroid-resistant clinical material, and with the finding that cells with lower receptor site content more frequently tend to be steroid-resistant. They show that nuclear transfer alone, without a standard of reference, is not a certain indication of functional receptors. The fact that the receptors from the resistant CEM cells are more labile than wild type with respect to steroid binding suggests that it is the receptor function which remains the primary determinant of steroid sensi-tivity in human ALL cells. However, the usual clinical research measurement of receptors, whole-cell binding assays, would not be sufficient to distinguish sensitive from resistant cells. Either fairly elaborate cell-free biochemical analyses of receptor properties may be necessary, or a functional test of receptors in whole cells is needed. The latter would offer many advantages in following clinical situations.

GLUTAMINE SYNTHETASE IS A MARKER FOR RECEPTOR FUNCTION IN CEM CELLS

Because of the above-stated reasoning, we have screened CEM cells for a number of potentially steroid-inducible enzymes which might serve as markers for receptor function. In CEM cells, glutamine synthetase appears to be such an enzyme (20). It is induced before cell killing starts, and its induction correlates with receptor occupancy. In a number of other cell systems, glucocorticoid induction of glutamine synthetase has been observed, and in some cells this induction has been demonstrated to be due to increased production of enzyme protein and the accumulation of its mRNA (1,2,7,10,36,46). When we examined our steroid-resistant, receptor-containing clones for glutamine synthetase, all were found to contain basal levels of enzyme which were not induced by steroid. We have not yet adequately tested this enzyme in ALL patients' cells, but hope that glutamine synthetase induction may prove useful as a marker for functional glucocorticoid receptors. Some indication that this may be so, at least in certain diseases, is given by our studies on a limited number of patients with Sézary syndrome. In these patients, high receptor content and steroid sensitivity appeared to correlate with glutamine synthetase induction (45).

SUMMARY AND DISCUSSION

In sum, CEM cells appear to represent a useful model system in which to explore certain elements of steroid hormone actions on ALL cells. The major points of relevance to clinical thinking, highlighted above, are listed in Table 2. We call attention to items 5–7 of the table in particular. The consensus at the recent Leukemia Workshop (52) was that the assay of choice for glucocorticoid receptors was the whole-cell assay. It has the advantages of applicability to small samples, speed, simplicity, and avoidance of underestimating receptors/cell through failing to consider nuclear sites and through losses in the cell-free environment. But such assays would fail to demonstrate that our steroid-resistant CEM cells have altered, non-functional receptors. They contain measurable receptors which are capable of undergoing some nuclear transfer. We know, of course, that they are quantitatively deficient in both receptor content and nuclear transfer, because we have wild-type, sensitive clones against which to compare. Without the sensitive parent cells for comparison (as would be the case in a patient whose leukemic cell population had already converted to steroid resistance) there would be no basis for showing that the receptor concentration per cell and percentage nuclear translocation were low for that particular individual. This is so because it does not seem, from the data at hand, that a specific number of sites/cell can be correlated with sensitivity. The reported ranges of sites/cell are too broad to allow, at present, absolute conclusions to be drawn for a specific patient. Thus there seems a need, whenever possible (and as mentioned in the Leukemia Workshop Report, ref. 52) to carry out cell-free studies

TABLE 2. *Some properties of CEM cells and their implications for steroid effects in clinical situations*

Property in tissue culture	Clinical implication
1. Contain glucocorticoid receptors whose occupancy by steroid correlates with direct cell killing.	1. A major therapeutic effect of glucocorticoids is similarly mediated by glucocorticoid receptors in ALL blast cells. Pharmacologic dose of glucocorticoid must be adequate to produce blood/tissue levels sufficient to saturate these receptors.
2. A delay of $\sim$ 24 hr occurs after addition of steroid to culture before cell kill begins.	2. Receptor-saturating dose must be maintained long enough (probably several days) to produce cell kill.
3. Glucocorticoids cause irreversible block in G_1.	3. Glucocorticoids should not protect cells against cycle-specific drugs, but the latter might protect some cells against steroids.
4. Steroid-resistant cells arise spontaneously at a rate of $\sim 10^{-5}$ per cell per generation.	4. Permanent remissions to steroid therapy will be rare.
5. Spontaneous steroid-resistant clones usually have reduced numbers of receptors with steroid affinity similar to sensitive cells.	5. Presence of high affinity receptors does not guarantee steroid sensitivity. Low concentration/cell overall correlates with reduced sensitivity, but in a given individual is not a reliable index.
6. Resistant cells show reduced nuclear transfer of steroid–receptor complex.	6. No nuclear transfer indicates steroid resistance, but some transfer uninterpretable, because percentage transfer level for "wild-type" cells from a given patient whose cells have become resistant is unobtainable for comparison.
7. Receptors of resistant cells more labile than those of sensitive cells, in cell-free extracts.	7. Simple whole-cell receptor assays may be inadequate to judge steroid sensitivity.
8. Glutamine synthetase induction correlates with steroid sensitivity, functional receptors.	8. Glutamine synthetase induction may provide a simple test for steroid responsiveness.

as well, and to apply tests of receptor function, such as glutamine synthetase induction.

Despite the several obvious virtues of this cell system, this chapter would be incomplete unless some of the limitations were pointed out as well. The most important of these is that this is only one cell system, from one patient; indeed, much of the work has been done with a few sensitive clones. Other human leukemia cell lines need to be explored in similar detail, to see whether clinical generalities can be made with more confidence. For example, will the high rate of spontaneous conversion to resistance seen in CEM cells be the rule for ALL cells? Other obvious limitations are that use of tissue culture systems avoids critical considerations of drug metabolism and excretion, of cell–cell and cell–tissue interactions, and of the effects of the hormone on general and specific growth factors. Nevertheless, we feel that with these limitations constantly kept in mind, the CEM cell system is of considerable usefulness.

ACKNOWLEDGMENTS

The authors wish to thank Mrs. Jean Regan for her editorial assistance in the preparation of this paper. T. Schmidt is the recipient of an NIH postdoctoral fellowship (1 F32 CA05447–01) awarded by the National Cancer Institute, DHEW.

REFERENCES

1. Alescio, T., and Moscona, A. A. (1969): *Biochem. Biophys. Res. Commun.,* 34:176–182.
2. Barnes, P. R., Hersh, R. T., and Kitos, P. A. (1974): *In Vitro,* 9:230–238.
3. Baxter, J. D., Harris, A. W., Tomkins, G. M., and Cohn, M. (1971): *Science,* 171:189–191.
4. Bell, P. A., and Borthwick, N. M., editors (1979): *Glucocorticoid Action and Leukemia.* Alpha Omega Publishing, Cardiff.
5. Bernard, J., Boiron, M., Weil, M., Levy, J. P., Seligman, M., and Najear, Y. (1962): *Nouv. Rev. Fr. Hematol.,* 2:195–222.
6. Bourgeois, S., Newby, R. F., and Huet, M. (1978): *Cancer Res.,* 38:4279–4284.
7. Chader, G. J., and Reif-Lehrer, L. (1972): *Biochim. Biophys. Acta.,* 264:186–196.
8. Claman, H. N. (1972): *N. Engl. J. Med.,* 287:388–397.
9. Crabtree, G., Smith, K., and Munck, A. (1978): *Cancer Res.,* 38:4268–4272.
10. Crook, R. B., Louie, M., Deuel, T., and Tomkins, G. M. (1978): *J. Biol. Chem.,* 253:6125–6131.
11. Dougherty, T., and White, A. (1945): *Am. J. Anat.,* 77:81–116.
12. Duval, D., Dausse, J. P., and Dardenne, M. (1976): *Biochim. Biophys. Acta,* 451:82–91.
13. Evans, H. M., Moon, H. D., Simpson, M. E., and Lyons, W. J. (1938): *Proc. Soc. Exp. Biol. Med.,* 38:419–420.
14. Fessas, P., Wintrobe, M., Thompson, R., and Cartwright, G. (1954): *Arch. Intern. Med.,* 94:384–401.
15. Foley, G. E., Lazarus, H., Farber, S., Uzman, B. G., Boone, B. A., and McCarthy, R. E. (1965): *Cancer,* 18:522–529.
16. Frei, E., III, and Freireich, E. J. (1965): *Adv. Chemotherapy,* 2:269–298.
17. Goldin, A., Sandberg, J. S., Henderson, E. S., Newman, J. W., Frei, E., III, and Holland, J. F. (1971): *Cancer Chemother. Rep.,* 55:309–401.
18. Granville, N., Rubio, F., Jr., Vnugur, A., Schulman, E., and Dameshek, W. (1958): *N. Engl. J. Med.,* 259:207–213.
19. Harmon, J. M., Norman, M. R., Fowlkes, B. J., and Thompson, E. B. (1979): *J. Cell Physiol.,* 98:267–278.
20. Harmon, J. M., Schmidt, T. J., and Thompson, E. B. (1978): *J. Cell Biol.,* 79 (No. 2, Part 2):HM 1244.
21. Homo, F., Duval, D., Thierry, C., and Serron, B. (1979): *J. Steroid Biochem.,* 10:609–613.
22. Kaiser, N., Milholland, R. J., and Rosen, F. (1974): *Cancer Res.,* 34:621–626.
23. Kaplan, J., Mastrangelo, R., and Peterson, W. (1974): *Cancer Res.,* 34:521–525.
24. Konior-Yarbro, G. S., Lippman, M. E., Johnson, G. E., and Leventhal, B. G. (1977): *Cancer Res.,* 37:2688–2695.
25. Lampkin, B. C., Nagao, T., and Mauer, A. M. (1969): *J. Clin. Invest.,* 48:1124–1130.
26. Lampkin, B. C., Nagao, T., and Mauer, A. M. (1971): *J. Clin. Invest.,* 50:2204–2214.
27. Leikin, S. L., Brubaker, C., Hartmann, J. R., Murphy, M. L., Wolff, J. A., and Perrin, E. (1968): *Cancer,* 21:346–351.
28. Levisohn, S. R., and Thompson, E. B. (1972): *Nature (New Biol.),* 235:102–104.
29. Lippman, M., and Barr, R. (1977): *J. Immunol.,* 118:1977–1981.
30. Lippman, M. E., Halterman, R., Leventhal, B., Perry, S., and Thompson, E. B. (1973): *J. Clin. Invest.,* 52:1715–1725.
31. Lippman, M. E., Halterman, R. H., Perry, S., Leventhal, B., and Thompson, E. B. (1973): *Nature (New Biol.),* 242:157–158.
32. Lippman, M. E., Perry, S., and Thompson, E. B. (1974): *Cancer Res.,* 34:1572–1576.
33. Lippman, M. E., and Thompson, E. B. (1973): *Lancet,* 1 (1713):1198.

34. Makman, M. H., Nakagawa, S., and White, A. (1967): *Recent Prog. Horm. Res.,* 23:195–227.
35. Moon, H. (1937): *Proc. Soc. Exp. Biol. Med.,* 37:34–36.
36. Moscona, A. A., Moscona, M. H., and Saenz, N. (1968): *Proc. Natl. Acad. Sci. USA,* 61:160–167.
37. Munck, A., and Leung, K. (1977): In: *Receptors and Mechanism of Action of Steroid Hormones, Part II,* edited by Jorge R. Pasqualini, pp. 311–397. Dekker, New York.
38. Munck, A., and Wira, C. (1971): In: *Advances in the Biosciences, No. 7: Schering Workshop on Steroid Hormone Receptors,* edited by G. Raspe, pp. 301–330. Pergamon, Oxford.
39. Nicholson, M. L., and Young, D. A. (1978): *Cancer Res.,* 38:3673–3680.
40. Norman, M. R., Harmon, J. M., and Thompson, E. B. (1978): *Cancer Res.,* 38:4273–4278.
41. Norman, M. R., and Thompson, E. B. (1977): *Cancer Res.,* 37:3785–3791.
42. Pearson, O., and Eliel, L. (1950): *JAMA,* 144:1349–1353.
43. Roath, S., Israels, M., and Wilkinson, J. (1964): *Q. J. Med.,* 33:257–283.
44. Schmidt, T., Harmon, J., and Thompson, E. B. (1980): *Nature (in press).*
45. Schmidt, T. J., and Thompson, E. B. (1979): *Cancer Res.,* 39:376–382.
46. Schwartz, R. J. (1972): *Nature (New Biol.),* 237:121–125.
47. Selye, H. (1937): *Endocrinology,* 21:169–188.
48. Shanbrom, E., and Miller, S. (1962): *N. Engl. J. Med.,* 266:1354–1358.
49. Simpson, M. E., Li, C. H., Reinhardt, W. O., and Evans, H. M. (1943): *Proc. Soc. Exp. Biol. Med.,* 54:135–137.
50. Smith, K. A., Crabtree, G. R., Kennedy, S. J., and Munck, A. U. (1977): *Nature,* 267:523–526.
51. Smith, R., Blaese, R., Hathcock, K., Buell, D., Edelson, R., and Lutzner, M. (1974): In: *Lymphocyte Recognition Effector Mechanisms,* edited by K. Lindahl-Kiessling and D. Osoba, pp. 127–146. Academic, New York.
52. Thompson, E. B. (1979): *Cancer Treatment Rep.,* 63:189–195.
53. White, A., and Dougherty, T. F. (1944): *Proc. Soc. Exp. Biol. Med.,* 56:26–27.
54. Wolff, J., Brubaker, C., Murphy, M., Pierce, M., and Severo, N. (1967): *J. Pediatr.,* 70:626–631.
55. Yamamoto, K. R., Gehring, U., Stampfer, M. R., and Sibley, C. H. (1976): *Recent Prog. Horm. Res.,* 32:3–32.

Hormones and Cancer, edited by S. Iacobelli et al.
Raven Press, New York © 1980.

The Regulation of Transcription in Lymphocytes by Glucocorticoids

P. A. Bell, N. M. Borthwick, and T. C. Dembinski

*Tenovus Institute for Cancer Research, Welsh National School of Medicine,
Cardiff CF4 4XX, Wales*

Although the profound growth-suppressive and cytotoxic effects of glucocorticoids on lymphoid cells have long been appreciated (13), the mechanisms by which they are produced remain obscure. Over the past 10 to 15 years, however, extensive studies with steroid-sensitive normal and malignant rodent lymphoid cells have provided much information on the metabolic responses of these cells to glucocorticoids and on the intracellular fate of the administered hormone. In such cells, functions inhibited by glucocorticoids include the transport of glucose (26) and α-aminoisobutyric acid (AIB) (41) and oxidative adenosine triphosphate (ATP) production (30), the last leading in turn to inhibitory effects on nucleoside transport and protein synthesis (41). It has been suggested by Nordeen and Young (30) that the suppressive effects of glucocorticoids on energy metabolism may be responsible for their growth-inhibitory actions. Yet another effect of glucocorticoids on lymphoid cells is the decreased resistance of nuclei to hypo-osmotic shock ("nuclear fragility"), reported by Giddings and Young (14). Since the first visible effects of the lethal actions of glucocorticoids are seen in the nuclear membranes and chromatin (7,38), it is probable that enhanced "nuclear fragility" represents an early manifestation of the lytic action of these steroids.

Differences in the time of appearance of these effects, together with varying requirements for the presence of energy-yielding substrates for their expression, suggest that they may be produced via separate pathways. Nevertheless, they share in common a dependence on continuing RNA and protein synthesis, in that the inhibitory effects of the steroid are abolished in the presence of compounds such as actinomycin D, α-amanitin, cordycepin (3′-deoxyadenosine), or cycloheximide (1,14,16,23,25,40). Furthermore, for each effect the period of sensitivity to cycloheximide corresponds with the course of emergence of the effect at the cellular level (16,23). Such circumstantial evidence has led to the hypothesis that glucocorticoids act in lymphoid cells to initiate or stimulate the synthesis of regulatory proteins responsible for producing the observed inhibitory effects. Thus, the primary action of glucocorticoids in tissues where the ultimate response is inhibitory is viewed as being essentially the same as that

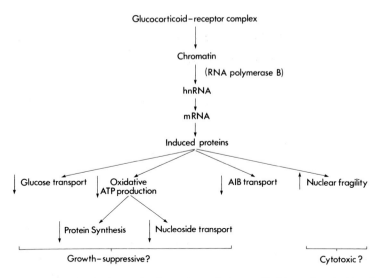

FIG. 1. Hypothetical scheme for the actions of glucocorticoids on lymphoid cells.

in tissues where the ultimate response is anabolic, as in the liver, and indeed the same as that of other steroid hormones which produce stimulatory responses in their respective target tissues.

The hypothesis is indirectly supported by evidence that in this system, as in virtually all other steroid hormone-responsive systems, the magnitude and specificity of the responses are closely related to the extent of interaction of an activated glucocorticoid–receptor complex with nuclear chromatin. The interaction of glucocorticoids with a specific intracellular receptor protein appears to be the initial obligatory step in the production of many, if not all, of the effects of these hormones. After this primary interaction, the steroid-receptor complex undergoes a temperature- and ionic strength-dependent activation process, possibly a change in conformation, as a result of which the affinity of the receptor for binding sites in chromatin is increased (27). This interaction of the steroid–receptor complex with chromatin is believed to result, in some as yet unknown way, in the transcription of genes for regulatory proteins responsible for producing the ultimate physiological effects (Fig. 1). Thus one approach to the evaluation of the mechanism of action of glucocorticoids may be through an analysis of their effects at the transcriptional level.

GLUCOCORTICOID EFFECTS ON RNA POLYMERASE ACTIVITY

In early studies of the effects of glucocorticoids on transcription in lymphoid cells, Nakagawa and White (28) observed that the DNA-dependent RNA polymerase activity of isolated rat thymus nuclei was inhibited by 25 to 30% 3 hr after the injection of cortisol into intact rats. The observations were subsequently confirmed with an aggregated chromatin preparation (29); inhibition of enzyme activity by cortisol was seen in the presence of magnesium ions at low ionic strength and also in presence of manganese ions at high ionic strength, suggesting that both hnRNA and pre-rRNA synthesis were affected by the steroid.

We have studied the early effects of glucocorticoids on RNA polymerase activity in rat thymus nuclei in some detail, using α-amanitin to resolve the activities of the different enzymes (31), and have confirmed and extended these early observations. RNA polymerase B (or II) activity, believed to be that responsible for hnRNA synthesis, was determined at high ionic strength in the presence of manganese ions and was inhibited by 1.25 µg/ml α-amanitin. RNA polymerase A (or I) activity, responsible for 45S rRNA synthesis, was measured under low salt conditions in the presence of magnesium ions and was resistant to 1.25 µg/ml α-amanitin; this activity was also resistant to an α-amanitin concentration of 125 µg/ml, indicating that the contribution of RNA polymerase C (or III) activity to that measured as RNA polymerase A was negligible. The enzyme activities were determined in nuclei isolated at various times up to 3 hr after the addition of 1 µM dexamethasone to thymus cell suspensions obtained from 7 to 8-week-old adrenalectomized rats and incubated *in vitro*.

The results obtained (4) are summarized in Fig. 2. Steroid treatment produced an early, transient rise in the activity of RNA polymerase B. Enzyme activity

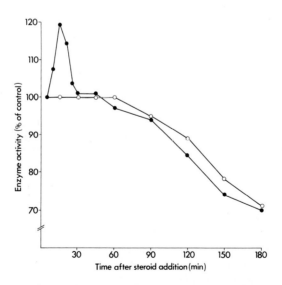

FIG. 2. Effect of 1 µM dexamethasone *in vitro* on the activity of RNA polymerase A *(open circles)* and RNA polymerase B *(closed circles)* in rat thymus cells. (Reproduced, with permission of Pergamon Press, from ref. 3.)

was increased within 10 min of the time of steroid addition, reached a maximum at 15 min, and was back to control levels at 30 min. This effect represents one of the earliest, and one of the few stimulatory, responses of rat thymus cells to glucocorticoids. The kinetics of appearance of the effect are compatible with the kinetics of nuclear accumulation of the steroid–receptor complex and with the kinetics of the sensitivity of a variety of metabolic effects to inhibitors of RNA synthesis (27), suggesting that the effect may well reflect the synthesis of hnRNA destined to produce the species of mRNA involved in the generation of the metabolic effects of the glucocorticoids. Although the peak stimulation of about 20% is substantial, the net increase in nucleotide incorporation over the first 30 min of steroid treatment only amounts to 7%. A stimulation of this magnitude probably could not be detected by precursor incorporation studies with intact cells and, indeed, radioactivity profiles of total cellular or polysomal RNA, pulse-labeled with [^{3}H]uridine at early times after the addition of dexamethasone to rat thymus cells and analyzed on sucrose gradients, have shown no obvious qualitative or quantitative changes.

The early stimulation of RNA polymerase B activity was followed by a progressive decline in enzyme activity below control levels, the inhibition reaching 30% by 3 hr after steroid addition. The activity of RNA polymerase A was unchanged over the first hour of steroid treatment but then declined in parallel with the decrease in activity of RNA polymerase B. Identical results were obtained following the administration of dexamethasone *in vivo,* confirming the physiological relevance of the effects. Biphasic changes in RNA polymerase B activity coupled with monophasic changes in RNA polymerase A activity have also been observed as a consequence of estrogen action in the uterus (6,15), although the second phase of the response in that tissue was a stimulatory one.

These effects of glucocorticoids on RNA polymerase activity were unaffected by nucleotide pool size and appeared to reflect the further elongation *in vitro* of RNA chains initiated and partly elongated in the intact cell. The magnitudes of the inhibitory effects are likely to be underestimates, since the nuclei of cells in which the hormone effects are most advanced will be the ones least able to survive the preparation procedures due to increased "nuclear fragility" (14).

The early stimulation of RNA polymerase B activity and the subsequent inhibition of the activities of both enzymes A and B were glucocorticoid-specific effects (5). They could be elicited by active glucocorticoids such as cortisol or dexamethasone, with dexamethasone being more potent than cortisol by an order of magnitude, and the concentration ranges over which they were produced were similar to those for receptor occupancy and for the generation of the metabolic effects of glucocorticoids in these cells. Neither cortexolone (11-deoxy-cortisol) nor progesterone had any effect on RNA polymerase activity, but cortexolone functioned as an antiglucocorticoid in relation to the RNA polymerase response as in relation to other responses (27), in that a 10-fold excess of cortexolone blocked the RNA polymerase response to cortisol.

PRIMARY OR SECONDARY NATURE OF TRANSCRIPTIONAL EFFECTS

In order to determine whether any of the effects of dexamethasone on RNA polymerase activities were secondary effects mediated by prior RNA or protein synthesis, experiments were performed in which inhibitors of RNA and protein synthesis were added to cells before the addition of dexamethasone. The results obtained (5) indicate that the effects of glucocorticoids on RNA polymerase A and B activities are mediated by different mechanisms. Pretreatment of thymus cells with α-amanitin, cordycepin, or cycloheximide abolished the inhibitory effect of dexamethasone on the form A enzyme activity, but was without effect on the control level over the period studied. In contrast, cycloheximide had no effect on either the basal activity of the form B enzyme or the early stimulation or later inhibition produced by dexamethasone. The concentration of cycloheximide used (0.1 mM) was capable of inhibiting protein synthesis by more than 95% within 5 min of addition.

The ability of these inhibitors of RNA and protein synthesis to block the effects of dexamethasone on RNA polymerase A activity was confined to the first few minutes after steroid addition. When α-amanitin or cordycepin was added to cell suspensions 15 min after dexamethasone, the steroid-induced inhibition of activity developed normally and was maintained at normal levels for up to 3 hr (5). A detailed time-course study of the influence of cycloheximide on the development of the steroid effect at 3 hr indicated that the inhibitor could block the expression of the effect only if it was added within 10 to 20 min of the steroid. The period of sensitivity to inhibitors corresponds to the time during which the form B enzyme activity is stimulated by glucocorticoids, suggesting that the inhibitory effect of these steroids on rRNA synthesis, unlike that on hnRNA synthesis, is a secondary one and depends on the synthesis of a species of mRNA and on its translation. Since the experiments resulted in the reversal of an inhibitory action, with no effects of the agents on the control enzyme activity, it is unlikely that nonspecific toxic effects of these agents are responsible for the abolition of the hormone effect.

Differential effects on the steroid-mediated changes in RNA polymerase activity were also observed in response to energy deprivation. Omission of glucose and amino acids from the medium in which the cells were incubated resulted in the abolition of the glucocorticoid effect on the form A, but not the form B, activity (2). Glucose deprivation had no effect on the control RNA polymerase A activity, making it unlikely that the steroid effect on rRNA synthesis is secondary to effects on ATP production; instead it seems probable that the glucose dependence is an indirect effect arising from the requirement for an energy source for continued protein synthesis in rat thymus cells (41).

RELATIONSHIPS BETWEEN TRANSCRIPTIONAL EFFECTS AND OTHER CELLULAR EFFECTS

If, as indicated earlier, the incorporation of nucleotides into RNA chains by isolated nuclei (the RNA polymerase assay) represents the elongation of nascent RNA chains initiated in the intact cell, it is pertinent to enquire into the relationship between these transcriptional effects and other actions of gluco-corticoids on rat thymus cells.

The kinetics of the early rise in RNA polymerase B activity are, as mentioned previously, compatible with it reflecting the synthesis of precursors to mRNA species coding for regulatory proteins responsible for producing many of the ultimate metabolic effects of the glucocorticoids. To investigate this possibility, poly(A)-rich mRNA has been isolated from control and dexamethasone-treated rat thymus cells by oligo(dT)-cellulose chromatography at early times after steroid addition. The electrophoretic analysis of the cell-free translation products of these fractions may indicate whether new mRNA species are produced in response to dexamethasone. Hybridization analysis of these RNA fractions is unlikely to provide useful information, since it is probable that any induced species of mRNA coding for regulatory proteins will be present in low abundance.

When glucocorticoid-treated lymphoid cells are examined microscopically, the first signs of the lethal action are observed in the nuclear membranes and chromatin (7,37). In particular, the characteristic structure of chromatin disappears, and nuclei become structurally homogeneous (pyknotic). It is tempting to associate this phenomenon with the progressive inhibition of RNA polymerase B activity which becomes apparent from about 1 hr after steroid addition. In keeping with the hypothesis are the observations that glucocorticoid-induced cytolysis, nuclear fragility, and the inhibition of the form B enzyme are all glucose-independent processes (14,34,37). On the other hand, glucocorticoid-induced nuclear fragility and pyknosis in thymus cells appear to be processes that are dependent on protein synthesis for their expression (14,37), whereas the inhibition of the form B enzyme activity is unaffected by the presence of inhibitors of protein synthesis (5). Clearly, if these observations are correct, neither process can be secondary to the other. One possible explanation is that the events mediated by protein synthesis occur at the level of the nuclear membrane in parallel to, but independent of, direct effects of the steroid–receptor complex on the structure of chromatin, but further investigations are obviously required to reconcile these observations.

The inhibitory effect of glucocorticoids on the activity of RNA polymerase A clearly appears to be a secondary effect mediated by some induced protein. This inhibition would be expected to have little effect on resting lymphocytes, since the rate of transcription of 45S ribosomal precursor RNA is not the rate-limiting step in rRNA synthesis in these cells, but would effectively prevent the increase in rRNA synthesis following growth stimulation, a condition in which the rate of transcription does become rate limiting (8). Such an effect could be expected to contribute to the growth-inhibitory effects of the glucocorticoids, since the initiation of DNA synthesis in lymphocytes can be prevented by the selective inhibition of rRNA synthesis (19).

The relationship between inhibitory effects of glucocorticoids on RNA polymerase activity and effects on the incorporation of precursors into RNA in intact cells is complicated by the fact that these steroids also inhibit nucleoside transport. Young et al. (41) concluded that the effects of cortisol on the incorporation of nucleosides into RNA 2 hr after steroid addition do not reflect changes in the rate of RNA synthesis but rather effects on nucleoside transport secondary to the cortisol-induced inhibition of ATP production. However, other studies have provided evidence which suggests that the effects of glucocorticoids on RNA polymerase activity in isolated nuclei do relate to RNA synthesis in the intact cell. In particular, Makman et al. (23) showed that an inhibitory effect of cortisol on the incorporation of orotic acid into acid-insoluble material could be observed in the absence of an effect on acid-soluble pools after 4 hr of incubation. Furthermore, an effect on the incorporation of uridine into acid-insoluble material in the absence of any effect on acid-soluble incorporation was observed in the presence of puromycin.

MECHANISMS OF TRANSCRIPTIONAL EFFECTS OF GLUCOCORTICOIDS

Although the mechanisms responsible for their production may differ, it is unlikely that the inhibitory effects of glucocorticoids on RNA polymerase activities represent changes in the total cellular levels of these enzymes. The effects occur rapidly, yet the turnover of the enzymes appears to be slow. It is probable that the changes observed in the activity of RNA polymerase B in rat thymus nuclei in response to dexamethasone reflect differences in the level of initiation of the enzyme on chromatin, since they were detected under high salt conditions where elongation rates are probably maximal and reinitiation is at a minimum. Preliminary results of the analysis of elongation rates and levels of initiation by hydrolysis of the reaction products and the determination of uridine:uridine monophosphate ratios (9,10) tend to support these conclusions. Thus, it is likely that steroid treatment is affecting the level of transcription of certain DNA sequences, but whether these include specific structural sequences remains to be determined. For the chick oviduct, there is evidence that ovalbumin gene products induced by estrogens in the intact cell are also present in the nascent RNA chains completed by incubation of nuclei *in vitro* (35).

The magnitude of the early stimulation of RNA polymerase B activity by dexamethasone in rat thymus cells is much larger than might be expected if the only effect of the steroid was to activate the transcription of a few specific genes for regulatory proteins. A possible explanation for this discrepancy is provided by the model for glucocorticoid hormone action proposed by Yamamoto and Alberts (39). They have suggested that the glucocorticoid–receptor complex may interact relatively nonspecifically with a variety of sites in chromatin to cause a local structural disturbance. The concentration or clustering of complexes is required for the activation of a complete structural gene, but the local disturbance caused by interaction of individual complexes at "nonspecific" sites may be sufficient to cause activation of certain, albeit short, sequences. This model can account for both the extent of interaction of glucocorticoid–receptor complexes with chromatin and also the considerable changes in "template activity," measured with exogenous enzymes that are observed in a variety of steroid-responsive systems (11,17,33). If "nonspecific" interactions of the glucocorticoid–receptor complex with chromatin in the intact cell can cause local relaxations of chromatin structure so that RNA polymerase B molecules can initiate, perhaps correctly, at a variety of sites but only elongate along portions of the complete structural sequences, then the model can also account for the present observations. The bulk of the hnRNA synthesized in response to dexamethasone would then be expected to be composed of relatively short sequences destined for destruction rather than conversion to mRNA.

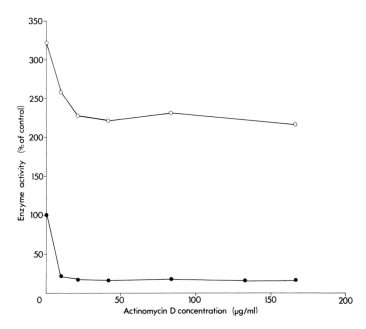

FIG. 3. Assay of free and engaged RNA polymerase A activity in rat thymus nuclei. Enzyme activity in the absence *(closed circles)* or presence *(open circles)* of an exogenous poly[d(A-T)] template (30 μg/ml) was determined in the presence of increasing concentrations of actinomycin D.

The steroid–receptor complex might produce local changes in the structure of chromatin either by virtue of some inherent catalytic function or by activation of chromatin-associated enzymes or other factors. The phenotype of the cell might well determine the direction and extent of such changes and, indeed, studies using bacterial RNA polymerase as a probe for chromatin structure have demonstrated that the direction of changes in template capacity as a result of glucocorticoid treatment depends both on the cell type and the metabolic state of the cell (17,18). It is possible that the inhibitory effect of glucocorticoids on RNA polymerase B activity reflects a direct action of this kind which, as a result of the phenotypic programming of the cell, is irreversibly destructive.

The inhibitory effect of glucocorticoids on RNA polymerase A activity in rat thymus cells, unlike the effects on RNA polymerase B, appears to be secondary to effects on mRNA and protein synthesis. In this respect the effect mirrors the stimulatory action of glucocorticoids on RNA polymerase A activity and rRNA synthesis in liver (43). Recent investigations of the control of rRNA synthesis have revealed that eukaryotic cells contain two discrete pools of RNA polymerase A activity. One pool exists as a tightly bound transcription complex

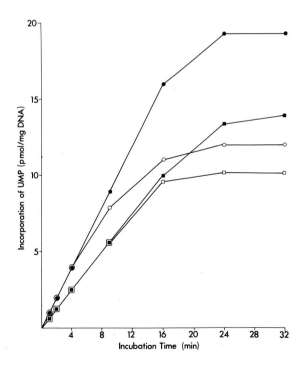

FIG. 4. Effects of dexamethasone and rifamycin AF/0–13 on RNA polymerase A activity in rat thymus nuclei. Nuclei from cells incubated for 3 hr in the absence *(circles)* or presence *(squares)* of 1 μM dexamethasone were assayed for RNA polymerase A activity in the absence *(closed symbols)* or presence *(open symbols)* of rifamycin AF/0–13 (200 μg/ml). (Reproduced, with permission of the Biochemical Society, from ref. 12.)

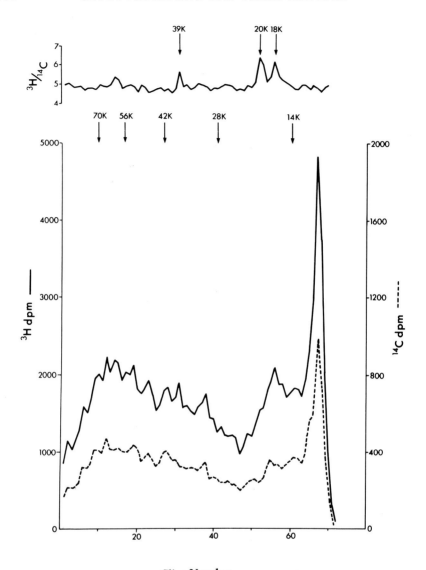

FIG. 5. Electrophoretic separation and analysis of labeling patterns for nonhistone chromatin proteins from dexamethasone-treated and control rat thymus cells. Cells were incubated with 1 μM dexamethasone and ^{3}H-amino acids or with ^{14}C-amino acids alone for 1 hr at 37°C and subsequently combined *(left panel)*. In a control experiment dexamethasone was omitted *(right panel)*. Following the preparation of chromatin and removal of histones, total nonhistone chromatin proteins were solubilized and electrophoresed on 10% acrylamide gels containing 0.1% SDS. *Arrows* indicate the positions of molecular weight markers and the steroid-induced protein peaks. (Reproduced, with permission of Pergamon Press, from ref. 3.)

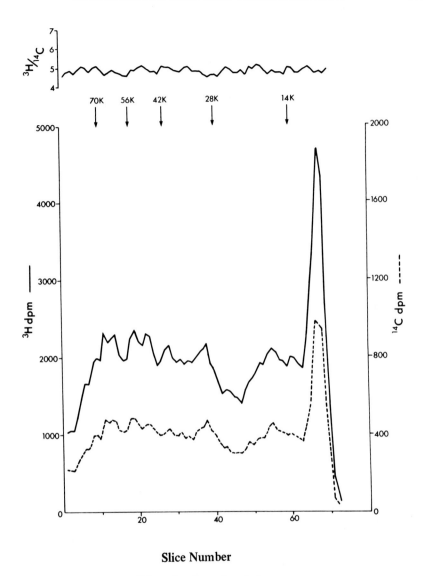

Slice Number

FIG. 5. See legend on facing page.

and is probably RNA polymerase A_{II} (I_A) (20), whereas the other pool is "free" with regard to its ability to transcribe exogenous templates in the presence of actinomycin D (42) and is believed to be RNA polymerase A_I (I_B) (20). The two forms of the enzyme appear to differ in respect of the presence of one polypeptide component or subunit (31) and since, in rat liver, engaged enzyme activity is tightly coupled to protein synthesis and energy metabolism, the redistribution of enzyme between free and engaged pools has been proposed as a mechanism for the modulation of the rate of pre-rRNA synthesis (21). Glucocorticoids might produce their effects either by directly mediating the synthesis of some component of the engaged enzyme (43) or by indirect control over the synthesis or degradation of some such component by a mechanism similar to that proposed for the regulation of amino acid transport in hepatoma tissue culture cells (24).

To investigate these various possibilities, we have determined the activity of the free form of RNA polymerase A, simultaneously with that of the engaged form, in rat thymus nuclei and cytosol, in the presence of actinomycin D (to inhibit engaged enzyme) and an exogenous poly[d(A-T)] template. In contrast with the findings of Kellas et al. (20) with rat liver nuclei, rat thymus nuclei prepared by hypo-osmotic lysis of cells contained a substantial pool of RNA polymerase A activity capable of transcribing a poly[d(A-T)] template in the presence of high concentrations of actinomycin D (Fig. 3). Treatment of the cells with 1 μM dexamethasone for 3 hr resulted in inhibition of activity of the engaged form of the enzyme by $30.0 \pm 5.4\%$, inhibition of the nuclear free form by $11.2 \pm 9.0\%$, and inhibition of free activity in cytosol by $8.3 \pm 2.4\%$ (12).

The failure to detect an increase in the activity of the free pool after steroid treatment suggests that the inhibitory effect on the engaged activity was not due to a decrease in the number of enzyme molecules initiated. Support for this conclusion was obtained from experiments using rifamycin AF/0–13 to suppress reinitiation of RNA polymerase A in the assay *in vitro*. Figure 4 shows the activity of the engaged enzyme in nuclei from rat thymus cells treated with dexamethasone for 3 hr. In the absence of rifamycin, the initial enzyme activity in nuclei from steroid-treated cells was 62.5% of that in nuclei from control cells. Rifamycin AF/0–13 did not affect initial synthetic rates, but prevented reinitiation by binding enzyme released following termination of the polynucleotide chains. In the presence of rifamycin, the effect of dexamethasone on the plateau level of incorporation was much less ($7.3 \pm 1.4\%$ in three experiments) than that on the initial rate, suggesting that the primary effect is on the elongation rate rather than on the number of enzyme molecules initiated (12). Preliminary results of measurements of the numbers of transcribing enzyme molecules and of elongation rates (9,10) tend to support these conclusions. It remains to be determined whether the change in elongation rate represents an action on the enzyme or template; in liver there is evidence to suggest that glucocorticoid treatment alters the catalytic activity of the enzyme (32,36). The effect does seem to be mediated via protein synthesis and in this respect it is interesting that Lindell et al. (22) have obtained data that suggest a relation between the synthesis of rapidly labeled nuclear proteins and the modulation of pre-rRNA transcription. Using double-labeling amino acid incorporation techniques, we have been able to demonstrate glucocorticoid-specific changes in the labeling pattern of chromatin-associated nonhistone proteins within 1 hr of steroid addition (3) (Fig. 5) and it is possible that these steroid-regulated proteins are localized in the nucleolus.

CONCLUSIONS

The results reviewed here indicate that glucocorticoids have major effects on the transcription process in rat thymus lymphocytes. Both the early stimulatory and later inhibitory effects on the activity of RNA polymerase B appear to be direct effects produced by the steroid–receptor complex modifying the structure of chromatin in some as yet undetermined way. Insight into these actions might be obtained from studies of the effects of glucocorticoids on processes likely to modify chromatin structure such as protein acetylation or phosphorylation, or nuclease, protease, or phosphatase activity. Glucocorticoids also have an inhibitory effect on RNA polymerase A activity, but this action appears to be secondary to the induction by the steroid of some regulatory protein which in turn mediates the effect. The elucidation of the mechanism of this effect may well offer important insights into the mechanisms regulating ribosomal RNA synthesis in general.

ACKNOWLEDGMENTS

The authors acknowledge with gratitude the continuing financial support provided by the Tenovus Organization.

REFERENCES

1. Baran, D. T., Lichtman, M. A., and Peck, W. A. (1972): *J. Clin. Invest.*, 51:2181–2189.
2. Bell, P. A., and Borthwick, N. M. (1976): *J. Steroid Biochem.*, 7:1147–1150.
3. Bell, P. A., and Borthwick, N. M. (1979): *J. Steroid Biochem.*, 11:381–387.
4. Borthwick, N. M., and Bell, P. A. (1975): *FEBS Lett.*, 60:396–399.
5. Borthwick, N. M., and Bell, P. A. (1978): *Mol. Cell. Endocrinol.*, 9:269–278.
6. Borthwick, N. M., and Smellie, R. M. S. (1975): *Biochem J.*, 147:91–101.
7. Burton, A. F., Storr, J. M., and Dunn, W. L. (1967): *Can. J. Biochem.*, 45:289–297.
8. Cooper, H. L. (1971): In: *The Cell Cycle and Cancer*, edited by R. Baserga, pp. 197–226. Dekker, New York.
9. Coupar, B. E. H., and Chesterton, C. J. (1977): *Eur. J. Biochem.*, 79:525–533.
10. Cox, R. F. (1976): *Cell*, 7:455–465.
11. Davies, P., Thomas, P., Giles, M. G., Boonjawat, J., and Griffiths, K. (1979): *J. Steroid Biochem.*, 11:351–360.
12. Dembinski, T. C., Borthwick, N. M., and Bell, P. A. (1979): *Biochem. Soc. Trans.*, 7:1297–1298.
13. Dougherty, T. F., and White, A. (1945): *Am. J. Anat.*, 77:81–116.
14. Giddings, S. J., and Young, D. A. (1974): *J. Steroid Biochem.*, 5:587–595.
15. Glasser, S. R., Chytil, F., and Spelsberg, T. C. (1972): *Biochem. J.*, 130:947–957.
16. Hallahan, C., Young, D. A., and Munck, A. (1973): *J. Biol. Chem.*, 248:2922–2927.
17. Johnson, L. K., and Baxter, J. D. (1978): *J. Biol. Chem.*, 253:1991–1997.
18. Johnson, L. K., Baxter, J. D., and Rousseau, G. G. (1979): In: *Glucocorticoid Hormone Action*, edited by J. D. Baxter and G. G. Rousseau, pp. 305–326. Springer-Verlag, Berlin.

19. Kay, J. E., Leventhal, B. G., and Cooper, H. L. (1969): *Exp. Cell Res.,* 54:94–100.
20. Kellas, B. L., Austoker, J. L., Beebee, T. J. C., and Butterworth, P. H. W. (1977): *Eur. J. Biochem.,* 72:583–594.
21. Lampert, A., and Feigelson, P. (1974): *Biochem. Biophys. Res. Commun.,* 58:1030–1038.
22. Lindell, T. J., O'Malley, A. F., and Puglisi, B. (1978): *Biochemistry,* 17:1154–1160.
23. Makman, M. H., Nakagawa, S., Dvorkin, B., and White, A. (1970): *J. Biol. Chem.,* 245:2556–2563.
24. McDonald, R. A., and Gelehrter, T. D. (1977): *Biochem. Biophys. Res. Commun.,* 78:1304–1310.
25. Mosher, K. M., Young, D. A., and Munck, A. (1971): *J. Biol. Chem.,* 246:654–659.
26. Munck, A. (1968): *J. Biol. Chem.,* 243:1039–1042.
27. Munck, A., and Leung, K. (1977): In: *Receptors and Mechanism of Action of Steroid Hormones, Part II,* edited by J. R. Pasqualini, pp. 311–397. Dekker, New York.
28. Nakagawa, S., and White, A. (1967): *Endocrinology,* 81:861–870.
29. Nakagawa, S., and White, A. (1970): *J. Biol. Chem.,* 245:1448–1457.
30. Nordeen, S. K., and Young, D. A. (1976): *J. Biol. Chem.,* 251:7295–7303.
31. Roeder, R. G. (1976): In: *RNA Polymerase,* edited by R. Losick and M. Chamberlin, pp. 285–329. Cold Spring Harbor Laboratory, Cold Spring Harbor, New York.
32. Sajdel, E. M., and Jacob, S. T. (1971): *Biochem. Biophys. Res. Commun.,* 45:707–715.
33. Schwartz, R. J., Tsai, M.-J., Tsai, S. Y., and O'Malley, B. W. (1975): *J. Biol. Chem.,* 250:5175–5182.
34. Stevens, J., and Stevens, Y.-W. (1975): *J. Natl. Cancer Inst.,* 54:1493–1494.
35. Swaneck, G. E., Nordstrom, J. L., Kreuzaler, F., Tsai, M.-J., and O'Malley, B. W. (1979): *Proc. Natl. Acad. Sci. U.S.A.,* 76:1049–1053.
36. Todhunter, J. A., Weissbach, H., and Brot, N. (1978): *J. Biol. Chem.,* 253:4514–4516.
37. Waddell, A. W., Wyllie, A. H., Robertson, A. M. G., Mayne, K., Au, J., and Currie, A. R. (1979): In: *Glucocorticoid Action and Leukaemia, Proceedings 7th Tenovus Workshop,* edited by P. A. Bell and N. M. Borthwick, pp. 75–83. Alpha Omega Publishing, Cardiff.
38. Whitfield, J. F., Perris, A. D., and Youdale, T. (1968): *Exp. Cell Res.,* 52:349–362.
39. Yamamoto, K. R., and Alberts, B. M. (1976): *Annu. Rev. Biochem.,* 45:721–746.
40. Young, D. A., Barnard, T., Mendelsohn, S., and Giddings, S. J. (1974): *Endocrine Res. Commun.,* 1:63–72.
41. Young, D. A., Giddings, S., Swonger, A., Klurfeld, G., and Miller, M. (1971): In: *Proceedings 3rd International Congress on Hormonal Steroids,* edited by V. H. T. James and L. Martini, pp. 624–635. Excerpta Medica, Amsterdam.
42. Yu, F.-L. (1974): *Nature,* 251:344–346.
43. Yu, F.-L., and Feigelson, P. (1973): *Biochem. Biophys. Res. Commun.,* 53:754–760.

Hormones and Cancer, edited by S. Iacobelli et al.
Raven Press, New York © 1980.

Effects of Glucocorticoids on the Plasma Membrane of Rat Hepatoma Cells

*M. Verhaegen, **D. K. Granner, A. Amar-Costesec,
P. M. Edwards, and G. G. Rousseau

*International Institute of Cellular and Molecular Pathology B-1200 Brussels, Belgium;
and **Department of Internal Medicine and Biochemistry, University of Iowa College
of Medicine and Veterans Administration Hospital, Iowa City, Iowa 52242*

Rat hepatoma tissue culture (HTC) cells exhibit several plasma membrane-related properties which are considered typical of the "morphologic phenotype" of transformed cells (12). These include a decrease in cell surface adhesiveness, an increase in the density of microvilli and of net negative charges, and an increase in the membrane transport of amino acids and in the production of plasminogen activator. All these modifications are reversed by glucocorticoids (Table 1) (3,12). These hormones are thought to act by influencing the rate of synthesis of specific proteins, presumably by increasing the transcription of specific genes (22). In HTC cells, the number of glucocorticoid-sensitive genes

TABLE 1. *Effects of glucocorticoids in HTC cells*

Process	Effect	Refs.
Adhesiveness	↑	3
Surface antigens	↑	3
Net negative charge	↓	3
Surface microvilli	↓	12
Tyrosine aminotransferase induction by cyclic AMP	+	14
Mouse mammary tumor virus induction	+	20
Amino acid and hexose uptake	↓	21
Plasminogen activator	↓	29
Acid release	↑	This chapter
Enzymes		
Tyrosine aminotransferase	↑	4
Glutamine synthetase	↑	8
Ornithine decarboxylase	↑	7
Cyclic AMP phosphodiesterase	↓	19
Alkaline phosphodiesterase I	↑	This chapter
Nucleoside (ADP) diphosphatase	↓	This chapter

---

* Present address: Institut Pasteur du Brabant, B-1040 Brussels, Belgium.

appears to be quite limited (15). The most intensively studied of the induced proteins is tyrosine aminotransferase, and a selective increase in the mRNA for this enzyme has been measured in HTC cells (13).

The biochemical mechanisms involved in regulating the membrane-related processes are still unknown, although it has been suggested that the glucocorticoid-mediated changes in amino acid transport (12,21) and plasminogen activator (25) each involve at least one unidentified protein intermediate. We have identified two specific plasma membrane enzymes whose activities are altered by glucocorticoid hormones. These are alkaline phosphodiesterase I, which is stimulated, and nucleoside diphosphatase acting on adenosine diphosphate (ADP), which is inhibited. In the course of these studies, we also noted that glucocorticoids stimulate acid production by HTC cells. In this chapter, we will review these new findings and attempt to relate them to the previously noted membrane effects of glucocorticoids.

RESULTS

Alkaline Phosphodiesterase I

Stimulation by Dexamethasone

HTC cells grown in the presence of the synthetic glucocorticoid dexamethasone show the well-known increase in the cytosolic enzyme tyrosine aminotransferase (EC 2.6.1.5) and in cell adhesiveness to glass (Table 2). We found that, in addition, the activity of alkaline phosphodiesterase I (EC 3.1.4.1) is stimulated about threefold (23,24) (Table 2). In HTC cells (18) as well as in rat hepatocytes

TABLE 2. *Effects of dexamethasone in HTC cells*

	Dexamethasone	No. exp.	Mean ± SEM
Tyrosine aminotransferase	−	10	5.8 ± 1.0
	+		37.1 ± 9.3
Alkaline phosphodiesterase I	−	10	72.0 ± 5.2
	+		229 ± 6.6
Nucleoside diphosphatase	−	4	12.4 ± 0.3
	+		7.0 ± 0.4
Culture pH	−	9	7.44 ± 0.05
	+		7.22 ± 0.06
Cell adhesiveness	−	7	18.8 ± 4.6
	+		43.0 ± 7.2

HTC cell cultures were exposed for 24 hr (tyrosine aminotransferase, pH, cell adhesiveness) or 48 hr (other parameters) to either dexamethasone (0.1–1 μM) or an equal volume of the vehicle, ethanol. Enzyme activities were assayed as described (24) and are expressed as mU/mg protein. The mean pH of the culture medium was 7.8 at the beginning of the experiments. Adhesiveness to glass was assayed by decrease in turbidimetry of cell suspensions and is expressed as the percentage change in optical density caused by attachment.

(1,28), this enzyme is specifically associated with the plasma membrane. The time course of the effect shows a lag period followed by a progressive rise towards a new steady state and a reversibility upon removal of the hormone, which are characteristic features of the induction of enzymes by glucocorticoids. Stimulation of alkaline phosphodiesterase I can be detected 8 hr after the addition of dexamethasone and is maximal by 48 to 72 hr, depending on the feeding schedule of the culture. It is seen in both the absence and presence of serum. Cells in monolayer are as sensitive as suspension cultures.

Stimulation of alkaline phosphodiesterase I can be best demonstrated at dexamethasone concentrations (0.1 μM or above) which maximally induce tyrosine aminotransferase (4). However, the effect occurs with concentrations of dexamethasone as low as 2 nM. The dose–response curve is superimposable on that for induction of tyrosine aminotransferase (Fig. 1). The dependence of alkaline phosphodiesterase I activity on the concentration of substrate (*p*-nitrophenyl-thymidine-5′-phosphate) is exactly the same in dexamethasone-treated as in con-

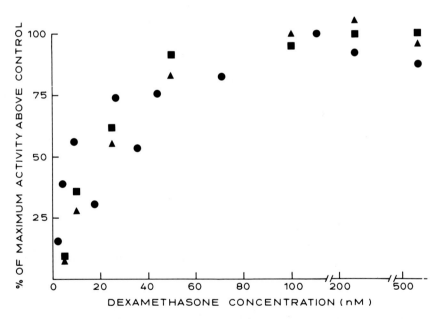

FIG. 1. Effect of various concentrations of dexamethasone on the activity of tyrosine aminotransferase *(triangles)*, alkaline phosphodiesterase I *(circles)*, and acid release *(squares)* in HTC cells. Cells were incubated in serum-free medium for either 24 hr *(triangles, squares)* or 32 hr *(circles)* in the presence of dexamethasone at the indicated concentrations. The activities of the two enzymes are expressed as a percentage of the maximum increase over the basal activity measured in the absence of dexamethasone. Acid release is expressed as a percentage of the difference between the pH (7.17) of the medium of cells treated with the highest dexamethasone concentration and the pH (7.5) of control cultures. Basal and maximum activities were 1.95 and 24.8 mU/mg protein for tyrosine aminotransferase and 102 and 237 mU/mg protein for alkaline phosphodiesterase I.

trol cells. Thus, the stimulation corresponds to an increase in the V_{max} of the enzyme without change in the K_m (0.55 mM). The other properties of alkaline phosphodiesterase I which are not changed by dexamethasone treatment include pH optimum (9.6), and dependence on zinc (maximum activity at 2 mM) and on temperature. The Arrhenius plot is biphasic with a breaking point (24°C) that is typical of several membrane enzymes (17). Both the transition temperature and the activation energies are similar in control and dexamethasone-treated cells, suggesting that the physicochemical environment of the enzyme remains unchanged. This is supported by studies on the subcellular distribution of alkaline phosphodiesterase I. Table 3 shows that, following stimulation by dexamethasone, the enzyme remains associated with the particulate fraction. Furthermore, upon isopyknic centrifugation analysis of the cell organelles (Table 4), we find that in dexamethasone-treated cells the gradient subfraction between densities 1.141 and 1.156 has the highest phosphodiesterase I specific activity with a fairly good yield (13%). The density of the subfraction corresponds to that observed for plasma membrane-related structures in rat liver (5). Finally, although alkaline phosphodiesterase I is thought to be located on the outer surface of the cell (9), none is released into the culture medium following stimulation by glucocorticoids.

Glucocorticoid induction of tyrosine aminotransferase is a characteristic shared by hepatocytes and HTC cells. We wondered whether glucocorticoids also stimulated alkaline phosphodiesterase I in rat liver. In adult rats, the basal activity of this enzyme is about twice as high as in HTC cells (Table 2 and Fig. 2). Following treatment with dexamethasone, alkaline phosphodiesterase I increases by only about 30% ($p < 0.001$). The natural glucocorticoid corticosterone has the same effect, while it increases tyrosine aminotransferase activity by about 300%. A slight but significant increase is also seen with deoxycorticosterone, a mineralocorticoid that does not stimulate tyrosine aminotransferase (Fig. 2). In these experiments, the steroids were administered over 5 days. Because alkaline phosphodiesterase I has a long half-life (see below) such a period would be required to reach maximal stimulation if the latter were the result of an increased rate of enzyme synthesis (6).

During development, several glucocorticoid-sensitive responses show a precocious rise to adult levels following treatment with dexamethasone (2). Newborn rats had low basal activities of both tyrosine aminotransferase and alkaline phosphodiesterase I (Fig. 2). Dexamethasone treatment influenced neither tyrosine aminotransferase activity, which is consistent with earlier work (2), nor alkaline phosphodiesterase I activity.

Specificity of the Effect

In addition to alkaline phosphodiesterase I, several enzymes in rat liver are considered to be specific constituents of the hepatocyte plasma membrane. We investigated whether their activity changed under conditions of alkaline phospho-

TABLE 3. *Lack of effect of dexamethasone on the distribution of alkaline phosphodiesterase I after differential centrifugation of HTC cell homogenates*

Constituent	Dex.	Amount in homogenate	Nuclear fraction (%)	Particulate fraction (%)	Final supernate (%)	% Recovery
Alkaline	−	4.33	7.3	91.4	1.3	104.3
Phosphodiesterase I	+	9.20	4.2	92.7	3.1	101.8
Protein	−	86.9	16.2	44.4	39.4	94.0
	+	82.1	8.4	50.7	40.9	103.5

HTC cells were homogenized and submitted to differential centrifugation as described for rat liver (1) except that the particulate fraction and final supernate were obtained by centrifuging the cytoplasmic extract at 39,000 rpm for 60 min. Values given are the means of two experiments with or without 1 μM dexamethasone (Dex.) for 24 hr. Tyrosine aminotransferase specific activity was 4.75 and 23.10 mU/mg protein in control and treated cells, respectively. The amount in homogenate is given in milliunits (enzyme) or mg (protein) per g cells. The distribution is in percentage of the sum over the quantity in whole homogenate. The recovery is in percentage of this sum of values found in the three fractions.

TABLE 4. *Biochemical composition of a gradient subfraction enriched in plasma membrane*

Constituent	Component	% Total activity	Relative specific activity
Protein		0.56	
Alkaline phosphodiesterase I	Plasma membrane	13.24	23.64
Galactosyltransferase	Golgi complex	5.90	10.54
NADPH cytochrome c reductase	Endoplasmic reticulum	1.44	2.57
Cytochrome oxidase	Mitochondria	0.41	0.13

HTC cells were exposed to 0.5 μM dexamethasone for 48 hr. A cell homogenate in 0.25 M sucrose, 3 mM imidazole, pH 7.4, was centrifuged at 30,000 rpm for 60 min in a Beckman rotor no. 30. The pellet, which contained the bulk of cellular organelles, was resuspended in sucrose at a final density of 1.25. This preparation was introduced under a linear sucrose gradient (density 1.24 to 1.10) and centrifuged for 16 hr at 24,000 rpm in a Beckman rotor SW 25.2. Seven gradient subfractions were obtained and analyzed for the constituents indicated above. The composition of the subfraction of mean density 1.15 is given here, each constituent as a percentage of the total activity in all gradient subfractions and original supernate.

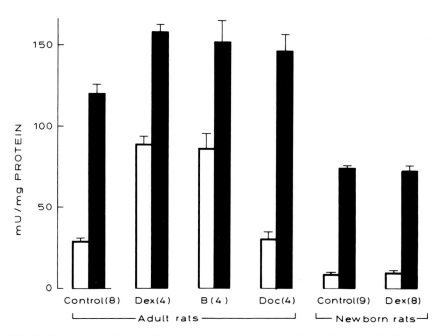

FIG. 2. Effect of steroids on rat liver tyrosine aminotransferase *(open bars)* and alkaline phosphodiesterase I *(closed bars)*. Adult male Wistar rats (200 g) were adrenalectomized and treated with five daily s.c. doses of dexamethasone (Dex; 0.1 mg/kg), corticosterone (B; 10 mg/kg) or deoxycorticosterone (DOC; 10 mg/kg). Newborn rats were treated daily from 1 to 10 days of age with dexamethasone (0.1 mg/kg/day). The final body weight was 22.4 ± 0.6 and 11.6 ± 0.5 g in control and treated newborn rats, respectively. Results are means ± SEM with the number of animals in parentheses.

diesterase I stimulation. The most typical of these enzymes is 5'-nucleotidase (EC 3.1.3.5). However, it is not detectable in HTC cells and does not appear following treatment with dexamethasone. Of the four other plasma membrane enzymes studied in HTC cells—alkaline phosphatase (EC 3.1.3.1), Mg^{2+} adenosine triphosphatase (ATPase; EC 3.6.1.3), aminopeptidase (EC 3.4.11.2), and nucleoside diphosphatase acting on ADP—none is stimulated by dexamethasone. Actually, the latter enzyme is inhibited (see below). Therefore, the stimulatory effect of dexamethasone appears to be specific for alkaline phosphodiesterase I.

Steroids other than glucocorticoids, such as progesterone, estradiol, methyltestosterone, or an inactive glucocorticoid metabolite, do not increase alkaline phosphodiesterase I activity in HTC cells (Fig. 3). The effect of various steroids alone or in combination is consistent with their interaction with the glucocorticoid receptor present in these cells (22). Thus, an excess of estradiol (a glucocorticoid antagonist) or of deoxycorticosterone (a partial agonist–antagonist) inhibits the stimulatory effect of dexamethasone (Fig. 3).

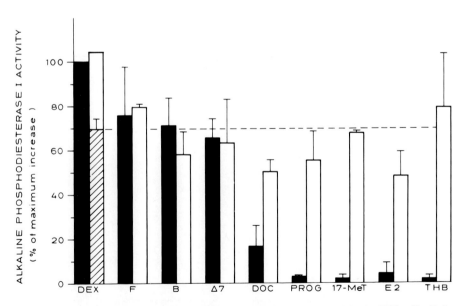

FIG. 3. Effect of various steroids on alkaline phosphodiesterase I activity in HTC cells. Cells in serum-free medium were exposed for 48 hr either to 5 μM of one of the steroids indicated *(closed bars)* or to 25 nM dexamethasone *(hatched bars)* or to *(open bars)* both 25 nM dexamethasone and 5 μM of the following steroids: dexamethasone (DEX), cortisol (F), corticosterone (B), Δ7-prednisolone (Δ7), deoxycorticosterone (DOC), progesterone (PROG), 17α-methyltestosterone (17-MeT), estradiol (E2) or tetrahydrocorticosterone (THB). Mean and range of two experiments.

Mechanisms of the Stimulation

Neither dexamethasone nor cortisol at concentrations up to 10 μM influence alkaline phosphodiesterase I activity of cell extracts *in vitro*. In intact cells, the dose–response curve and the effect of different steroids both indicate that the stimulation of alkaline phosphodiesterase I by dexamethasone results from its interaction with the receptor involved in tryosine aminotransferase induction. When extracts from dexamethasone-treated and control cells are mixed in various proportions, alkaline phosphodiesterase I activity in the mixture exactly corresponds to the sum of activities in the original extracts. This makes it unlikely that dexamethasone stimulates an activator or inactivates an inhibitor of this enzyme. Thus, it is probable that increased alkaline phosphodiesterase I activity also results from an induction phenomenon, i.e., an increase in the number of enzyme molecules (11). This is also consistent with the increase in V_{max} and with the time course of the effect.

If this induction is secondary to an increased rate of synthesis, one would predict from the slower rate of increase in alkaline phosphodiesterase I activity,

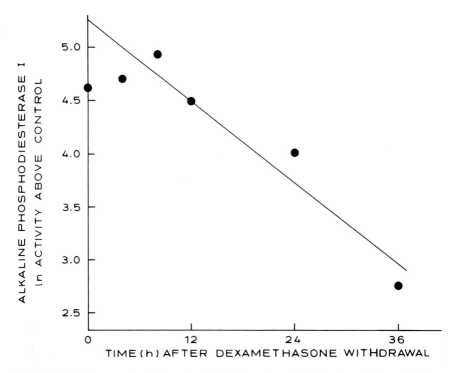

FIG. 4. Rate of decrease in alkaline phosphodiesterase I activity following withdrawal of dexamethasone. After 48 hr of pretreatment with 0.1 μM dexamethasone the cells were washed and resuspended in steroid-free medium at 0 time. Maximum enzyme activity was 180 mU/mg protein as compared with 78 mU/mg protein in the control culture.

as compared with tyrosine aminotransferase upon dexamethasone stimulation, that the phosphodiesterase has a longer half-life than the aminotransferase (6). This is the case. Following removal of dexamethasone from a stimulated culture, alkaline phosphodiesterase I activity returns to the control value with a half-life of about 11 hr (Fig. 4) as compared with 2 to 3 hr for tyrosine aminotransferase (26). Finally, the effect of dexamethasone is blocked by cycloheximide and by actinomycin D, inhibitors of protein and RNA synthesis, respectively.

Nucleoside Diphosphatase

While only one of all the plasma membrane-related enzymes examined in this study is stimulated, another one, nucleoside diphosphatase acting on ADP is inhibited (Table 2). In certain cell lines a function which is stimulated by glucocorticoids in growing cultures can become inhibited by these hormones under nutritional deprivation. This is the case for growth hormone production by rat pituitary GC cells (16). In HTC cells, however, nucleoside diphosphatase is reproducibly inhibited by dexamethasone in the same culture where tyrosine aminotransferase and alkaline phosphodiesterase I are stimulated. This observation requires further study, since preliminary experiments suggest that in addition to authentic nucleoside diphosphatase another enzyme may contribute to the ADP hydrolysis. Moreover, upon isopyknic centrifugation, the distribution profile of nucleoside diphosphatase is less typical of plasma membrane enzymes than that of alkaline phosphodiesterase I.

Acid Release

The growth of HTCs is accompanied by an acidification of the medium. Depending on cell density, the initial pH of the medium (7.8) can fall by up to 0.8 units over a 48-hr period. This release of acid due to metabolic activity does not require cell multiplication, as it takes place in stationary cultures at high cell density or in serum-free medium where cells do not divide. We have observed a reproducible increase of acid release from HTC cells treated with dexamethasone (Table 2). The pH of the culture is 0.22 ($\pm$ 0.03 SEM, nine experiments) units lower than in control cells 24 hr after addition of the glucocorticoid; the difference is 0.31 ($\pm$ 0.05 SEM, six experiments) pH units after 48 hrs. This effect becomes apparent between 4 and 8 hr following glucocorticoid treatment.

Dexamethasone stimulation of acid release is specific. The dose–response curve is superimposable on that of stimulation of tyrosine aminotransferase and alkaline phosphodiesterase I (Fig. 1). Moreover, the effect of various steroids is consistent with a receptor-mediated event (Fig. 5). The glucocorticoids cortisol and corticosterone also stimulate acid release; the partial agonist Δ7-prednisolone has an intermediate effect; the partial antagonist deoxycorticosterone inhibits the effect of dexamethasone. The other steroids do not increase acid production by the

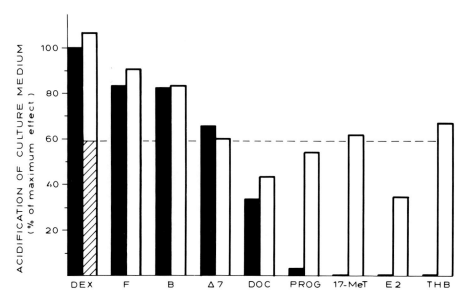

FIG. 5. Effect of various steroids on the pH of HTC cell suspension cultures. Cells in serum-free medium were exposed for 48 hr to different steroids as described in the legend of FIG. 3. The final pH of the culture containing 5 μM dexamethasone was 7.31 as compared with 7.8 for the control culture.

cells. However, some of these (progesterone, estradiol) display the antagonistic effect also seen on induction of tyrosine aminotransferase (22).

DISCUSSION

In HTC cells, less than 1% of the genes appear to be under glucocorticoid control (15). By two-dimensional gel electrophoresis, seven peptides, two of which are associated with the plasma membrane, are reproducibly induced by dexamethasone; a few peptides are also repressed. These dexamethasone-sensitive peptides characterize the so-called glucocorticoid domain (15). Several cell membrane-related properties are altered by glucocorticoids in these cells (Table 1). Thus, the HTC system is an appropriate model for studying the biochemical basis of plasma membrane functions. On the one hand, the role of alkaline phosphodiesterase I and of nucleoside disphosphatase in the liver cell is unknown. On the other, with respect to adhesiveness stimulation, the time course, the steroid dose and structural requirements, and the need for RNA and protein synthesis all suggest that glucocorticoids induce either a membrane enzyme or a structural membrane protein (3). Concerning the reversible inhibition of the alanine-preferring transport system, the data are consistent with a rapid

(30-min lag period), receptor-mediated induction of a factor which either decreases the synthesis or increases the degradation of a rate-limiting protein component of the transport mechanism (12). As to the inhibition of plasminogen activator release, it results from the rapid stimulation (60-min lag period) by the steroid of an inhibitor of intracellular plasminogen activator (25). How all these phenomena are related to enzyme activity remains unknown.

This question could be investigated, first, by identifying in HTC cells the few proteins of the glucocorticoid domain. It was known that tyrosine aminotransferase, glutamine synthetase (8), and ornithine decarboxylase (7) are stimulated, while cyclic nucleotide phosphodiesterase is inhibited (19). We now find that alkaline phosphodiesterase I is stimulated and nucleoside diphosphatase is inhibited and these are two enzymes that belong to the plasma membrane. Secondly, we can take advantage of variant HTC cell lines which have lost one or several of the glucocorticoid responses (27). Work with such variants has already shown that plasminogen activator does not play an important role in the regulation of cell-substrate adhesiveness (10). Thus, glucocorticoid hormones become a very selective tool to correlate enzyme activities with cellular functions. Concerning the latter, this work also contributes to a better definition of the glucocorticoid domain of responses, as it is shown here that dexamethasone increases acid release by the cells in a specific way.

The functional and structural integrity of the plasma membrane is essential for normal cell growth, differentiation, and recognition. Our studies on glucocorticoid-sensitive membrane properties should help to elucidate the molecular mechanisms of the alterations in membrane function seen in transformed cells.

ACKNOWLEDGMENTS

The assistance of C. Turu and M. A. Gueuning is gratefully acknowledged. We thank Prof. M. De Visscher for continuous support and interest. D.K.G. is a Medical Investigator of the Veterans Administration and is supported in part by research funds from the US Veterans Administration and USPHS (AM24037). P.M.E. was the recipient of an ICP Fellowship. G.G.R. is Maître de Recherches of the F.N.R.S. (Belgium) and supported in part by F.R.S.M. Grant 3.4514.75. A.A.C. is supported by grants from the FRFC (2.4533.76) and SPPS (Belgium). We thank Th. Lambert for secretarial help.

REFERENCES

1. Amar-Costesec, A., Beaufay, H., Wibo, M., Thinès-Sempoux, D., Feytmans, E., Robbi, M., and Berthet, J. (1974): *J. Cell. Biol.*, 61:201–212.
2. Ballard, P. L. (1979): In: *Monographs on Endocrinology, Vol. 12: Glucocorticoid Hormone Action*, edited by J. D. Baxter and G. G. Rousseau, pp. 493–515. Springer Verlag, Berlin, Heidelberg, New York.
3. Ballard, P. L., and Tomkins, G. M. (1970): *J. Cell Biol.*, 47:222–234.
4. Baxter, J. D., and Tomkins, G. M. (1970): *Proc. Natl. Acad. Sci. USA*, 65:709–715.

5. Beaufay, H., Amar-Costesec, A., Thinès-Sempoux, D., Wibo, M., Robbi, M., and Berthet, J. (1974): *J. Cell Biol.,* 61:213–231.
6. Berlin, C. M., and Schimke, R. T. (1965): *Mol. Pharmacol.,* 1:149–156.
7. Canellakis, Z. N., and Theoharides, T. C. (1976): *J. Biol. Chem.,* 251:4436–4441.
8. Crook, R. B., Louie, M., Deuel, T. F., and Tomkins, G. M. (1978): *J. Biol. Chem.,* 251:6125–6131.
9. Evans, W. H. (1974): *Nature,* 250:391–394.
10. Fredin, B. L., Seifert, S. C., and Gelehrter, T. D. (1979): *Nature,* 277:312–313.
11. Gelehrter, T. D. (1976): *N. Engl. J. Med.,* 294:522–526.
12. Gelehrter, T. D. (1979): In: *Monographs on Endocrinology, Vol. 12: Glucocorticoid Hormone Action,* edited by J. D. Baxter and G. G. Rousseau, pp. 561–574. Springer Verlag, Berlin, Heidelberg, New York.
13. Granner, D. K., Diesterhaft, M., Noguchi, I., Olson, P., Hargrove, J., and Volentine, G. (1979): In: *Hormones and Cell Culture,* The Sixth Cold Spring Harbor Conference on Cell Proliferation, edited by R. Ross and G. Sato. Cold Spring Laboratory Press, Cold Spring Harbor, New York.
14. Granner D. K., Lee, A., and Thompson, E. B. (1977): *J. Biol. Chem.,* 252:3891–3897.
15. Ivarie, R. D., and O'Farrell, P. H. (1978): *Cell,* 13:41–57.
16. Johnson, L. K., Baxter, J. D., and Rousseau, G. G. (1979): In: *Monographs on Endocrinology, Vol. 12: Glucocorticoid Hormone Action,* edited by J. D. Baxter, and G. G. Rousseau, pp. 305–326. Springer Verlag, Berlin, Heidelberg, New York.
17. Kimelberg, H. K. (1977): In: *Dynamic Aspects of Cell Surface Organization,* edited by G. Poste and G. L. Nicholson, pp. 205–293. Elsevier North Holland, New York.
18. Lopez-Saura, P., Trouet, A., and Tulkens, P. (1978): *Biochim. Biophys. Acta,* 543:430–449.
19. Manganiello, V., and Vaughan, M. (1972): *J. Clin. Invest.,* 51:2763–2767.
20. Ringold, G. M., Cardiff, R. D., Varmus, H. E., and Yamamoto, K. R. (1977): *Cell,* 10:11–18.
21. Risser, W. L., and Gelehrter, T. D. (1973): *J. Biol. Chem.,* 248:1248–1254.
22. Rousseau, G. G. (1975): *J. Steroid Biochem.,* 6:75–89.
23. Rousseau, G. G., Amar-Costesec, A., Gueuning, M. A., and Granner, D. K. (1979): *Arch. Int. Physiol. Biochim.,* 87:207–208.
24. Rousseau, G. G., Amar-Costesec, A., Verhaegen, M., and Granner, D. K. (1980): *Proc. Natl. Acad. Sci. USA,* 77:1005–1009.
25. Seifert, S. C., and Gelehrter, T. D. (1978): *Proc. Natl. Acad. Sci. USA,* 75:6130–6133.
26. Steinberg, R. A., Levinson, B. B., and Tomkins, G. M. (1975): *Cell,* 5:29–36.
27. Thompson, E. B., Granner, D. K., Gelehrter, T. D., Simons, S. S., and Hager, G. L. (1979): In: *Hormones and Cell Culture,* The Sixth Cold Spring Harbor Conference on Cell Proliferation, edited by R. Ross and G. Sato. Cold Spring Laboratory Press, Cold Spring Harbor, New York.
28. Touster, O., Aronson, N. N., Dulaney, J. T., and Hendrickson, H. (1970): *J. Cell Biol.,* 47:604–618.
29. Wigler, M., Ford, J. P., and Weinstein, I. B. (1975): In: *Proteases and Biological Control,* edited by E. Reich, D. B. Rifkin, and E. Shaw, pp. 849–856. Cold Spring Laboratory Press, Cold Spring Harbor, New York.

Hormones and Cancer, edited by S. Iacobelli et al.
Raven Press, New York © 1980.

Glucocorticoid Control of T-Cell Proliferation

Kendall A. Smith, *Gerald R. Crabtree, Steven Gillis,
and *Allan Munck

*The Hematology Research Laboratory, Departments of Medicine and *Physiology,
Dartmouth Medical School, Hanover, New Hampshire 03755*

Early studies on the physiological action of glucocorticoid hormones indicated that they exerted a strict regulatory control on the lymphoid system (for review, see refs. 7,22). The control appeared to be in the form of a tonic suppression which governed the total lymphoid cell mass. Evidence in support of this concept has accumulated from many different disciplines, but perhaps the most striking demonstrations of glucocorticoid control are the observations made in situations of glucocorticoid deficiency or excess. In disease states or experimental conditions which resulted in adrenocortical hormone deficiency, a noticeable finding was lymphoid hyperplasia. In fact, generalized lymphadenopathy was one of the prominent clinical manifestations of adrenal insufficiency originally described by Addison (1). In contrast, during situations of glucocorticoid excess, lymphopenia and lymphoid organ wasting occurred (10,11). These findings led to the generally accepted belief that glucocorticoids suppressed both lymphocyte number and function, and as a result, adrenocorticotrophic hormone and glucocorticoids were employed as immunosuppressive agents and as chemotherapeutic agents in the treatment of lymphoid malignancies. It was readily established that these agents were very effective in both areas.

As detailed studies of the mechanism of action of glucocorticoids began to accumulate, it became apparent that the glucocorticoid effect in a variety of cell types was mediated after hormone binding to specific cytoplasmic receptors, and glucocorticoid receptors were soon demonstrated in lymphocytes from all lymphoid sites and in all species examined (22,23). The effect of glucocorticoid receptor binding in lymphocytes was observed to be of a catabolic nature; for example, glucocorticoids were found to rapidly inhibit glucose uptake, suppress transcription and translation, and ultimately cause cytolysis of rat thymocytes (19,22,23). Subsequent studies on human peripheral blood lymphocytes revealed similar effects, although they were of less magnitude and occurred more slowly than the changes observed in rat thymocyte metabolism (24). Thus, these observations seemed to explain the generalized tonic suppressive physiological and pharmacological effects of glucocorticoids on the lymphoid system. It quickly became appreciated, however, that the sensitivity of lymphocytes to glucocorticoid suppression was dependent on many variables, most notably the maturational state of the cell, and the stage of immunological activation. Immature, immunoincompetent cortical thymocytes were found to be much more susceptible to the catabolic and cytolytic effects of glucocorticoids than were mature, immunocompetent, medullary thymocytes, or peripheral thymic-derived lymphocytes (T-cells) (7). Additionally, it was observed *in vivo,* that glucocorticoid-induced immunosuppression was much more effective if glucocorticoids were administered prior to antigenic challenge, than if they were administered after an ongoing immune response had become established (5,20). These observations led to the hypothesis that glucocorticoid-resistant and -sensitive stages existed among lymphocytes (4,7). Because glucocorticoid receptors had been shown to be obligatory for a hormone-mediated effect in glucocorticoid-sensitive tissues, initial studies centered on attempts to uncover differences in hormone–receptor binding. Although it remains unresolved, detailed studies have failed to find differences in receptor binding, or hormone–receptor complex function between resistant and sensitive cells (18,27). Thus, such an approach has not yielded useful information to explain the observed differences in glucocorticoid sensitivity among lymphocytes.

Recently, it has been suggested that lymphocyte maturation, proliferation, differentiation, and function may be controlled by a separate class of hormone-like factors. This concept arose in part through the discovery by Morgan et al. (21) and Ruscetti et al. (26) that lectin-activated normal human T-cells could be maintained in indefinite exponential proliferative culture with the aid of a T-cell growth factor (TCGF)[1] derived from lectin-stimulated mononuclear cell-conditioned medium. Subsequent studies have revealed that antigen-specific cytolytic T-cells could also be selected, maintained, and cloned in TCGF (IL2)-dependent proliferative culture (2,12–14,17). Furthermore, such T-cell lines retained the immunologic function and specificity originally present at the initiation of long-term growth.

Studies designed to probe the biological significance of TCGF (IL2) indicated that this mitogenic factor was not merely an interesting biological phenomenon that accompanied T-cell activation, but that it was an obligatory growth hormone that mediated the proliferative expansion, and allowed the subsequent differentiation of antigen-specific cytolytic T-cell clones (3). These observations prompted us to reevaluate the role of glucocorticoid hormones in the control of T-cell proliferation and function. In this chapter, we have summarized the results of experimentation which suggest that glucocorticoids may influence lymphocyte proliferation by a dual mechanism; a direct catabolic effect on lymphocytes resulting from hormone–receptor interaction, and indirectly through the control of lymphocyte hormone release.

---

[1] A revised nomenclature for T-cell growth factor was proposed at the recent *Second International Lymphokine Workshop* (Ermatigen, Switzerland, May, 1979). The revised name for TCGF is Interleukin 2. To avoid confusion, the term IL2 will be initially assimilated into the literature by using both acronyms as follows: TCGF (IL2).

IN VITRO MODELS OF THE IMMUNE RESPONSE

Early immunological studies revealed that ligand-driven lymphocyte proliferation was central to the generation of immune responses. *In vitro* models provided the means to study such responses, and a variety of antigenic and mitogenic agents were identified which would activate lymphocytes to undergo morphological blastic transformation prior to DNA synthesis and mitosis. Subsequent studies revealed that these changes were obligatory for the expression of lymphocyte immune function (e.g., cytolysis or antibody secretion).

Soon after the discovery of ligand-induced lymphocyte transformation and mitosis, glucocorticoids were shown to specifically inhibit both the morphological changes of blast transformation and concomitantly, cellular proliferation as measured by increased cell numbers, mitoses, and the incorporation of radiolabeled nucleic acid precursors into DNA (25,31). Early studies indicated that for maximum suppression, glucocorticoids were required at the initiation of the response (25,31). If the addition of hormone was delayed for as little as 12 hr after mitogen sensitization, markedly less inhibition of proliferation was observed. These results, combined with similar *in vivo* observations (5,20), led to the generally accepted concept that glucocorticoid sensitivity varied with the state of immunological activation of the cell. Lymphocytes were thought to be insensitive to the catabolic effects of glucocorticoids until they were stimulated by specific antigen or lectin. Stimulation was thought to induce a glucocorticoid-sensitive phase which ended once the activated cell underwent full morphological blast transformation and mitosis (4,7).

Based on this hypothesis, we performed a series of experiments to determine the mechanism of the changes in glucocorticoid sensitivity as the lymphocyte underwent activation. Our initial studies explored the glucocorticoid receptor since it appeared likely that glucocorticoid-resistance might be related to initial stages of hormone action. Specifically, we hypothesized that ligand stimulation of lymphocytes might induce a change in glucocorticoid receptor binding after sensitization, and this might account for an early glucocorticoid-sensitive phase followed by a return to glucocorticoid resistance once the changes associated with blastic transformation had taken place. We found that indeed there was a two- to threefold increase in the number of receptors per cell 12 to 24 hr after lectin or antigen stimulation (27). Subsequent studies revealed that the increased receptors functioned in every way as did receptors in unsensitized lymphocytes. Further studies revealed that increased glucocorticoid receptors occurred after antigen sensitization *in vivo* (8), and cell separation studies performed *in vitro* indicated that the receptor number varied with the cell cycle (9). Similar results were reported for other cell types (6) and thus, it appeared that glucocorticoid receptors increased in late G_1 as the cells were preparing for DNA synthesis and mitosis. Thus, if glucocorticoid sensitivity correlated directly with the absolute number of receptors, we thought we might find a glucocorticoid-sensitive phase after ligand stimulation.

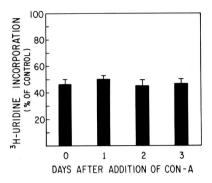

FIG. 1. Effect of dexamethasone (10^{-7} M) on unstimulated and Concanavalin A (Con-A)-stimulated human peripheral blood mononuclear cell [³H]uridine incorporation. [³H]uridine incorporation was determined after a 1-hr pulse 19 hr after the addition of dexamethasone. Depicted are the mean + 1 SEM of quadruplicate cultures where the [³H]uridine incorporation in dexamethasone-treated cultures is expressed as a percentage of the [³H]uridine incorporation in the absence of dexamethasone.

When examined directly, however, human peripheral blood lymphocytes were found to be equally sensitive to glucocorticoids regardless of the state of activation of the cell (27). Figure 1 depicts a typical experiment in which human lymphocytes were studied for the rate of radiolabeled uridine incorporation before, and at daily intervals after, stimulation by Concanavalin A. At the times indicated, dexamethasone (10^{-7} M) was added to the cultures and [³H]uridine incorporation was measured 19 hr later. As depicted, there was no difference in the inhibitory effects of glucocorticoids regardless of the state of cellular activation. Similar results were obtained when glucose uptake, leucine incorporation, and thymidine incorporation were measured (27). Because these observations indicated that lymphocytes were equally sensitive to glucocorticoid-induced inhibition of cellular metabolism before, and at all stages after activation, the mechanism of glucocorticoid-induced suppression of lymphocyte proliferation and the loss of this suppression upon delayed addition of the hormone was left unexplained.

T-CELL GROWTH FACTOR AND THE CONTROL OF T-CELL PROLIFERATION

It had been assumed that the signal which triggered T-cell DNA synthesis and mitosis was delivered to the cell by lectin or antigen-binding to specific cell membrane receptors. Recently, however, it has become apparent that lectin- or antigen-induced T-cell proliferation is actually mediated by a soluble T-cell growth factor [TCGF (IL2)], released after ligand-membrane binding (28,30). This conclusion was based on the following observations: (a) Inhibition of TCGF (IL2) production (by removal of adherent cells) completely suppressed T-cell proliferation despite ligand–T-cell membrane binding (28,29); and (b) purified TCGF (IL2) sustained continuous T-cell proliferation, whereas lectin or antigen did not (30).

Further experimentation indicated that TCGF (IL2) was an obligatory growth hormone for the generation of a T-cell immune response. It appeared that at least two different subsets of T-cells were involved; one subset, upon lectin/

antigen binding released TCGF (IL2), and a second subset of T-cells responded to the proliferative effect of TCGF (IL2). TCGF (IL2)-producer cells were found only among mature T-cell populations (30), and were demonstrated to express Lyl surface antigens (32). TCGF (IL2)-responder cells were found among both immature (i.e., nude mouse splenocyte and normal mouse thymocyte) and mature T-cell populations (17,30), and were demonstrated to express Ly 23 surface antigens (32). T-cells which had not been exposed to a lectin or antigen were not responsive to TCGF (IL2), whereas cells activated by a ligand were found to absorb TCGF (IL2) and to proliferate indefinitely as long as the cultures were supplemented by TCGF (IL2) (30).

Based on these observations, a model for T-cell activation and proliferation was proposed (29) as depicted in Fig. 2. Subsequent to lectin/antigen binding and a signal derived from macrophages, a subset of T-cells [TCGF (IL2)-producer cells] release TCGF (IL2). A separate subset of T-cells (TCGF (IL2)-responder cells] bind TCGF (IL2) and proliferate. Once the initial activation signal has been received by the TCGF (IL2)-responsive subset of T-cells, the lectin/antigen is no longer necessary. The initial cell population and all subsequent daughter cells retain TCGF (IL2) responsiveness, thereby ensuring their maintenance in proliferative culture solely by the continuous addition of TCGF (IL2).

Because it was evident that T-cell proliferation after ligand sensitization was driven by TCGF (IL2), it followed that TCGF (IL2) was a key hormone-like substance which regulated T-cell immune responses. It was also evident that *both* TCGF (IL2) production and TCGF (IL2) responsiveness were required. Therefore, anything that enhanced TCGF (IL2) production or responsiveness

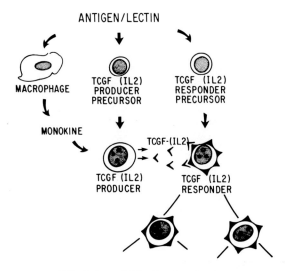

FIG. 2. A model for T-cell activation.

would lead to an augmentation of T-cell proliferation, and anything that suppressed TCGF (IL2) production or responsiveness would lead to an inhibition of T-cell proliferation. Therefore, when viewed from the standpoint of glucocorticoids, it appeared that the inhibitory effects of these hormones might be manifested at either of two levels; TCGF (IL2) production or TCGF (IL2) responsiveness.

EFFECT OF GLUCOCORTICOIDS ON TCGF (IL2) RESPONSIVENESS

Since glucocorticoid-specific receptors appeared to be obligatory for a hormone effect, we first examined TCGF (IL2)-responsive cells for the presence of these receptors. At saturating concentrations of dexamethasone, TCGF (IL2)-responsive cells were found to contain approximately 5,600 nuclear glucocorticoid binding sites (15), a concentration similar to that which we had previously found as typical for both lectin- and antigen-activated lymphocytes (27). The association constants for binding, cytoplasmic to nuclear translocation, and binding specificity behaved in all respects like those found for glucocorticoid receptors in normal lymphocytes, whether stimulated with lectin/antigen or unstimulated.

We next studied the effects of glucocorticoids on the TCGF (IL2)-mediated proliferation of T-cells. The results were similar when the response was quantified by either tritiated thymidine incorporation or by determination of viable cell number. For example, as shown in Fig. 3, there was a 25 to 30% inhibition

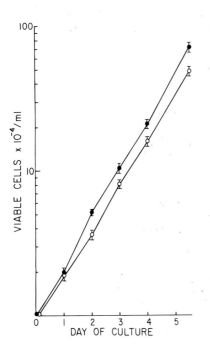

FIG. 3. Proliferation of murine TCGF (IL2)-dependent T-cells in the presence *(open circles)*, and absence *(closed circles)* of 10^{-7} M dexamethasone.

of cellular proliferation when the cells were exposed to saturating concentrations (10^{-7} M) of dexamethasone. It was of interest that there did not appear to be a direct cytolytic effect of glucocorticoids as long as TCGF (IL2) was present. If TCGF (IL2) was removed, however, proliferation ceased and cell death occurred rapidly.

The observation that the cells were not lysed by glucocorticoids as long as TCGF (IL2) was present, was distinctly different from our previous observations on rat or human lymphocytes cultured in the absence of TCGF (IL2) (19,24). It appeared that TCGF (IL2) in some way protected the cells from the catabolic effects of glucocorticoids, which in the absence of TCGF (IL2) led to cell lysis. These results prompted us to examine the effect of glucocorticoids on the immunologic function of TCGF (IL2)-responsive T-cells. Although there was only a slight inhibition of proliferation and no apparent cytolytic effect, it remained possible that glucocorticoids might inhibit the effector function of differentiated T-cells. Therefore, to investigate the effect of glucocorticoids on T-cell-mediated cytolysis, TCGF (IL2)-dependent antigen-specific murine and human cytolytic T-cells were exposed to dexamethasone (10^{-10}–10^{-6} M) for 48 hr prior to testing for cytolytic efficiency. As displayed in Fig. 4, there was no effect of glucocorticoids on the cytolytic function of either murine (Fig. 4A) or human (Fig. 4B) cytolytic T-cells (16). Thus, the profound antiproliferative and immunosuppressive effects of glucocorticoids could not be explained by a direct action on TCGF (IL2)-responsive cells.

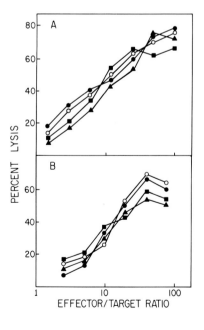

FIG. 4. Effect of dexamethasone on CTLL-mediated cytolysis. **A:** Murine CTLL lysis of allogeneic P815 target cells. **B:** Human CTLL lysis of allogeneic peripheral blood mononuclear target cells. CTLL were grown in the absence *(open circles)* and presence of 10^{-6} M *(closed circles)*, 10^{-8} M *(triangles)*, and 10^{-10} M *(squares)* dexamethasone prior to testing for cytolytic activity.

THE EFFECT OF GLUCOCORTICOIDS ON TCGF (IL2) PRODUCTION

In experimentation designed to determine the kinetics of TCGF (IL2) release after ligand sensitization, we found that measurable TCGF (IL2) activity first appeared 6 hr after the initiation of the culture, and peak levels occurred after 18 to 36 hr (14). In addition, from the work of Wagner and Rollinghoff (32), transcription and translation appeared to be required for TCGF (IL2) release after ligand sensitization. Therefore, if glucocorticoids suppressed T-cell proliferation by an inhibition of TCGF (IL2) production, it was possible to understand why delayed addition of glucocorticoids would abrogate their suppressive effects: The synthesis and release of the proliferation-inducing agent [i.e., TCGF (IL2)] would already have occurred. To examine the effects of glucocorticoids on TCGF (IL2) production, rat, mouse, and human lymphocytes were sensitized by T-cell lectins and antigens in the presence of dexamethasone (10^{-10}–10^{-6} M). We found that glucocorticoids exerted a dose-dependent suppression of TCGF (IL2) release so that complete inhibition occurred at saturating concentrations. In addition, inhibition of the T-cell proliferative response paralleled the degree of inhibition of TCGF (IL2) production (15).

If the primary inhibitory action of glucocorticoids was mediated by a suppression of TCGF (IL2) production, rather than by an effect on TCGF (IL2)-responsive cells, then one would predict that TCGF (IL2) supplementation of the cultures might overcome the antiproliferative glucocorticoid effect. A representative experiment where we tested this hypothesis is shown in Fig. 5. Murine splenocytes were stimulated with allogeneic irradiated splenocytes in a mixed

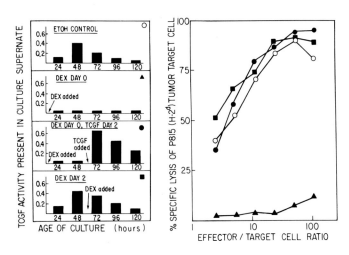

FIG. 5. The effect of dexamethasone (10^{-7} M) on murine MLC (C57B1/6 × BALB/C$_x$) TCGF production **(left)** and the generation of cytolytic effector cells **(right)**. Control MLC *(open circles)*, dexamethasone added to MLC on day 0 *(triangles)*, TCGF (IL2) added on day 2 *(closed circles)*, dexamethasone added to MLC on day 2 *(squares)*. (From Gillis et al., ref. 16, with permission.)

lymphocyte culture (MLC) for 5 days; on each day of culture, an aliquot of culture medium was removed and tested for TCGF (IL2) activity (left panel). At the end of the culture period, the cells were harvested and tested for cytolytic activity on appropriate allogeneic target cells (right panel). When dexamethasone (10^{-7} M) was added at the initiation of the culture, there was a complete inhibition of TCGF (IL2) release, and the generation of cytolytic T-cells. However, when the cultures were supplemented with exogenous TCGF (IL2) on the second day of culture, the number and efficiency of cytolytic T-cells generated, equaled those observed in the control (nondexamethasone-treated) cultures. As a further indication that the dexamethasone-induced suppression of MLC-generated cytolytic immune reactivity could be traced to an inhibition of TCGF (IL2) production and subsequent TCGF (IL2) mediated proliferation, we noted that the addition of dexamethasone after peak levels of TCGF (IL2) production had already occurred (48 hr after the onset of the MLC) had little effect on the caliber of cytolytic reactivity subsequently generated. This observation is also consistent with the lack of a significant inhibition of TCGF (IL2)-responder cells as detailed above.

Although the suppressive effect of glucocorticoids appears to occur at the level of TCGF (IL2) production, the target cell of the glucocorticoids and the mechanism of its inhibitory action remain to be delineated. As mentioned above, the TCGF (IL2)-producer T-cell subset requires two signals for TCGF (IL2) release; lectin/antigen binding and a signal contributed by a soluble factor derived from macrophages. Thus, it is quite possible that the effect of glucocorticoids, which is manifested by the suppression of T-cell proliferation, may actually be mediated at the level of the macrophage as a suppression of the release of the monokine which is required to signal T-cells to release TCGF (IL2). Thus, the tonic regulatory control that glucocorticoids exert on lymphocytes may actually occur indirectly by the regulation of accessory cells.

CONCLUSIONS

Several of the results of the above-detailed experimentation require emphasis. First, lymphocytes were found to be equally sensitive to glucocorticoid-induced catabolism regardless of the state of immunological activation. Secondly, despite glucocorticoid-induced inhibition of cellular metabolism, the immunological function of differentiated cytolytic effector T-cells was not reduced. Thirdly, although the decreased cellular metabolism promulgated by glucocorticoids resulted in a reduced proliferative rate, a cytolytic effect of glucocorticoids was not apparent as long as cells were exposed to TCGF (IL2). Finally, glucocorticoids were demonstrated to completely inhibit the release of TCGF (IL2), resulting in the complete abrogation of the antigen/lectin-induced T-cell proliferative response. Together, these observations imply that glucocorticoids exert a generalized tonic suppressive control over lymphocyte number and function by a dual mechanism; a direct inhibition of lymphocyte cellular metabolism, and indirectly through the regulation of *other* hormones which control lymphopoiesis. Therefore, glucocorticoids may serve as important probes which may allow for experimentation to define the nature of the lymphocyte regulatory molecules.

ACKNOWLEDGMENTS

This work was supported in part by NCI Grants CA-17643, CA-17323, CA-23108, NCI Contract No. 1-CB-74141, and a grant from The National Leukemia Association, Inc. S. Gillis is a Fellow of The Leukemia Society of America.

REFERENCES

1. Addison, T. (1855): *Lond. Med. Gaz.,* 43:517.
2. Baker, P. E., Gillis, S., Ferm, M., and Smith, K. A. (1978): *J. Immunol.,* 121:2168–2173.
3. Baker, P. E., Gillis, S., and Smith, K. A. (1979): *J. Exp. Med.* 149:273–278.
4. Baxter, J. D., and Harris, A. W., (1975): *Transplant. Proc.,* 7:55–65.
5. Billingham, R. E., Krohn, P. L., and Medawar, P. B. (1951): *Bri. Med. J.,* 1:1157.
6. Cidlowski, J. A., and Michaels, G. A. (1977): *Nature,* 266:643–645.
7. Clamon, H. N. (1972): *N. Engl. J. Med.,* 287:388–397.
8. Crabtree, G. R., Munck, A., and Smith, K. A.: *Submitted.*
9. Crabtree, G. R., Munck, A., and Smith, K. A.: *Submitted.*
10. Dougherty, T. F., and White, A. (1944): *Endocrinology,* 35:1014.
11. Dougherty, T. F., and White, A. (1947): *J. Lab. Clin. Med.,* 32:584–605.
12. Gillis, S., and Smith, K. A. (1977): *Nature,* 268:154–156.
13. Gillis, S., Baker, P. E., Ruscetti, F. W., and Smith, K. A. (1978): *J. Exp. Med.,* 148:1093–1098.
14. Gillis, S., Ferm, M. M., Ou, W., and Smith, K. A. (1978): *J. Immunol.,* 120:2027–2032.
15. Gillis, S., Crabtree, G. R., and Smith, K. A. (1979): *J. Immunol.,* 123:1624–1631.
16. Gillis, S., Crabtree, G. R., and Smith, K. A. (1979): *J. Immunol.,* 123:1632–1638.
17. Gillis, S., Union, N. A., Baker, P. E., and Smith, K. A. (1979): *J. Exp. Med.,* 149:1460–1476.
18. Homo, F., Duval, D., Hatzfeld, J., and Evrard, C. (1979): *J. Steroid Biochem. (in press).*
19. Leung, K., and Munck, A. (1975): *Endocrinology,* 97:744–748.
20. Medawar, P. B., and Sparrow, E. M. (1956): *J. Endocrinol.,* 14:240–256.
21. Morgan, D. A., Ruscetti, F. W., and Gallo, R. (1976): *Science,* 193:1007–1008.
22. Munck, A., and Young, D. A. (1975): In: *Handbook of Physiology, Section 7: Endocrinology, Vol. VI: Adrenal Gland,* edited by S. R. Geiger, pp. 231–243. American Physiological Society, Washington, D.C.
23. Munck, A., and Leung, K. (1977): In: *Receptors and Mechanism of Action of Steroid Hormones Part II,* edited by J. R. Pasqualini, pp. 311–397. Dekker, New York.
24. Munck, A., Crabtree, G. R., and Smith, K. A. (1978): *J. Toxicol. Environ. Health* 4:409–425.
25. Nowell, P. C. (1961): *Cancer Res.,* 21:1518–1521.
26. Ruscetti, F. W., Morgan, D. A., and Gallo, R. C. (1977): *J. Immunol.* 119:131–138.
27. Smith, K. A., Crabtree, G. R., Kennedy, S. J., and Munck, A. (1977): *Nature,* 267:523–526.
28. Smith, K. A., Gillis, S., and Baker, P. E. (1979): In: *The Molecular Basis of Immune Cell Function,* edited by J. G. Kaplan, pp. 223–237. Elsevier/North-Holland, Amsterdam.
29. Smith, K. A., Gillis, S., Baker, P. E., McKenzie, D., and Ruscetti, F. W. (1979): *Ann. N.Y. Acad. Sci.,* 332:423–432.
30. Smith, K. A., Baker, P. E., Gillis, S., and Ruscetti, F. W. (1979): *Mol. Immunol. (in press).*
31. Tormey, D. C., Fudenberg, H. H., and Kamin, R. M. (1967): *Nature,* 213:218–219.
32. Wagner, H., and Rollinghoff, M. (1978): *J. Exp. Med.,* 148:1523–1538.

Hormones and Cancer, edited by S. Iacobelli et al.
Raven Press, New York © 1980.

Mechanisms Involved in the Generation of the Metabolic and Lethal Actions of Glucocorticoid Hormones in Lymphoid Cells

Donald A. Young, Mary L. Nicholson, Bruce P. Voris, and Robert T. Lyons

The E. Henry Keutman Laboratories, Division of Endocrinology and Metabolism, Department of Medicine, University of Rochester School of Medicine and Dentistry, Rochester, New York 14642

During the past decade much of our research has been aimed at sorting out the various biological effects of glucocorticoid hormones on lymphocytes, particularly thymic lymphocytes, in an attempt to gain insights about mechanisms of glucocorticoid hormone action at the biochemical and molecular levels. More recently we have also been interested in the actions of glucocorticoids on hormone-sensitive and -resistant lymphosarcoma cells. Here the aim has been to understand mechanisms of hormone-induced cell killing, with particular emphasis on the resistance to cell killing that usually emerges upon the repeated use of glucocorticoids clinically for suppression of malignant tumors. It is my intention to summarize here some of our findings that provide insights into four topics that are relevant to hormone actions on cancer cells.

METHODS

Most of the studies presented have been carried out by incubating surviving cells, either rat thymus cells or P1798 mouse lymphosarcoma cells, for a few hours. Thymuses or tumors are removed from the animal and cells rapidly disbursed by gentle homogenization. Incubations are carried out in multiple Erlenmeyer flasks, in either Krebs-Ringer bicarbonate buffer or RPMI-1640 medium, to which physiological levels of glucocorticoid hormones (biological activity equivalent to 10^{-6} M cortisol or less) and various nutrients have been added when appropriate (cf. 18,20).

RESULTS AND DISCUSSION

Two Kinds of Hormone Actions: Metabolic Suppression and Lymphocytolytic Attack at the Level of the Nuclear Membrane

Metabolic Effects

Figure 1 attempts to summarize the evolution of those biological effects of glucocorticoids that appear when the hormones are added to incubated thymic lymphocytes. It also illustrates causal relationships where they exist. The solid lines show the evolution of metabolic inhibitions and their relative magnitude. The inhibition of glucose transport clearly precedes those other hormone actions shown, becoming nearly maximal by 30 min. As the largest and most rapidly evolving metabolic event, the effect on glucose has attracted much attention as a focus for understanding mechanisms, and as a potential cause of those later metabolic suppressions that develop (15). There is, however, a second metabolic inhibition, a suppression of mitochondrial adenosine triphosphate (ATP) production (20), which evolves separately and somewhat more slowly. This inhibition may be measured by decreased incorporation of carbon atoms from pyruvate into CO_2, by an increase in cellular lactate production when low levels of glucose are provided, or when adenosine is substituted for glucose as an energy source (20). [Adenosine is rapidly metabolized to inosine which is then taken into the cell and its ribose utilized for energy production (21).] Figure 1 shows the time course of effects on ATP; these parallel the emergence of effects on energy charge, CO_2 production, and lactate (20,29,33).

Recent studies by Foley et al. (5) have also demonstrated a reduction in acetate incorporation into fatty acids that parallels the effect on glucose uptake in time course and magnitude; they suggest a direct regulatory influence of glucose uptake on fatty acid synthesis. Pyruvate also supports the incorporation, but when pyruvate is substituted for glucose, a hormone effect on acetate incorporation is not seen. The physiological significance of this effect to the cell is not yet clear. As will be mentioned later, lethal hormone effects emerge in the absence of glucose, so it would seem that a decrease in lipid synthesis is not required to generate the lethal action.

Before leaving the effect on glucose it is also worth pointing out that lymphocytes, at least thymic lymphocytes, are particularly dependent on exogenous glucose. Studies done in collaboration with Giddings nearly 10 years ago showed that small amounts of glucose seemed to be essential for the selective support of nuclear protein synthesis (6). The evidence suggested that these special effects of glucose might be a consequence of an essential role for it in nuclear energy production. It is of interest in this regard that the studies by Foley et al. show that, in the presence of glucose, the glucocorticoid inhibition of acetate incorporation is most marked in lipid isolated from the nuclear fraction. It is worth

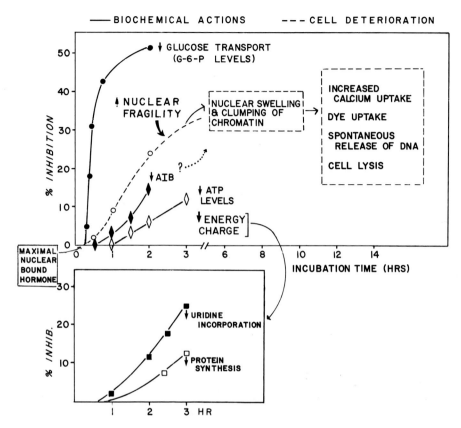

FIG. 1. Comparison of time of onset and magnitude of several cortisol effects in thymus cells. *Open circles* represent nuclear fragility measured as nonsedimentible DNA from cells lysed in a hypotonic solution (1.5 mM $MgCl_2$). *Closed circles* represent glucose 6-P levels 5 min after glucose is added to cells incubated without substrate. *Closed diamonds* represent effects on AIB accumulation when ^{14}C-AIB (20 µg/ml) was present from the start. *Open diamonds* represent ATP levels from cells incubated in the presence of adenosine (2.5 mM). *Closed squares* represent the incorporation of [^{3}H]uridine (0.06 mg/ml) into RNA. *Open squares* represent the incorporation of [^{14}C]valine (0.5 mg/ml) into cellular proteins (label was added at the start of the incubation). *Diamonds* represent the adenylate energy charge, calculated as ([ATP] + [ADP])/([ATP] + [ADP] + [AMP]). In all instances cortisol was added at the start of the incubation. The specific binding of cortisol to thymus cells and transfer to the nucleus is maximal by 5–10 min. Each point represents the mean of five to six flasks. [From ref. 7, Giddings, S. J., and Young, D. A. (1974): *J. Steroid Biochem.,* 5:587.]

noting that we find that the hormonal inhibition of glucose transport is not in itself sufficient to deprive the cells of that small amount of glucose that is needed for maximal rates of protein synthesis when energy metabolism is sustained by pyruvate. Yet the studies by Foley et al. suggest that the inhibition of glucose uptake is sufficient to limit fatty acid synthesis.

Some metabolic hormone effects related to small suppressions in energy production

We have accumulated considerable evidence that it is the hormone effect on mitochondrial ATP production that is responsible for a small hormone-induced steady state reduction that is seen in the cellular adenylate energy charge (20,33). Careful measurements reveal about a 5 to 10% decline in ATP by 2 hr, associated with a 10 to 20% rise in adenosine monophosphate (AMP). The studies by Nordeen show that the reduction in glucose transport by itself is neither sufficient nor responsible for this reduction in energy charge. Yet, the reduced glucose uptake may possibly be essential for preventing the cells from overriding the consequences of the inhibition of mitochondrial ATP production via a compensatory increase in glycolytic ATP (20).

We have also explored the relationships between emerging hormone actions on energy metabolism and those on other metabolic parameters (6,20–22,29–32). It appears that the gradually emerging inhibition on protein synthesis (29, 30,32,33) and probably inhibitions on nucleic acid synthesis (13,20,30,32,33) are the consequences of the hormone-induced limitations on energy production. Apparently, cellular processes related to growth and development are quite sensitive to very small changes in the adenylate energy charge. They are quickly reduced to low levels when energy charge is less than optimal, thus preserving ATP for more immediately essential processes such as ion pumping. According to this formulation, the well-known tonic suppression of the growth and development of immunologically noncommitted thymus cells by normal levels of glucocorticoids is the consequence of the operation of such normal mechanisms for the reordering of metabolic priorities (20,33) in the face of a hormone-induced suppression of energy production. The hormones appear to have "tricked" the cells into believing that they are in a stringent environment.

Since these ideas have been published on several occasions, the supporting data has been omitted. However, it is worth considering here the high degree of sensitivity of steady state rates of protein biosynthesis to small changes in the cellular energy charge. In Fig. 2 energy charge has been manipulated by a variety of means including starvation, readdition of nutrients (with differing abilities to restore synthesis), addition of rotenone (an inhibitor of mitochondrial ATP production), and the presence of glucocorticoids. What is apparent is that regardless of the means of changing adenine nucleotide ratios, the quantitative response of overall rates of protein biosynthesis is similar and predictable. Figure 3 provides evidence that this regulation (which is probably mediated by the changes in AMP) is achieved at the level of the initiation reaction; dexamethasone has no effect when cells are starved, but limits the ability of added glucose to increase the number of initiated ribosomes (8–10,21).

A recent effort in our laboratory has also been to look for possible energy charge-related changes in the kinds of proteins made by using two-dimensional gel electrophoretic separations. There is a pattern of changes that occurs when glucose is omitted: As the energy charge is reduced slightly, the synthesis of

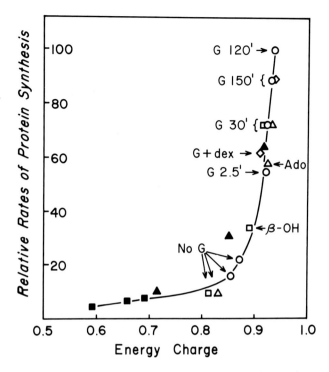

FIG. 2. Rates of protein synthesis vs. energy charge. Each of the four types of symbols represents data from one experiment. Experiment 1 *(open circles):* glucose for 120 and 150 min, no glucose for 120 and 150 min, or glucose for 2.5 and 30 min after 120 min without. Rates of protein synthesis are expressed as percentage of rates in cells incubated with glucose (5.5 mM) for 2 hr. Experiment 2 *(open diamonds):* glucose or glucose + dexamethasone (10⁻⁷ M) for 150 min. Experiment 3 *(open and closed squares):* β-hydroxybutyrate (5.5 mM), glucose, or glucose + rotenone *(filled symbols;* 350, 535, or 720 nM) added at 120 min. Incubation ended at 150 min. Experiment 4 *(open and closed triangles):* same protocol as experiment 3 except adenosine (2.5 nM) replaced β-hydroxybutyrate, and rotenone levels were 70, 140, or 280 nM. [From ref. 13, Mendelsohn, S., Nordeen, S. K., and Young, D. A. (1977): *Biochem. Biophys. Res. Commun.,* 79:53–60.]

most proteins declines to very low levels. However, a few (designated by the arrows in Fig. 4) go against the trend and increase. While these increases can be prevented by glucose (and adenosine), pyruvate is not effective. Within the first 2 hr the overall hormonal suppression of protein synthesis appears to be uniform (data not shown), which is consistent with an overall effect on energy charge. But the hormone-induced limitation on glucose uptake is not sufficient to cause the changes in those few "glucose-related" proteins that appear when glucose is omitted; a small amount of glucose uptake is sufficient to prevent these.

While a thorough exploration of all of these metabolic interrelationships is not possible here, several are worth noting. A feature of the hormonal suppression

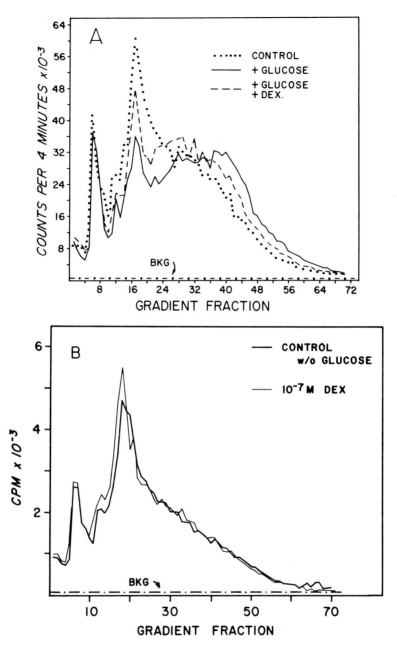

FIG. 3. Ability of dexamethasone to inhibit the redistribution of [³H]uridine-labeled ribosomes when energy-providing substrate (glucose) is added to steroid cells. Rat thymus cells (2 ml/ flask of a suspension containing 24% cells by volume) were incubated in Krebs-Ringer bicarbonate buffer at 37°C with 100 μCi/ml [³H]uridine for 2 hr in order to label ribosomal RNA; dexamethasone (10⁻⁷ M) was added to two of the flasks from the start where indicated. **A:** Glucose was added at 120 min to some flasks and sucrose gradient analyses of polyribosome profiles were performed 20 min later to measure the distribution of labeled ribosomes. **B:** Incubations were continued without glucose for a total of 3 hr and similar gradient analyses were performed. [From ref. 33, Young, D. A., Nicholson, M. L., Guyette, W. A., Giddings, S. J., Mendelsohn, S. L., Nordeen, S. K., and Lyons, R. T. (1979): In: *Glucocorticoid Action and Leukaemia, Proceedings 7th Tenovus Workshop,* edited by P. A. Bell and N. M. Borthwick, pp. 53–68. Alpha Omega Publishing, Cardiff.]

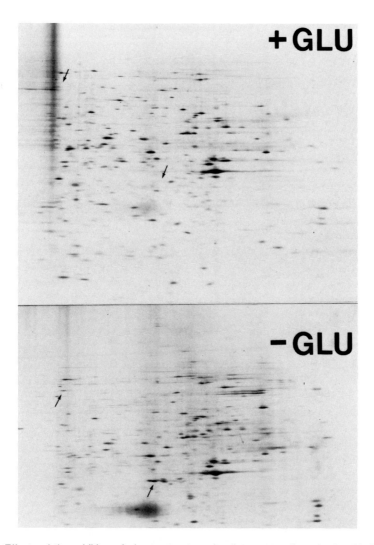

FIG. 4. Effects of the addition of glucose to starved cells on rate of synthesis of individual proteins. Suspensions of rat thymus cells (5×10^7 cells/ml) were incubated for 100 min in Krebs-Ringer bicarbonate (KRB) at 37°C. At 100 min [^{35}S]methionine was added to each flask (100 μCi/100 μl of cell suspension). After 20 min, cells received either glucose (final conc. 1 mg/ml) or H_2O, and were incubated an additional 1 hr. Cells were then washed in KRB and lysed; proteins were separated via two-dimensional electrophoresis (23). *Upward arrows* indicate proteins whose rate of synthesis has increased; *downward arrows* indicate proteins whose rate of synthesis has decreased. The *arrows* indicate those consistent differences seen in separate experiments.

on RNA, DNA, and protein synthesis in studies from a number of laboratories has been the requirement for an external energy source such as glucose or pyruvate (12,20,29,30), or in special cases (where cells are adapted to derive energy from amino acids) for amino acids (27). Should this energy source already be sufficiently restricted to produce those declines in energy charge that reduce synthetic rates (as in Fig. 3B), then further hormonal suppressions on energy charge and macromolecular synthesis are not seen. Thus glucocorticoids appear to dampen growth processes when they are rapid, but not when they have already been slowed. Other regulatory mechanisms that allow utilization of sufficient intracellular substrates to support basal energy requirements intervene.

Hormone-Induced Cell Killing

A different kind of hormone action, the ability of high levels of glucocorticoids to kill some lymphocytes is of special interest to those interested in cancer chemotherapy. The dashed lines in Fig. 1 illustrate the evolution of the lethal action in rat thymus cells. Earlier ideas had attributed this effect to suppressions on either glucose uptake or macromolecular synthesis. However, we have come to view the lethal effect as a separate action. The reason for this decision has been the ability to produce lethal actions under conditions of stringent substrate supply (mentioned above) where the metabolic effects of the hormones on energy metabolism and macromolecular synthesis are not seen (6,18,33). When viewed electron microscopically the lethal actions begin by an alteration in chromatin after about 6 hr. They culminate with the inability to exclude dyes and cellular lysis seen at 12 hr.

In order to study mechanisms further, we have sought some earlier measure of onset of these lytic effects. We have come to rely on early changes in the osmotic fragility of nuclei as a reliable measure of the incipient lethal actions (see Fig. 5). The method measures number of nuclei that survive when the whole cells are lysed in hypotonic medium. Nuclei may be counted directly, or broken nuclei estimated from DNA released (7). When thymus or lymphosarcoma cells are incubated during the first 2 hr, almost all nuclei remain intact after cellular lysis; but if glucocorticoids are added, there are marked hormone-induced increases in the tendency of nuclei to lyse.

Mechanisms of Hormone-Induced Cell Killing

The nuclear fragility assay has allowed us to draw some conclusions about mechanisms responsible for the lethal actions (18,19,33). First, the lethal effect is receptor-mediated since it is blocked by large amounts of the antagonist cortexolone. Second, it requires RNA and protein synthesis. It is of special interest that reducing rates of protein synthesis by starvation does not lead to lysis. Indeed, a total block in protein synthesis protects the cells from the lethal actions. This appears to rule out the possibility that lethal actions are the conse-

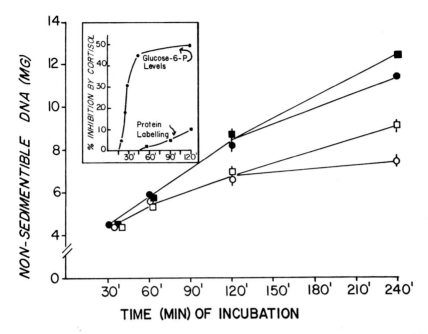

FIG. 5. Time course of the development of the effect of cortisol increasing nuclear fragility in the presence and absence of added glucose. Cell suspensions (0.5 ml) were incubated with or without cortisol (10^{-6} M) and with or without glucose (1 mg/ml) for 240 min. Aliquots of cell suspensions were lysed at the times indicated in the figure. *Closed circles* represent the amount of DNA recovered in supernatant fractions of cells incubated with glucose and with cortisol; *open circles,* with glucose and without cortisol; *closed squares* without glucose and with cortisol; *open squares,* without glucose or cortisol. Data presented are the means of determinations from five flasks $\pm$ 1 SE. The *insert,* included for comparison, shows the time of onset and course of development of effects of cortisol on glucose transport (levels of glucose-6-phosphate) and on rates of incorporation of radiolabeled valine into protein. The difference between cortisol and controls is significant at the $p < 0.05$ level by 60 min, at the $p < 0.01$ level by 2 hr and at the $p < 0.001$ level by 4 hr, both in the presence and in the absence of added glucose. The difference between glucose and no glucose, either in the presence or absence of cortisol, does not become significant until 4 hr, when the difference is significant at $p < 0.01$ level. [From ref. 7, Giddings, S. J., and Young, D. A. (1974): *J. Steroid Biochem.,* 5:587–595.]

quence of a generalized reduction in rates of protein synthesis, or of the impaired synthesis of an essential growth factor. Third, the initial appearance of the lethal effect is not much influenced by changes in the energy charge of the magnitude produced by the hormone. For example, lowering the energy charge by other means does not (over the first 2 hr) produce changes in nuclear fragility. Fourth, hormone effects on nuclear fragility occur within 2 hr. This is prior to any detectable changes in calcium uptake, which appear after 5 hr (Fig. 6). They also appear both in the absence of calcium and in the presence of EGTA (Fig. 7). Thus, we seem to be able to rule out the hormone-induced increases in calcium uptake as the initiating events in the lethal mechanism. Finally,

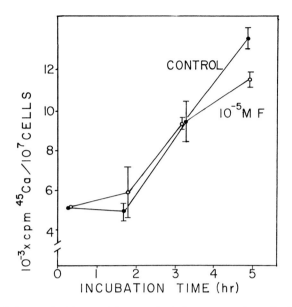

FIG. 6. Effect of glucocorticoids on calcium uptake in P1798-sensitive cells. Cell suspensions were incubated in RPMI-1640 with or without 10^{-6} M cortisol for up to 5 hr prior to the addition of ^{45}Ca. Calcium uptake was measured following a 60-min pulse with ^{45}Ca after washing cells four times in 0.9% NaCl. The data are the means of determinations from three flasks ± SEM. The difference between cortisol-treated and control is significant ($p < 0.02$) only at 5 hr. [From ref. 19, Nicholson, M. L., and Young, D. A. (1979): *J. Supramol. Struct.,* 10:165–174.]

there is a metabolic action—the decrease in α-aminoisobutyric acid (AIB) concentrating ability—which is possibly a membrane-related phenomenon; its emergence parallels the action on nuclear fragility (31,33). It is possible, if not likely, that both represent the same or similar hormone actions: an attack on the integrity of cellular membranes (18,33).

Hormone-Induced mRNAs and Proteins as Initiators of all Biological Effects

Much indirect evidence suggests that the glucocorticoid hormone–receptor complex leads to the transcription of hormone-induced messenger RNAs, and that these in turn induce proteins that produce the biological actions. As might be expected, where the effect itself is a large increase in a protein, increases in the respective associated message have been observed (4). Moreover, studies from our laboratory and Munck's (sometimes in collaboration) on thymic lymphocytes, and also those of Stevens on lymphosarcoma cells, have suggested that both the metabolic, (10,20,14,26,32,33) and the lethal actions (7,18) require new mRNA and protein synthesis. With thymus cells the message that generates the inhibition on glucose appears almost simultaneously with hormone binding, i.e., within the first 10 min, since periods of susceptibility of the hormone action

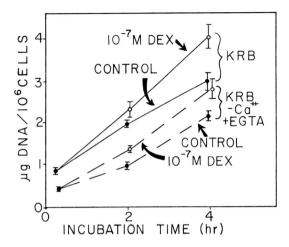

FIG. 7. Calcium independence of the glucocorticoid effect on nuclear fragility in rat thymus cells. Cell suspensions were prepared in Krebs-Ringer bicarbonate (KRB; 2.5 mM Ca, 1.2 mM Mg) and cells were resuspended in either KRB or KRB − calcium + EGTA (0 mM Ca, 3.7 mM Mg, 0.5 EGTA). Cell suspensions were added to flasks containing dexamethasone (final concentration 10^{-7} M) or water and incubated for 15 min, 2 hr, or 4 hr. Aliquots (20 μl) were taken for determination of prelysis and postlysis DNA at the times indicated in the figure. The data are presented as micrograms DNA released per 10^6 cells and are the means of determinations from five to six flasks ± SEM (two to three flasks for 15-min incubation time). Dexamethasone-treated (compared with control) represents an increase of 18 and 35% at 2 and 4 hr, respectively. The difference between dexamethasone-treated and control is significant at 2 hr (KRB − Ca + EGTA, $p < 0.002$) and at 4 hr (KRB − Ca + EGTA, $p < 0.01$; KRB, $p < 0.009$). [From ref. 19, Nicholson, M. L., and Young, D. A. (1979): *J. Supramol. Struct.,* 10:165–174.]

on glucose to inhibitors of mRNA synthesis (14) and poly(A) addition to message (31) are restricted to the first few minutes. At somewhat later times inhibitors of protein biosynthesis block all of the emerging hormone actions, with the time of sensitivity to the inhibitor generally corresponding with that of the emergence of the effect (reviewed in ref. 33). Other support comes from observations that glucocorticoids can induce viral mRNAs within the first 15 min (26) and increase RNA polymerase B activity (1). Changes in synthesis in some classes of nuclear nonhistone proteins have also been reported (2).

Yet all of this notwithstanding, it should be pointed out that this general thesis can only be regarded as a working hypothesis. Over the past 2 years we have attempted to utilize techniques of two-dimensional gel electrophoresis to seek those hypothetical hormone-induced proteins whose rate of synthesis might change within the first hour of hormone addition. Initially we utilized the two-dimensional gel system developed by O'Farrell. This method allows the detection of about 700 proteins (see Fig. 8A). Although our gels were very satisfactory we found no early changes in proteins (Voris and Young, *unpublished*) nor did we find changes in nuclear acidic proteins within the first hour (Fig. 9). We then enlarged the dimensions to create "giant" two-dimensional

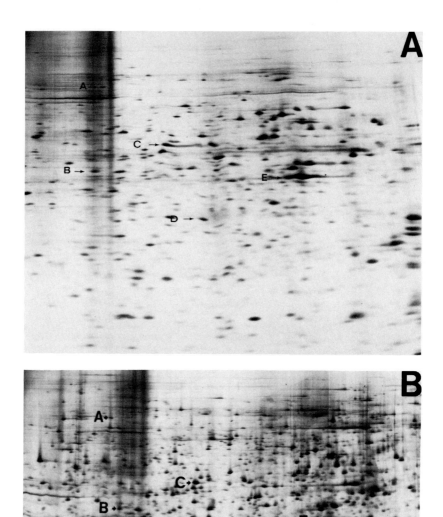

FIG. 8. Comparison of small **(A)** vs. large **(B)** gel separations of [³⁵S]methionine-labeled whole rat thymus cell proteins. Suspensions of rat thymus cells (5×10^7 cells/ml) were labeled in Krebs-Ringer bicarbonate (KRB) with [³⁵S]methionine (spec. act. > 500 Ci/mmole; 500 μCi/ml of cell suspension) for 1 hr at 37°C. Cells were washed in KRB and resuspended in cell lysis buffer [9.5 M urea, 2% Nonidet P-40, 2% ampholines (comprised of 1.6% pH range 5–7 and 0.4% pH range 3–10), and 5% 2-mercaptoethanol]. The sample applied to the small gel **(A)** contained 500,000 cpm in 1.7 μg protein and was focused 14 hr at 400 V followed by 1 hr at 800 V. The sample applied to the large gel **(B)** contained 5×10^6 cpm in 20 μg protein and was focused for 34 hr at 1,155 V. Autoradiograms were exposed for 2 weeks. Peaks marked *A–E* indicate corresponding proteins in small and large gels.

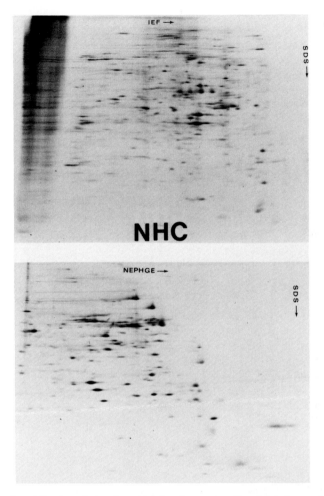

FIG. 9. Two-dimensional analysis of nonhistone chromosomal proteins from rat thymus cell. Suspensions of rat thymus cells (5×10^7 cells/ml) were incubated for 1 hr with [^{35}S]methionine (spec. act. > 500 Ci/mmole; 250 μCi/ml). Cells were lysed by a 25-fold dilution into ice-cold 3mM MgCl$_2$, and nuclei were pelleted at $1,800 \times g$ for 5 min. Nonhistone chromosomal proteins were prepared for electrophoresis (25), and were separated by isoelectric focusing (IEF) and nonequilibrium pH gradient (NEPHGE) two-dimensional electrophoresis (23,24). Both IEF and NEPHGE gels received 4×10^5 cpm and were exposed for 10 days.

gel separations. This system (developed by Voris) accepts about 10-fold more sample and yields at least a 3-fold increase in the proteins detectable (see Fig. 8B), up to 2,000 in thymus and lymphosarcoma cells, when the results from nonequilibrium gels are included (28). Yet to date we have still not found evidence for hormone-induced proteins within the first hour. I have included these negative results here to emphasize the fact that the most widely accepted hypothesis for the mechanism of hormone actions is still far from proven. We have found selective glucocorticoid effects on the kinds of proteins made (Fig. 10) at later times (4–6 hr), but these cannot be *initiating events* for the early metabolic effects. Our continuing efforts here will be aimed at examining membrane and mitochondrial proteins, since changes in these could possibly account for inhibitions on glucose uptake, on mitochondrial ATP, and possibly also for the lethal effects that may occur through altered membrane function.

Emergence of Resistance to Glucocorticoid Killing

The clinical usefulness of glucocorticoids to suppress lymphoid tumors is usually limited by the emergence of cells that are resistant to glucocorticoid-induced killing. In some instances, especially in tumors that have been adapted for growth in tissue culture, such as the S49 cell, resistance occurs via mutation to receptorless cells, or to cells with deficient receptor-related mechanisms (see ref. 11). It has become appreciated, however, that many if not most tumors growing in the host that are resistant when steroids are administered nevertheless exhibit a variety of metabolic effects of glucocorticoids, and can by no means be considered as receptorless (3). This is true of the mouse P1798 lymphosarcoma cells (generously supplied to us by Fred Rosen from nearby Roswell Park). We have applied our nuclear fragility assay to those tumors that are sensitive or highly resistant to glucocorticoid killing when the hormone is administered to the host animal. When examined within the first 2 hr the *in vivo* sensitivity can be predicted by the hormone action on nuclear fragility; little effect is seen in steroid-resistant cells (Fig. 11). A somewhat unexpected finding, however, was that the nuclei of the sensitive cells spontaneously deteriorate more rapidly during the course of further incubation than those of resistant cells, so much so that one can predict steroid sensitivity in the absence of hormone. Furthermore, highly steroid-resistant cells incubated for additional hours to the point that they exhibit the same basal increase in nuclear fragility now exhibit further hormone-directed increases in fragility of the same magnitude as the sensitive cells (18). The results from such experiments, and others, suggest that steroids may perform their intracellular destructive effects within both sensitive and resistant cells. It seems that resistance to hormone-directed cell killing emerges not by the absence of the initial events in hormone action, but instead via the

---

FIG. 10. Long-term effects of dexamethasone on rat thymus cell proteins. Suspension of rat thymus cells (5×10^7 cells/ml) were incubated at 37°C in RPMI-1640 ([methionine] = 6 μM) in the presence (10^{-6} M) **(A)** or absence **(B)** of dexamethasone. After 4 hr of incubation, [^{35}S]methionine was added to each flask (50 μCi/100 μl of cell suspension). At 6 hr, cells were washed once in Krebs-Ringer bicarbonate and lysed with cell lysis buffer. Whole cell proteins were then subjected to giant two-dimensional electrophoresis (28); 5×10^6 cpm was applied to each gel. Autoradiograms were exposed to the dried gel for 10 days. *Upward arrows* indicate proteins with increased synthetic rate; *downward arrows* indicate proteins with a decreased synthetic rate.

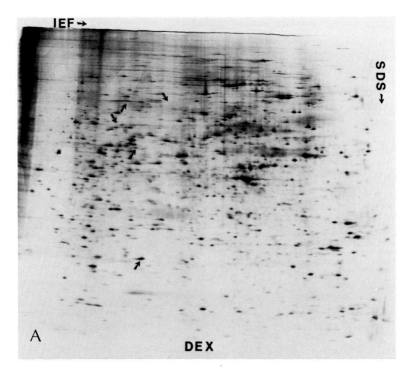

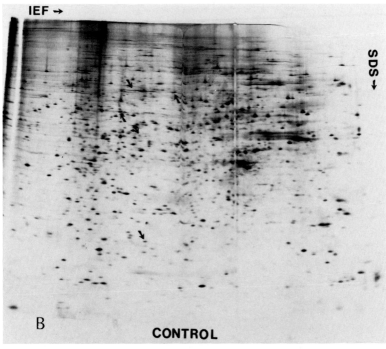

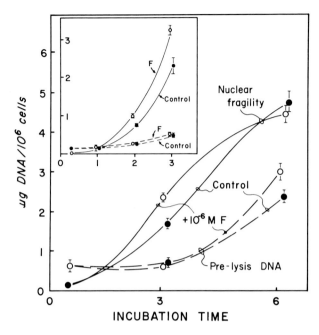

FIG. 11. Time course of the development of the cortisol effect on nuclear fragility of the P1798 lymphosarcoma cells. Cell suspensions were incubated in RPMI-1640 with or without cortisol (F) (10^{-6} M) for up to 6 hr. Aliquots (50 μl) were taken for determination of prelysis DNA by 20-fold dilution into RPMI-1640. Prelysis DNA was subtracted from total postlysis DNA to obtain the quantity of DNA released as a result of the rupture of nuclei as cells are lysed. The *insert* is a typical experiment demonstrating the onset of the cortisol effect on nuclear fragility in the sensitive line. The data represent the means of determinations for five to six flasks ± SEM. The difference between the cortisol-treated and control for the sensitive line is significant ($p < 0.001$) only at the 2-hr and 3-hr points, and for the resistant line it is significant ($p < 0.006$) only at the 6-hr point. [From ref. 18, Nicholson, M. L., and Young, D. A. (1978): *Cancer Res.,* 38:3673–3680.]

selection of those cells with hardier membranes, i.e., those that are better able to withstand the intracellular consequences of hormonal attack (18,19,33).

Another approach to understanding the hormone-resistant state has been to search for changes in the kinds of proteins made by the cell. When resistant P1798 lymphosarcoma cells are compared with sensitive cells, the proteins made in each case are remarkably similar. Yet a few changes are present, and these appear to be highly reproducible in experiments repeated many times (see Fig. 12). Some proteins are decreased and a few are increased. Using a comparative method for estimating spot density, plots can be made of these changes. A striking feature of these plots is that the changes become pronounced only when the cells are extremely resistant to glucocorticoid killing. In these studies there is one spot that exhibits the largest change, that is no. 110 on Fig. 12. It is absent in the sensitive cells and becomes a substantial peak in the highly resistant state (17).

Recent studies in our lab by Nicholson and Voris have applied this same

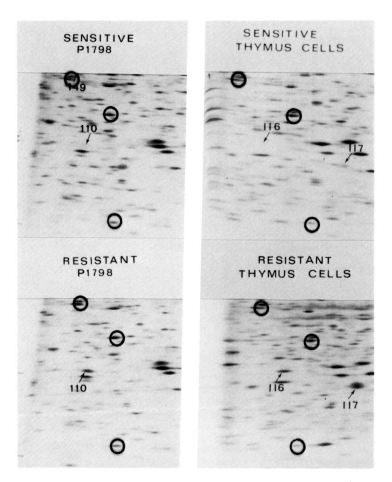

FIG. 12. In both P1798 lymphosarcoma cells and normal rat thymus cells resistance to glucocorticoid hormone-induced cell killing is associated with the increased synthesis of similar proteins. Thymus cells were selected for resistance by treating rats with 10 mg/kg/day dexamethasone (suspended in tricaprylin) for 3 days, followed by 2 days untreated. Suspensions of both thymus (1% packed cell volume) and tumor cells (5 × 10⁷ cells/ml) were labeled in Krebs-Ringer bicarbonate or RPMI-1640, respectively, with [³⁵S]methionine (100 μCi/100 ml cell suspension, 500–1,200 Ci/mmole) for 1 hr at 37°C. Cells were washed in their respective incubation media and resuspended in cell lysis buffer. Samples applied to the gels contained 500,000 cpm and were focused for 4 hr at 400 V. The figures are enlarged segments of the autoradiograms from nonequilibrium gels of glucocorticoid-sensitive and -resistant P1798 lymphosarcoma cells *(left)* and sensitive and resistant normal thymus cells *(right)*. The pH increases from left to right. This section of the gel spans a MW range from ≈60,000 *(top)* to 25,000 *(bottom)*. *Circled proteins* are invariant peaks used here for orientation. *Upward arrows* indicate consistent increases in the density of the protein spot.

approach to resistant normal thymus cells. After several days of steroid injection most cells are killed. It has been known for some time that some cells survive and those that do are immunologically competent ones (see ref. 16). In our experiments rats were injected for 3 days with glucocorticoids, and the kinds

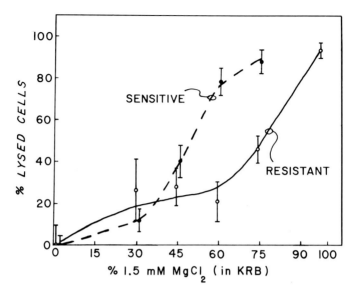

FIG. 13. Plasma membrane fragility in glucocorticoid-sensitive and -resistant thymus cells. Thymus cells are selected for resistance by treating rats with 10 mg/kg body wt/day of dexamethasone suspended in tricaprylin (s.c. injections), followed by 2 days untreated. Since only 5% of the thymus (by weight) survives this treatment, normal thymus is considered sensitive. Cell suspensions were prepared in Krebs-Ringer bicarbonate (KRB). Cells were resuspended at 1% packed cell volume in KRB and glucose (1 mg/ml), and maintained at 37°C in a shaking incubator. Randomized aliquots, taken at 5-min increments, were diluted 1:20 into solutions of varying hypotonicity. These solutions span a range from being isotonic to the cells (KRB) to being almost pure water (1.5 mM $MgCl_2$ for maintenance of nuclear integrity). After 10 min at 22°C, Trypan Blue Viability stain is added to diluted cells and 5 min later both live unlysed cells and swollen, lysed cells are counted microscopically. In this figure the percentage of lysed cells is plotted against the hypotonicity of the solution (isotonic on *left* and very hypotonic on *right*). The data, pooled from three experiments, have been corrected for variations (between experiments) in live cell number and are plotted as mean ± SEM.

of proteins made were compared with those made by normal thymus cells from sham-injected controls. Once again the differences between the resistant and sensitive cells were minimal. However, to our surprise a protein (peak 116 in these gels; see Fig. 12) located at the same position as spot 110 in lymphosarcoma cells also appears in these resistant thymus cells. So far we have little information about the nature of this protein other than the observation that proteins from resistant lymphosarcoma and normal thymus cells coelectrophorese. From such considerations it seems at least possible that resistance to glucocorticoid killing occurs via an increase in synthesis of a few cellular proteins (21).

    The hypothesis mentioned earlier, that resistance occurs via the selection of cells with hardier membranes, evolved from studies on nuclear fragility in which all of the cells were lysed by hypotonic shock. From such considerations one might suspect that the hardier membrane referred to nuclear membrane. Recently we have begun to examine the fragility of cells themselves by using osmotic gradients. The experiments were done by a series of dilutions of balanced salt solutions by millimolar magnesium chloride. The function of magnesium chloride is to maintain the integrity of the nuclear structures in the lysed cells. Fig. 13 shows the curve obtained from normal thymus cells. In general we observed that prolonged incubation leads to a shift to the left. We then examined the osmotic fragility of the cells obtained after 3 days of glucocorticoid treatment. These results indicate that the cells resistant to glucocorticoid killing are also relatively more resistant to osmotic lysis. Although these conclusions are preliminary, they encourage us in the thought that resistance to glucocorticoid killing may indeed involve structural changes in cell membranes that are generalized and not restricted to the nucleus.

Some Potential Therapeutic Implications Related to Cancer Chemotherapy

The mixed chemotherapeutic approach that has achieved moderate success in certain lymphoid and related neoplasms often includes high levels of glucocorticoids. However, in most instances there is no attempt at timing the administration of glucocorticoids relative to the other agents. Our finding that when cells begin to deteriorate (on prolonged incubation), those that are normally highly resistant to glucocorticoids become sensitive does have some potential therapeutic possibilities. It suggests that if steroids are administered when cells are maximally weakened by other agents, then there may be an increase in the steroid action to encompass cells that might otherwise be resistant. The possibility of resistance to glucocorticoids via selection of cells with hardier membranes of course also suggests the possible usefulness of agents that might selectively weaken membranes, or enhance glucocorticoid action at the membrane level by other means.

SUMMARY AND CONCLUSIONS

1. Both the rapidly evolving metabolic effects of glucocorticoids and the more slowly developing lethal actions appear to be initiated by the synthesis of new mRNAs and proteins. However, this concept should still only be regarded as a working hypothesis since changes in mRNAs and proteins have yet to be detected.

2. The chronic suppression of cell growth may be the consequence of a small steady state suppression of cellular energy production, a hormone action at the level of the mitochondria. The inhibition of glucose transport may also play a role in preventing a compensatory increase in glycolytic ATP production.

3. Small steady state hormone-induced changes in ratios of adenine nucleotides (suppression of cellular energy charge) lead to a larger suppression in overall rates of protein synthesis by actions (probably related to the increase in AMP) on the rate of peptide initiation.

4. Cell killing is not the result of suppression of protein synthesis or of hormone-induced increases in calcium uptake. While the mechanisms are unknown,

the increase in nuclear fragility, and possibly the decrease in AIB concentrating ability, appear to be the earliest measures of their operation.

5. In tumor cells, resistance to the lethal actions of glucocorticoids appears to emerge via the selection of cells with hardier membranes, those that are better able to withstand the intracellular destructive events set in motion by high levels of glucocorticoids.

6. Resistance to cell killing in immunologically committed normal thymus cells is associated with increased resistance to osmotic lysis. These latter two phenomena suggest changes in all cellular membranes.

7. In both tumor cells and normal thymus cells resistance is also associated with the increased synthesis of a few proteins, one of which is similar in both types of cells.

ACKNOWLEDGMENTS

This research was supported by NIH Grants AM 16177, CA-25665, GM-07136, and AM-07092 and grants from the United Cancer Council of Rochester and the American Cancer Society. We are grateful to Mary Wilkey for her invaluable help in typing the manuscript and to David A. Taylor and Ingrid E. Wood for their excellent technical assistance.

REFERENCES

1. Bell, P. A., and Borthwick, N. M. (1976): *J. Steroid Biochem.,* 7:1147–1150.
2. Borthwick, N. M. (1979): In: *Glucocorticoid Action and Leukaemia, Proceedings 7th Tenovus Workshop,* edited by P. A. Bell and N. M. Borthwick, pp. 41–53. Alpha Omega Publishing, Cardiff.
3. Crabtree, G. R., Smith, K. A., and Munck, A. (1978): *Cancer Res.,* 38:4268–4272.
4. Feigelson, P., Beato, M., Colman, P., Kalimi, M., Killewich, L. A., and Schutz, G. (1975): *Recent Prog. Horm. Res.,* 31:213–242.
5. Foley, J. E., Jeffries, M., and Munck, A. U. (1980): *J. Steroid Biochem.,* 12:231–243.
6. Giddings, S. J., and Young, D. A. (1974): *J. Cell. Physiol.,* 83:409–417.
7. Giddings, S. J., and Young, D. A. (1974): *J. Steroid Biochem.,* 5:587.
8. Guyette, W. A., and Young, D. A. (1974): *Fed. Proc.,* 33:1667.
9. Guyette, W. A., and Young, D. A. (1976): *Endocrinology [Suppl.],* 98:244.
10. Hallahan, C., Young, D. A., and Munck, A. (1973): *J. Biol. Chem.,* 248:2922–2927.
11. Higgins, S. J., and Gehring, U. (1978): *Adv. Cancer Res.,* 28:313–397.
12. Makman, M. H., Dvorkin, B., and White, A. (1966): *J. Biol. Chem.,* 241:1646–1648.
13. Mendelsohn, S. L., Nordeen, S. K., and Young, D. A. (1977): *Biochem. Biophys. Res. Commun.,* 79:53–60.
14. Mosher, K. M., Young, D. A., and Munck, A. (1971): *J. Biol. Chem.,* 246:654–659.
15. Munck, A. (1971): *Perspect. Biol. Med.,* 14:265–289.
16. Munck, A., and Young, D. A. (1972): In: *Handbook in Physiology: Endocrinology and Adrenal Cortex,* pp. 231–243, American Physiological Society, Washington, D.C.
17. Nicholson, M. L., Voris, B. P., and Young, D. A. (1980): *Cell (submitted for publication).*
18. Nicholson, M. L., and Young, D. A. (1978): *Cancer Res.,* 38:3673–3680.
19. Nicholson, M. L., and Young, D. A. (1979): *J. Supramol. Struct.,* 10:165–174.
20. Nordeen, S. K., and Young, D. A. (1976): *J. Biol. Chem.,* 251:7295–7303.
21. Nordeen, S. K., and Young, D. A. (1977): *J. Biol. Chem.,* 252:5324–5331.
22. Nordeen, S. K., and Young, D. A. (1978): *J. Biol. Chem.,* 243:1234–1239.
23. O'Farrell, P. H. (1975): *J. Biol. Chem.,* 250:4007–4021.

24. O'Farrell, P. H., Goodman, H. M., and O'Farrell P. H. (1977): *Cell,* 12:1133–1142.
25. Peterson, J. L., and McConkey, E. H. (1976): *J. Biol. Chem.,* 251:584–554.
26. Ringold, G. M., Yamamoto, K. R., Bishop, J. M., and Varmus, H. E. (1977): *Proc. Natl. Acad. Sci. USA,* 74:2879–2883.
27. Stevens, J., and Stevens, Y. W. (1975): *Cancer Res.,* 35:2145–2153.
28. Voris, B. P., and Young, D. A. (1980): *Anal. Biochem.,* 104:478–484.
29. Young, D. A. (1969): *J. Biol. Chem.,* 244:2210–2217.
30. Young, D. A. (1970): *J. Biol. Chem.,* 245:2747–2752.
31. Young, D. A., Barnard, T., Mendelsohn, S., and Giddings, S. (1974): *Endocrine Res. Commun.,* 1:63–72.
32. Young, D. A., Giddings, S., Swonger, A., Klurfeld, G., and Miller, M. (1971): In: *Proceedings 3rd International Congress Hormonal Steroids,* edited by V. H. T. James and L. Martini, pp. 624–635. Excerpta Medica, Amsterdam.
33. Young, D. A., Nicholson, M. L., Guyette, W. A., Giddings, S. J., Mendelsohn, S. L., Nordeen, S. K., and Lyons, R. T. (1979): In: *Glucocorticoid Action and Leukaemia, Proceedings 7th Tenovus Workshop,* edited by P. A. Bell and N. M. Borthwick, pp. 53–68. Alpha Omega Publishing, Cardiff.

Hormones and Cancer, edited by S. Iacobelli et al.
Raven Press, New York © 1980.

Effects of Glucocorticoids on Fc Receptors of a Human Granulocytic Cell Line

*Gerald R. Crabtree, Kendall A. Smith, Paul Guyre,
and Allan Munck

Departments of Physiology and Medicine, Dartmouth Medical School,
Hanover, New Hampshire 03755*

Since the discovery of Fc receptors 20 years ago by Boyden and Sorkin (4,5) evidence has accumulated indicating that these receptors are involved in a number of immunologic processes. These include phagocytosis, antibody-dependent cellular cytotoxicity, placental transfer of maternal immunoglobulin, and regulation of immunoglobulin synthesis. The possibility that some of these processes may be important in killing tumor cells makes the topic of Fc receptors and their hormonal regulation relevant to this volume on hormones and cancer.

Present knowledge of Fc receptors indicates that they are a heterogenous class of membrane structures capable of binding the Fc but not the Fab region of immunoglobulin (for review, see refs. 15,33). Several different types of Fc receptors have been defined by their immunoglobulin specificity and biologic function. For example, receptors for IgE on mast cells mediate histamine release, while receptors for IgG on macrophages and granulocytes initiate phagocytosis by binding antibody-coated particles to their surfaces. Although Fc receptors have been described for IgM (19,29) and IgA (26), their biologic significance is as yet uncertain. This chapter deals with the effects of glucocorticoid hormones on receptors having specificity for IgG.

The IgG-Fc receptor appears to be a protein of about 40,000 to 80,000 molecular weight (1,16,32). In partially purified preparations it retains its ability to bind immunoglobulin (1,14,28) and is destroyed by treatment with trypsin (2,8), papain (1), pronase (1,32), or phospholipase (1,16). It generally shows high affinity binding of human immunoglobulins IgG_1 and IgG_3, while IgG_2 and IgG_4 bind with less affinity (21,23,25).

The clearest function of IgG-Fc receptors is their role in binding antibody-coated particles to the surface of phagocytic cells (15,23). In this way they promote the phagocytosis and destruction of foreign materials recognized by the immune system. Enhancement of phagocytosis by antibody shows immunoglobulin subclass specificity which is similar to that of the Fc receptor. Thus, IgG_1 and IgG_3 which bind to the Fc receptor with greatest affinity are most

---

* Present address: National Cancer Institute, National Institutes of Health, Bethesda, Maryland 20205.

effective in promoting binding and phagocytosis (23). The importance of this class of Fc receptor in mediating phagocytosis *in vivo* is indicated by the clinical observation that autoantibodies of subclasses IgG_1 and IgG_3 directed against red cell antigens are much more frequently associated with extravascular hemolysis.

Possibly the simplest way in which Fc receptors could be involved in host defenses against malignancy is by promoting the phagocytosis of tumor cells covered with antibodies. This mechanism would require a humoral response to a tumor antigen. Although in model systems animals frequently form antibodies to virally induced tumors, there is less support for production of antibodies to naturally occurring human tumors.

Another more complex and apparently conflicting way in which Fc receptors could be involved in host–tumor relationships is the phenomenon of immunologic enhancement (13,14,22). Immunologic enhancement refers to increased rates of tumor growth accompanying antibody formation. Although the mechanism of enhancement is not known, the involvement of Fc receptors is inferred from the requirement for an intact Fc portion of the enhancing antibody (13).

A puzzling, but possibly relevant observation is the fact that many human as well as animal tumors appear to express Fc receptors (7,15,24,28,31). They have been reported on a variety of tumors which are not derived from cells normally expressing Fc receptors, including epithelial carcinomas and soft tissue sarcomas (31). The possible significance of these receptors to tumor growth is unknown.

We were led to study the effects of glucocorticoids on Fc receptors by the clinical observation that when patients with autoimmune thrombocytopenia or autoimmune hemolytic anemia (diseases in which antibodies are formed to autologous platelets or red cells) are treated with glucocorticoids, they often improve dramatically long before antibody titers began to fall (30). Platelet or red cell destruction in these diseases occurs primarily by phagocytosis by macrophages in the spleen and other reticuloendothelial organs (2,3,27,30), and evidence indicates that the therapeutic effect of glucocorticoids is due to inhibition of phagocytosis of antibody-coated cells (2). Thus the Fc receptor, which is important in initiating phagocytosis, was a reasonable place to begin looking for an explanation of the therapeutic effects of glucocorticoids in these diseases. That a reduction in Fc receptors might be responsible for the rapid cessation of platelet or red cell destruction associated with steroid therapy had been suggested by clinical observers (3,20).

Fc receptors are commonly measured by rosetting or fluorescence techniques in which cells bearing Fc receptors in excess of some detectable threshold are distinguished by binding antibody-coated red cells or fluorescent-labeled immune complexes. These techniques are useful for enumerating Fc receptor-bearing cells among a heterogenous population such as lymph node or bone marrow cell suspensions. However, to study hormonal regulation of Fc receptors among a homogenous cell line a more quantitative method for measuring these receptors is necessary. In our studies we have determined the mean number of Fc receptors per cell by analysis of the binding of an iodinated IgG_1 to the surface of a human progranulocytic cell line. (The details of the assay are given below in the legend to Fig. 1.) We have chosen to use a monoclonal myeloma protein since it was available in large quantities, could be purified to near homogeneity, and would permit study of the binding of a single immunoglobulin subclass.

The HL-60 cell line was felt to be particularly appropriate to the study of Fc receptors since it maintains a high degree of differentiation in culture—to the extent that it is capable of phagocytosing antibody-coated particles. This cell line was derived from the peripheral blood of a patient with acute promyelocytic leukemia and was initially described by Collins et al. (8) in 1977. Morphologically and histochemically these cells resemble promyelocytes, the precursors of polymorphonuclear leukocytes. A remarkable characteristic of this cell line is its ability to differentiate to a relatively mature polymorphonuclear leukocyte after 5 to 7 days' culture with 1.3% dimethylsulfoxide (9). As previously described (11), binding of IgG to HL-60 cells is entirely specific for the Fc portion of the immunoglobulin molecule, and is specific for immunoglobulin of subclasses IgG_1 and IgG_3. Human IgG_2 and IgG_4 bind with reduced affinity, while IgM, IgA, and IgE do not compete with IgG_1 for binding sites.

Figure 1 illustrates the effects of dexamethasone (200 μM, 72 hr) on Fc receptors, viable cell counts, and rates of leucine incorporation in HL-60 cells. Within 24 hr there is a significant reduction in Fc receptors which by 48 to 72 hr falls to 40 to 75% of controls without dexamethasone. With the continued presence of dexamethasone the levels stay low for at least 8 days, but return to normal within 48 hr of removing the hormone. As indicated by the upper two lines of Fig. 1, cells incubated with dexamethasone grew slightly more rapidly and had slightly increased rates of leucine incorporation over controls grown in the absence of dexamethasone. Thus, the reduction in Fc receptors is not associated with cytotoxic effects or a general decrease in rates of protein synthesis.

The affinity of the Fc receptor for IgG_1 was similar in cells incubated with dexamethasone and controls. In each case the dissociation constant was approximately 5 to 10 nM (Fig. 2).

The reduction in Fc receptors was specific for glucocorticoids (Fig. 3). Dexamethasone, prednisolone, and cortisol at 1 μM reduced the number of Fc receptors from about 14,000 sites per cell to about 8,000 sites per cell after 48 hrs incubation, while estradiol and progesterone had no effect. Cortexolone (1 μM) produced a small reduction in Fc receptors. This latter effect is consistent with our unpublished observations that cortexolone at high concentrations produces glucocorticoid effects in human lymphocytes.

In studies of the dose–response relationships for this effect, dexamethasone was found to produce a half-maximal response at 10^{-8} M, similar to other cellular effects of dexamethasone (data not shown). The dose–response relationship and specificity suggest that the effect may be mediated by the glucocorticoid receptor,

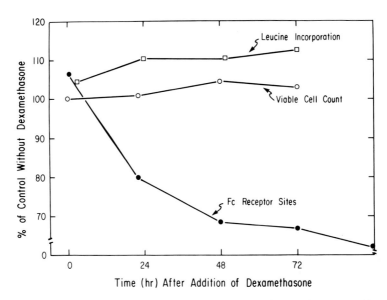

Time (hr) After Addition of Dexamethasone

FIG. 1. Time course with HL-60 cells of the effect of 200 nM dexamethasone on Fc receptor sites per cell *(closed circles),* leucine incorporation *(squares),* and viable cell counts *(open circles).* HL-60 cells were cultured in RPMI-1640 (GIBCO) with 10% fetal calf serum, penicillin (50 units/ml) and gentamycin (50 μg/ml) at 37°C in humidified room air containing 5% CO_2. Dexamethasone dissolved in medium at 0.1 mM was added at time zero to three flasks containing 50 ml cell suspension (2×10^{-5} cells/ml). An equivalent amount of medium was added to three control flasks. At 15 min and 24, 48, and 72 hr, 4×10^6 cells were removed and washed twice with 15 ml Dulbecco's phosphate-buffered saline (PBS; GIBCO) containing 1 mg/ml bovine serum albumin (BSA; 2× recrystallised, Calbiochem) at room temperature. The cells were incubated for 30 min in 15 ml PBS-BSA ($2–8 \times 10^5$ cells/ml) at 37°C with 60 cpm shaking to dissociate endogenous immunoglobulins in fetal calf serum from the Fc receptors. They were then resuspended in PBS-BSA at 5×10^7 cells/ml, and 20 μl aliquots were incubated in duplicate with 20 μl of ^{125}I-labeled IgG_1 (40 nM), with and without unlabeled IgG_1 (1 μM) in albuminized 1.5-ml conical polypropylene Eppendorf centrifuge tubes (Brinkman) for 30 min at 37°C with 60 cpm shaking. At the end of the incubation the cell suspension was pipetted over 350 μl fetal calf serum at 0°C in 400-μl Microfuge tubes (Brinkman) and centrifuged for 30 sec at $10,000 \times g$. The supernatant was rapidly aspirated and the tips of the tubes containing the cell pellet counted in a gamma counter at an efficiency of 70% for ^{125}I. The difference between the cpm bound in the presence (an almost negligible amount, as shown in Fig. 2) and absence of 1 μM competing unlabeled IgG_1 (that is, the cpm corresponding to saturably bound IgG_1) was calculated as molecules per cell. Since at 40 nM IgG_1 nearly saturates the Fc receptor sites (see Fig. 2) this value gives a close estimate of the total number of Fc receptor sites per cell. Leucine incorporation was measured by removing 100-μl aliquots from each of the flasks and incubating for 4 hr at 37°C under 5% CO_2 in humidified room air in microtiter plates (Costar) with 100 μl of a solution (3 μCi/ml) of [^{3}H]leucine (NEN, 297 Ci/mole) in GIBCO minimum essential medium. Cells were collected on glass fiber filters using a multiple automated sample harvester, and after drying were counted in a toluene-based scintillation fluid at an efficiency of 50% for ^{3}H. Viable cell counts were determined as the product of the fraction viable by Trypan blue exclusion and the cell count determined with a Coulter counter. Viabilities of control and dexamethasone-treated cells were not significantly different, and always remained above 95%. Each point represents the mean for determinations on three control flasks and three flasks with dexamethasone. For the controls, the number of Fc receptor sites remained essentially constant at about 16,000 sites per cell over the whole time period; the rates of leucine incorporation increased slightly, and the viable cell counts increased from 200 to 650 cells per μl. (From Crabtree et al., ref. 11, with permission.)

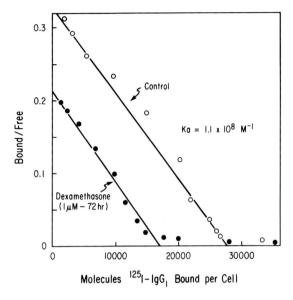

FIG. 2 Scatchard plot of binding of IgG$_1$ to Fc receptors of HL-60 cells after incubation with 1 μM dexamethasone. *Open circles,* controls without dexamethasone; *closed circles,* cells incubated with 1 μM dexamethasone. Cells were incubated with or without dexamethasone for 96 hr and washed in PBS-BSA as described for Fig. 1. They were then resuspended at 1.6 × 10^8 cells/ml in PBS-BSA. Aliquots were incubated as described for Fig. 1 with ^{125}I-labeled IgG$_1$ at 12 concentrations from 100 pM to 1 μM. After the incubation the tubes were centrifuged at 10,000 × g for 10 sec and 20 μl supernatant removed and counted to determine the final concentration of free labeled IgG$_1$. The tubes were then cooled to 3°C, 1.2 ml of PBS-BSA at 0°C was added, and the cells were resuspended. After 5 min the tubes were centrifuged at 12,000 × g for 4 min, the supernatant aspirated, and the tips counted as described for Fig. 1 to determined bound ^{125}I-labeled IgG$_1$. Nonsaturably bound IgG$_1$ was not subtracted for these results. Bound IgG and free IgG on the ordinate are given in units of cpm/20 μl of cell suspension; the values on the ordinate therefore represent the bound IgG$_1$ as a fraction of the free IgG$_1$ at equilibrium. (From Crabtree et al., ref. 11, with permission.)

and in separate experiments we have found that HL-60 cells contain approximately 1,500 glucocorticoid receptor sites per cell with a dissociation constant of 10^{-8} M.

The importance of these observations is that they provide a molecular mechanism for some of the immunosuppressive actions of glucocorticoids and suggest the generalization that these effects are related to inhibition of synthesis of immunologically important proteins. Although these immunosuppressive effects have commonly been attributed to killing of lymphocytes, little lympholytic effect is observed in humans with physiologic or pharmacologic concentrations of glucocorticoids (6,12). In separate studies we have shown that inhibition of mitogen- or antigen-induced proliferation is very likely related to the inhibition of production of specific growth factors necessary for lymphocyte proliferation (see Smith et al., *this volume;* 10,17,18). Taken together, these observations suggest that the immunosuppressive actions of glucocorticoids are due to the

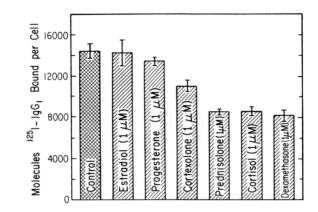

FIG. 3. Effects of steroids on number of Fc receptor sites on HL-60 cells. HL-60 cells were cultured as described in Fig. 1 for 48 hr with the steroids indicated above at a final concentration of 1 μM. Fc receptors were assayed as described in Fig. 1. The *points* and *bars* represent the mean ± 1 SEM of three flasks for each steroid.

inhibition of production of proteins that are essential for normal immune responses and are not related to a generalized lympholytic effect.

ACKNOWLEDGMENTS

We thank Dr. Gibbons Cornwell for the myeloma serum and Drs. Collins, Gallo, and Gallagher for the HL-60 cell line. These studies were supported in part by Grants CA 17323, AM 03535, and CA 17643 from the National Institutes of Health and by the Core Grant (CA 23108) of the Norris Cotton Cancer Center.

REFERENCES

1. Anderson, C. L., and Grey, H. M. (1977): *J. Immunol.,* 118:819–824.
2. Atkinson, J. P., and Frank, M. M. (1974): *Blood,* 44:629–637.
3. Atkinson, J. P., Schreiber, A. D., and Frank, M. M. (1973): *J. Clin. Invest.,* 52:1509–1517.
4. Boyden, S. V., and Sorkin, E. (1960): *Immunology,* 3:272–783.
5. Boyden, S. V., and Sorkin, E. (1961): *Immunology,* 4:244–250.
6. Claman, H. N. (1972): *N. Engl. J. Med.,* 287:388–401.
7. Cohen, D., Gurner, B. W., and Coombs, R. R. A. (1971): *Br. J. Exp. Pathol.,* 52:447–455.
8. Collins, S. J., Gallo, R. C., Gallagher, R. E. (1977): *Nature,* 270:347–349.
9. Collins, S. J., Ruscetti, F. W., and Gallagher, R. E., and Gallo, R. C. (1979): *J. Exp. Med.,* 149:969–974.
10. Crabtree, G. R., Gillis, S., Smith, K. A., and Munck, A. (1980): *J. Steroid Biochem.,* 12:445–449.
11. Crabtree, G. R., Munck, A., and Smith, K. A. (1979): *Nature,* 279:338–339.
12. Crabtree, G. R., Smith, K. A., and Munck, A. (1978): *Cancer Res.,* 38:4268–4272.
13. Cruse, J. M., Forbes, J. T., Gillespie, G. Y., Lewis, G. K., Scales, R. W., Shivers, B. R., Fields, J. F., Hester, R. B., Watson, E. S., and Whitten, H. D. (1972): *Z. Immunitaetsforsch.,* 143:43–49.
14. Cruse, J. M., Whitten, H. D., Lewis, G. K., and Watson, E. S. (1973): *Transplant. Proc.,* 5:961–968.

15. Dickler, H. B. (1976): In: *Advances in Immunology, Vol. 24,* edited by F. J. Dixon and H. G. Kunkel, pp. 167–215. Academic Press, New York.
16. D'Urso-Coward, M., and Cone, R. E. (1978): *J. Immunol.,* 121:1973–1980.
17. Gillis, S., Crabtree, G. R., and Smith, K. A. (1979): *J. Immunol.,* 123:1624–1631.
18. Gillis, S., Crabtree, G. R., and Smith, K. A. (1979): *J. Immunol.,* 123:1632–1638.
19. Grossi, C. E., Webb, S. R., Zicca, A., Lydyard, P. M., Moretta, L., Mingari, M. C., and Cooper, M. D. (1978): *J. Exp. Med.,* 144:1405–1417.
20. Handin, R. I., and Storrel, T. P. (1978): *Blood,* 51:771–776.
21. Hay, F. C., Torrigiani, G., and Roitt, I. M. (1972): *Eur. J. Immunol.,* 2:257–261.
22. Hellstrom, K. E., and Hellstrom, I. (1970): *Annu. Rev. Microbiol.,* 24:298–373.
23. Huber, H., and Fudenberg, H. H. (1968): *Int. Arch. Allergy Appl. Immunol.,* 34:18–31.
24. Kerbel, R. S., and Davis, J. S. (1974): *Cell,* 3:105–112.
25. Lawrence, D. A., Weigle, W. O., and Spiegelberg, H. L. (1975): *J. Clin. Invest.,* 55:368–376.
26. Lum, L. G., Muchmore, A. V., O'Connor, N., Strobber, W., and Glaese, R. M. (1979): *J. Immunol.,* 123:714–721.
27. Van Der Meulen, F. W., Van Der Hart, M., Fleer, A., Von Dem Borne, A. E. G. Kr., Engelfriet, C. P., and Van Loghem, J. J. (1978): *Br. J. Haematol.,* 38:541–549.
28. Milgrom, F., Humphrey, L. J., Tondor, O., Yasuda, J., and Witebsky, E. (1968): *Int. Arch. Allergy,* 33:478–482.
29. Morretta, L., Webb, S. R., Grossi, C. E., Lydyard, P. M., and Cooper, M. D. (1977): *J. Exp. Med.,* 146:184–195.
30. Swisher, S. N., and Burka, E. R. (1977): In: *Hematology, 2nd ed.,* edited by W. J. Williams, E. Beutler, A. J. Ersleu, and R. W. Rundles, pp. 585–596. McGraw-Hill, New York.
31. Tondor, O., and Thunold, S. (1973): *Scand. J. Immunol.,* 2:207–215.
32. Yagawa, K., Onoue, K., and Yoshitomi, A. (1979): *J. Immunol.,* 122:366–373.
33. Zuckerman, S. H., and Douglas, S. D. (1979): *CRC Crit. Rev. Microbiol.,* 7:1–26.

Hormone Action in Normal and Neoplastic Tissues: Protein Hormones

Hormones and Cancer, edited by S. Iacobelli et al.
Raven Press, New York © 1980.

Neurohypophysial Hormones and Cancer

M. E. Monaco, *W. R. Kidwell, P. H. Kohn, J. S. Strobl, and
M. E. Lippman

*Medicine Branch and *Laboratory of Pathophysiology, National Cancer Institute, National
Institutes of Health, Bethesda, Maryland 20205*

A number of hormones have been implicated in the etiology and growth of a variety of tumors. These hormones include estrogens, androgens, progestins, glucocorticoids, insulin, prolactin, and peptide growth factors. For many years the actions of the neurohypophysial hormones oxytocin and vasopressin were thought to be limited to a few discrete loci: oxytocin was believed to function solely as a myotonic factor, stimulating uterine and mammary gland contraction; and vasopressin, primarily as an antidiuretic, although pharmacologic concentrations exhibited pressor activity. Recently, other activities for both these hormones have been described. Oxytocin has been shown to increase the conversion of glucose to CO_2 by rat adipocytes. This effect of oxytocin is additive with that of insulin. In addition, specific, high-affinity receptors for oxytocin can be demonstrated on the adipocyte. Evaluation of dose–response relationships suggests that the binding may be related to the biological response: the K_D for binding $(5 \times 10^{-9}$ M) coincides with the concentration required for a half-maximal response (3). Whether or not this action of oxytocin has physiological significance remains to be determined.

Vasopressin has recently been shown to possess a wide range of activities in addition to its pressor and antidiuretic functions. Its ability to stimulate *in vivo* adrenocorticotropic hormone (ACTH) secretion in both man and animals has been well documented (6). Furthermore, several studies indicate that vasopressin stimulates the adenohypophysis directly (21). The ability of vasopressin to alter memory and/or learning in rats has been described by Walter et al. (20): a single injection of vasopressin increases resistance to extinction of a pole-jumping avoidance response in rats. A variety of metabolic functions in the liver can be altered by vasopressin, including glucose and lipid metabolism as well as the activities of pyruvate dehydrogenase and glycogen phosphorylase (7,8,10–12). These actions of vasopressin do not appear to be mediated by changes in cyclic adenosine monophosphate (AMP) concentrations.

Although oxytocin is generally considered the myotonic hormone, vasopressin has also been shown to stimulate milk-ejection (18) and uterine contraction (5). In fact, the nonpregnant uterus is sensitive to vasopressin rather than oxytocin (5). It has recently been suggested that the response to oxytocin is dependent on the concentration of specific oxytocin receptors, which appears to increase during pregnancy and/or lactation (14,17). Lastly, vasopressin has been reported to possess mitogenic properties when added to certain cell culture systems. Physiologic concentrations of vasopressin increase the growth rate of Hela cells (1) as well as 3T3 fibroblasts (16). The effect on Hela cells is decreased in the presence of glucocorticoids. These data suggested a clinical protocol involving vasopressin and glucocorticoids which appeared to result in the palliation of advanced breast cancer (2). We have recently reported the establishment of a cell line (WRK-1) from a dimethylbenz[a]anthracene (DMBA)-induced rat mammary tumor which responds to vasopressin and oxytocin (9,13). We would like to review the nature of this response in more detail.

WRK-1 CELLS

WRK-1 is a cloned cell line in continuous tissue culture derived from a (DMBA)-induced rat mammary tumor (9). The cells have epithelial morphology and many features characteristic of secretory cells of rodent mammary glands, such as tight junctions and gap junctions; however, they lack a significant number of desmosomes. Their ability to utilize D-valine in the absence of L-valine further supports their epithelial nature. Although the cells do not form tumors when injected into nude mice, they appear to be transformed. They have a modal chromosome number of 80 and do not exhibit contact inhibition. WRK-1 were initially cultured in medium supplemented with 10% fetal bovine serum and 5% rat serum. The cells have retained the requirement for both these sera throughout subculturing. Omission of either results in the death of the cells. The requirement for rat serum appears, at least in part, to be related to the high concentration of linoleic acid present in this serum (19 times that found in fetal bovine serum). In fact, replacement of rat serum with pure linoleic acid results in a growth rate approximately 75% of that seen with rat serum. Experiments with serum from hypophysectomized rats suggest that some pituitary factor may also affect the growth of WRK-1 cells, either directly or indirectly.

EFFECTS OF "PROLACTIN" ON WRK-1 CELLS

Because a majority of DMBA-induced rat mammary tumors are sensitive to prolactin, we initially tested this hormone for activity on WRK-1 cells. Figure 1 illustrates the effect of various concentrations of rat prolactin (B-1; obtained from A. F. Parlow, NIH) on acetate incorporation into lipids by WRK-1 cells. However, there were certain problems with the data: (a) The range of the dose–response curve was higher than that seen physiologically; (b) no binding of ^{125}I-labeled prolactin to WRK-1 cells could be detected; and (c) bovine growth hormone was as potent as prolactin in stimulating WRK-1 cells. Furthermore, activity of both prolactin and growth hormone was inversely related to the purity of the preparation. Further investigation indicated that it was not the

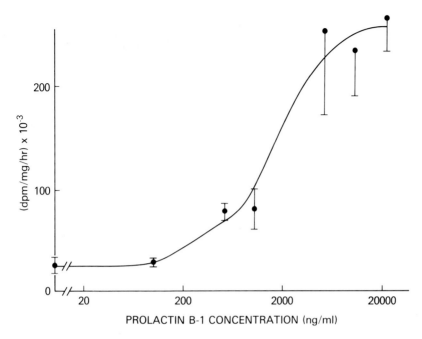

FIG. 1. Effect of rat "prolactin" preparation B-1 on incorporation of radioactate into lipids by WRK-1 cells. Values represent the means of triplicate determinations ± 1 SD. (From Monaco et al., ref. 13, with permission.)

prolactin, but rather the neurohypophysial hormone contamination of the prolactin preparation that was responsible for the observed activity (13). When low molecular weight components (<10,000 MW) were removed from the prolactin preparation by filtration, the residue had no activity, while all the original activity was recovered in the low molecular weight fraction. Furthermore, the activity of the low molecular weight fraction could be mimicked by vasopressin or oxytocin.

EFFECTS OF VASOPRESSIN ON WRK-1 CELLS

Figure 2 illustrates three effects of vasopressin on WRK-1 cells, namely (a) increased incorporation of [^{14}C]acetate into lipids, (b) increased incorporation of [^{32}P]orthophosphate into lipids, and (c) increased protein accumulation. While the effects on protein accumulation and acetate incorporation are delayed, the effect on orthophosphate incorporation is rapid. Concentrations of vasopressin required to elicit a response are in the range of 10^{-11} to 10^{-10} M. When the radiolabeled lipids from control and vasopressin-treated cells are analyzed, no difference is found in the distribution of individual fatty acids. In both cases, C-16 (50%) and C-18 (35%) fatty acids predominate (9). Furthermore, the majority of the labeled lipids are present as phospholipids (70%) rather than as the triglycerides characteristic of the lactating mammary gland. When the

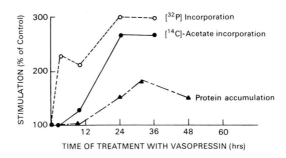

FIG. 2. Some effects of vasopressin on WRK-1 cells. Shown are incorporation of [^{32}P]orthophosphate and [^{14}C]acetate into lipids and accumulation of protein. Means ± SD (*N* = 3).

phospholipids are examined in detail by two-dimensional thin-layer chromatography, a greater degree of stimulation by vasopressin is routinely observed in the phosphatidylinositol and phosphatidylethanolamine fractions, than in the phosphatidylcholine fraction. The mechanisms by which vasopressin increases the labeling of WRK-1 lipids is not clear. Increases in the activities of both the fatty acid synthetic enzymes, acetyl CoA carboxylase and fatty acid synthetase, can be observed. Preliminary results indicate that stimulation of these enzyme activities occurs several hours before acetate incorporation is stimulated. Furthermore, while the presence of rat serum, or the lipid fraction from rat serum, inhibits the stimulatory effects of vasopressin on acetate incorporation, activities of fatty acid synthetic enzymes are maximal in serum.

SPECIFICITY OF THE RESPONSE OF WRK-1 CELLS TO VASOPRESSIN

To analyze the specificity of the response of WRK-1 cells to vasopressin, several other peptides were tested which are either structurally or bioactively similar to vasopressin. Results are seen in Fig. 3. Compounds of equal and maximal activity include lysine vasopressin, arginine vasopressin, and arginine vasotocin. Oxytocin is approximately 100 to 1,000 times less active than vasopressin. 1-Desamino-8-D-arginine-vasopressin (DDAVP), which has an antidiuretic to pressor ratio of 4,000 (15), is inactive on WRK-1 cells, as is the potent pressor peptide, angiotensin II. Both these compounds have previously been reported to lack milk-ejection activity (4,19). The findings suggest that the WRK-1 cells are myoepithelioid in nature.

IS VASOPRESSIN A MITOGEN FOR WRK-1 CELLS?

Growth effects of vasopressin have been described for Hela cells (2) and 3T3 cells (16). Although vasopressin increases protein accumulation and ^{32}P-

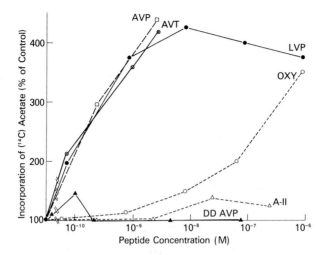

FIG. 3. Specificity of the response of WRK-1 cells to vasopressin. AVP, arginine vasopressin; LVP, lysine vasopressin; AVT, arginine vasotocin; DDAVP, 1-desamino-8-D-arginine-vasopressin; OXY, oxytocin; A-II, angiotensin II.

incorporation into phospholipids by WRK-1 cells, no mitogenic properties of the hormone have been noted. The growth rate of the cells is the same in rat serum obtained from rats with hereditary diabetes insipidus as it is in normal rat serum. To eliminate the possibility that unidentified serum factors were masking a mitogenic effect of vasopressin, a series of experiments was carried out in serum-free medium under conditions identical with those employed for stimulation experiments. Since the cells do not divide in the absence of serum, parameters other than cell number were used to assess mitogenicity. These included mitotic index and the incorporation of 5-bromo-2′-deoxyuridine (BUdR) into DNA as assessed by a differential staining technique. That new DNA is indeed synthesized under these conditions is suggested by two facts: (a) BUdR incorporation into DNA increases with time, and (b) ploidy increases with time. No effect of vasopressin is seen on either mitotic index or BUdR incorporation. Under identical conditions, insulin increases both these parameters in WRK-1 cells. Further experimentation will be necessary to determine the exact nature of the stimulatory effects of vasopressin on WRK-1 cells.

SUMMARY

Neurohypophysial hormones, particularly vasopressin, appear to have activities other than those traditionally ascribed to them. One of these involves interactions with mammary cancer cells, WRK-1. Whether or not these phenomena have any physiological significance remains to be determined. Initially, assessment of receptor binding activity in tumor samples will be investigated as a means of answering this question.

REFERENCES

1. Bernard-Weil, E., and da Lage, C. (1968): *Experientia,* 24:1001.
2. Bernard-Weil, E., and Pilleron, J. P. (1973): *Oncology,* 28:492–508.
3. Bonne, D., and Cohen, P., (1975): *Eur. J. Biochem.,* 56:295–303.
4. Brovetto, J., Olhaberry, J., Gioia de Coch, M. N., Coda, H., Fielitz, C., Cabot, H. M., Fraga, A., and Coch, J. A. (1967): *J. Endocrinol.,* 38:355–356.
5. Coutinho, E. M., and Lopes, A. V. C. (1968): *Am. J. Obstet. Gynecol.,* 102:479–489.
6. Gwinup, G. (1965): *Metabolism,* 14:1282–1286.
7. Hems, D. A., and Whitton, P. D. (1973): *Biochem. J.,* 136:705–709.
8. Hems, D. A., Whitton, P. D., and Ma, G. Y. (1975): *Biochim. Biophys. Acta,* 411:155–164.
9. Kidwell, W. R., Monaco, M. E., Wiche, M., and Smith, G. (1978): *Cancer Res.,* 38:4091–4100.
10. Kirk, C. J., and Hems, D. A. (1974): *FEBS Lett.,* 47:128–131.
11. Kirk, C. J., Rodrigues, L. M., and Hems, D. A. (1979): *Biochem. J.,* 178:493–496.
12. Kirk, C. J., Verrinder, T. R., and Hems, D. A. (1977): *FEBS Lett.,* 83:267–271.
13. Monaco, M. E., Lippman, M. E., Knazek, R. A., and Kidwell, W. R. (1978): *Cancer Res.,* 38:4101–4104.
14. Nissenson, R., Flouret, G., and Hechter, O. (1978): *Proc. Natl. Acad. Sci. USA,* 75:2044–2048.
15. Robinson, A. G. (1976): *N. Engl. J. Med.,* 294:507–511.
16. Rozengurt, E., Leggs, A., and Pettican, P. (1979): *Proc. Natl. Acad. Sci. USA,* 76:1284–1287.
17. Soloff, M. S., Alexandrova, M., and Feinstrom, M. J. (1979): *Science,* 204:1313–1314.
18. van Dongen, C. G., and Marshall, J. M. (1967): *Nature,* 213:632–633.
19. Vávra, I., Machová, A., Holeček, V., Cort, J. H., Zaoral, M., and Sorm, F. (1968): *Lancet,* 1:948–952.
20. Walter, R., VanKee, J. M., and de Wied, D. (1978): *Proc. Natl. Acad. Sci. USA,* 75:2493–2496.
21. Yasuda, N., Greer, M. A., Greer, S. E., and Panton, P., (1978): *Endocrinology,* 103:906–911.

Hormones and Cancer, edited by S. Iacobelli et al.
Raven Press, New York © 1980.

Control of Prolactin Receptors in Normal and Neoplastic Tissue

Paul A. Kelly, Lucile Turcot-Lemay, Lionel Cusan, Carl Séguin, Fernand Labrie, and *Jean Djiane

*MRC Group in Molecular Endocrinology, Hospital Center of the University of Laval, Quebec G1V 4G2, Canada; and *Laboratory of the Physiology of Lactation, National Institute of Agronomy Research, 78350 Jouy-en-Josas, France*

Prolactin, a pituitary hormone with numerous reported actions (8) is most commonly known for its stimulatory action on the mammary gland including mammogenesis, lactogenesis, and galactopoiesis. In addition to these well-known effects, prolactin has been characterized as a luteotrophic hormone involved in the maintenance of the corpus luteum in many species.

Binding of prolactin to specific receptors located in the plasma membrane of the cell is the first event in the action of this and other polypeptide hormones. Specific prolactin binding has been identified in crude membrane fractions of a number of tissues including chorioid plexus of the brain, liver, kidney, mammary gland, mammary tumor, adrenal, ovary, testis, prostate, seminal vesicle, and uterus (12,27,46,59,70,71).

In this chapter, we will describe the self-regulatory effect of prolactin on its own receptor and discuss mechanisms by which treatment with luteinizing hormone-releasing hormone (LHRH) and its agonistic analogs reduce the growth of mammary tumors.

PROLACTIN RECEPTORS IN NORMAL MAMMARY GLANDS

The mammary gland is the primary target organ of prolactin. This tissue was in fact chosen for the development of a radioreceptor assay for lactogenic hormones (66). Prolactin receptors from the rabbit mammary gland were subsequently characterized (62), and solubilized and purified (63). One of the actions of prolactin in the mammary gland is the production of milk proteins. In both rabbit (20) and rat (53) mammary gland, prolactin has been shown to stimulate the production of casein messenger RNA. Antiserum prepared against purified prolactin receptors has been shown to inhibit by more than 90% the binding of [125I]prolactin to rabbit mammary tissue (65) as well as to prevent the prolactin-induced synthesis of casein from rabbit mammary explants (64). These studies

171

demonstrate the functional importance of the binding of prolactin to a specific receptor as the central event leading to hormone action.

Assay of Prolactin Receptors

For determining receptor density in a tissue, crude plasma membrane fractions are prepared by differential centrifugation, and ovine prolactin (oPRL) is iodinated to a low specific activity (20–60 μCi/μg). Prolactin binding is assayed by incubating receptors with labeled prolactin in the absence or presence of excess unlabeled prolactin and is often reported as a percentage of the total counts added. In addition, saturation or displacement curves can be derived from experiments on representative membrane preparations, and transformed data plotted according to Scatchard (61) yield affinity constants and binding capacities of the membranes.

In addition to the classic approach to measuring prolactin receptors, which involves differential centrifugation of a tissue homogenate and subsequent binding to the particulate membrane fraction, alternative approaches which allow determinations to be made on small biopsies have emerged. Costlow et al. (14) reported the use of 0.5-mm thick slices of tumor tissue. Even smaller samples can be utilized if frozen "microslices" are used (32). This involves cutting 20-μm slices of tumor on a cryostat and incubation of approximately eight slices (0.5 mm^2) with [^{125}I]oPRL as described for membrane fractions (39). Ongoing studies in our laboratory indicate that this technique is applicable to repeated determinations in the same tumor (Turcot-Lemay and Kelly, *unpublished observations*).

Receptor Levels During Pregnancy and Lactation

The concept that hormone receptors are not static systems, but change with the physiological state of the animal, is important in terms of the control of cellular activity. Recently, we measured prolactin receptors in the mammary gland of pregnant rabbits which had been pretreated for a 36-hr period with the dopamine agonist CB-154 (Sandoz Ltd., Basle) to lower circulating prolactin (24). This technique was effective because the rabbit does not produce a placental lactogen (36,47). Measurement of receptor levels revealed a gradual increase in receptor concentration until day 22 of gestation followed by a decline until parturition, and a marked increase in early lactation (24). Prolactin binding to rat mammary gland decreased between day 30 and 100 of age in virgin glands. Binding was low during pregnancy and increased during early lactation and declined following removal of litters (29). It has been demonstrated, however, that by simply removing the ovaries and the uterus (including placentae) 24 hr prior to sacrifice, a marked increase in prolactin binding was observed, indicating that a large proportion of receptors are saturated by the high levels of circulating placental lactogen (31). Prolactin binding under these circumstances increases as pregnancy progresses and remains elevated during lactation. Other groups reported a peak of prolactin binding on day 2 of lactation, after which receptor levels declined rapidly (9).

PROLACTIN RECEPTORS IN MAMMARY TUMORS

Binding sites for prolactin have been identified in the particulate membrane fraction of dimethylbenz[a]anthracene (DMBA) mammary tumors (39,70). These binding sites are specific for prolactin or other lactogenic hormones and have an affinity similar to that of the mammary gland. We have previously reported that higher prolactin binding was observed in those DMBA tumors that show the greater growth response to injected prolactin, suggesting that the level of the receptor may be important in determining the tissue response to prolactin.

In contrast to the importance of the pituitary for the maintenance of prolactin binding sites in rat liver (44,58), there was only a slight reduction in prolactin receptors from tumors of hypophysectomized, DMBA-treated rats (14).

Holdaway and Friesen (32) reported that it was not possible to differentiate prolactin-responsive from prolactin-dependent tumors by prolactin-receptor determination of biopsy samples, but that following either prolactin administration or prolactin suppression, prolactin-responsive tumors had higher prolactin-receptor levels. A combination of estradiol and prolactin-receptor levels has also been reported to predict the responsiveness to endocrine ablation more accurately than either receptor level alone (18).

In addition to DMBA-induced tumors, prolactin receptors have been identified and characterized in nitrosomethylurea (NMU)-induced mammary tumors (68,69). Prolactin receptors decline following ovariectomy and after treatment with antiestrogens, as we have shown to be true also in DMBA-induced tumors (37,38). Prolactin binding sites have also been measured in tumors from R3230AC rats (70) and GR mice (15).

If prolactin does stimulate human mammary tumors, the tissue should contain prolactin receptors, as is the case for other prolactin responsive tissues as well as for experimental mammary tumors (12,27,59,70,71). Holdaway and Friesen (33) have reported on the specific binding of prolactin to human breast tumors. Specific binding exceeding 1% of the added radioactivity (which the authors considered significant) occurred in 8 of 41 tumors (19.5%). For one tumor, enough material was present to perform a Scatchard plot analysis, and an affinity constant similar to that of other prolactin receptors was found (45,59).

Morgan et al. (54) have reported that out of 55 human breast tumors, 15 (27%) showed specific prolactin binding; of these tumors, 64% were prolactin-dependent in culture. Prolactin binding sites in human breast tumors were also localized immunohistochemically. Of 80 cases studied, 45 were prolactin-dependent in culture, whereas 30 showed positive staining for prolactin binding (19). In another study of 20 tumors, 70% were reported to have measurable prolactin binding capacity (67).

In our laboratory, we have examined over 500 biopsies of human mammary carcinoma, including both primary lesions and metastases. Our results indicate that slightly less than 50% of the tumors are potentially "prolactin-responsive" in the sense that they possess prolactin receptors. The role of prolactin in tumor development has recently been reviewed (41).

TUMOR GROWTH AND LHRH AGONISTS

LHRH and its agonistic analogs have potent pre- and postcoital contraceptive activity in female rats (5,7,11,34) and rabbit (30). We have previously shown that treatment of adult male rats with LHRH or its agonists leads to a marked loss of testicular LH and prolactin receptors accompanied by decreased testis, seminal vesicle, and prostate weight, as well as lowered testosterone levels (3, 4,51,56). It therefore occurred to us that the antifertility effects of LHRH agonists could also be mediated by a desensitization of the ovary. We confirmed the antifertility activity of the potent LHRH agonist [D-Ala^6,des-Gly-NH$_2$^{10}]LHRH ethylamide. Animals injected starting on day 7 of pregnancy four times a day with 25 μg of the LHRH agonist showed an almost complete loss of ovarian LH receptors measured on days 10, 12, and 18, and a 45 to 60% decline in plasma progesterone levels coincident with an almost complete resorption of fetuses (48). A similar inhibitory effect of the LHRH agonist on ovarian gonadotropin receptors was observed in cycling female rats (49).

In view of the fact that LHRH agonists have been shown to be as effective as ovariectomy or antiestrogen treatment in reducing the growth and devel-

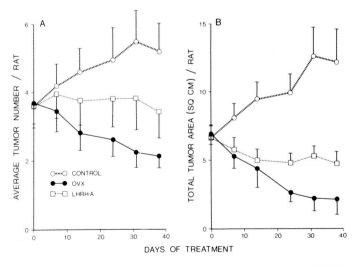

FIG. 1. Effect of ovariectomy (OVX) or treatment with 1 μg/day of an LHRH-like agonist (LHRH-A) on average tumor number **(A)** and total tumor mass **(B)** in rats with established DMBA-induced mammary tumors. Treatment was continued for 38 days (for details see text).

opment of DMBA-induced mammary tumors in the rat (16,17,25,35,55), we investigated the mechanisms by which a potent LHRH agonist [D-Ala[6],des-Gly-NH$_2$[10]]LHRH ethylamide induced a regression of tumor growth.

Rats with established DMBA-induced tumors (120 days after carcinogen administration) were divided into three groups, each with approximately equal tumor number and size. One group of 17 rats served as a control, a second group of 16 rats was ovariectomized and the final group (17 rats) received daily subcutaneous injections of the LHRH analog at a dose of 1 μg/day in 1% gelatin—0.9% NaCl for 38 days.

Figure 1 shows the effect of ovariectomy and treatment with the LHRH agonist on tumor number (Fig. 1A) and total tumor size per rat (Fig. 1B). Tumor number and size of control rats increased steadily throughout the study. Ovariectomy resulted in a marked reduction in both tumor number and total mass. Administration of the LHRH agonist also caused a reduction in tumor number and a 60% reduction in total mass compared with control values. When only primary tumors are considered, the LHRH agonist resulted in a 38% reduction in the number of tumors present at the beginning of the study, compared with a 45% decline in the ovariectomized group (data not shown).

The hormone responsiveness of the tumors was assessed by measuring receptor concentrations for estradiol, progesterone, and prolactin in tumor tissue (2). Ovariectomy resulted in a marked reduction in the number of receptors for these three hormones (Fig. 2). Treatment with the LHRH-like agonist was

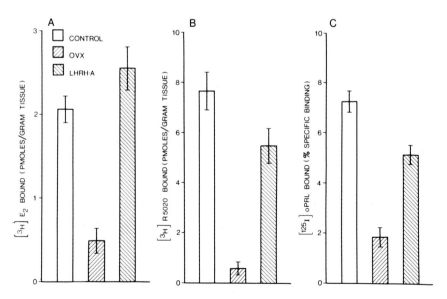

FIG. 2. Effect of ovariectomy (OVX) or treatment with LHRH-A (1 μg/day) on the specific binding of [^{3}H]E$_2$ **(A)**, [^{3}H]R5020 **(B),** and [^{125}I]oPRL **(C)** to DMBA-induced mammary tumors from rats treated for 38 days.

without significant effect on binding of $[^3H]E_2$ (Fig. 2A), whereas $[^3H]R5020$ binding (Fig. 2B) was reduced from 7.6 ± 0.7 to 5.5 ± 0.7 pmoles/g tissue ($p < 0.05$) and $[^{125}I]oPRL$ binding (Fig. 2C) declined from 7.2 ± 0.4 to $5.1 \pm 0.4\%$ ($p < 0.05$).

The reduction in tumor growth in response to treatment with LHRH-like agonists (see above) may partially be explained by these reductions in the concentration of progesterone and prolactin receptors in the tumors. However, a more direct effect of the LHRH-like agonist involves a desensitization effect at the pituitary and ovarian levels. A marked decrease in ovarian LH and follicle stimulating hormone (FSH) receptor levels was accompanied by a decline in circulating estradiol and progesterone, as well as a reduction in circulating prolactin concentrations (data not shown).

These studies confirm the antitumor effect of LHRH agonists on the growth of DMBA-induced mammary tumors. The mechanism of the inhibitory effect appears to be a "functional castration" subsequent to ovarian desensitization.

DISSOCIATION OF BOUND ENDOGENOUS PROLACTIN

As a result of elevated plasma levels of prolactin or other lactogenic hormones, often exceeding 1 μg/ml, during pregnancy (36,47) or during a spontaneous afternoon surge (43), a certain fraction of the prolactin receptors in a target cell may be occupied with endogenous prolactin. Although the procedure of homogenization and membrane fractionation offers the opportunity for prolactin to dissociate from its binding sites, a large portion of the prolactin still remains bound to the receptors. It thus became of interest to develop a technique to remove bound endogenous prolactin.

Two possible approaches have been developed. The first involved an *in vivo* desaturation of the prolactin receptor by lowering the circulating level of plasma prolactin for a short period of time prior to removal of the tissue. We have successfully applied this approach to the quantitation of prolactin receptors in the mammary gland of the rabbit during pregnancy (24).

The second technique involves an *in vitro* dissociation of the hormone from the receptor (42). Several chiotropic agents were examined, including high molar concentrations of magnesium chloride, manganous chloride, ammonium thiocyanate and sodium trifluoroacetate, as well as urea or acidic or basic pH. Most of these agents were capable, with greater or lesser effectiveness, of removing $[^{125}I]$-labeled prolactin from the receptors. Few, however, maintained the integrity of the receptor. Magnesium chloride at a concentration of 3 to 4 M was capable of removing 90 to 95% of the labeled hormone from rabbit mammary gland or rat liver prolactin receptors. When the receptors are reexposed to fresh labeled prolactin, they retained their ability to specifically bind prolactin (42). This procedure may also be useful for the quantification of prolactin receptor levels in situations where levels of lactogenic hormones are sufficiently high to interfere with prolactin binding.

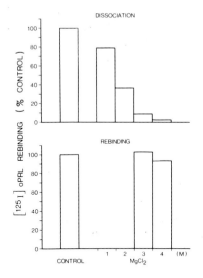

FIG. 3. Effect of increasing concentrations of MgCl$_2$ on the dissociation **(top)** and rebinding **(bottom)** of [^{125}I]oPRL to DMBA-induced mammary tumors. Crude membrane fractions (300 μg protein) were incubated with 104,000 cpm labeled prolactin of which 8,200 cpm were specifically bound by the control (H$_2$O-treated) tubes. Dissociation and rebinding were performed within the same tube.

The technique is effective in removing endogenous prolactin from liver or mammary tissue, as well as from mammary tumors. The effect of increasing concentrations of MgCl$_2$ on the dissociation and rebinding of prolactin receptors in DMBA-induced mammary tumors is shown in Fig. 3. Concentrations of 3 or 4 M were most efficient in removing bound [^{125}I]oPRL (Fig. 3, *top*). The 3 M concentration was slightly less damaging to the receptor in that maximal rebinding with fresh [^{125}I]oPRL was observed at this molarity (Fig. 3, *bottom*).

EFFECT OF PROLACTIN ON ITS OWN RECEPTOR

Up-Regulation

The hormonal regulation of prolactin receptors is complex (40). Estradiol injection into male or female rats leads to an increase in hepatic prolactin binding sites (44,57). Prolactin binding can be stimulated by estrogens, changes with the stage of the estrous cycle, and is reduced by ovariectomy. These findings imply a direct physiological involvement of estradiol.

The loss of prolactin binding in rat liver following hypophysectomy implied the importance of a pituitary factor in the maintenance of these binding sites (44,57). A direct effect of prolactin on its own receptor was first implied when we demonstrated that prolactin binding to rat liver in hypophysectomized rats given a pituitary implant under the kidney capsule began to increase approximately 3 days following the increase in serum prolactin levels (58). Costlow et al. (13) have also shown that direct administration of 2 mg prolactin to hypophysectomized female rats increased prolactin binding in rat liver.

The effect of androgen administration to both males and females results in a reduction of prolactin binding to rat liver (43). In that study, testosterone and dihydrotestosterone (DHT) reduced basal as well as estrogen-stimulated prolactin binding without affecting plasma prolactin levels.

Other groups have failed to see a stimulatory effect of estrogens on mammary gland prolactin receptors (31) whereas prolactin itself has been shown to stimulate, and progesterone to inhibit, prolactin binding in lactating rabbit mammary glands (23).

This discussion has dealt primarily with prolactin receptors in mammary gland and rat liver. However, the control of prolactin receptors is not uniform in all prolactin-responsive tissues. This point is best illustrated by the rat ventral prostate, which has abundant prolactin receptors (61). Castration of male rats results in a reduction of prolactin receptor number in the prostate (1,50) but an increase in the liver, and androgens have been shown to be inhibitory to hepatic prolactin binding (43). On the other hand, prolactin receptors in the prostate are enhanced in animals injected with testosterone proprionate or DHT (10,50) and hepatic prolactin binding is reduced (43).

Down-Regulation

Using 4 M MgCl$_2$ to dissociate bound prolactin from its receptor, we have investigated the short-term action of prolactin on its receptor in target tissues with the goal of evaluating whether prolactin, in addition to its ability to up-regulate prolactin receptors (23,58), is capable, like most other hormones studied thus far (28,52), of inducing a down-regulation of its own receptor. This in turn would lend some support to recent views (60) contending that down-regulation (and possibly up-regulation as well) are ubiquitous events which might be intimately linked to the very mechanism of hormone action.

Lactating New Zealand rabbits were injected every 12 hr over a 36-hr period with 2 mg of the dopamine agonist CB-154 (Sandoz Ltd.) to lower circulating prolactin levels (24) and were then anesthetized with 50 mg/kg of sodium pentobarbital. Three milligrams bovine prolactin was injected intravenously and 2-g biopsies of mammary gland tissue were removed at the times indicated in Fig. 4, between 0 and 30 hr after prolactin injection. As seen in Fig. 4, injection of 3 mg of prolactin led to a maximal occupancy of free rabbit mammary gland prolactin receptors 15 min after the intravenous injection. The highest serum prolactin levels were seen 1 min after injection, with values rapidly declining thereafter (data not shown). Although saturating concentrations of circulating prolactin were present 15 min after injection, 20% of the prolactin receptors remained free to bind [^{125}I]oPRL. This could be due to an inaccessibility of the receptors to the circulating prolacton or to some dissociation occurring while membranes were isolated from the tissues.

Somewhat surprisingly, total prolactin receptor levels assayed following *in vitro* desaturation with 4 M MgCl$_2$ declined progressively up to 6 hr after the intravenous injection of prolactin and returned to normal at 24 to 30 hr. The

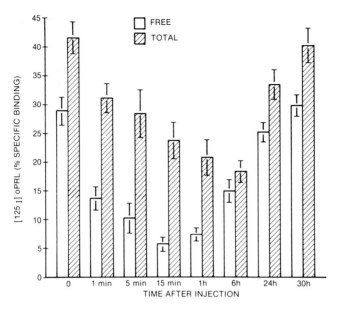

FIG. 4. Effect of an i.v. injection of 3 mg bovine prolactin on prolactin receptors in rabbit mammary glands. The rabbits were pretreated for 36 hr with CB-154 (Sandoz, Ltd.). Biopsies (2 g) were removed at the indicated times after prolactin injection from lactating rabbits. Free and total (MgCl$_2$-treated) prolactin receptor levels were determined. Binding is expressed as percentage of specific binding per 400 μg protein. Values are means $\pm$ SEM of 7 animals.

difference in total prolactin binding between time 0 and 6 hr was statistically significant ($p < 0.01$). A difference was observed between the time-course of changes in occupancy (i.e., proportion of free receptors) and of the down-regulation reflected by total receptor concentration: free receptors increased between 1 and 6 hr, whereas total receptors continued to decline until 6 hr (21).

It has been well established that the mammary gland can be maintained in organ culture and responds well to hormones (6,26). In addition, mammary explants can be used as an experimental model to study the steps involved in the mechanisms of hormone action (20). The following study was undertaken to verify the maintenance of prolactin receptors in mammary glands in organ culture, to assess the apparent turnover of receptors and to describe the effect of large doses of prolactin on the levels of its own receptor.

Figure 5A illustrates the maintenance of prolactin receptors (measured using [^{125}I]hGH) in mammary gland explants cultured in the presence of insulin. Binding increased slightly during the first 12 hr and remained constant to 48 hr (22). Addition of cycloheximide (1 μg/ml) resulted in a rapid decline of binding during the first 6 hr to a low level maintained until 48 hr. Figure 5B shows another experiment and demonstrates the reversibility of the effect of cycloheximide (1 μg/ml). In the presence of insulin only, the level of receptors was maintained up until 48 hr as shown previously. The addition of cyclohexi-

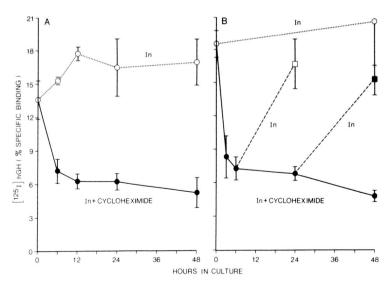

FIG. 5. Maintenance of prolactin receptors and the effect of cycloheximide on prolactin receptors in rabbit mammary gland explants. **A:** Mammary explants were cultured for different times in the presence of insulin (In) or In + cycloheximide. **B:** Mammary explants cultured in the presence of In + cycloheximide after which media were changed at 6 or 24 hr and the cycloheximide was removed. Prolactin receptors were measured using [^{125}I]hGH. Values are means ± SEM of three cultures.

mide resulted in a rapid decrease of receptors approaching a minimum at 3 hr. Removal of cycloheximide from the culture medium at either 6 or 24 hr resulted in a return of prolactin binding to near control levels within 18 to 24 hr.

A down-regulation of prolactin receptors in rabbit mammary gland in organ culture has also been observed. Inclusion of prolactin (5 µg/ml) in the incubation medium resulted in 80% saturation of free receptors. As observed *in vivo*, total receptor concentration measured following treatment of the membranes with 4 M $MgCl_2$ was markedly reduced, viz. from 12.3 ± 1.3 to 4.4 ± 0.8%, suggesting a down-regulation of prolactin receptors by prolactin (data not shown).

SUMMARY

Prolactin receptors are abundant in normal mammary tissue as well as in several experimental mammary tumor models. Hormone-dependent DMBA-induced mammary tumors are one of the most well-characterized models. Potent agonistic analogs of LHRH have been shown to markedly reduce tumor growth and development, similar to results seen following ovariectomy or antiestrogen treatment. The present studies confirm the antitumor activity of LHRH-like agonists and indicate that the mechanism by which these agonists inhibit tumor growth involves a "functional castration" subsequent to ovarian desensitization.

The regulation of prolactin receptor concentrations in various target tissues is complex. Prolactin has been clearly shown to have an up-regulatory or stimulatory activity on its own receptor level in both rabbit mammary gland and rat liver. Following the development of a technique to remove endogenous prolactin from receptors without destroying receptors, we have been able to demonstrate a transient down-regulation of prolactin receptors both *in vivo* and *in vitro*. In addition, using mammary explants, we have shown that prolactin receptors appear to have a relatively rapid rate of turnover, based on the rate of receptor replenishment following removal of cycloheximide. The role of this rapid turnover as well as the down-regulation and possible internalization of prolactin receptors remains to be elucidated.

REFERENCES

1. Aragona, C., and Friesen, H. G. (1975): *Endocrinology,* 97:677–684.
2. Asselin, J., Kelly, P. A., Caron, M. G., and Labrie, F. (1977): *Endocrinology,* 101:666–671.
3. Auclair, C., Kelly, P. A., Coy, D. H., Schally, A. V., and Labrie, F. (1977): *Endocrinology,* 101:1890–1893.
4. Auclair, C., Kelly, P. A., Coy, D. H., and Schally, A. V. (1977): *Biochem. Biophys. Res. Commun.,* 76:855–862.
5. Banik, U. K., and Givner, M. L. (1975): *J. Reprod. Fertil.,* 44:87–94.
6. Barnawell, E. B. (1965): *J. Exp. Zool.,* 160:189–206.
7. Beattie, C. W., and Corbin, A. (1977): *Biol. Reprod.,* 16:333–339.
8. Bern, H. A., and Nicoll, C. S. (1968): *Recent Prog. Horm. Res.,* 24:681–713.
9. Bohnet, H. G., Gomez, F., and Friesen, H. G. (1977): *Endocrinology,* 101:1111–1121.
10. Charreau, E. H., Attramadal, A., Torjesen, P. A., Calandra, R., Purvis, K., and Hanson, V. (1977): *Mol. Cell. Endocrinol.,* 7:1–7.
11. Corbin, A., Beattie, C. W., Yordley, J., and Toell, T. J. (1976): *Endocrine Res. Commun.,* 2:359–376.
12. Costlow, M. E., Buschow, R. A., and McGuire, W. L. (1974): *Science,* 184:85–86.
13. Costlow, M. E., Bushcow, R. A., and McGuire, W. L. (1975): *Life Sci.,* 14:1457–1466.
14. Costlow, M. E., Buschow, R. A., and McGuire, W. L. (1976): *Cancer Res.,* 36:3941–3943.
15. Costlow, M. E., Sluyser, M., and Gallagher, P. E. (1977): *Endocrine Res. Commun.,* 4:285–294.
16. Danguy, A., Legros, N., Heuson-Stiennon, J. A., Pasteels, J. L., Atassi, G., and Heuson, J. C. (1977): *Eur. J. Cancer,* 13:1089–1094.
17. DeSombre, E. R., Johnson, E. S., and White, W. F. (1976): *Cancer Res.,* 36:3830–3833.
18. DeSombre, E. R., Kledzik, G. S., Marshall, S., and Meites, J. (1976): *Cancer Res.,* 36:354–358.
19. De Souza, I., Hobbs, J. R., Morgan, L., and Salih, H. (1977): *J. Endocrinol.,* 73:71P.
20. Devinoy, E., Houdebine, L. M., and Delouis, C. (1978): *Biochim. Biophys. Acta,* 517:360–366.
21. Djiane, J., Clauser, H., and Kelly, P. A. (1979): *Biochem. Biophys. Res. Commun.,* 90:1371–1378.
22. Djiane, J., DeLouis, C., and Kelly, P. A. (1979): *Proc. Soc. Exp. Biol. Med.,* 162:342–345.
23. Djiane, J., and Durand, P. (1977): *Nature,* 266:641–643.
24. Djiane, J., Durand, P., and Kelly, P. A. (1977): *Endocrinology,* 100:1348–1356.
25. Dutta, A. S., Furr, B. J. A., Giles, M. B., Valcaccia, B., and Walpole, A. L. (1978): *Biochem. Biophys. Res. Commun.,* 81:382–390.
26. Forsyth, I. A. (1971): *J. Dairy Res.,* 28:419–444.
27. Frantz, W. L., MacIndoe, J. H., and Turkington, R. W. (1974): *J. Endocrinol.,* 60:485–497.
28. Gavin, J. R., Roth, J., Neville, D. M., De Meytes, P., and Buell, D. N. (1974): *Proc. Natl. Acad. Sci. USA,* 71:84–88.
29. Hayden, T. J., Bonney, R. C., and Forsyth, I. A. (1979): *J. Endocrinol.,* 80:259–269.
30. Hilliard, J., Pang, C. N., and Sawyer, C. H. (1976): *Fertil. Steril.,* 27:421–425.

31. Holcomb, H. H., Costlow, M. E., Buschow, R. A., and McGuire, W. L. (1976): *Biochim. Biophys. Acta,* 428:104–112.
32. Holdaway, I. M., and Friesen, H. G. (1976): *Cancer Res.,* 36:1562–1567.
33. Holdaway, I. M., and Friesen, H. G. (1977): *Cancer Res.,* 37:1946–1952.
34. Humphrey, R. R., Windsor, B. L., Bousley, F. G., and Edgren, R. A. (1976): *Contraception,* 14:625–629.
35. Johnson, E. S., Seely, J. H., White, W. F., and De Sombre, E. R. (1976): *Science,* 194:329–330.
36. Kelly, P. A. (1976): In: *Proceedings of the Vth International Congress of Endocrinology, Vol. 2,* edited by V. H. T. James, pp. 298–302. Excerpta Medica, Amsterdam.
37. Kelly, P. A., Asselin, J., Caron, M. G., Labrie, F., and Raynaud, J. P. (1977): *J. Natl. Cancer Inst.,* 58:623–628.
38. Kelly, P. A., Asselin, J., Caron, M. G., Raynaud, J. P., and Labrie, F. (1977): *Cancer Res.,* 37:76–81.
39. Kelly, P. A., Bradley, C., Shiu, R. P. C., Meites, J., and Friesen, H. G. (1974): *Proc. Soc. Exp. Biol. Med.,* 146:816–819.
40. Kelly, P. A., Ferland, L., and Labrie, F. (1978): In: *Progress in Prolactin Physiology and Pathology,* edited by C. Robyn and M. Harter, pp. 59–68. Elsevier/North-Holland, Amsterdam.
41. Kelly, P. A., Labrie, F., and Asselin, J. (1979): In: *Influences of Hormones in Tumor Development,* edited by J. A. Kellen and R. Hilf, pp. 157–194. CRC Press, Boca Raton, Florida.
42. Kelly, P. A., Leblanc, G., and Djiane, J. (1979): *Endocrinology,* 104:1631–1638.
43. Kelly, P. A., Leblanc, G., Ferland, L., Labrie, F., and De Léan, A. (1977): *Mol. Cell. Endocrinol.,* 9:195–204.
44. Kelly, P. A., Posner, B. I., and Friesen, H. G. (1975): *Endocrinology,* 97:1408–1515.
45. Kelly, P. A., Posner, B. I., Tsushima, T., and Friesen, H. G. (1974): *Endocrinology,* 96:532–539.
46. Kelly, P. A., Posner, B. I., Tsushima, T., Shiu, R. P. C., and Friesen, H. G. (1974): In: *Advances in Human Growth Hormone Research,* edited by S. Raiti, pp. 567–584. Government Printing Office, Washington, D.C.
47. Kelly, P. A., Tsushima, T., Shiu, R. P. C., and Friesen, H. G. (1976): *Endocrinology,* 99:765–774.
48. Kledzik, G. S., Cusan, L., Auclair, C., Kelly, P. A., and Labrie, F. (1978): *Fertil. Steril.,* 29:560–564.
49. Kledzik, G. S., Cusan, L., Auclair, C., Kelly, P. A., and Labrie, F. (1978): *Fertil. Steril.,* 30:348–353.
50. Kledzik, G. S., Marshall, S., Campbell, G. A., Gelato, M., and Meites, J. (1976): *Endocrinology,* 98:373–378.
51. Labrie, F., Auclair, C., Cusan, L., Kelly, P. A., Pelletier, G., and Ferland, L. (1978): *Int. J. Androl. [Suppl.],* 2:303–318.
52. Lesinak, M. A., and Roth, J. (1976): *J. Biol. Chem.,* 251:3720–3729.
53. Matusik, R. J., and Rosen, J. M. (1978): *J. Biol. Chem.,* 253:2343–2347.
54. Morgan, L., Raggatt, P. R., de Souza, I., Salih, H., and Hobbs, J. R. (1977): *J. Endocrinol.,* 73:17P.
55. Nicholson, R. I., Finney, E. J., and Maynard, P. V. (1978): *J. Endocrinol.,* 79:51P–52P.
56. Pelletier, G., Cusan, L., Auclair, C., Kelly, P. A., Désy, L., and Labrie, F. (1978): *Endocrinology,* 103:641–643.
57. Posner, B. I., Kelly, P. A., and Friesen, H. G. (1974): *Proc. Natl. Acad. Sci. USA,* 71:2407–2410.
58. Posner, B. I., Kelly, P. A., and Friesen, H. G. (1975): *Science,* 187:57–59.
59. Posner, B. I., Kelly, P. A., Shiu, R. P. C., and Friesen, H. G. (1974): *Endocrinology,* 96:521–531.
60. Posner, B. I., Raquidan, D., Josefsberg, Z., and Bergeron, J. M. (1978): *Proc. Natl. Acad. Sci. USA,* 75:3302–3306.
61. Scatchard, G. (1949): *Ann. NY Acad. Sci.,* 51:660–672.
62. Shiu, R. P. C., and Friesen, H. G. (1974): *Biochem. J.,* 140:301–311.
63. Shiu, R. P. C., and Friesen, H. G. (1974): *J. Biol. Chem.,* 249:7902–7911.
64. Shiu, R. P. C., and Friesen, H. G. (1976): *Science,* 192:259–261.
65. Shiu, R. P. C., and Friesen, H. G. (1976): *Biochem. J.,* 157:619–626.

66. Shiu, R. P. C., Kelly, P. A., and Friesen, H. G. (1973): *Science,* 180:698–971.
67. Stagner, J. I., Jochimsen, P. R., and Sherman, B. M. (1977): *Clin. Res.,* 25:302A.
68. Turcot-Lemay, L., and Kelly, P. A. (1980): *Cancer Res. (in press).*
69. Turcot-Lemay, L., and Kelly, P. A. (1980): *submitted for publication.*
70. Turkington, R. W. (1974): *Cancer Res.,* 34:758–763.
71. Walsh, R. J., Posner, B. I., Kopriwa, B. M., and Brawer, J. R. (1978): *Science,* 201:1041–1043.

Hormones and Cancer, edited by S. Iacobelli et al.
Raven Press, New York © 1980.

Protein Hormones and Prostatic Cancer

K. Griffiths, *W. B. Peeling, G. V. Groom, P. E. C. Sibley,
and M. E. Harper

*Tenovus Institute for Cancer Research, Welsh National School of Medicine, Cardiff
CF4 4XX, Wales; and *Department of Urology, St. Woolos Hospital,
Newport, Gwent, Wales*

The basis of most endocrine studies concerning the prostate gland has been the fact that its growth, maintenance, and functional activity are largely dependent on androgenic hormones secreted by the testis. Despite experimental work with animals which has suggested that pituitary hormones may influence prostatic growth and function, their involvement in tumor development is unproven. Certainly there is little direct evidence to implicate hormones in the initiation of prostatic cancer (6,21). One approach to the study of the interrelationships of protein hormones to prostatic tumors has been an examination of their effects on prostatic tissue biochemistry. An alternative approach more amenable to studies with the human has been to compare plasma hormone concentrations and their changes in response to various stimuli in patients with benign and malignant prostatic tumors and in asymptomatic controls of similar age. Inherent in all such studies is the possibility that endocrine factors influencing the course of the disease may have been critically different at a time long before the patient is seen in the clinic.

DIRECT EFFECTS ON THE PROSTATE GLAND

Early studies in animals indicated that pituitary hormones could influence prostatic growth and functioning. A greater degree of atrophy of the gland was noted after combined hypophysectomy and castration than after castration alone (10,15). Impaired uptake of testosterone by the ventral prostate was observed in hypophysectomized rats (13). Some discrepancies then ensued as to which of the protein hormones were able to stimulate prostatic growth. Lostroh and Li (15) found growth hormone (GH) and adrenocorticotropic hormone (ACTH) to be active, but not luteinizing hormone (LH), follicle stimulating hormone (FSH), and prolactin, while Tullner's (19) experiments indicate a role for ACTH and prolactin as stimulators of rat prostatic growth. Grayhack and Lebowitz (5) observed an augmented increase in the fructose and citric acid content of rat prostate when prolactin and testosterone were administered compared with that caused by testosterone alone. GH appeared to be complementary to prolactin and testosterone in increasing prostate weight (2). It is possible that the differences observed by the various investigators were a reflection of the heterogeneity of the pituitary hormone preparations used at that time. Experiments in our laboratory failed to show an effect of 30 days' treatment with 2-Br-α-ergocryptine, a prolactin secretion inhibitor, on prostatic weight, but a marked decrease in prostatic zinc content and cellular distribution was noted. The latter observation was consistent with earlier work on the effect of prolactin on zinc uptake into the prostate gland (7). Studies by several groups (4,12,14) have indicated that prolactin could influence the uptake of steroids into prostatic tissue, a factor of some importance when treating prostatic cancer patients with various endocrine therapies. There is no evidence that LH or FSH directly effect the prostate gland, but they can indirectly alter its growth and maintenance through their influence on testosterone and estradiol-17β production. Prolactin also appears to work synergistically with LH to increase testicular androgen production (8) and, interestingly, prolactin receptors have been demonstrated in testicular tissue (1). Both prolactin and ACTH can increase the availability of steroids to the prostate by increasing adrenal steroid biosynthesis (3,11).

PLASMA HORMONE CONCENTRATIONS

Measurement of plasma hormone concentrations in patients with prostatic cancer or benign prostatic hypertrophy (BPH) and in asymptomatic controls of the same age have been carried out in an attempt to delineate an endocrine abnormality in the prostatic tumor patients if such should exist. In our original study (9) we noted no significant difference in the protein hormone concentrations of cancer patients when compared with controls. A significantly higher level of prolactin was seen, however, when the cancer patients were compared with the BPH group. Subsequent studies have not consistently shown elevated values of prolactin in the cancer group, so a more detailed study was undertaken in order to see if there was a relationship between the hormone values obtained and the clinical staging of the patients. Table 1 shows the results obtained when patients were staged according to the UICC classification (20). Prolactin values did not correlate with either the primary tumor stage or metastatic status. GH concentrations were significantly higher in the metastatic group, but whether this is a consequence of increased stress and debilitating disease in these patients or a preexisting condition conducive to metastatic spread warrants further study. A wide variation in hormone values was noticed in all these studies and might be due to single sample determination of parameters which exhibit circadian or periodic variations. Changes in hormone concentrations throughout the day or night were therefore undertaken in a few BPH and prostatic cancer patients, as few data are available in subjects of this age. Blood was withdrawn from patients via an indwelling catheter at 30-min intervals over 12- or 24-hr periods. Large subject-to-subject variation in hormone levels were also encountered in this multiple sampling study, even within the same age group and disease category. An example of the differences can be seen in Fig. 1 in which data for

TABLE 1. *Plasma hormone concentrations in patients with prostatic carcinoma classified according to UICC*

Patient category	Statistic[a]	Age (yr)	Plasma hormone concentration			
			LH (U/liter)	FSH (U/liter)	GH (mU/liter)	Prolactin (U/liter)
Primary tumor stage						
T0	Mean	71	6.4	15.5	3.1	0.1
	SD	9.04	5.33	13.05	3.72	0.13
	N	24				
T1	Mean	68	6.7	16.9	1.6	0.1
	SD	7.07	5.28	10.07	2.44	0.09
	N	14				
T2	Mean	71	5.4	15.1	3.8	0.1
	SD	9.23	4.13	14.03	7.06	0.10
	N	31				
T3	Mean	70	8.2	16.8	2.5	0.1
	SD	7.86	8.09	17.27	3.49	0.11
	N	73				
T4	Mean	68	6.5	14.6	3.7	0.1
	SD	7.43	7.15	22.46	4.85	0.11
	N	21				
Metastatic status						
M1	Mean	71	6.0	11	4.0	0.19
	SD	8.4	4.75	14.7	4.09	0.13
	N	118				
M0	Mean	70	8.1	15	2.6	0.17
	SD	8.5	9.54	18.2	2.68	0.16
	N	79	64	65	62	62

[a] N = number of patients.

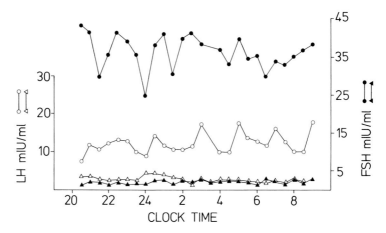

FIG. 1. Plasma gonadotropin concentrations measured at 30-min intervals in 2 patients with BPH: *circles,* patient H.R., age 71; *triangles,* patient S.B., age 69.

two patients with BPH are plotted. As prostatic tumor development is an age-dependent process, profound changes in hormone concentrations will occur because of testicular senescence, which in the human occurs over a large age range. Perhaps as a consequence of this, a comparison of rhythms and periodicity of plasma gonadotrophins in patients with prostatic cancer and BPH revealed no significant differences. This was also true of these patients' responses to LHRH injection.

PLASMA HORMONE CHANGES WITH ENDOCRINE THERAPY

Another aspect to be considered in the relationship of pituitary hormones and prostatic cancer is the alteration induced by various endocrine therapies which are designed to reduce androgen levels and thereby prostatic tumor growth (9). Typical profiles of testosterone and pituitary concentrations obtained with various therapies are illustrated in Fig. 2. It is interesting to consider that on one regimen, namely estrogen therapy (Fig. 2b), prolactin and GH levels are increased and gonadotropin levels are decreased, while on another regimen, orchidectomy (Fig. 2a), normal prolactin and GH concentrations exist but gonadotropins are significantly raised. The clinical response of patients in these two groups are similar, despite their vastly differing protein hormone milieux.

PROTEIN HORMONE LOCALIZATION IN PROSTATIC TISSUE

Another aspect of the association of pituitary hormones and prostatic tissue can be explored using immunocytochemistry. Visual localization of polypeptide

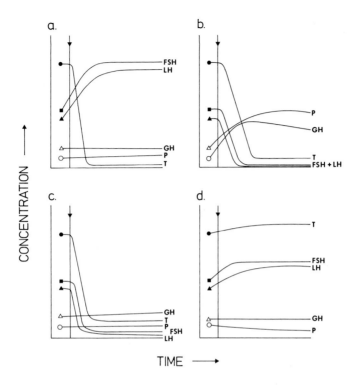

FIG. 2. General hormone profiles with various endocrine therapies. **a:** Orchidectomy; **b:** estrogen therapy; **c:** antiandrogen therapy; **d:** antiestrogen therapy. *Arrows* indicate commencement of therapy. P, prolactin; T, testosterone.

hormones in the pituitary gland by employing this technique is well established (16,17). Localization at the target tissue level is more difficult because of the much lower concentrations and success will largely depend on the specificity and titer of the antisera used. Results obtained using the method described by Sternberger (18) on sections of human prostate tumor with antisera raised against human FSH or GH or prolactin can be seen in Figs. 3 and 4. The staining obtained with the various antisera was different in tissue distribution. Staining with the FSH antiserum was mostly confined to the epithelial cell secretory margins and the prostatic secretion, while staining with the prolactin antiserum was present in some epithelial cells, and in stromal and blood cells. Predominantly stromal cell staining was obtained with the GH antisera, but occasionally a few cells were stained in the epithelial region. Only with the advent of monoclonal antisera raised against highly purified antigens will it be possible to equate staining with the presence of antigen at that site.

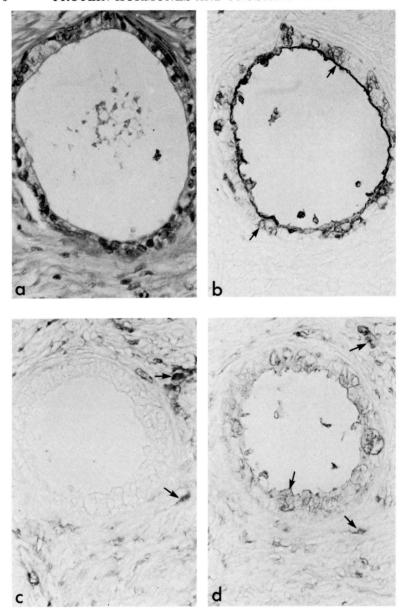

FIG. 3. Photomicrographs of consecutive sections of a single acinus from a patient with BPH (×289). **a:** Stained with hematoxylin and eosin. **b—d:** Immunocytochemical staining obtained with antisera raised against: **(b)** h.FSH (1/100), staining *(arrow)* seen predominantly in the epithelial cell region; **(c)** h.GH (1/100), staining seen in stromal cells; **(d)** h.Pr (1/500), staining appears in the cytoplasm of epithelial cells lining the acinus and also in the stroma.

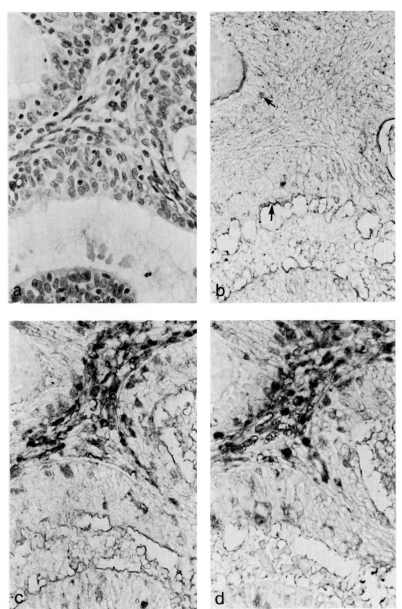

FIG. 4. Photomicrographs of consecutive sections of a block of tissue from a patient with benign, predominantly fibromuscular hypertrophy of the prostate (×289). **a:** Stained with hemotoxylin and eosin. **b—d:** Immunocytochemical staining obtained with antisera raised against **(b)** h.FSH, staining *(arrow)* associated with stromal areas and with the cell membrane; **(c)** h.GH, staining predominantly seen in cells of the stroma and occasionally in epithelial cells (stain also appears in the secretions); **(d)** h.Pr, distribution of stain as in (c).

ACKNOWLEDGMENTS

We are indebted to the Tenovus Organisation for financial support and also to the Gwent Hospital Contributory Fund for financial assistance in computer storage of data.

REFERENCES

1. Aragona, C., and Friesen, H. (1975): *Endocrinology,* 97:677–684.
2. Chase, M. D., Geschwind, I. I., and Bern, H. A. (1957): *Proc. Soc. Exp. Biol. Med.,* 94:680–683.
3. Cowley, T. H., Brownsey, B. G., Harper, M. E., Peeling, W. B., and Griffiths, K. (1976): *Acta Endocrinol. (Kbh.),* 81:310–320.
4. Farnsworth, W. E. (1975): *Urol. Res.,* 3:129–132.
5. Grayhack, J. T., and Lebowitz, J. M. (1967): *Invest. Urol.,* 6:87–94.
6. Griffiths, K., Davies, P., Harper, M. E., Peeling, W. B., and Pierrepoint, C. G. (1979): In: *Endocrinology of Cancer, Vol. 2,* edited by D. P. Rose, pp. 1–55. CRC Press, Boca Raton, Florida.
7. Gunn, S. A., Gould, T. C., and Anderson, W. A. D. (1965): *J. Endocrinol.,* 32:205–214.
8. Hafiez, A. A., Lloyd, C. W., and Bartke, A. (1972): *J. Endocrinol.,* 52:327–332.
9. Harper, M. E., Peeling, W. B., Cowley, T., Brownsey, B. G., Phillips, M. E. A., Groom, G., Fahmy, D. R., and Griffiths, K. (1976): *Acta Endocrinol. (Kbh.),* 81:409–426.
10. Huggins, C., and Russell, P. S. (1946): *Endocrinology,* 39:1–7.
11. Jones, T., Brownsey, B. G., Cowley, T. H., and Griffiths, K. (1974): In: *Tissue Culture in Medical Research,* edited by F. Facoby and K. T. Rajan, pp. 263–272. Heinemann, London.
12. Lasnitzki, I. (1972): In: *Prolactin and Carcinogenesis,* edited by A. R. Boyns and K. Griffiths, p. 200. Alpha Omega Alpha, Cardiff.
13. Lawrence, A. M., and Landau, R. L. (1965): *Endocrinology,* 73:1119–1125.
14. Lloyd, J. W., Thomas, J. A., and Mawhinney, M. G. (1973): *Steroids,* 22:473–483.
15. Lostroh, A. J., and Li, C. H. (1957): *Acta Endocrinol. (Kbh.),* 25:1–16.
16. Nakane, P. K. (1970): *J. Histochem. Cytochem.,* 18:1–20.
17. Sibley, P. E. C., Joyce, B., Groom, G. V., Chandler, J. A., and Griffiths, K. (1978): *J. Endocrinol.,* 77:58p–59p.
18. Sternberger, L. A. (1974): In: *Foundations of Immunology,* pp. 129–171. Prentice–Hall, Englewood Cliffs, New Jersey.
19. Tullner, W. W. (1963): In: *Nat. Cancer Inst. Monogr.,* 12:211–223.
20. Wallace, D. M., Chisholm, G. D., and Hendry, W. F. (1975): *Br. J. Urol.,* 47:1–12.
21. Wynder, E. L., Mabuchi, K., and Whitmore, W. F. (1971): *Cancer,* 28:344–360.

Hormones and Cancer, edited by S. Iacobelli et al.
Raven Press, New York © 1980.

Effects of Estradiol and Antiestrogens on Pituitary Hormone Production, Metabolism, and Pituitary Tumor Growth

*Ivan Nagy, Carlos A. Valdenegro, **Ivan S. Login, Frank A. Snyder, and Robert M. MacLeod

*Departments of Medicine and **Neurology, University of Virginia School of Medicine, Charlottesville, Virginia 22908*

That estradiol administration stimulates prolactin production has been well established. Studies from our laboratory (22) and others (5,9,30) have shown that estradiol increases *de novo* prolactin synthesis and secretion, probably by acting directly on the pituitary as well as on the hypothalamus. In more recent studies, estradiol increased both preprolactin mRNA and prolactin synthesis simultaneously and before increasing prolactin secretion (37–39). We have previously observed that pituitary prolactin synthesis and release are greatly decreased in rats bearing transplanted prolactin-secreting pituitary tumors, and that estradiol restores prolactin and RNA synthesis (27,28) and stimulates pituitary gland metabolism (31) in these rats. It is widely believed that estradiol promotes these effects by binding to specific estradiol receptor sites in steroid-sensitive tissue.

Antiestrogens are thought to block estrogens from binding to receptors, thus preventing the stimulating action of the steroid (2,8,12). Although the effects of nonsteroidal antiestrogens have been studied in several tissues (2,8,12,13, 18,33), their effects on pituitary hormone secretion have not been established. These drugs seem not to affect basal prolactin secretion (10,33), although they inhibit the estradiol-mediated and proestrous increases in hormone release (10,11,14,15). The studies described below further examine the effects of estrogens and antiestrogens on prolactin production by and some enzymatic parameters in normal pituitary glands and prolactin-secreting pituitary tumor cells.

MATERIALS AND METHODS

Animals and Treatments

Mature Sprague-Dawley rats were housed in a constant temperature room (22–23°C) under artificial illumination (6 A.M.–6 P.M.). Estradiol-17β (provided

---

* On leave from the Central Laboratory of the Pal Heim Pediatric Hospital, Budapest, Hungary.

by Cancer Chemotherapy National Service, Bethesda, Maryland) was dissolved in absolute ethanol and diluted with normal saline to final 10% ethanol concentration, and 2.0 μg in 0.2 ml was injected. Polyestradiol phosphate (Estradurin, Ayerst Laboratories, Inc., New York, New York) stock solution was diluted with normal saline and 100.0 μg in 0.2 ml was injected. A combination of estradiol and polyestradiol phosphate was injected to obtain an immediate and sustained effect of estrogens.

Nitromifene citrate (CI-628: 1,2-[p-α-(p-methoxyphenyl)-β-nitrostyrylphenoxy]ethyl-pyrolidine monocitrate; provided by Parke-Davis and Co., Ann Arbor, Michigan) was dissolved in water and 1.75 mg in 0.2 ml was injected. Tamoxifen   (1-p-β-dimethylaminoethoxyphenyl-trans-1,2-diphenylbut-1-ene; provided by Lois Trench, ICI Americas Inc., Wilmington, Delaware, and F. Borvendég, Pharmaceutical Research Institute, Budapest, Hungary) was dissolved in a small volume of absolute ethanol containing 10% Triton X-100, and diluted with sesame oil to a final concentration of 50 μg in 0.1 ml, at which the tamoxifen formed a homogeneous suspension of microcrystals. The antiestrogens were injected prior to estrogen administration to provide the best possible opportunity for them to compete for estrogen-sensitive sites.

Twenty-four hours after the last injection the animals were decapitated, their trunk blood collected for prolactin radioimmunoassay, and the pituitaries removed for *in vitro* study of prolactin and growth hormone production or biochemical analysis.

In Vitro Study of Prolactin and Growth Hormone Biosynthesis

After decapitation the anterior pituitaries were immediately bisected and incubated in 1.0 ml tissue culture Medium 199 with Hanks' balanced salt solution and l-glutamine modified with 1.4 sodium bicarbonate per liter (Microbiological Associates, Walkersville, Maryland) containing 10 μCi [4,5-³H]leucine (Amersham, Arlington Heights, Illinois) for 5 hr at 37°C under 95% O_2, 5% CO_2(vol/vol) in a Dubnoff shaker. After the incubation, aliquots of the medium and pituitary homogenates were separated on 7.5% acrylamide gel columns and the radioactivity of the prolactin, albumin, and growth hormone fractions was counted in a Beckman LS-233 liquid scintillation spectrometer. The total newly synthesized prolactin and growth hormone was computed as the sum of the amount released into the medium and that found in the pituitary tissue.

Radioimmunoassays

The prolactin contents of the serum, the incubated medium, and the incubated tissue were measured by a double antibody radioimmunoassay using materials and protocols supplied by the NIAMDD Rat Pituitary Hormone Distribution Program, using RP-1 prolactin as reference hormone.

Biochemical Analyses

Pituitary homogenate was prepared in ice-cold 0.05 M triethanolamine-HCl buffer, pH 7.5, for analyses as reported earlier (31). Kinetic measurements at 25°C based on the nicotinamide-adenine dinucleotide/reduced NAD (NAD/NADH) or nicotinamide-adenine dinucleotide phosphate/NADP hydrogenase (NADP/NADPH) transformations (3) were used to determine the activity of the following dehydrogenases: G6P-dehydrogenase (G6P-DH; D-glucose-6-phosphate: NADP oxidoreductase, EC 1.1.1.49), [pyruvate kinase (PK); adenosine triphosphate (ATP): pyruvate 2-o-phosphotransferase, EC 2.7.1.40], lactate dehydrogenase (LDH; L-lactate: NAD oxidoreductase, EC 1.1.1.27), isocitric dehydrogenase (ICDH; threo-D_s-isocitrate: NADP oxidoreductase, EC 1.1.1.42), and malate dehydrogenase (MDH; L-malate: NAD oxidoreductase, EC 1.1.1.37). Tartarate-inhibited acid phosphatase (orthophosphoric monoester phosphohydrolase, EC 3.1.3.2) was determined by a two-point method (3) using p-nitrophenylphosphate as substrate after 30 min incubation at 25°C. Coomassie brilliant blue G-250 was used for protein determinations (4).

Biochemical compounds were purchased from Boehringer Mannheim Company (Mannheim, West Germany) and Sigma Chemical Company (St. Louis, Missouri).

Tumor Cell Dispersions

Female Buffalo rats were inoculated with 7315a tumor homogenates in the scapular region as previously described (22). Isolated tumor cells were prepared by mincing 7315a tumor tissue in a Teflon® beaker containing 10 ml of Eagle basal solution (EBS), 5 μM dopamine, 57 μM ascorbic acid, and 20 mg trypsin (Worthington, Freehold, New Jersey) and stirred constantly with a teflon paddle at 350 to 400 rpm for 20 min at 37°C. The cell suspension supernatant was removed and the residue was treated again. The overall procedure was carried out four times. The cell suspensions were centrifuged at room temperature at 32 × g (400 rpm) for 45 min. The supernatant was discarded and the cells suspended in 1.0 ml of a solution of 0.4 mg/ml lima bean trypsin inhibitor (Worthington), 5 μM dopamine, and 57 μM ascorbic acid in EBS. Debris was removed by filtration through a nylon gauze (1 μm) and the cells were allowed to settle for 30 to 40 min. The supernatant was withdrawn carefully and the remaining cells were suspended in a total volume of 10 ml Medium 199. This procedure was repeated and the cells were resuspended in 5 ml of the same medium and filtered again through nylon gauze. The cells were suspended in Medium 199 and were counted in a Newbauer counting chamber; their viability was determined by trypan blue exclusion. To 1-ml aliquots of cell suspension, 10 μg bacitracin was added, and the cell suspensions were incubated in a Dubnoff shaker at 37°C in an atmosphere of 95% O_2, 5% CO_2. After incubation the medium and cells were separated by centrifugation at 3,500 × g for 10 min.

[³H]Estradiol Binding Studies

Rats were decapitated and the anterior pituitaries were removed and homogenized immediately in a 1-ml glass homogenizer with 0.5-ml TTG buffer (10 ml Tris-HCl and 10 ml thioglycerol, pH 7.4) in an ice bath as previously described (35) in preparation for estrogen receptor determination. Homogenates were centrifuged at 127,000 $\times$ g for 45 min and pellets discarded.

A specimen of tumor (0.5–0.8 g) was removed and frozen immediately by immersion in liquid nitrogen. The tissue was shattered at liquid nitrogen temperature and then homogenized with four times its weight of TTG buffer (pH 7.4) at 4°C. The homogenization was carried out for three 10-sec periods, allowing temperature to equilibrate with ice bath for 60 sec between pulses. Homogenates were centrifuged at 4,000 $\times$ g for 10 min at 4°C and pellets were discarded. Supernatant was centrifuged at 127,000 $\times$ g for 45 min and again pellet was discarded.

Aliquots (0.150 ml) of the cytosols were incubated at 4°C with either 0.45 pmole [³H]estradiol-17β, specific activity 141.67 Ci/mmole (New England Nuclear Corporation, Cambridge, Massachusetts) or 0.42 pmole [³H]estrogen-17β and 50 pmoles diethylstilbestrol in a total volume of 250 μl for 4 hr.

The incubations were quantitatively transferred with 0.1 ml TTG wash to tubes containing the pellet derived from 0.5 ml of a dextran-coated charcoal (DCC) suspension (0.024% dextran, 0.25% Norit A in TTG). Tubes were vortexed, incubated at 4°C for 10 min, and centrifuged at 250 $\times$ g for 10 min. Aliquots (0.10 ml) of supernatant were placed into Bio-Vials (Beckman) and dissolved in 3 ml triton-toluene scintillation counting fluid (5.5 g PPO, 0.15 g POPOP, 666 ml toluene, 333 ml Triton X-100). Counting efficiency was 50%.

In other studies aliquots of the cytosol after treatment with DDC were carefully layered on a 5-ml 10 to 30% sucrose gradient and centrifuged at 250,000 $\times$ g for 18 hr. Gradients were divided into 25 0.2-ml fractions, which were collected in Bio-Vials to which 3 ml of Triton-toluene scintillation fluid was added. The radioactivity in the tumor preparations was located entirely in the 8S region.

Results are expressed in femtomoles estradiol per milligram cytosol protein or femtomoles estradiol per milligram pituitary gland. Protein concentration was determined by the method of Waddell (40). All results are expressed as mean $\pm$ SEM and evaluated by analysis of variance.

RESULTS

Studies were designed to measure the binding of [³H]estradiol to rat pituitary glands and tumor cytosol protein, and where possible to correlate these findings with prolactin synthesis and release by a method previously described (1). These findings, expressed as femtomoles [³H]estradiol per milligram cytosol protein,

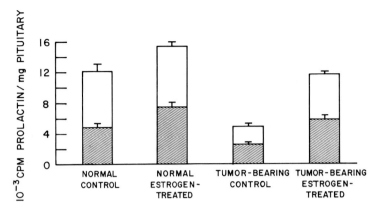

FIG. 1. Stimulation of *in vitro* prolactin synthesis *(shaded columns)* and release *(open columns)* in the anterior pituitary following estradiol injection. Female Buffalo rats were implanted with pituitary tumor 7315a. Six weeks later the rats were injected with 1 μg estradiol-17β and 100 μg polyestradiol phosphate and sacrificed 72 hr later. Pituitary glands were incubated with [³H]leucine; the incorporation of radioactive leucine into prolactin was measured as described in the text. Vertical brackets, SEM.

showed that pituitary gland and pituitary tumor 7315a bound 83.0 ± 12.8 and 101.5 ± 5.1, respectively. These pituitary tumors can be very large, weighing up to several grams. Thus they may provide a reservoir or "sink" for endogenous estradiol. Pituitary gland cytosol from pituitary tumor-bearing rats had 197.0 ± 11.2 fmoles [³H]estradiol/mg cytosol protein, 130% more than [³H]estradiol binding to control pituitary gland receptors ($p < 0.01$). This may help explain why pituitary glands from tumor-bearing rats synthesize and release less prolactin than do pituitary glands from normal rats.

The data in Fig. 1 show that pituitary glands from rats with 7315a tumors synthesize 60% less ($p < 0.01$) and release 76% less ($p < 0.01$) [³H]prolactin than do control glands. Treatment of nontumor rats with estradiol increased [³H]prolactin synthesis 26% ($p < 0.05$). This change represents [³H]prolactin retained within the pituitary; the steroid did not increase prolactin release. In contrast, estradiol treatment of rats with transplanted pituitary tumors increased synthesis and release of prolactin by 140% ($p < 0.01$). We believe that these findings are related to the increased ability of this tissue to bind estradiol. It is currently unknown whether this reflects an increase in the number of estrogen receptors in this gland or whether the large pituitary tumor, which functions as a "sink" for endogenous estrogen, deprives the pituitary gland of the steroid, thus causing the observed reduction in prolactin synthesis and release.

It has long been known that estradiol administration to rats increases serum prolactin concentration. We observed an increase from 51 ± 12 to 119 ± 18 ng/ml on day 3 following 1 μg estradiol-17β and 100 μg polyestradiol phosphate to intact female rats. The prolactin concentration in serum of rats with 7315a tumors was $2,080 \pm 285$ ng/ml; surprisingly, estrogen treatment as above in-

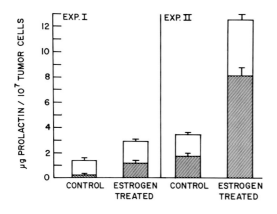

FIG. 2. Effect of *in vivo* estradiol injection on the prolactin concentration in pituitary tumor 7315a cells *(shaded columns)* and incubation medium *(open columns)* following incubation *in vitro* for 5 hr.

creased serum prolactin to 15,070 ± 3,410 ($p < 0.01$). This finding shows that estradiol can directly affect prolactin secretion by transplanted pituitary tumors.

The effect of estradiol administration on *in vitro* prolactin release by pituitary tumor cells was also studied. Pituitary tumor 7315a was cut into 1-mm³ pieces and further dispersed using trypsin. After harvesting and washing, the cells were incubated in tissue culture Medium 199 and radioimmunoassayable prolactin in medium and tumor cells was determined. The data in Fig. 2 show that tumor cell prolactin content and the amount released into the medium were significantly greater in cells obtained from estradiol-treated animals. Hence, one can conclude that estradiol stimulates normal and tumorous pituitary cells to synthesize and release prolactin.

To study the possible role of antiestrogens as modifiers of prolactin synthesis and release, tamoxifen and nitromifene citrate alone and in combination with estradiol were administered to male rats as described in Table 1. None of the treatments changed pituitary gland weight significantly. Estradiol produced a slight but significant ($p < 0.01$) increase in serum prolactin concentration. Nitromifene citrate did not affect basal serum prolactin, and reduced the increase

TABLE 1. *Schedule of estrogen and antiestrogen treatments to male rats[a]*

	Day of treatment					
Group	1	2	3	4	5	6
1. Control	—	—	—	—	—	Sacrifice
2. Estrogen	—	—	E_2	—	—	Sacrifice
3. Nitromifene citrate	—	NC	—	—	—	Sacrifice
4. Tamoxifen	TX	TX	TX	TX	TX	Sacrifice
5. Estrogen + nitromifene citrate	—	NC	E_2	—	—	Sacrifice
6. Estrogen + tamoxifen	TX	TX	TX + E_2	TX	TX	Sacrifice

[a] Injections were given s.c. at doses indicated in the text. Where no treatment is indicated, the animals received 0.1 ml sesame oil. NC, nitromifene citrate; TX, tamoxifen; E_2, estradiol.

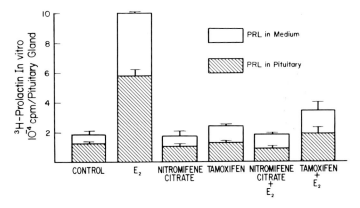

FIG. 3. Effect of *in vivo* estradiol and antiestrogen administration on the *in vitro* synthesis and release of [³H]prolactin by the anterior pituitary.

produced by estradiol slightly and insignificantly. Tamoxifen had no effect either on basal serum prolactin or on the increase produced by estradiol.

Figure 3 presents data on the effect of antiestrogens on [³H]prolactin synthesis and release in these rats. In contrast to the moderate estradiol-induced stimulation of [³H]prolactin synthesis in female rats, hormone synthesis by pituitary glands from male rats was increased fivefold. Although the treatment stimulated primarily [³H]prolactin synthesis, *in vitro* release of the radioactive hormone was also significantly increased. Radioimmunoassayable prolactin contained in the pituitary gland and that released into the incubation medium were also stimulated by the steroid (Fig. 4). Neither nitromifene citrate nor tamoxifen altered basal prolactin synthesis and release at the doses used in these studies. However, both of these antiestrogens markedly inhibited the stimulation of prolactin synthesis and release produced by estradiol. Higher doses of these drugs

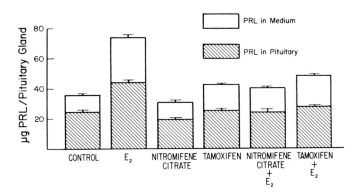

FIG. 4. Effect of *in vivo* estradiol and antiestrogen administration on the *in vitro* synthesis and release of radioimmunoassayable prolactin by the anterior pituitary.

TABLE 2. *Effect of estrogen and antiestrogen administration on growth hormone synthesis and release* in vitro, *measured by [³H]leucine incorporation*[a]

Group	10^{-3} cpm/mg Anterior pituitary		
	Pituitary gland	Medium	Total synthesis
1. Control	17.9 ± 1.6	1.6 ± 0.05	19.5 ± 1.6
2. Estrogen	16.2 ± 0.7	1.4 ± 0.05	17.6 ± 0.7
3. Nitromifene citrate	12.5 ± 0.6[b]	2.2 ± 0.2[c]	14.7 ± 0.8[b]
4. Tamoxifen	13.5 ± 0.8	1.6 ± 0.1	15.1 ± 0.9[b]
5. Estrogen + nitromifene citrate	10.3 ± 0.7[d,e]	1.8 ± 0.1[e]	12.1 ± 0.9[c]
6. Estrogen + tamoxifen	12.3 ± 1.5[c,d]	1.4 ± 0.1	13.7 ± 1.5[c,e]

[a] Mean $\pm$ SEM. Statistical analysis by analysis of variance. Three hemipituitaries per flask, four flasks per group.
[b] $p < 0.05$ versus controls.
[c] $p < 0.01$ versus controls.
[d] $p < 0.05$ versus estrogen group.
[e] $p < 0.01$ versus estrogen group.

produced a significant stimulation of prolactin synthesis and release, indicating that they have significant inherent estrogenic properties.

The effects of estradiol and antiestrogens on growth hormone contrast with those on prolactin. The data in Table 2 show that estradiol injection to male rats did not influence *in vitro* synthesis or release of growth hormone. Pituitary glands from nitromifene citrate- but not tamoxifen-treated rats showed significantly reduced growth hormone synthesis. When injected in combination with estradiol, both antiestrogens caused a significant decrease in growth hormone synthesis. The present findings contrast with those of others who reported that antiestrogenic agents increase growth hormone production in pituitary glands (11) and in clonal strains of rat pituitary cells (6). The reason for this discrepancy is unknown.

We next examined pituitary tumor sensitivity to antiestrogens. Animals bearing pituitary tumors were injected with 25 μg/100 g body weight tamoxifen daily for several days. Rate of tumor growth decreased in rats receiving this treatment (Fig. 5). However, no significant decrease in serum prolactin concentration was observed. The data in Fig. 6 show that dispersed tumor cells from tamoxifen-treated rats contain slightly less prolactin than do controls (the difference is not significant). Tamoxifen had no effect on *in vitro* prolactin release by pituitary tumor cells.

An attempt was made to correlate these estrogen-induced endocrinological changes with metabolic markers in pituitary gland and tumors. Normal female rats and females bearing prolactin-secreting tumor 7315a were injected with 1.0 μg estradiol-17β and 100 μg polyestradiol phosphate and sacrificed 72 hr later. The data in Table 3 show that the weight of the glands from normal

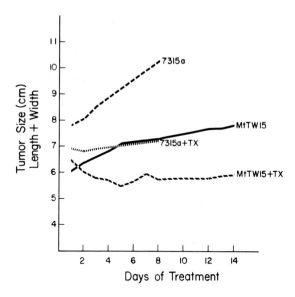

FIG. 5. Effect of tamoxifen (TX) on growth of transplantable pituitary tumors. Each group contained 6 rats injected with 25 μg tamoxifen/day.

and tumor-bearing rats increased slightly after estradiol treatment. This was accompanied by a slight decrease in water-soluble protein concentration. A slight and insignificant increase in tumor weight was also observed.

The effects of estradiol treatment on pituitary gland and tumor activities of G6P-DH, PK, and LDH are summarized in Table 3. Estradiol administration increased G6P-DH activity by 56%, PK by 12%, and LDH by 37% (mU/mg protein) in pituitary glands from nontumor rats. With the exception of PK, enzyme activities in the pituitary glands from untreated tumor-bearing rats were significantly lower than in controls. This finding correlates with the decreased production of prolactin in these glands. Estrogen treatment of tumor-

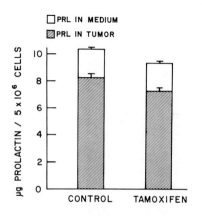

FIG. 6. Effect of tamoxifen administration on the *in vitro* synthesis and release of prolactin (PRL) by pituitary tumors.

TABLE 3. Effect of estradiol administration on pituitary gland and tumor weight, protein concentration, and enzyme activities in rat anterior pituitary glands and 7315a pituitary tumors[a]

Group	Tissue	Pituitary wt (mg)	Tumor wt (g)	ng Prot./mg tiss.	G6P-DH (mU/mg prot.)	PK (mU/mg prot.)	LDH (mU/mg prot.)
Controls	Gland	10.75 ± 0.37	—	125.8 ± 3.4	45.6 ± 4.8	201.9 ± 24.5	771.3 ± 43.1
Estradiol-treated	Gland	13.79 ± 0.70	—	119.6 ± 5.9	71.2 ± 3.1[b]	226.7 ± 14.4[c]	1,056.7 ± 37.4[b]
Tumor-bearing controls	Gland	7.42 ± 0.23[b]	—	117.5 ± 4.6	24.7 ± 3.1[b]	228.1 ± 15.8	557.3 ± 28.7[b]
Tumor-bearing estradiol-treated	Gland	8.24 ± 0.53	—	107.6 ± 11.2	56.9 ± 2.7[f]	308.9 ± 31.6[e]	928.4 ± 60.0[f]
Controls	Tumor	—	24.7 ± 3.7	93.7 ± 1.7	44.4 ± 1.5	295.8 ± 20.6[f]	1,488.9 ± 50.6[f]
Estradiol-treated	Tumor	—	30.4 ± 3.1	91.5 ± 2.5	82.0 ± 3.1[d]	282.1 ± 11.6	1,503.6 ± 47.0

[a] Rats were injected s.c. with 1.0 μg estradiol-17β and 100 μg polyestradiol phosphate and sacrificed 72 hr later. Data are derived from six pools each containing two glands or tumors. All values are mean ± SEM.

[b] $p < 0.01$ versus controls.

[c] $p < 0.05$ versus controls.

[d] $p < 0.01$ versus tumors from controls.

[e] $p < 0.05$ versus glands from tumor controls.

[f] $p < 0.01$ versus glands from tumor controls.

TABLE 4. Activity of anterior pituitary glycolytic enzymes after estrogen and antiestrogen treatment[a]

Group	G6P-DH mU/mg Protein	G6P-DH mU/Anterior pituitary	PK mU/mg Protein	PK mU/Anterior pituitary	LDH mU/mg Protein	LDH mU/Anterior pituitary
1. Control	37.3 ± 1.4	38.9 ± 2.5	171.7 ± 13.5	181.3 ± 18.6	497.6 ± 25.0	522.0 ± 38.8
2. E_2	54.5 ± 1.9^b	62.0 ± 3.6^b	214.4 ± 18.2	245.1 ± 23.3	662.7 ± 14.6^b	762.6 ± 61.7^b
3. NC	31.3 ± 0.6^b	29.6 ± 1.8^c	117.5 ± 7.1^b	118.5 ± 10.8^b	411.5 ± 11.1^c	390.4 ± 30.5^c
4. TX	35.9 ± 1.6	29.6 ± 2.8^c	124.2 ± 13.5^c	100.6 ± 12.7^b	534.2 ± 21.1	431.8 ± 31.9
5. E_2 + NC	$31.6 \pm 0.7^{b,d}$	$31.1 \pm 1.9^{c,d}$	$124.3 \pm 9.7^{b,d}$	$120.6 \pm 8.1^{b,d}$	429.8 ± 24.6^d	424.0 ± 35.1^d
6. E_2 + TX	37.7 ± 0.9^d	32.5 ± 3.6^d	$146.9 \pm 13.2^{b,d}$	$121.4 \pm 8.5^{b,d}$	597.7 ± 33.0^c	482.2 ± 18.4^d

[a] Mean ± SEM. Statistical analysis by analysis of variance. Seven animals per group. E_2, estrogen; TX, tamoxifen; NC, nitromifene citrate.
[b] $p < 0.01$ versus controls.
[c] $p < 0.05$ versus controls.
[d] $p < 0.01$ versus estrogen group.

bearing rats increased G6P-DH by 131%, PK by 36%, and LDH by 20% (mU/mg protein). Similar increases in enzyme activity were found when the data were expressed as milliunits per milligram tissue. The activities of PK and LDH in tumor tissue were greater than observed in normal glandular tissue. It is interesting that estradiol treatment increased only G6P-DH activity in tumor tissue.

The enzyme activities of MDH and ICDH were similar in normal pituitary and tumor tissue, and remained essentially unchanged following estradiol treatment. A significant decrease was observed in total acid phosphatase and a slight decrease in the tartarate-inhibited enzyme in the pituitary glands of tumor-bearing rats. Estradiol treatment, however, had no influence on these activities. Phosphatase activity in pituitary tumor preparations was significantly less (30–40%, $p < 0.01$) than the activity found in normal pituitary tissue, but estradiol had no effect on this enzyme.

The effects of antiestrogens in combination with estradiol on the activity of pituitary gland enzymes was also studied; Table 1 presents the injection schedule. Once again, estradiol stimulated the enzyme activities of G6P-DH, PK, and LDH (Table 4). In contrast, nitromifene citrate significantly reduced the basal activities of these enzymes, and completely blocked the estradiol-induced increase in each case. Tamoxifen alone decreased the activities of G6P-DH and PK without affecting LDH activity. Tamoxifen treatment also completely blocked the estradiol-mediated increase in these enzymes.

DISCUSSION

Estradiol stimulation of prolactin synthesis and release is well established (5,9,22,30,37–39). Recently a series of excellent studies has demonstrated that the steroid acts directly on pituitary cells to increase the generation of prolactin mRNA, subsequently increasing the rate of prolactin synthesis (37–39). Estradiol is presumed initially to bind to specific cytoplasmic receptors which are subsequently translocated into the nucleus (20,34), thereby stimulating the synthesis of mRNA and ultimately of prolactin. Our finding that cytosol from pituitary glands of prolactin-secreting tumor-bearing rats binds greater amounts of [³H]estradiol than do cytosol preparations of pituitary glands from normal animals correlates well with the finding of increase pituitary prolactin synthesis following estradiol administration to tumor-bearing rats.

Because the large mass of tumor tissue has a high affinity for [³H]estradiol, the tumor may preferentially compete with the gland for endogenous estradiol. Our data, however, do not distinguish between the potentially increased number of new estradiol receptor sites and the increased availability of nonsaturated sites. Whether the pituitary gland in tumor-bearing animals is deprived of estrogenic stimulation and whether that effect is instrumental in causing the atrophy and the decreased prolactin synthesis and release can only be conjectured at this time.

The concept that estrogen deprivation due to tumor mass may contribute to a decrease in prolactin synthesis by the glandular tissue may also contribute to the understanding of dopamine's action to inhibit prolactin secretion. This relates to our previous finding that the decrease in prolactin synthesis and release in tumor-bearing rats can be completely reversed by dopamine receptor antagonists (26). Although it was demonstrated that hyperprolactinemia due to transplanted pituitary tumors increased hypothalamic dopamine synthesis (36) and thereby contributed to prolactin suppression, we postulate that the increased dopaminergic tone may be even more effective in pituitary glands deficient in estrogen. Several studies have demonstrated that dopamine and its agonists are less effective in decreasing prolactin secretion in preparations stimulated by estradiol (19,23,25).

The molecular mechanism of the antiestrogenic effect is not completely established, but it is well documented that the antiestrogens strongly inhibit estrogen uptake by the endocrine-hypothalamus and anterior pituitary (21), and hence also estrogen-dependent functions. Jordan et al. (14,15) and Heuson et al. (10) showed that synthetic triphenylethylene compounds inhibit the estrogen-induced serum prolactin increase. Nicholson and Golder (33) demonstrated that these drugs did not influence serum prolactin concentration either in ovariectomized or in normal cycling female rats. In the present experiments we used male rats, the estrogen sensitivity of whose nervous system is widely documented. Neither nitromifene citrate nor tamoxifen influenced *in vivo* prolactin secretion in these rats. Nitromifene citrate suppressed the serum prolactin stimulatory effect of estrogen only slightly, while tamoxifen was completely ineffective.

In these animals the pretreatment with nitromifene citrate did not affect either total *in vitro* synthesis or release of prolactin. The amount of prolactin retained in pituitaries from nitromifene citrate-treated rats decreased slightly but significantly; the biological significance of this effect is uncertain. Tamoxifen pretreatment stimulated *in vitro* prolactin synthesis slightly but significantly, perhaps as a consequence of its mild time- and dose-dependent estrogenic activity (2,18). As observed previously (1,22,30,37–39), estrogen priming dramatically increased *in vivo* and *in vitro* synthesis and release of prolactin. Nitromifene citrate completely abolished this effect and tamoxifen partially suppressed it. In spite of the endogenous effect of tamoxifen at this level (2,18), it did not increase estrogen's effect. This coincides with our hypothesis that estrogen primarily stimulates the synthesis of prolactin (24) and only secondarily its release, and strongly supports the hypothesis that the antiestrogens inhibit the binding of estrogen to its receptor and hence its biological effects (2,8,12).

Alternatively, since estrogen stimulates the receptor binding of prolactin in various organs (7,16,17,29), and the appearance of prolactin receptors in the liver is estrogen-dependent (17), antiestrogens could decrease prolactin binding in the different organs, so that a decreased binding and/or utilization may cause an apparent increase in serum prolactin concentration. Although antiestrogens decreased the growth rate of transplanted prolactin-secreting pituitary tumors, the drugs affected neither the extremely high serum prolactin levels in these rats nor prolactin content and release by tumor cells *in vitro.* These findings support the thesis that these drugs have little or no effect on prolactin release.

The administration of estrogen in small doses does not influence rat pituitary growth hormone production (22). In the present experiments estrogen did not influence growth hormone synthesis, but the antiestrogens caused a decrease. Jacobi and Lloyd (11) found increased pituitary and serum growth hormone concentrations after administration of nafoxidine. Dannies et al. (6) reported that antiestrogens stimulate growth hormone production in clonal strains of rat pituitary cells. Further experiments are needed for unambiguous conclusions concerning the effect of antiestrogens on growth hormone production.

The antiestrogens have a clear effect on anterior pituitary estrogen-dependent metabolic functions. In addition to strongly blocking the effect of estrogen on gonadotropin and prolactin production (10,14,15), nonsteroidal antiestrogens strongly inhibit the hexosemonophosphate shunt activity (21) and DNA synthesis (11) in the anterior pituitary. The present experiments show that nitromifene citrate and tamoxifen inhibit the estrogen stimulation of pituitary pentose phosphate shunt and anaerobic glycolytic activity as measured by G6P-DH, PK, and LDH. Numerous morphological, physiological, and biochemical data support the hypothesis that enzyme activities in anterior pituitary homogenates reflect the metabolic activity of the lactotrophs. In the present experiments the antiestrogens effectively inhibited both prolactin production and glycolytic activity in the pituitary gland.

The present results suggest that antiestrogens affect pituitary cell function by inhibiting the mechanisms through which estrogen stimulates their hormone-producing and metabolic functions. Hence these compounds may provide a useful means for investigating estrogen's role in regulating pituitary functions, as described concurrently in another publication (32).

ACKNOWLEDGMENTS

This research was supported by USPHS Research Grant CA-07535-16.

REFERENCES

1. Augustine, E. C., and MacLeod, R. M. (1975): *Proc. Soc. Exp. Biol. Med.,* 150:551–556.
2. Baulieu, E. E. (1978): In: *Cell Membrane Receptors for Drugs and Hormones: A Multidisciplinary Approach,* edited by R. W. Straub and L. Bolis, pp. 129–149. Raven Press, New York.
3. Bergmeyer, H. U., and Gawehn, K. (1974): *Methods of Enzymatic Analysis, Vol. 2, 2nd English ed.* Verlag Chemie Weinheim, Academic Press, New York.
4. Bradford, M. M. (1976): *Anal. Biochem.,* 72:248–254.
5. Chen, C. L., Amenomori, Y., Lu, K. H., Voogt, J. L., and Meites, J. (1970): *Neuroendocrinology,* 6:220–227.
6. Dannies, P. S., Yen, P. M., and Tashjian, A. H., Jr. (1977): *Endocrinology,* 101:1151–1156.
7. Gelato, M., Marshall, S., Boudreau, M., Bruni, J., Campbell, G. A., and Meites, J. (1975): *Endocrinology,* 96:1292–1296.

8. Gorski, J., Toft, D., Shyamala, G., Smith, D., and Notides, A. (1968): *Recent Prog. Horm. Res.,* 24:45–80.
9. Haug, E., and Gautvik, K. M. (1976): *Endocrinology,* 99:1482–1489.
10. Heuson, J. C., Waelbroek, C., Legros, N., Gallez, G., Robyn, C., and L'Hermite, M. (1971/1972): *Gynecol. Invest.,* 2:130–137.
11. Jacobi, J. M., and Lloyd, H. M. (1978): *J. Endocrinol.,* 76:555–556.
12. Jensen, E. V., Suzuki, T., Kawashima, T., Stumpf, W. E., Jungblut, P. W., and DeSombre, E. R. (1968): *Proc. Natl. Acad. Sci. USA,* 59:632–638
13. Jordan, V. C., and Dowse, L. J. (1976): *J. Endocrinol.,* 68:297–303.
14. Jordan, V. C., and Koerner, S. (1976): *J. Endocrinol.,* 68:305–311.
15. Jordan, V. C., Koerner, S., and Robinson, C. (1975): *J. Endocrinol.,* 65:151–152.
16. Josefsberg, Z., Posner, B. I., Patel, B., and Bergeron, J. J. M. (1979): *J. Biol. Chem.,* 254:209–214.
17. Kelly, P. A., Ferland, L., Labrie, F., and DeLean, A. (1976): In: *Hypothalamus and Endocrine Functions,* edited by F. Labrie, J. Meites, and G. Pelletier, pp. 321–335. Plenum Press, New York.
18. Koseki, Y., Sava, D. T., Chamnes, G. C., and McGuire, W. L. (1977): *Endocrinology,* 101:1104–1110.
19. Labrie, F., Beaulieu, M., Caron, M. G., and Raymond, V. (1978): In: *Progress in Prolactin Physiology and Pathology,* edited by C. Robyn and M. Harter, pp. 121–136. Elsevier/North-Holland, Amsterdam.
20. Leavitt, W. W., Friend, J. P., and Robinson, J. A. (1968): *Science,* 165:496–498.
21. Luine, V. N., and McEwen, B. S. (1977): *Endocrinology,* 100:903–910.
22. MacLeod, R. M., Abad, A., and Eidson, L. L. (1969): *Endocrinology,* 84:1475–1483.
23. MacLeod, R. M., and Lamberts, S. W. J. (1979): In: *Neuroendocrine Correlates in Neurology and Psychiatry,* edited by E. E. Müller and A. Agnoli, pp. 89–102. Elsevier/North-Holland, Amsterdam.
24. MacLeod, R. M., Lamberts, S. W. J., Nagy, I., Login, I. S., and Valdenegro, C. A. (1980): In: *Pituitary Microadenomas,* edited by G. Faglia, M. A. Giovanelli, and R. M. Macleod, pp. 37–54. Academic Press, London.
25. MacLeod, R. M., and Lehmeyer, J. E. (1971): In: *CIBA Foundation Symposium on Lactogenic Hormones,* edited by G. E. W. Wolstenholme and J. Knight, pp. 53–82. Churchill Livingstone, Edinburgh.
26. MacLeod, R. M., and Lehmeyer, J. E. (1974): *Cancer Res.,* 34:345–350
27. MacLeod, R. M., and Lehmeyer, J. E. (1974): *J. Natl. Cancer Inst.,* 52:823–828.
28. MacLeod, R. M., Smith, M. C., and DeWitt, G. W. (1966): *Endocrinology,* 79:1149–1156.
29. Marshall, S., Bruni, J. F., and Meites, J. (1978): *Proc. Soc. Exp. Biol. Med.,* 159:256–259.
30. Maurer, R. A., and Gorski, J. (1977): *Endocrinology,* 101:76–84.
31. Nagy, I., and MacLeod, R. M. (1979): *Mol. Cell. Endocrinol.,* 13:317–332.
32. Nagy, I., Valdenegro, C. A., and MacLeod, R. M. (1980): *Neuroendocrinology,* 30:389–395.
33. Nicholson, R. I., and Golder, M. P. (1975): *Eur. J. Cancer,* 11:571–579.
34. Notides, A. C. (1970): *Endocrinology,* 87:987–992.
35. Panko, W. B., and MacLeod, R. M. (1978): *Cancer Res.,* 38:1948–1951.
36. Perkins, N. A., Westfall, T. C., Paul, C. V., MacLeod, R. M., and Rogol, A. D. (1979): *Brain Res.,* 160:431–444.
37. Seo, H., Refetoff, S., Martino, E., Vassart, G., and Brocas, H. (1979): *Endocrinology,* 104:1083–1090.
38. Shupnik, M. A., Baxter, L. A., French, L. R., and Gorski, J. (1979): *Endocrinology,* 104:729–735.
39. Vician, L., Shupnik, M. A., and Gorski, J. (1979): *Endocrinology,* 104:736–743.
40. Waddell, W. J. (1956): *J. Lab. Clin. Med.,* 48, 311–314.

Hormones and Cancer, edited by S. Iacobelli et al.
Raven Press, New York © 1980.

Initiation of Meiotic Maturation in *Xenopus laevis* Oocytes by Insulin

M. El Etr, *S. Schorderet Slatkine, and E. E. Baulieu

*Hormone Laboratory, Unit 33, INSERM, 94270 Bicêtre, France; and *Department of Obstetrics and Gynecology, University of Geneva, Geneva, Switzerland*

Progesterone and several other steroids can induce meiotic maturation of *Xenopus leavis* oocytes *in vitro*, triggering the process at surface membrane sites (1). As many membrane-active nonsteroid agents which also can promote meiosis, steroids seem to work via calcium movements and/or translocation from membrane stores (18). Cholera toxin, which increases cyclic adenosine monophosphate (AMP) in oocytes, or cyclic AMP derivatives injected into egg cytoplasm hinder progesterone-induced meiosis *in vitro* (9) by interfering with the formation/activity of the MPF (maturation promoting factor) that develops after progesterone exposure of oocytes and, in turn, provokes the germinal vesicle breakdown (GVBD) and related phenomena of oocyte maturation (12, 13,15). It is now reported that insulin can mimic the effect of progesterone on oocyte maturation. This newly discovered action of insulin may bring about further understanding of its involvement in the processes of cell division.

Ovarian tissues were removed from *X. laevis* females through a small lateral incision in the lateral abdominal wall. Full-grown oocytes free of follicle cells were obtained from ovaries with collagenase (15) and incubated at room temperature with different concentrations of insulin (monocomponent, Pork insulin, 24 U/ml, Novo, stored in 10 mM HCl) added to Barth medium. Groups of 50 oocytes were scored for GVBD following various times of incubation.

A systematic study with 35 nM to 7 μM insulin (5 mU/ml–1 U/ml) showed a dose–effect relationship with an apparent ED 50 of 2 μM (Table 1 and Fig. 1). The efficacy of 7 μM insulin remained less pronounced than that of progesterone used in appropriate concentrations. This was observed even when insulin concentration was raised to 70 μM, when the oocytes were obtained under various conditions of collagenase treatment, or when the ovaries were dissected manually (data not shown). It is not unlikely that the polysaccharide vitelline membrane impaired access of insulin to the oocyte surface or that insulin was progressively degraded during the time of incubation, as observed in many culture systems. Experiments were, therefore, performed by fractionally adding insulin at different times of incubation, such as 0, 2, 4, and 6 hr instead of incorporating the total amount of insulin at time 0. The percentage of GVBD

TABLE 1. *Insulin-induced maturation in* X. laevis *oocytes*[a]

	Individual (incubation time, hr)						
Dose	A 24	B 24	C 20	D 25	E 30	F 20	G 33
Insulin							
35 nM	2	3	0	4			
70 nM	12		0	4			
0.14 µM				6			
0.35 µM	12	11	10	14	44		
1.4 µM [b]	14			16	58		15
3.5 µM	26	23	18	32	62	48	23
7 µM			26	58	64	86	28
Progesterone							
10 µM	94	70	98	98	98	100	100

[a] Results are expressed in percent GVBD after the indicated incubation time. In each case, two to three batches of 50 oocytes of the same female were incubated with various concentrations of insulin and 10 µM progesterone. The efficacy of insulin differed greatly among individuals, a result which is also commonly observed with progesterone, even if the use of a large dose of progesterone and the fact that GVBD is read at > 20 hr give a standardized 100% response of oocytes to the steroid.

[b] At 0.7 µM, percent GVBD was 9.

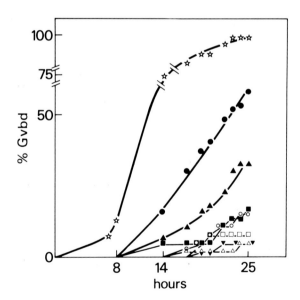

FIG. 1. Effect of various doses of insulin on *X. laevis* oocyte maturation. All tests were performed with batches of 50 oocytes from the same female (D). A control test was performed with progesterone 1 µM *(stars)*. Insulin: *closed circles,* 7 µM; *closed triangles,* 3.5 µM; *closed squares,* 1.4 µM; *open circles,* 0.35 µM; *open squares,* 0.14 µM; *open triangles,* 70 nM; *closed inverted triangles,* 35 nM.

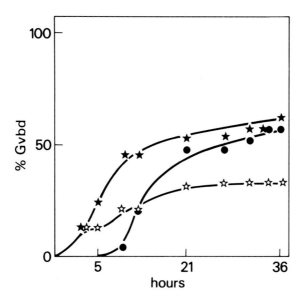

FIG. 2. A comparison between progesterone and insulin action on *X. laevis* oocyte maturation. Pools of 50 oocytes from the same female were exposed to various doses of insulin and progesterone and percentage GVBD was scored after different incubation periods. The three curves reported have been selected because, in this particular case, 50 nM progesterone and 3.5 μM insulin gave the same plateau value after 21 hr of incubation, thus allowing a straight comparison of the first part of the response curve of percentage GVBD. Progesterone-induced GVBD occurred earlier than insulin-induced GVBD, and this result was also observed when the plateau value obtained with 10 nM progesterone was inferior to the one reached with insulin. *Open stars:* 10 nM progesterone, *closed stars:* 50 nM progesterone; *circles:* 3.5 μM insulin.

counted after 20 hr of incubation was found to be 50% greater, suggesting a progressive time-dependent destruction of the hormone. Still, the efficacy of insulin remained lower than that of progesterone, even for periods of incubation up to 30 to 35 hr (data not shown), although it is known that oocytes become altered after such long periods. Another observation was that maturation proceeded faster with progesterone than with insulin (Fig. 2), suggesting that the two hormones trigger meiotic division by two different mechanisms (see below).

Further experiments were carried out to verify the appearance of a "true" maturation in insulin-exposed oocytes. First, a similar typical profile of labeled proteins was found after electrophoresis (16). Second, MPF was also formed, since 50 nl of cytoplasm of insulin-treated oocytes introduced into recipient oocytes provoked 100% GVBD after 2 to 3 hr. Third, as observed for progesterone (1,12,19), no maturation occurred when insulin was injected into the oocyte (final intracellular concentration up to 70 μM) or when 3 μg/ml cycloheximide was added together to incubated 7 μM insulin. Fourth, 50 pM cholera toxin was also able to antagonize the maturation induced by insulin (up to 7 μM) added 30 min after the toxin (Table 2). Finally, in most cases histochemistry

TABLE 2. *Effect of cholera toxin on insulin-induced maturation in X. laevis oocytes[a]*

Dose	% GVBD
Insulin (3.5 μM)	48
Insulin (7 μM)	86
Insulin[b] + Cholera toxin (50 pM)	0
Insulin[b] + Cholera toxin (5 pM)	0
Insulin[b] + Cholera toxin (1 pM)	0
Progesterone[c]	100
Progesterone[c] + Cholera toxin (50 pM)	0
Progesterone[c] + Cholera toxin (5 pM)	14
Progesterone[c] + Cholera toxin (1 pM)	74

[a] All results were obtained with the same female (F) and
percent GVBD read after 20 hr.
[b] Experiments with 3.5 and 7 μM.
[c] 10 μM.

of insulin-exposed oocytes revealed the existence of a single and normal spindle moving to the cortex (not shown); it is worthy of note, however, that a double spindle could also be observed in some insulin-exposed oocytes, as was also the case in oocytes exposed to nonsteroid inducers (17).

The next series of experiments was undertaken in order to verify the specificity of insulin effect on oocyte maturation, since in most target cells [such as mammalian hepatocytes, adipocytes or muscular cells (4,14,18)], the apparent affinity of the hormone is $\sim 10^3$ times more elevated than that observed in the present system. However, the micromolar range is itself 10^3 times smaller than the millimolar range at which nonsteroidal drugs are usually active. Denatured insulin did not provoke meiotic maturation. Denaturation was achieved by treating the hormone overnight at room temperature in the presence of 10 mM mercaptoethanol (11). After dialysis a radioimmunoassay showed > 99% denaturation (J. Kervran, *personal communication*). Two modified insulins were prepared by D. Brandenburg: 7242 [A1-B29-adipoylinsulin (2)] and 7207 [A1-B29-bis(*tert*-butyloxicarbonyl-Trp) insulin *(unpublished)*]. They display 1 to 2% of the affinity of insulin for usual receptors (6,8) and showed no maturational activity even at concentrations up to 7 μM. Negative effects were also obtained when oocytes were exposed to growth factors EGF or FGF (gifts of D. Gospodarowicz), each used at concentrations of 0.1, 1, and 10 μg/ml in bovine serum albumin (BSA) containing buffer (5 mg/ml). In contrast to the above data, chick insulin (gift of J. Simon) applied at concentrations of 3.5 and 7 μM displayed the same effect as pork insulin. Finally, proinsulin (gift of P. Freychet) had a constantly lower activity than insulin on oocyte maturation (Fig. 3), a result comparable to those obtained with proinsulin in other systems (7). Thus, a large body of experimental evidence seems to demonstrate a true correlation between the effects of insulin derivatives on mammalian metabolic systems and on *X. leavis* oocyte maturation. It is therefore possible that the insulin action

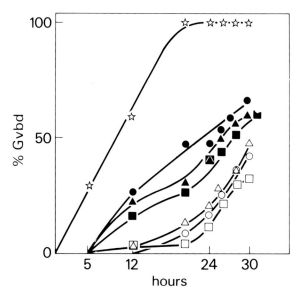

FIG. 3. Effect of proinsulin on *X. laevis* maturation. Batches of 50 oocytes all coming from the same female were exposed to three different corresponding concentrations of insulin and proinsulin. A control test was performed with 1 μM progesterone *(star)*. Insulin: *Closed circle,* 7 μM; *closed triangle,* 3.5 μM; *closed square,* 1.4 μM. Proinsulin: *Open circle,* 7 μM; *open triangle,* 3.5 μM; *open square,* 1.4 μM.

for triggering amphibian meiosis is mediated by a receptor mechanism, although such a receptor has not yet been described in amphibian oocyte membrane. Recent studies using high resolution chromatography have indicated that most insulin preparations are not homogenous (R. Guillemin, *personal communication*), but purer insulins have recently become available and we are planning to use them as soon as possible.

The last part of this chapter deals with the study of a synthetic estrogen, 17α-ethynyl-estradiol (17α-EE), simultaneously applied on *X. laevis* oocytes. It was found previously that 17α-EE was a very weak agonist as compared with progesterone and was an antagonist of progesterone when the two agents competed for possible "steroid sites" located on the oocyte membrane (1). Interestingly, when insulin was substituted for progesterone, no antagonistic effect of 17α-EE was found (Table 3). Rather, we observed that 17α-EE potentiated the effects of insulin in a dose-dependent manner and in two different ways. First, the efficacy of insulin became comparable to that of progesterone. Second, the lag between insulin application and the first GVBD became similar to that of progesterone. If we accept that 17α-EE interacts with the steroid sites (1) and insulin with a typical insulin receptor, both in the oocyte membrane, then there might be some interactions between these two loci or some cooperation between effects initiated at two separate places. Studies are in progress to check

TABLE 3. *Potentiation of insulin-induced maturation in* X. laevis *oocytes by 17α-EE[a]*

	Hours of incubation			
Dose	8	10	16	33
Insulin				
3.5 μM	0	0	0	23
1.4 μM	0	0	0	15
0.7 μM	0	0	0	9
17α-EE				
10 μM	2	2	2	2
5 μM	0	0	0	0
Insulin (3.5 μM) + 17α-EE (10 μM)	6	12	44	97
Insulin (3.5 μM) + 17α-EE (5 μM)	0	0	5	59
Insulin (1.4 μM) + 17α-EE (10 μM)	7	12	37	92
Insulin (1.4 μM) + 17α-EE (5 μM)	0	0	0	45
Insulin (0.7 μM) + 17α-EE 10 μM	7	7	10	80
Progesterone 50 nM	2	10	28	94

[a] All results are expressed in percent GVBD and were obtained with the same female (G).

the presence of insulin receptors, and to determine the number of available binding sites, eventually in the presence of 17α-EE.

It has been suggested that in "metabolic" target cells calcium may play the role of second messenger in insulin action(s) (3) and/or that cyclic AMP levels decrease as a response of insulin (10). These two possibilities are interesting to consider, since Ca^{2+} released from membrane sites (1) and cyclic AMP levels at the stage of MPF formation (18) have been found to be linked to progesterone reinitiation of meiosis. The meiotic process observed in amphibian oocytes may serve (unexpectedly) as a model system for the study of mechanism(s) of the poorly understood insulin effect on cell division.

REFERENCES

1. Baulieu, E. E., Godeau, F., Schorderet, M., and Schroderet-Slatkine, S. (1978): *Nature,* 275:593–598.
2. Brandenburg, D. (1972): *Hoppe Seylers Z. Physiol. Chem.,* 353:869–873.
3. Clausen, T., Elbrink, S., and Martin, B. R. (1974): *Acta Endocrinol. (Suppl.),* 191:137–143.
4. Cuatrecasas. P., Hollenberg, M. D., Chang, K. J., and Bennett, V. (1975): *Recent Prog. Horm. Res.,* 31:37–94.
5. Czech, M. P. (1977): *Annu. Rev. Biochem.,* 46:359–384.
6. Freychet, P., Aranderburg, D., and Wollmer, A. (1974): *Diabetologia,* 10:1–5.
7. Freychet, P. (1974): *J. Clin. Invest.,* 54:1020–1031.
8. Gliemann, J., and Gammeltoft, S. (1974): *Diabetologia,* 10:105–113.
9. Godeau, F., Boquet, P., Schorderet, M., Schorderet-Slatkine, S., and Baulieu, E. E. (1978): *C.R. Acad. Sci. Ser. D,* 286:685–688.
10. Jefferson, L. S., Exton, J. H., Butcher, R. W., Sutherland, E. W., and Park, C. R. (1968): *J. Biol. Chem.,* 243:1031–1038.

11. Loten, E. G. (1970): *Biochem. J.,* 120:187–193.
12. Masui, Y., and Markert, C. L. (1971): *J. Exp. Zool.,* 177:129–146.
13. Reynhout, J. K., and Smith, L. D., (1974): *Dev. Biol.,* 38:394–400.
14. Roth, J., Kahn, C. R., Lesniak, M. A., Gorden, P., De Meyts, P., Megyesi, K., Neville, D. M., Jr., Gavin, J. R., III, Soll, A. H., Freychet, P., Goldfine, I. D., Bar, R. S., and Archer, J. A. (1975): *Recent Prog. Horm. Res.,* 31:95–139.
15. Schorderet-Slatkine, S. (1972): *Cell Diff.,* 1:179–189.
16. Schorderet-Slatkine, S., and Baulieu E. E. (1977): *Ann. NY Acad. Sci.,* 286:421–433.
17. Schorderet-Slatkine, S., Schorderet, M., and Baulieu, E. E. (1977): *Differentiation,* 9:67–76.
18. Schorderet-Slatkine, S., Schorderet, M., Boquet, P., Godeau, F., and Baulieu, E. E. (1978): *Cell,* 15:1269–1275.
19. Smith, L., and Ecker, R. (1971): *Dev. Biol.,* 25:232–247.

Advances in Receptor Measurement

Hormones and Cancer, edited by S. Iacobelli et al.
Raven Press, New York © 1980.

Theoretical Considerations in Assessing Steroid Hormone–Receptor Interactions: How Do Slow Kinetics Influence the Results of Equilibrium Measurements?

Péter Arányi*

*2nd Institute of Biochemistry, Semmelweis University Medical School,
1088 Budapest, Puskin u.9, Hungary*

The presence of a specific receptor protein in the cytoplasm of the target cells is required for steroid hormone action. According to the current view, the hormone enters the cell, associates with the receptor, and the latter mediates the hormone response by translocating into the nucleus and presumably participating in a series of poorly understood molecular events. The initial hormone–receptor interaction is characterized by high affinity and hormone specificity, which closely correlate with the physiological potency of the steroid molecules (3,7–9,17).

Receptors for different steroid hormones are present in a wide variety of normal and malignant tissues and cell cultures (6,10,12,13,18). Determinations of their affinity and specificity for the hormones are the most commonly used methods of receptor characterization. Screening steroids for their ability to bind to receptors has a great value in drug design. A full understanding of the steroid–receptor interaction is, therefore, desirable. Reports from different laboratories have pointed out clearly that dissociation constants determined in saturation experiments may strongly differ from the ratio of rate constants. This discrepancy was always characteristic of steroids whose receptor complex exhibited very low dissociation rates. Moreover, it has recently been shown that measured equilibrium dissociation constant decreased from 4.6 to 0.44 nM as equilibration time was varied between 2 and 15 hr (14). Pertinent to my subject are other findings demonstrating that the competition pattern of a series of steroids depends on the incubation time and temperature (11). The very slow dissociation of the steroid–receptor complex is discussed in this chapter, since it is clearly a cause of many artifacts in such studies.

---

* Present address: Department of Cell Growth and Regulation, Sidney Farber Cancer Institute, Charles A. Dana Cancer Center, Boston, Massachusetts 02115.
[1] A glossary of symbols is given at the end of this chapter.

RESULTS AND DISCUSSION

Saturation Analysis in the Absence of Competitor

In order to understand how a possible lack of equilibrium would be reflected in saturation curves, one has to resort to kinetics. I try to make assumptions that are simple, but that still apply to situations met frequently in steroid receptor research. A $1:1$ stoichiometry is assumed for the steroid–receptor interaction, and nonspecific binding is neglected. It does not exclude receptors with multiple binding sites from consideration, but the deductions can be only applied to them if the binding sites are uniform and do not interact with one another. This assumption is met in most cases. There are important exceptions, however, that require a more refined model.

The system is characterized by the following stoichiometric equation[1]

$$H + R \underset{k_{-1}}{\overset{k_1}{\rightleftharpoons}} B \tag{I}$$

and the time course of complex formation is given by Eq. 1 (see ref. 1 for details).

$$[B(t)] = \frac{e^{-pk_1t} - e^{-qk_1t}}{\dfrac{1}{p} e^{-pk_1t} - \dfrac{1}{q} e^{-qk_1t}} \tag{1}$$

The steroid receptors are particularly labile *in vitro*. They have to be kept at low temperatures, need different protecting agents such as mercaptoethanol, glycerol, ethylene diaminetetraacetic acid, and the like (4,16,19,20). They tend to lose their steroid binding ability even under optimal conditions, but they are strongly stabilized by their ligands, the respective steroids.

The mineralocorticoid and the androgen receptors are probably the most labile in the absence of hormone, with half-lives of approximately 1 hr or less; glucocorticoid receptors display intermediate stability, whereas progesterone and estradiol receptors are fairly stable. That is why a model incorporating receptor inactivation has also been considered as an alternative to the simplest model.

To describe this system another stoichiometric equation (II) should be added to (I) and the formation of B complex also follows an altered kinetics (1,4) as given by Eq. 2.

$$R \xrightarrow{k_d} D \tag{II}$$

$$[B(t)] = \frac{\alpha}{\mu - \lambda} (e^{\mu t} - e^{\lambda t}) \tag{2}$$

The time course of complex formation is shown in Fig. 1.

I want to underline here the feature that, due to the second-order association kinetics, the initial hormone concentration determines not only the equilibrium value of the bound hormone, but the rate at which equilibrium is approached as well.

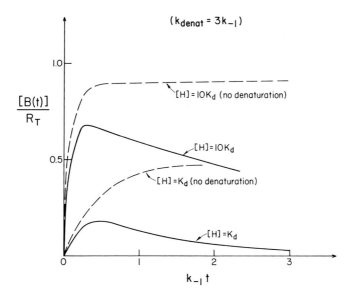

FIG. 1. Time course of steroid binding to receptor. *Solid lines:* labile receptor $k_d = 3k_{-1}$; *broken lines:* stable receptor. $R_T = 0.1K_d$. (Replotted from ref. 1 with the permission of the copyright holder.)

In the time required to achieve almost complete equilibration at high initial steroid concentration, only half complete equilibration is reached if 10-fold lower initial steroid concentration is used. For construction of saturation curves steroid concentration is varied over a fairly broad range, generally over two to three orders of magnitude, sometimes even more, and equilibration times are usually determined at the highest steroid concentration as one gets the most radioactivity counts in this case.

Binding of steroid to a labile receptor won't reach any true equilibrium. Rather, the time course displays a maximum value, then a slow decay can be observed. The time when maximum binding is achieved depends not only on the rate constants, but on the initial concentrations as well. The maximum value may be much less than the equilibrium value would be if denaturation rate were reduced to zero (broken line).

Equilibrium constants are calculated from data that are usually obtained as bound hormone at different concentrations of free hormone, with incubation times fixed rather than variable.

The association equilibrium constant is defined by the expression on the left side of Eq. 3 if the concentrations at equilibrium are put into it, i.e., if t, the time of incubation with hormone, tends to infinity.

$$\frac{[B(t)]}{[H(t)]\,(R_t - [B(t)])} \simeq \begin{cases} k_1 t, \text{ short incubation} \\ K_a, \text{ long incubation, stable receptor} \\ 0, \text{ long incubation, labile receptor} \end{cases} \quad (3)$$

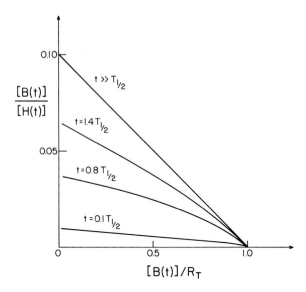

FIG. 2. Scatchard analysis of binding data in case of stable receptor. [B(t)] was calculated according to eq. 1. $R_t = 0.1 K_d$. (Reproduced from ref. 1 with the permission of the copyright holder.)

However, if incubation time is short, i.e., shorter than the half-life of the complex, then the value of that ratio becomes time dependent and for very short incubation times strictly proportional to the incubation time and independent of dissociation rate constant (1). This time dependence is, of course, reflected in the slope of Scatchard curves (Fig. 2). Interestingly, the Scatchard curves are also almost linear even when equilibrium has not been reached. They have only a very small curvature at the high concentration end, which is difficult, if not impossible, to observe experimentally.

Lack of proper equilibration results in apparent association constants that may be wrong by several orders of magnitude, since the half-life of the hormone–receptor complex can be as long as several days, and incubation time as short as 2 to 4 hr in practice. Total amount of receptor protein can be more accurately determined since at high steroid concentration equilibrium is approached more rapidly. In the case of the labile receptor, short incubations may give apparent association constants that are quite inaccurate. Long incubation times are not possible because the receptor disappears (Eq. 3).

Competition Analysis

Competition analysis is an important and widely used method of receptor characterization and drug design. However, it is also subject to error related to incomplete equilibrium.

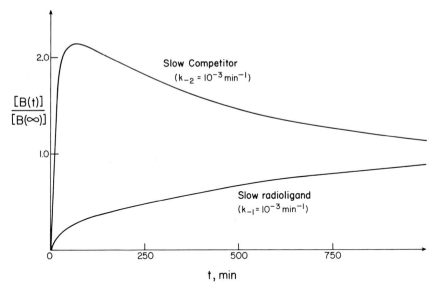

FIG. 3. Time course of radioligand binding in the presence of competitor. The amount of bound radioligand hormone is expressed as fraction of the equilibrium value. Parameters used for calculation: $[H] = 4.8 \times 10^{-7}$ M, $[C] = 10^{-7}$ M, $k_{-1} = 10^{-2}$ min^{-1}, $k_{-2} = 10^{-3}$ min^{-1} for slowly dissociating competitor, and $[H] = 3 \times 10^{-7}$ M, $[C] = 3 \times 10^{-6}$ M, $k_{-1} = 10^{-3}$ min^{-1}, $k_{-2} = 10^{-2}$ min^{-1} for slowly dissociating radioligand curves, respectively. $R_T = 2 \times 10^{-9}$ M, $k_1 = k_2 = 10^5$ M^{-1} min^{-1} for both curves.

For description of this system Eqs. I and III are used.

$$H + R \underset{k_{-1}}{\overset{k_1}{\rightleftharpoons}} B \qquad\qquad\qquad (I)$$

$$C + R \underset{k_{-2}}{\overset{k_2}{\rightleftharpoons}} B' \qquad\qquad\qquad (III)$$

Figure 3 shows the time course of formation of the labeled complex.

If the competitor dissociates more slowly from the receptor than the labeled hormone, the fraction of the bound radioligand displays a maximum in time. Again, the time of maximum and the speed at which equilibrium is approached depend on the initial concentrations. In competition experiments the fraction of bound hormone is generally measured at a fixed time and data are displayed as displacement curves on a semilog scale, or are linearized. Displacement curves are shifted parallelly along the concentration axis if incubation time increases (Fig. 4). In case of slow radioligand dissociation there is a shift to the higher concentration values at very short incubation times. Moderately short incubation time would result in binding affinity that was too large. If, however, the competitor dissociates slower than the radioligand, the apparent relative binding affinity of the competitor increases with the incubation time. That can be seen as a

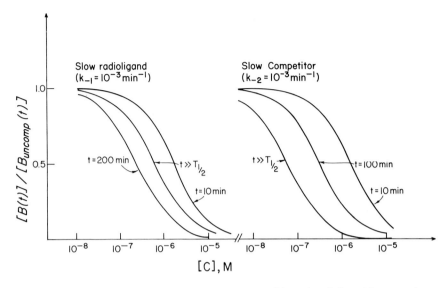

FIG. 4. Radioligand displacement curves. The amount of bound radioligand hormone is expressed as a fraction of bound hormone in the absence of competitor. **Left:** Slowly dissociating radioligand. **Right:** Slowly dissociating competitor. Parameters used for calculation: $[H] = 4.8 \times 10^{-8}$ M, $k_{-1} = 10^{-3}$ min^{-1}, $k_{-2} = 10^{-2}$ min^{-1}, and $[H] = 4.8 \times 10^{-7}$ M, $k_{-1} = 10^{-2}$ min^{-1}, $k_{-2} = 10^{-3}$ min^{-1} for left and right panels, respectively. $R_T = 2 \times 10^{-9}$ M, $k_1 = k_2 = 1 \times 10^5$ M^{-1} min^{-1} for both panels.

left shift of the competition curve. While the shape of the displacement curve does not reveal that equilibrium has not been reached, it is not apparent from linearized displacement curves, either.

On the basis of a long series of experiments, Ojasoo and Raynaud (15) and Bouton and Raynaud (5) have recently warned that relative binding affinities are dependent on incubation time and temperature, and have suggested that competition experiments should be done both at elevated temperature with longer incubation time and at low temperature with short incubation time. However, at high temperature, denaturation of the receptor prevents one from obtaining good estimation of the total receptor concentration. It is questionable, therefore, on the basis of the above analysis that one can accurately estimate the relative binding affinities when receptor denaturation is significant.

A quite thorough preliminary kinetic study seems to be required, therefore, to determine an optimal incubation time that allows equilibration but prevents extensive denaturation of the receptor protein. To meet both requirements may be difficult, if not impossible, with certain systems, e.g., if one of the ligands dissociates very slowly or the receptor is very labile. I suggest that an alternative approach would be to determine the rate constants of association and dissociation, if needed, separately. Equilibrium constants can be obtained using them. Numerous examples show that it is feasible at least in case of labeled ligands.

Rate Constants of Reactions of the Nonlabeled Ligand

A close examination of the time course of competition permits us also to establish conditions for the determination of rate constants of reactions of nonlabeled competitions. To determine the association rate constant, essentially a competition experiment is performed. Add both labeled and nonlabeled ligand to receptor at the same time. It is conceivable that the rate of occupation of binding sites on the receptor, and consequently the rate of labeled complex formation, depends on both k_1 and k_2. If the concentration of the ligands is high enough, association proceeds rapidly and a measurable amount of B forms within a period during which dissociation can be neglected. In this case, $[B(t)]$ is given by the following equation (2) (for short incubation):

$$[B(t)] = \frac{R_T[H]k_1}{[H]k_1 + [C]k_2} \{1 - \exp[-([H]k_1 + [C]k_2)t]\} \tag{4}$$

As R_T and k_1 can be determined in an independent experiment and $[H]$ and $[C]$ are approximately equal to the total concentration of the labeled and nonlabeled ligand, respectively, k_2 can be determined by nonlinear curve fitting to early time points in the competition experiment.

It is the dissociation rate constants that really set the time scale in saturation and competition experiments. For nonlabeled ligands they can be determined in the following manner. Add a saturating concentration of the nonlabeled ligand to the receptor and then separate the complex from excess free ligand and add radioligand at a concentration that would allow fast equilibration if free receptor were present. Continuous dissociation of the nonlabeled competitor–receptor complex generates free receptor at a rate determined by k_{-2} and that reacts instantaneously with the labeled steroid. Formation of the labeled complex as a function of time can then be determined.

Stoichiometric equations corresponding to the above ligand–receptor interactions give rise to a simple time course of labeled complex formation (Eq. 5).

$$[B(t)] = R_T[1 - \frac{1}{[H]k_1 - k_2}([H]k_1 e^{-k_{-2}t} - k_{-2}e^{-[H]k_1 t})] \approx R_T(1 - e^{-k_{-2}t}) \tag{5}$$

If the concentration of the labeled hormone is high enough, one gets a single exponential. Concentration of the labeled complex increases in time to the value of total receptor concentration at a rate determined by k_{-2}. The slope of a semilogarithmic plot gives us the required rate constant (Fig. 5).

CONCLUSION

Reported dissociation rate constants for different steroid–receptor complexes indicate that proper equilibration may take as long as several days in cell-free systems at low temperature. It has been known theoretically and is supported by experimental data cited above that lack of equilibration results in apparent

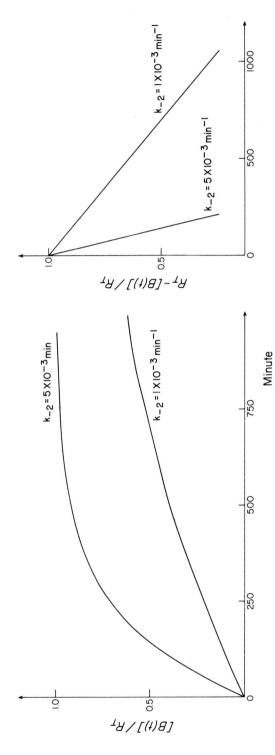

FIG. 5. Time course of competitor–receptor complex dissociation. Curves were calculated according to Eq. 5. See text for further explanation.

"equilibrium constants" that probably have nothing to do with the true ones.

Therefore, kinetic measurements should be an alternative or a compulsory supplementation to equilibrium analysis. The methods of determination of rate constants of the reactions of labeled ligands with receptor protein are well known, and here I gave the theoretical outlines for kinetic measurements with nonlabeled ligands. Experimental verification of the latter methods will be given elsewhere (2). Kinetic analysis is especially useful if one is not sure that equilibrium has been reached at *all* hormone concentrations. It is inevitable if receptor inactivation or hormone metabolism is appreciably fast. Moreover, it may reveal secondary transformation of the hormone–receptor complex that may give a deeper insight into the mechanism of hormone action. By use of these measurements, thermodynamic parameters can also be obtained that may help drug design.

GLOSSARY OF SYMBOLS

B	Radiolabeled steroid–receptor complex
B′	Nonlabeled steroid–receptor complex
C	Nonlabeled competitor
D	Denatured receptor
H	Radiolabeled steroid hormone
R	Receptor
K_a	Equilibrium association constant of the B complex
K_d	$1/K_a$
k_1, k_2	Second-order association rate constants
k_{-1}, k_{-2}	First-order dissociation rate constants
k_d	Denaturation rate constant of the receptor
$p, q, \alpha, \lambda, \mu$	Constants, algebraic expressions of rate constants and initial hormone and receptor concentrations
t	Time
T (subscript)	Total amount (of receptor)
[ ]	Concentration

REFERENCES

1. Arányi, P. (1979): *Biochim. Biophys. Acta,* 584:529–534.
2. Arányi, P., and Quiroga, V. (1980): *J. Steroid Biochem. (in press).*
3. Baxter, J. D., and Tomkins, G. M. (1970): *Proc. Natl. Acad. Sci. USA,* 65:709–715.
4. Bell, Ph. A., and Munck, A. (1973): *Biochem. J.,* 136:97–107.
5. Bouton, M. M., and Raynaud, F. P. (1977): *J. Steroid Biochem.,* 9:9–15.
6. Crabtree, G. R., Smith, K. A., and Munck, A. (1978): *Cancer Res.,* 38:4268–4272.
7. Dausse, J. P., Duval, D., Meyer, P., Gaignault, J. C., Marchandeau, C., and Raynaud, J. P. (1977): *Mol. Pharmacol.,* 13:948–953.
8. Edelman, I. S. (1975): *J. Steroid Biochem.,* 6:147–159.
9. Feldman, D., Funder, J. W., and Edelman, I. S. (1972): *Am. J. Med.,* 53:545–560.
10. Lippman, M., and Huff, K. A. (1976): *Cancer,* 38:868–874.
11. MacDonald, R., and Cidlowski, J. A. (1979): *J. Steroid Biochem.,* 10:21–29.

12. McGuire, W. L., Horwitz, K. B., Zava, D. T., Garola, R. E., and Chamness, G. C. (1978): *Metabolism,* 27:487–501.
13. McGuire, W. L., Raynaud, J. P., and Baulieu, E. E., editors (1977): *Progesterone Receptors in Normal and Neoplastic Tissues.* Raven Press, New York.
14. Murakami, T., Brandon, D., Rodbard, D., Loriaux, D. L., and Lipset, M. B. (1979): *J. Steroid Biochem.,* 10:475–481.
15. Ojasoo, T., and Raynaud, J. P. (1978): *Cancer Res.,* 38:4186–4198.
16. Rafestin-Oblin, M. E., Michaud, A., Claire, M., and Corrol, P. (1977): *J. Steroid Biochem.,* 8:19–23.
17. Rousseau, G. G., and Schmit, J. P. (1977): *J. Steroid Biochem.,* 8:911–919.
18. Wagner, R. K., Schulze, K. H., and Jungblut, P. W. (1975): *Acta Endocrinol. [Suppl.] (Copenh.),* 193:52.
19. Walters, M. R., and Clark, J. N. (1977): *J. Steroid Biochem.,* 8:1137–1144.
20. Wilson, E. M., and French, F. S. (1976): *J. Biochem. Chem.,* 251:5620–5629.

Hormones and Cancer, edited by S. Iacobelli et al.
Raven Press, New York © 1980.

Hormone Receptor Cytochemistry in Human Breast Cancer

Italo Nenci, Guidalberto Fabris, Andrea Marzola,
and Elisabetta Marchetti

Institute of Pathology, University of Ferrara, 44100 Ferrara, Italy

The main goal of the cytochemical investigation of steroid–cell interactions is to achieve the possibility of interfacing biochemical findings with biological processes at the level of individual morphologic units. This, in turn, depends on the opportunity of localizing the biochemical constituents and the related biochemical events in cellular structures. This opportunity is most valuable when dealing with the hormonal control of heterogeneous tissues such as cancer tissues. Actually, in spite of extensive investigation (see ref. 7 for review), the prediction of hormone responsiveness of neoplasia is often burdened with uncertainty. This may reflect in part the inadequacy of an approach dependent on destruction of the cell identity, such as the quantification of cytoplasmic receptors for steroid hormones by biochemical means that do not take into account the constitutive heterogeneity of tumors.

Therefore, it is important to devise alternative techniques to study the uptake, binding, and distribution of steroid hormones in intact cells. The advent of cytochemical tracer techniques has provided some of these alternative means to visualize steroid localization and activities in biological structures, thus contributing to close the gap between *in vitro* biochemistry and *in vivo* cell biology.

APPLIED METHODOLOGY

Several approaches have recently been set up to visualize steroid binding sites at the microscopic level. Since a technique that actually measures the receptor protein itself was not available until recently, it was previously necessary to exploit steroid binding properties in order to trace steroid binding sites in cell and tissue preparations (Table 1).

Molecular Cytochemistry

17β-Fluorescent Estradiol

For the purpose of visualizing steroid binding sites, a useful tool has been found in steroids linked to a fluorescein moiety which allows a direct tracing

TABLE 1. *Steroid receptor cytochemistry*

---

1. *Molecular cytochemistry*
with labeled steroids

STEROID ∗∗ RECEPTOR

2. *Immunocytochemistry*
(a) with steroid antibodies   (b) with receptor antibodies

---

of the hormone in cells and tissues. One of the newly synthesized fluorescent estradiol derivatives is 1-*(N)*-fluoresceinylestrone thiosemicarbazone (FE). Its relative binding affinity for specific cytosol receptors is sufficient to compete with estradiol to the same extent as estriol, with binding constants in the same range as those of estradiol (1).

Incubation of isolated target cells with FE has permitted the dynamic monitoring of hormone uptake, retention, and distribution. When breast cancer cells were incubated with 1×10^{-7} to 4×10^{-8} M FE at 4°C, they appeared to concentrate and retain the labeled hormone from the medium, with a heavy staining of the cytoplasmic area. Once taken up by target cells incubated at 4°C, the bound FE was translocated into the nucleus at permissive temperature much like the native hormone (Fig. 1a and b). As expected, only the nuclear localization was apparent in cells incubated from the start at 37°C, with any aspecific cytoplasmic positivity left after prolonged washing. It is noteworthy that the nucleolus appeared to be a main localization site of the translocated hormone.

Several control tests have verified that the observed positivity was issuing from specific interaction of FE with cytosol estradiol receptors. The differential dissociation of specific and unspecific complexes facing dilution due to prolonged washing in cold phosphate-buffered saline has permitted the removal of rapidly dissociating low-affinity complexes without involving loss of the receptor-bound fluorescent estradiol.

The specificity of binding to cytoplasmic sites withstanding dissociation during the prolonged cold washing step has been confirmed by competition experiments. In fact, no positivity was observed when cells had been pretreated with native estradiol or diethylstilbestrol and then incubated with the fluorescent derivative together with an excess of the native hormone (1×10^{-5} M) (Fig. 1c).

Estrogen nontarget cells, e.g., mouse fibroblast, BHK, and HEp-2 cell lines, have always failed to show any positivity after incubation with FE (Fig. 1d). In conclusion, the binding sites for this estradiol derivative appear to conform to the properties of estradiol receptors.

Besides contributing to the further elucidation of the steps of steroid-cell interaction in intact target cells, under proper conditions this fluorescent probe might be a reliable, simple, rapid, and inexpensive tool that is useful in establishing the steroid binding capacity of target tissues. In fact, when cryostatic sections of both normal and neoplastic breast specimens were incubated with FE, a

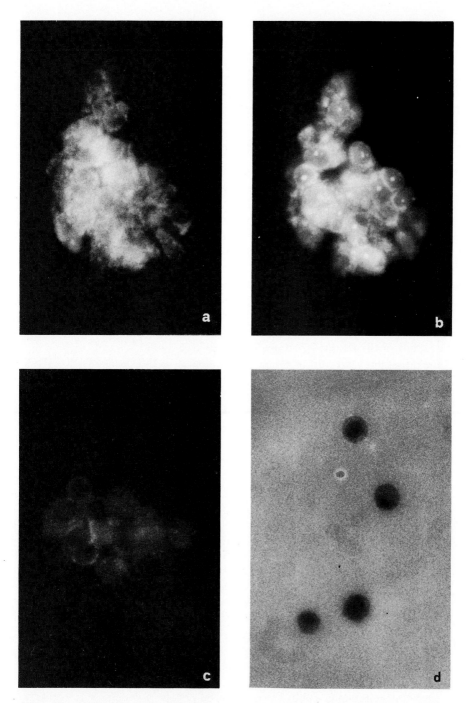

FIG. 1. Clustered breast cancer cells incubated with FE at 4°C display a cytoplasmic positivity only **(a);** when, after being photographed, they have been postincubated briefly at 37°C, the bound FE appears to translocate into the nuclear compartment **(b).** If the cells have been preincubated in "cold" estradiol, the positivity is manifestly prevented **(c).** Nontarget cells do not take up the fluorescent estradiol **(d).**

specific staining of the epithelial structures could be observed which could be prevented if binding sites had been saturated by previous incubation with specific competitors. The binding specificity has also been confirmed by the lack of positivity of nontarget cells and connective components (Fig. 2).

17β-Estradiol-Bovine Serum Albumin-Fluorescein Isothiocyanate

Other fluorescent estradiol conjugates are macromolecular steroid derivatives (4,17,18), such as 17β-estradiol-6-carboxymethyloxime-bovine serum albumin-fluorescein isothiocyanate (E-BSA-FITC). This highly fluorescent analog has been obtained by covalently linking estradiol to BSA that had previously been substituted with FITC. This macromolecular analog is hindered by its size from permeating the plasma membrane, so that it does not enter intact target cells; nevertheless, this bulky size has been an advantage in establishing the specific binding capacity on cryostatic tissue sections (Fig. 3), because of the high molecular steroid∶protein (E_2∶BSA = 24) and fluorescein∶protein (FITC∶BSA = 11) ratios. Thus, the issuing amplification of the fluorescent display could partially offset the possible decrease of total binding due to some receptor loss and to the carboxymethyloxime (CMO)-substitution of estradiol.

Careful studies have given satisfactory evidence of the specificity of E-BSA-FITC binding. The persisting reaction with estradiol antibody has offered reliable proof that the covalently bound estradiol keeps its functional groups intact; only the previous blocking of the estradiol reactive groups by specific estradiol antibody has prevented the binding of the hormone derivative to binding sites of tissue sections. Moreover, competition binding studies have shown that the fluorescent staining was prevented successfully when tissue sections had been preincubated with polyestradiol phosphate (25 µg/ml).

Immunocytochemistry

Another set of cytochemical techniques is available with several variations. These techniques involve the use of specific steroid antibodies (Table 2).

The first technique devised is a labeled antibody method, in which a primary specific antibody directed against steroid molecules is initially applied, followed by a fluorescein- or horseradish peroxidase-conjugated antibody against primary immunoglobulins. This technique has occasionally been challenged by the reported steric hindrance of steroid molecules on reaction with receptors, but it can be maintained that, at least in immunocytochemical preparations, the specifically bound steroids are not sterically hindered and can still be recognized by the antibody (3,8,12,15).

This double antibody method, the technical details of which have repeatedly been reported, has many advantages. It has also been applied successfully to the study of the dynamic monitoring of estradiol uptake, retention, and distribution in isolated breast cancer cells at the electron microscopic level (14).

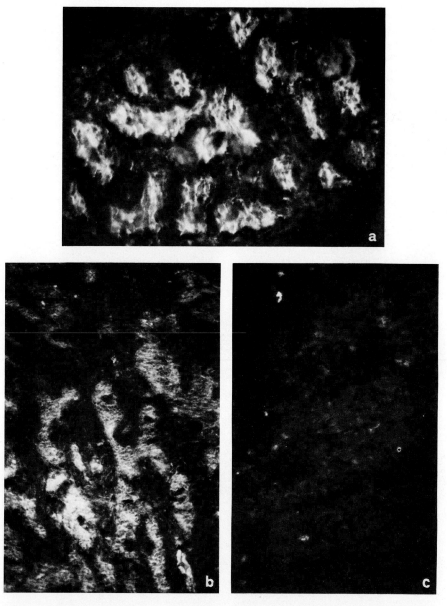

FIG. 2. Cryostatic sections of normal **(a)** and neoplastic **(b)** breast tissue treated with fluorescent estradiol display a bright cytoplasmic positivity of epithelial cells. Preincubation with diethylstilbestrol prevents the binding of fluorescent hormone **(c)**.

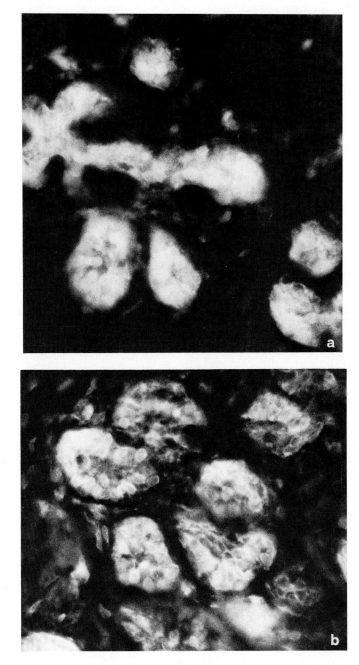

FIG. 3. Cryostatic sections of normal **(a)** and neoplastic **(b)** breast tissue treated with E-BSA-FITC. An intense fluorescence is displayed by epithelial cells that have bound the macromolecular estradiol analog.

TABLE 2. *Immunocytochemistry of specific[a] steroid binding*

Hormone	Bound by	Traced with	Surveyed by	Refs.
Native steroid	Intact cells	Steroid antibodies	Immunofluorescence Immunoperoxidase	8,12,14,15
Native steroid	Tissue fragments, then processed for inclusion	Steroid antibodies	PAP technique[b]	3
Polymeric steroid	Cryostat tissue sections	Steroid antibodies	Immunofluorescence	16
Polymeric steroid immuno-complexed with steroid antibodies	Crysostat tissue sections	—	Immunofluorescence Immunoperoxidase	13

[a] Inhibited by hormone competitors.
[b] PAP, peroxidase–antiperoxidase.

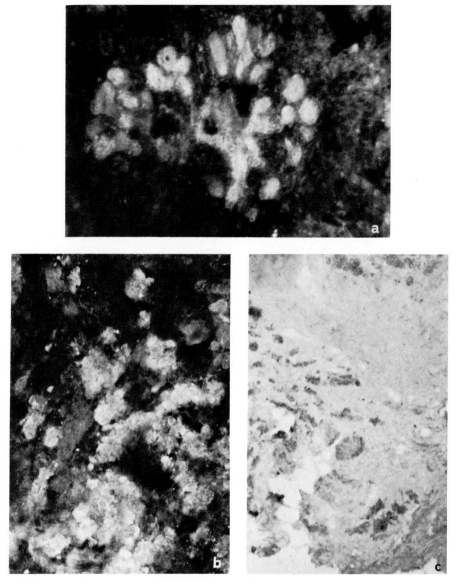

FIG. 4. Immunocomplexed polyestradiol is localized on epithelial structures of normal **(a)** and neoplastic breast tissue sections **(b,c)**. **a,b:** Immunofluorescence; **c:** Immunoperoxidase.

Among the technical variations in immunocytochemistry, an interesting one has been introduced involving a polymeric estradiol either alone (16) or reacted with specific estradiol antibody to obtain soluble polyestradiol–antibody immunocomplexes. The persistence of estradiol reactive groups in the immunocomplexed polyestradiol has been tested by the double immunodiffusion technique. This has shown that the complex maintains estradiol groups reactive with estradiol antibody, with identity lines also with native polyestradiol (13).

This macromolecular estradiol derivative cannot permeate the plasma membrane of vital cells, but it has proved to be a reliable tool in establishing the specific steroid binding capacity on cryostatic tissue sections, where it can be traced by a second anti-antibody labeled with fluorescein (Fig. 4a and b) or horseradish peroxidase (Fig. 4c).

The binding specificity has been assessed by inhibition experiments exploiting antiestrogens and diethylstilbestrol. It has been confirmed further by the lack of positivity obtained when the immunocomplex is built with an overly large antigen excess. In these instances, a competitive inhibitory effect on the finite binding capacity is caused by the excessive amount of polyestradiol.

HETEROGENEITY IN CELL HORMONE RECEPTIVITY

The cytochemical approach to specific estradiol binding has been particularly useful when focused on the problem of predicting endocrine responsiveness of breast cancer (10,11).

First of all, hormone uptake has been proved to vary considerably among individual cells of each tumor. This is not unexpected, since the cells of normal breast tissue also often show a large range of positivity. Moreover, breast cancer looks like a pool of cells, some of which bear receptors and some of which are devoid of receptors (Fig. 5).

The dynamic monitoring of hormone intracellular distribution has shown that many tumors contain a certain number of cells that fail to translocate the bound hormone into the nucleus despite normal cytoplasmic uptake (10,11).

Both fluorescent estradiol analog and immunocytochemical methods have revealed this cell heterogeneity in hormone receptivity. It appears so constitutive of breast cancer that it stands out as a biological constant of these tumors.

Fewer than 10% of the investigated tumors (approximately 150 cases) were found to be completely receptor-positive or -negative.

If the threshold of cytochemical–receptor positivity is fixed arbitrarily at 20% of the cell population of a given tumor, then the results of the cytochemical assays agree, in our experience and that of others (16–18), with those of the conventional dextran technique in more than 80% of cases. It follows that, in tumors considered positive by biochemical receptor assays, hormone responsiveness could actually be restricted to one-fifth of their cell population. This possibility must be taken into consideration when dealing with the problem of clinical management.

Generally, this cell heterogeneity in receptor content and dynamics is not reflected by distinctive morphological features. Nevertheless, in several instances a relationship between the presence of estrogen receptors and the cell functional differentiation has been recognized at the cytological level. In fact, it often occurs that the differentiated cell population of a tumor displays an evident

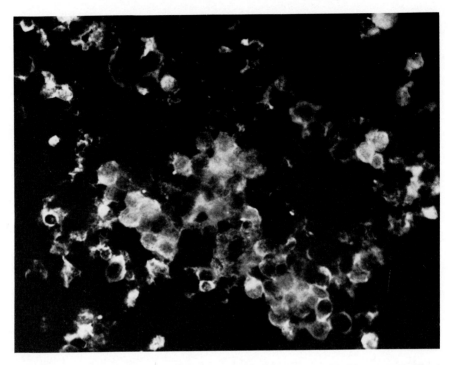

FIG. 5. Manifest heterogeneity in estradiol uptake by breast cancer cells. Fluorescent antibody technique.

estradiol uptake and nuclear translocation, while the undifferentiated cell component of the same tumor appears negative (Fig. 6).

As a general rule, in breast cancer cells in which estradiol cytoplasmic receptors have been traced, differentiated features can be recognized. This does not rule out the possibility that steroid receptors may be detected in undifferentiated cells.

Although it is not possible to define when this cell heterogeneity arises in neoplastic transformation, the available data suggest that breast cancer is a very complex entity from its first detectable expression. Since in *in situ* breast carcinomas the cytochemical methods have also displayed the presence of both receptor-positive and receptor-negative cells (Fig. 7), it seems that the heterogeneous hormone receptivity is connatural to the incipient tumor.

CONCLUDING COMMENTS

At present, although the mechanisms giving rise to the resistant phenotype are not known, this cell heterogeneity is so characteristic that it seems to be relevant to the understanding of tumor progression.

Since receptor-negative cells appear to be present in breast cancer from its

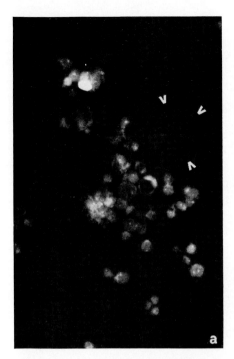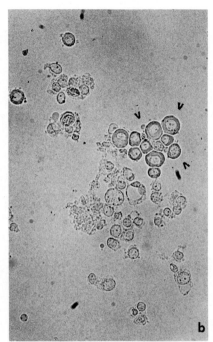

FIG. 6. Isolated cells from a signet ring lobular carcinoma of the breast treated at 37°C with FE. Differentiated cells (signet ring) have taken up and translocated the fluorescent estradiol into the nucleus **(a)**, while the anaplastic cells do not display any binding capacity and are recognizable only at phase contrast *(arrowheads)* **(b)**.

inception and, on the other hand, tumor progression leads to the final hormone unresponsiveness, receptor-negative cells appear to be favored by evolutionary intratumoral selective pressure. This, in turn, appears to signify that estradiol receptors do not provide cells with a selective growth advantage, so that the receptor mechanism could not be directly involved in the positive control of cell proliferation by estrogen. Moreover, as receptors have more often been traced in cells in which differentiated features were recognizable, it seems that the presence of receptors correlates better with the positive control of cell differentiation by estrogens.

This possibility is supported also by the demonstrated inverse relationship between receptor levels and growth rate parameters, such as the labeling index (9,19), and by the earlier recurrence (2,6) and the higher sensitivity to chemotherapy (5) of breast tumors without estrogen receptors.

In view of these data, some mechanisms other than receptors should be sought to explain how cell proliferation is controlled by estrogens. In this respect, meaningful outlooks could be afforded by the demonstrated presence of binding sites for estrogens on the plasma membrane of target cells (13).

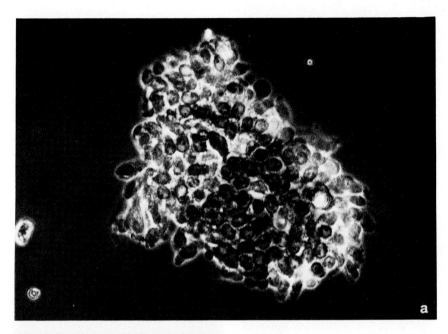

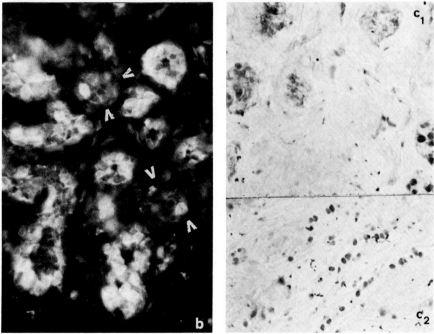

ACKNOWLEDGMENTS

The authors thank Prof. G. B. Lanza, Director of the Institute of Pathology, University of Ferrara, for institutional support. This study was supported in part by Progetto Finalizzato del C.N.R.: Controllo della Crescita Neoplastica. Sottoprogetto: Controllo Endocrinologico. Dr. Elisabetta Marchetti is the recipient of a fellowship from Fondazione Anna Villa Rusconi, Varese, Italy.

REFERENCES

1. Dandliker, W. B., Brawn, R. J., Hsu, M.-L., Brawn, P. N., Levin, J., Meyers, C. Y., and Kolb, V. M. (1978): *Cancer Res.*, 38:4212–4224.
2. Knight, W. A., III, Livingston, R. B., Gregory, E. J., and McGuire, W. L. (1977): *Cancer Res.*, 37:4669–4671.
3. Kurzon, R. M., and Sternberger, L. A. (1978): *J. Histochem. Cytochem.*, 26:803–808.
4. Lee, S. H. (1978): *Am. J. Clin. Pathol.*, 70:197–203.
5. Lippman, M. E., Allegra, J. C., Thompson, E. D., Simon, R., Barlock, A., Green, L., Huff, K. K., Do, H. M. T., Aitken, S. C., and Warren, R. (1978): *N. Engl. J. Med.*, 298:1223–1228.
6. Maynard, P. V., Blamey, R. W., Elston, C. W., Haybittle, J. L., and Griffiths, K. (1978): *Cancer Res.*, 38:4292–4295.
7. McGuire, W. L., editor (1978): *Hormones, Receptors, and Breast Cancer.* Raven Press, New York.
8. Mercer, W., Wahl, T., Carlson, C., and Teague, P. (1978): *Fed. Proc.*, 37:246 (Abstr.).
9. Meyer, J. S., Bauer, M. C., and Rao, B. R. (1978): *Lab. Invest.*, 39:225–235.
10. Nenci, I. (1978): *Cancer Res.*, 38:4204–4211.
11. Nenci, I., Beccati, M. D., and Arslan-Pagnini, C. (1978): *Tumori*, 64:161–174.
12. Nenci, I., Beccati, M. D., Piffanelli, A., and Lanza, G. (1976): *J. Steroid Biochem.*, 7:505–510.
13. Nenci, I., Fabris, G., Marchetti, E., and Marzola, A. (1980): In: *Perspectives in Steroid Receptor Research*, edited by F. Bresciani, pp. 61–72. Raven Press, New York.
14. Nenci, I., Fabris, G., Marzola, A., and Marchetti, E. (1980): In: *Pharmacological Modulation of Steroid Action*, edited by E. Genazzani, F. DiCarlo, and W. I. P. Mainwaring, pp. 99–110. Raven Press, New York.
15. Nenci, I., Piffanelli, A., Beccati, M. D., and Lanza, G. (1976): *J. Steroid Biochem.*, 7:883–891.
16. Pertschuk, L. P., Tobin, E. H., Brigati, D. J., Kim, D. S., Bloom, N. D., Gaetjens, E., Berman, P. J., Carter, A. C., and Degenshein, G. A. (1978): *Cancer*, 41:907–911.
17. Pertschuk, L. P., Tobin, E. H., Gaetjens, E., Degenshein, G. A., Antuoro, L. M., Brigati, D. J., Bloom, N. D., Carter, A. C., and Rainford, E. A. (1979): *Res. Commun. Chem. Pathol. Pharmacol.*, 23:635–638
18. Pertschuk, L. P., Zava, D. T., Gaetjens, E., Macchia, R. J., Brigati, D. J., and Kim, D. S. (1978): *Res. Commun. Chem. Pathol. Pharmacol.*, 22:427–430.
19. Silvestrini, R., Daidone, M. G., and Di Fronzo, G. (1979): *Cancer*, 44:665–670.

FIG. 7. Heterogeneity in incipient tumors of the breast. **a:** Cell cluster of an *in situ* papillary carcinoma of mammary ducts. Only part of the cells display an evident binding of FE. **b:** *In situ* lobular carcinoma. The binding of E-BSA-FITC is varying among neoplastic cells; some neoplastic ductules are plugged by cells for the most part negative *(arrowheads)*. **c:** Lobular carcinoma, *in situ* **(1)** and infiltrating **(2),** treated with immunocomplexed polyestradiol and then with horseradish peroxidase-labeled anti-IgG. The cells of the *in situ* area are highly dissimilar in binding capacity for the estradiol analog.

Hormones and Cancer, edited by S. Iacobelli et al.
Raven Press, New York © 1980.

Effects of Pyridoxal 5'-Phosphate on Estrogen–Receptor Activation and Nuclear Binding

R. Enzio Müller, Abdulmaged Traish, and H. Herbert Wotiz

*Department of Biochemistry, Boston University School of Medicine,
Boston, Massachusetts 02188*

On entry into uterine cells, estradiol (E_2) binds to specific cytoplasmic receptor proteins to form a receptor–estradiol complex (RE_2) which is rapidly translocated to the nucleus. Within the nucleus, RE_2 is thought to initiate those reactions which will eventually lead to the observed estrogen-induced alterations of the physiological state of the uterine tissue. Studies with cell-free systems have demonstrated that the cytoplasmic RE_2 complex formed at $0°C$ will only translocate to nuclei if a transformation of the complex has occurred; this transformed receptor is generally referred to as "activated" receptor. In this chapter R_iE_2 refers to the "inactive" state and R_aE_2 stands for activated state of the hormone–receptor complex. Activation can be induced by a variety of experimental manipulations, such as cytosol $(NH_4)_2SO_4$ precipitation (9), dialysis (13), gel filtration, dilution (7), and brief exposure to elevated temperatures (1). Any of these manipulations alters the physicochemical characteristics of the receptor; thus R_iE_2 sediments as a 4-S entity on 0.4 M KCl sucrose density gradients (SDG), whereas the R_aE_2 complex has a 5-S sedimentation constant; the MW of R_iE_2 is approximately 70,000, that of R_aE_2 is 130,000 (12); the R_iE_2 is a monomer, R_aE_2 is a dimer (hetero- or homodimer) (17); R_aE_2 induces RNA polymerase (9), binds to nuclei at $0°C$ during short-term incubations (4), and binds to polyanions (7). E_2 dissociates rapidly from R_iE_2, whereas the R_aE_2 complex dissociates at much slower rates (17). We have recently shown (16) that some of the above transformation reactions also occur in the intact uterine cells at 0 and $37°C$.

Since transformation–activation of R_iE_2 complexes is a prerequisite for their nuclear binding and, therefore, their biological activity, the study of these reactions is important for a better understanding of estrogen action. Recent studies have shown that pyridoxal 5'-phosphate (PLP) may be a useful compound for the chemical modification and characterization of the progesterone receptor (14) and of the glucocorticoid receptor (3,5). The studies reported here suggest that PLP inhibits nuclear binding of the uterine estrogen receptor by interfering with R_iE_2 transformation into activated R_aE_2 and with nuclear retention of R_aE_2.

MATERIALS AND METHODS

Animals

Immature 21- to 23-day-old female Sprague-Dawley CD rats were used in these studies.

Isotopes and Chemicals

[2,4,6,7-³H]Estradiol-17β (98–109 Ci/mmole) was obtained from Amersham/ Searle; diethylstilbesterol (DES) was obtained from Steraloids. All reagents were reagent grade obtained from commercial sources: dextran grade C (clinical grade) and sucrose, crystalline, RNase-free (Schwarz/Mann); hydroxylapatite (Bio-gel HTP) (Bio-Rad Laboratories); ethylenediaminetetraacetic acid (EDTA) (Eastman); Cleland reagent, A grade (dithiothreitol) (Calbiochem); PLP, pyridoxal, pyridoxine, L-lysine, and activated charcoal (Norit A) (Sigma Chemical Co.); and scintillation fluids (Liquiscint and Betafluor, National Diagnostics).

Buffers and Solutions

BSM buffer: 0.2 M boric acid, 0.25 M sucrose, 3 mM MgCl₂; pH 8.0 at 0°C. TED Buffer: 10 mM Tris, 1.5 mM EDTA, 0.5 mM dithiothreitol; pH 7.5 at 0°C. KRBG buffer: (calcium-free Krebs-Ringer bicarbonate buffer): 6.923 g/ liter NaCl, 0.353 g/liter KCl, 0.162 g/liter KH₂PO₄, 1 g/liter glucose, 2.1 g/ liter NaHCO₃; pH 7.4 at 25°C. BMK buffer: 0.2 M boric acid, 3 mM MgCl₂, 0.4 M KCl; pH 8.0 at 0°C. KCl/phosphate buffer: 5 mM NaH₂PO₄, 0.4 M KCl; pH 7.5 at 0°C.

PLP, pyridoxal, and pyridoxine were dissolved in KRBG buffer or BSM buffer and the pH adjusted at 0°C to 7.4 and 8.0 respectively; these solutions as well as the experimental incubations were always kept from exposure to light.

Preparation of Cytosol and Nuclear Fractions

All operations were done at 0 to 4°C, unless otherwise stated. Excised uteri were rinsed with BSM buffer and homogenized in this buffer (five uteri/ml). Preparation of nuclear and cytoplasmic fractions by centrifugation were performed exactly as described elsewhere (15).

Formation of Nonactivated and Temperature-Activated R[³H]E₂

Cytosol was incubated with [³H]E₂ for 1 hr at 0°C in the presence or absence of a 200-fold excess of unlabeled DES. [³H]E₂ was prepared in BSM buffer and 1 volume added to 9 volumes of cytosol to yield a final [³H]E₂ concentration of 1×10^{-8} M; protein concentrations ranged from 2 to 5 mg/ml. Temperature activation was achieved by incubating the R_iE_2 preparation at 28°C for 30 min.

Nuclear Binding of Activated RE₂

Unless otherwise stated, 1 volume of temperature-activated RE_2 was added to 1 volume of uterine nuclei suspended in BSM buffer. The incubation was performed at 0°C for 2 hr with frequent blending on a vortex mixer. Nuclei were then sedimented by centrifugation for 20 min at 800 $\times$ g and washed three times by resuspending the pellet in 3 ml of the same buffer followed by centrifugation for 10 min at 800 $\times$ g.

RE₂ Formation in Intact Uterine Tissue

Uteri was excised and placed in KRBG buffer at 0°C. The tissue was rinsed in that buffer and transferred to KRBG buffer (one uterus per milliliter) containing $[^3H]E_2$ (1×10^{-8} M) in the presence or absence of DES (2×10^{-6} M). The incubation was performed under air at 37°C for 1 hr. The tissue was then extensively rinsed in ice-cold BSM buffer and the cytoplasmic and nuclear fractions prepared as described above, except that the 800 $\times$ g supernatant of the tissue homogenate was used as a cytosol source without further centrifugation at 105,000 $\times$ g.

Assay of Nuclear-Bound and Cytoplasmic RE₂

The washed nuclear pellets were suspended in 1 ml of 95% ethanol and $[^3H]E_2$ extracted overnight at 22°C. The entire suspensions were transferred to scintillation vials, the test tubes rinsed with 1 ml of ethanol which was combined with the extracts, and radioactivity counted (2 ml ethanol: 10 ml Betafluor).

Cytoplasmic RE_2 was determined by the dextran-coated charcoal technique (11) or by the hydroxylapatite technique (18).

Throughout this study specific estrogen binding was assessed by subtracting $[^3H]E_2$ bound in the presence of an excess of unlabeled DES (nonspecific binding) from $[^3H]E_2$ bound in parallel incubations in the absence of unlabeled DES (total binding). The data shown in this chapter represent only specifically bound $[^3H]E_2$.

DNA was determined by the method of Burton (2) using calf thymus DNA as a standard. Protein was determined by the procedure of Lowry et al. (6), using bovine serum albumin as a standard.

Sucrose Density Gradients

Linear 5 to 20% or 10 to 30% sucrose gradients in the appropriate buffer (3.8 ml) were prepared in polyallomer tubes and kept at 0°C for 1 to 2 hr before use. Samples of 0.2 ml were layered on each gradient and 20 μl of a mixture of [^{14}C]bovine serum albumin and [^{14}C]γ-globulin (New England Nuclear Corp.) were added to each sample as sedimentation markers (4.6 S and 7 S, respectively). The gradients were centrifuged at 2°C in an SW 60 rotor (Beckman) using a Beckman L 5-75B ultracentrifuge. Unless otherwise specified, centrifugation was performed at an $\omega^2 t$ integrator setting of 174,000 (Radians^2/ sec × 10^7). Individual 0.1-ml fractions were collected and 4 ml of scintillation fluid was added and radioactivity counted.

Kinetics of RE₂ Dissociation

Cytoplasmic RE₂ formed at 0°C in BSM buffer (1 × 10^{-8} M [^{3}H]E₂) was incubated for 30 min at 0°C with BSM buffer containing PLP (1 vol cytosol: 1 vol buffer). Following temperature activation for 30 min at 28°C, the incubation was cooled to 0°C and added to a pellet of dextran-coated charcoal to remove most of the unbound and nonspecifically bound [^{3}H]E₂. After 15 min the sample was centrifuged and the supernatant removed and used for the dissociation kinetic studies. RE₂ dissociation was measured by adding to this cytosol unlabeled DES dissolved in BSM buffer containing the same PLP concentration as the cytosol (the final DES concentration was 2 × 10^{-6} M). At the desired time intervals duplicate samples (0.1 or 0.2 ml) were removed, added to an equal volume of an ice-cold dextran-coated charcoal suspension prepared in BSM buffer, and the specifically bound RE₂ was measured. All the data reported have been corrected for RE₂ instability (10–25% RE₂ loss over 120 min at 28°C) and for nonspecific binding.

RESULTS AND DISCUSSION

The Presence of PLP During Heat Activation of R$_i$E₂ Prevents Subsequent Nuclear Binding

Figure 1 (left) shows that cytoplasmic RE₂ heat activated for 30 min at 28°C binds to uterine nuclei at 0°C. In contrast, preincubation of the same cytosol RE₂ preparation with PLP (20 mM) at 0°C followed by heat activation inhibits nuclear binding by 86%. This inhibition is not due to a PLP-induced instability of RE₂, since at 28°C in the presence or absence of PLP RE₂ was equally stable (Fig. 1, *right*). Since PLP was present during the nuclear translocation assay, it was important to demonstrate that the observed inhibition was not due to a direct PLP effect on nuclear specific and nonspecific acceptor sites. Uterine nuclei were first treated with PLP with or without subsequent NaBH₄ reduction; nuclei were washed and heat-activated R$_a$E₂ was added. Figure 2 shows that PLP did not significantly alter nuclear acceptor capacity for R$_a$E₂, suggesting that the 86% inhibition of nuclear translocation described above (Fig. 1) was due to PLP reaction with the cytosol.

The inhibition of nuclear translocation could also have been the result of a

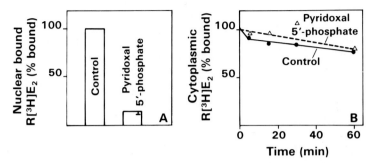

FIG. 1. Effect of PLP on nuclear binding of heat-activated $R[^3H]E_2$. **Left:** Aliquots of cytoplasmic RE_2 (3.6 mg/ml) were added to an equal volume of BSM buffer (control) or BSM buffer containing 40 mM PLP and kept at 0°C for 30 min followed by 30 min heat activation at 28°C. After cooling, 0.4 ml (620 fmoles RE_2) was added to 0.2 ml of nuclear suspension (150 μg DNA) and incubated for 2 hr at 0°C. Nuclear-bound RE_2 was measured and the data are expressed as percent of control. Nuclear-bound RE_2 in the control incubation was 127 fmoles/ 100 μg DNA. The data represent the mean of six separate experiments ± SEM. **Right:** Uterine cytosol RE_2 was added to an equal volume of BSM buffer or BSM buffer plus 40 mM PLP and incubated at 28°C; at the indicated time intervals aliquots were removed and RE_2 measured by the dextran-coated charcoal technique. 100% binding corresponded to 1.2 pmoles/ uterine equivalent and represents binding prior to incubation at 28°C.

direct effect of PLP on nuclear retention rather than inhibition of receptor activation and translocation. As shown in Fig. 3, 20 mM PLP extracted 34% of R_aE_2 from nuclei labeled in intact tissue. When nuclei were incubated with temperature-activated R_aE_2, the translocated complexes were more susceptible to PLP extraction. This suggests that, in the intact cell, RE_2 binding to nuclear acceptors is not identical to binding in a cell-free system, at least with regard to disruption of acceptor–receptor interactions by PLP. It is possible that a

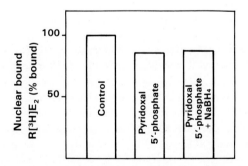

FIG. 2. Effects of PLP on uterine nuclei. One-half milliliter of nuclei (245 μg DNA) suspended in BSM buffer was mixed with an equal volume of the same buffer with or without (control) 40 mM PLP and incubated at 0°C for 15 min followed by 30 min at 28°C and 15 min at 0°C. At this point, 100 μl of NaBH₄ (1.1 M) in BSM buffer was added to one set of nuclei treated with PLP and the incubation kept at 0°C for 30 min. The other two sets received 100 μl of BSM buffer. Nuclei were then washed three times by centrifugation with BSM buffer and resuspended in 0.2 ml of BSM buffer. To each sample, 0.2 ml (2.5 mg protein/ml) of heat-activated RE_2 (550 fmoles) was added and nuclear binding performed at 0°C for 2 hr. Nuclear-bound RE_2 in the control group was equal to 200 fmoles/245 μg DNA.

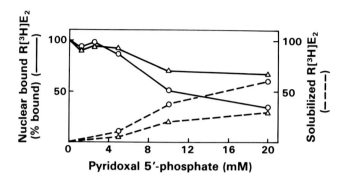

FIG. 3. Extraction of nuclear RE_2 by PLP. *Triangles:* Intact uteri were incubated at 37°C for 1 hr with $[^3H]E_2$ in the presence or absence of a 100-fold excess of unlabeled DES. Nuclei were prepared and extracted at 0°C for 1 hr with BSM buffer with the indicated concentrations of PLP (1 vol nuclear pellet : 6 vol buffer). RE_2 in the nuclei *(solid lines)* and in the extraction medium *(dashed lines)* was determined. *Circles:* Temperature-activated RE_2 was incubated at 0°C for 2 hr with uterine nuclei. Extraction of nuclear-bound RE_2 was performed as described above and RE_2 in the nuclei *(solid lines)* and in the extraction medium *(dashed lines)* was determined.

large fraction of the RE_2 solubilized in the cell-free system represents RE_2 which was bound to nonspecific acceptor sites. Alternatively, heating of cytoplasmic RE_2 complexes might yield activated RE_2 complexes that have lower affinity for nuclear binding sites than RE_2 translocated in the intact tissue. Indeed, with cell-free systems the efficiency of nuclear translocation of temperature-activated steroid–receptor complexes never exceeds 40% (4,8).

The PLP effect was due to solubilization of nuclear R_aE_2 and not to E_2 dissociation from the receptor, since the RE_2 was recovered from the extraction medium by adsorption to hydroxylapatite. Still, solubilization of nuclear-bound RE_2 only partially accounts for the 86% inhibition of nuclear binding shown in Fig. 1.

The binding of RE_2 to nuclear acceptor sites is reversible; therefore, the extraction of RE_2 by PLP could also be the result of PLP interaction with either unbound nuclear RE_2 or with RE_2 bound to nuclear acceptor sites with concomitant decreased affinity for nuclear acceptor sites and release of RE_2 into extraction medium. The effects of PLP cannot be explained on the basis of simple ionic interaction, since the ionic strength of at least 0.4 M KCl is required to achieve solubilization of nuclear RE_2.

PLP Inhibits the Temperature-Induced Transformation of R_iE_2 into R_aE_2

Transformation of R_iE_2 into R_aE_2 can be analyzed on SDG. On conventional Tris-EDTA-0.4 M KCl gradients, R_iE_2 sediments as a 4-S complex, whereas activated R_aE_2 has a sedimentation constant of 5 S. The reaction of PLP with proteins to form a Schiff's base is reversible; it was therefore important to include PLP in each gradient, to prevent its irreversible dissociation from the

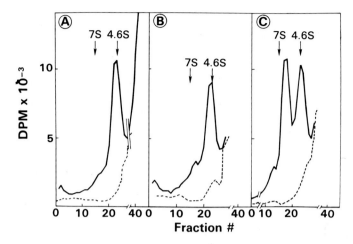

FIG. 4. PLP inhibition of RE₂ activation. Unactivated RE₂ (2.4 mg protein/ml) was incubated for 30 min at 0°C with an equal volume of BSM buffer containing 40 mM PLP. Aliquots **(A)** were kept at 0°C, or heat activated **(B)** and subjected to centrifugation on BSMK plus 20 mM PLP 10–30% sucrose gradients. **C:** A mixture of unactivated and activated untreated RE₂ (1:1, vol:vol) was centrifuged on BSMK gradients without PLP. The radioactivity profiles represent total binding **(solid line)** and nonspecific binding **(dashed line)**. Centrifugation was performed at an $\omega^2 t$ integrator setting of 174,000. [¹⁴C]γ-Globulin and [¹⁴C]bovine serum albumin were included in each gradient as internal 7-S and 4.6-S markers.

receptor during centrifugation. Furthermore, BSM or phosphate buffer had to be used, since the action of the nucleophilic -NH₂ groups in Tris-EDTA buffer may release PLP bound to receptors by transschiffization reaction.

Figure 4C demonstrates that control R_iE_2 and R_aE_2 (i.e., heat activated in the absence of PLP and centrifuged through BSMK gradients without PLP) sediment as 4.6-S and 6-S entities. Identical data were obtained when 20 mM PLP was included in these gradients. Thus the buffer composition slightly alters the sedimentation coefficients of the receptor states which, on conventional Tris-EDTA-KCl gradients, would have sedimented as 4-S (R_iE_2) and 5-S (R_aE_2) complexes. Figure 4B shows that RE₂ heat activated in the presence of PLP, sediments as a 4.6-S entity, exactly as the inactive R_iE_2 on panel A. Thus, the inhibitory effect of PLP on nuclear binding described above (Fig. 1) is due to PLP inhibition of R_iE_2 activation, and not to a PLP extraction effect on translocated R_aE_2. This latter possibility, which had to be considered since PLP was present during the translocation assay, is excluded by our findings (see Table 2) that if one reduces the unreacted PLP with NaBH₄ after the heat-activation step, an almost complete inhibition of nuclear binding is still observed.

The Effect of PLP is Specific and Concentration-Dependent

The specificity of the PLP effect was assessed by comparing the action of this reagent to that of pyridoxal and pyridoxine. As in the previous experiments,

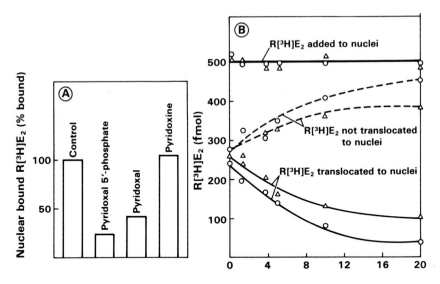

FIG. 5. Specificity and concentration dependence of the PLP effect on RE$_2$ binding to nuclei. **A:** Cytoplasmic RE$_2$ (4 mg protein/ml) was diluted with an equal volume of BSM buffer containing 40 mM PLP, pyridoxal, or pyridoxine and heat activated. Aliquots of 0.4 ml (450 fmoles RE$_2$) were added to 0.4 ml of nuclear suspension (115 μg DNA) and nuclear binding determined (control: 220 fmoles RE$_2$ bound/115 μg DNA). **B:** Cytoplasmic RE$_2$ (4.6 mg protein/ml was diluted with an equal volume of BSM buffer containing increasing concentrations of PLP or pyridoxal and heat activated. The final concentration of each reagent is given on the abscissa. Aliquots of 0.2 ml (500 fmoles RE$_2$) were added to 0.2 ml of nuclear suspension (154 μg DNA) and nuclear binding was determined (*circles:* PLP; *triangles:* pyridoxal).

the presence of 20 mM PLP inhibited nuclear binding (80% inhibition). At the same concentration, pyridoxal was less effective (60% inhibition), whereas pyridoxine was completely ineffective (Figure 5A), suggesting that positively charged groups on the receptor interact with the phosphate of PLP, thereby increasing its effective concentration at the site of Schiff's base formation. These specificity data correlate well with the capacity of each compound to interact with nucleophilic centers on the receptor, such as -NH$_2$ and -SH groups. As previously suggested for the glucocorticoid (3) and for the progesterone receptors (14), PLP is probably acting by Schiff's base formation with ε-amino groups of lysine. Figure 5B shows that the effect of these reagents was concentration-dependent and that the stability of temperature-activated RE$_2$ was not affected, since the RE$_2$ not translocated to the nuclei was recovered in the supernatant of the nuclear pellet by adsorption to hydroxylapatite.

The concentration dependence of the PLP effect is also seen in Figure 6. In this experiment R$_i$E$_2$ was heat activated in the presence of increasing concentrations of PLP (1.25, 5, and 10 mM) and subjected to SDG centrifugation analysis. The sedimentation profiles demonstrate that with increasing PLP concentration a higher fraction of RE$_2$ remains in the inactivated 4.6-S state. Similarly (10),

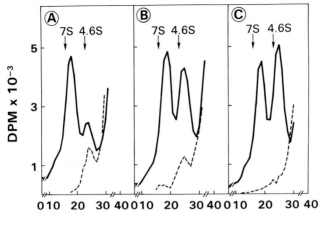

FIG. 6. Effects of increasing concentrations of PLP on RE₂ activation. Unactivated RE₂ (2.5 mg/ml) was diluted with an equal volume of BSM buffer containing 2.5 mM **(A)**, 10 mM **(B)**, and 20 mM **(C)** PLP. Following heat activation the samples were centrifuged on linear 5–20% BSMK gradients containing 1.25 mM **(A)**, 5 mM **(B)**, and 10 mM **(C)** PLP. Centrifugation conditions and symbols as in Fig. 4.

when the protein concentration of the cytoplasm was diluted and the PLP concentration kept constant, the fraction of inactivated R_iE_2 (4.6 S) increased with decreasing protein concentration.

PLP Reacts with R_iE_2 and R_aE_2

Since in the previous experiments PLP was added to R_iE_2 at 0°C and then the temperature of the incubation raised to 28°C, the inhibition of nuclear binding could have been the result of PLP binding to R_iE_2 with consequent inhibition of transformation as well as PLP binding to heat-activated R_aE_2. The SDG analysis data presented in Figs. 4 and 6 suggest that PLP prevents transformation of R_iE_2 into R_aE_2. However, it is also conceivable that those RE₂ complexes which sediment as activated 6-S R_aE_2 are modified by PLP through Schiff's base formation with amino acid residues that became accessible upon heat activation.

Table 1 summarizes the data obtained in two experiments in which PLP was added to the RE₂ preparation either before or after heat activation. PLP reacted with the heat-activated receptor to inhibit nuclear binding (inhibition is 64% in experiment 1 and 53% in experiment 2). The inhibition of nuclear binding was significantly higher when PLP was added before heat activation (80% in experiment 1 and 73% in experiment 2). This suggests that the compound also interacts with the inactive receptor.

TABLE 1. *Effects of PLP addition before and after heat activation on nuclear binding of RE₂*

| | Nuclear binding | |
| | --- | --- |
Exp. no.	PLP added before heat-activation (% bound)[c]	PLP added after heat-activation (% bound)
Exp. 1[a]	20	36
Exp. 2[b]	27	47

[a] Exp. 1. Cytoplasmic RE₂ was mixed with an equal volume of BSM buffer with or without (control) PLP, (40 mM), incubated for 30 min at 0°C followed by temperature activation, and the nuclear binding assay was performed. 489 fmoles RE₂ (1.7 mg protein/ml) were incubated with an equal volume of nuclear suspension (190 μg DNA). RE₂ binding in the control incubation was 200 fmoles.

[b] Exp. 2. Aliquots of cytoplasmic RE₂ were heat activated, cooled, and then diluted either with an equal volume of BSM buffer (control) or with BSM buffer containing 20 mM PLP. After 1 hr at 0°C the nuclear binding assay was performed.

[c] Data expressed as percent of control.

Reversibility of PLP Inhibition of RE₂ Activation

The data presented in Table 2 demonstrates that the nuclear binding capacity of PLP-treated RE₂ is partially restored if dithiothreitol or L-lysine is added to the incubation. However, when NaBH₄ reduction preceded addition of dithiothreitol or lysine, nuclear binding could not be restored, suggesting that a Schiff base had been formed between PLP and R₁E₂. Treatment of control cytosol with NaBH₄ had no effect on nuclear binding.

TABLE 2. *Reversibility of the PLP inhibition of RE₂ activation*[a]

Treatment of RE₂ formed at 0°C	RE₂ (fmoles) translocated to nuclei
1. 28°C (control incubation)	214
2. PLP → 28°C	13
3. 28°C → DTT 0°C	234
4. PLP → 28°C → DTT 0°C	96
5. 28°C → NaBH₄ 0°C	230
6. PLP → 28°C → NaBH₄ 0°C → DTT 0°C	30
7. 28°C → L-lysine 0°C	209
8. PLP → 28°C → L-lysine 0°C	134
9. PLP → 28°C → NaBH₄ 0°C → L-lysine 0°C	16

[a] Cytoplasmic RE₂ was formed at 0°C (4.2 mg protein/ml) and added to an equal volume of BSM buffer (no. 1), or BSM containing 40 mM PLP (no. 2). Aliquots were heat activated and treated for 30 min at 0°C with dithiothreitol (DTT) or L-lysine (final molarity 0.1 M) (nos. 3,4,7,8). Aliquots of no. 1 and no. 2 were also treated with NaBH₄ prior addition of DTT or L-lysine (nos. 5,6,9). Furthermore, the effects of each reagent on nuclear translocation of control RE₂ were examined (nos. 3,5,7). NaBH₄ reduction was performed at 0°C for 30 min at 0.1 M concentration.

Kinetics of E_2 Dissociation from Receptor Heat Activated in the Presence of PLP

E_2 dissociates from the activated R_aE_2 complex at a much slower rate than from the inactive R_iE_2 complex (17). Thus, analysis of dissociation kinetics provides a criterion to distinguish between the transformed and untransformed receptor states (R_aE_2 versus R_iE_2). Figure 7 demonstrates that heat activation of R_iE_2 in the presence of PLP yields two populations of RE_2 complexes with different affinity for E_2: the fast dissociating component represents R_iE_2; the slow dissociating component represents the activated high affinity state of RE_2, with a $t\ ½$ value of 85 min, identical to that of control R_aE_2. The ratio of fast to slow dissociating RE_2 states is a function of the PLP concentration; the slow dissociating component is detected at 2.5 mM PLP and progressively increases to reach a maximum at 10 mM PLP.

PLP and Pyridoxal (But Not Pyridoxine) Inhibit Nuclear Binding of RE_2

It was important to verify whether PLP and related compounds were also effective inhibitors of nuclear translocation when added to intact uteri. Uteri were incubated at 37°C for 30 min in calcium-free KRBG buffer containing either PLP, pyridoxal, or pyridoxine; RE_2 formation and nuclear translocation were then achieved by adding E_2 to the medium and continuing the incubation for 60 min at 37°C. The nuclear and cytoplasmic fractions were prepared and specifically bound E_2 was measured. The data on Table 3 show that similarly to the previous experiments with a cell-free system, PLP and Pyridoxal, but

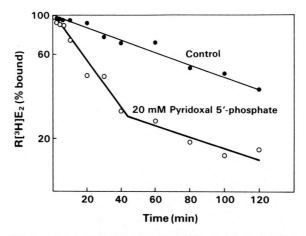

FIG. 7. Effect of PLP on dissociation kinetics of $R[^3H]E_2$. Unactivated $R[^3H]E_2$ complex was heat activated in the absence (control) or presence of 20 mM PLP. Dissociation of $[^3H]E_2$ was measured at 28°C by adding an excess of radioinert E_2 and specific binding measured as described. The data are expressed as percentage of 0 time binding, i.e., prior to addition of radioinert E_2. The data were corrected for nonspecific binding and RE_2 instability. Protein concentration in the dissociation incubation was 1 mg/ml.

TABLE 3. *Specificity of the PLP effect on nuclear binding of RE₂ in intact tissue[a]*

Experiment	fmoles Nuclear RE₂[b] (uterine equivalent)	fmoles Cytoplasmic RE₂ (uterine equivalent)	
		Direct assay	Assayed after 18 hr incubation at 0°C with [³H]E₂
Exp. 1			
Control	840 (100)	250	230
PLP	540 (64)	278	245
Pyridoxal	415 (49)	95	105
Pyridoxine	860 (102)	240	(not measured)
Exp. 2			
Control	640 (100)	200	185
PLP	420 (65)	150	140
Pyridoxal	300 (46)	100	90
Pyridoxine	668 (104)	260	(not measured)
Exp. 3			
Control	480 (100)	65	
PLP	350 (72)	63	
Exp. 4			
Control	760 (100)	150	
PLP	460 (60)	100	
Pyridoxal	240 (31)	45	

[a] Uteri (one uterus/ml) were preincubated under air for 30 min at 37°C in KRBG buffer, pH 7.4, containing the indicated compounds at a final concentration of 20 mM. To each group [³H]E₂ in KRBG buffer was added (final concentration 1×10^{-8} M) and the incubation extended for 60 min at 37°C. The uteri were extensively rinsed in ice-cold BSM buffer and homogenized in the same buffer (five uteri/ml). Nuclear and cytoplasmic fractions were then assayed for specifically bound [³H]E₂. To determine the presence of empty receptor sites, aliquots of cytosol were incubated at 0°C for 18 hr with [³H]E₂ and RE₂ measured by the dextran-coated charcoal technique.
[b] Numbers in parentheses are percentages.

not pyridoxine, are inhibitors of nuclear binding. At the molarity tested, the extent of the inhibition was less than that observed with the cell-free system. Surprisingly, the cytoplasmic fraction of those uteri in which inhibition of nuclear RE₂ binding was measured did not contain correspondingly higher amounts of RE₂, nor could empty receptor sites be detected by reincubation in BSM or TED buffer with [³H]E₂ (1×10^{-8} M) for 18 hr.

These data provide the first evidence for a possible role of PLP as a modulator of estrogen receptor activity in the intact tissue. The inhibition of nuclear binding was smaller than that observed with the cell-free system, and pyridoxal appeared to be somewhat more effective than PLP. Differences in the mechanism of uptake of these two compounds may alter their intracellular concentration and contribute to the quantitative differences in inhibition of nuclear RE₂ binding observed between cell-free system and intact tissue. The failure to detect untranslocated

RE$_2$ or unbound receptor cannot be explained at the moment and may represent an experimental artifact. This question is currently under investigation.

The scheme presented in Fig. 8 is based on the assumption that PLP inhibits nuclear binding of RE$_2$ by direct interaction with the receptor. Our data do not rule out the possibility that the decreased nuclear binding was due to PLP interference with the action of other cytoplasmic components (e.g., enzymes) required for receptor activation and nuclear binding; however, since such components have not as yet been identified, we will only discuss PLP action on the receptor.

We have demonstrated that PLP prevents nuclear binding of RE$_2$ in a cell-free system and in the intact tissue. This action was not due to PLP alteration of nuclear acceptor sites, nor to PLP-induced dissociation of E$_2$ from the receptor.

The first reaction in Fig. 8, i.e., E$_2$ binding to the receptor at 0°C to form R$_i$E$_2$, is not affected by PLP. It is likely that PLP reacts with nucleophilic centers of both R$_i$ and R$_i$E$_2$ to form a Schiff's base. Whether the same amino acid residues are involved in this reaction cannot be assessed at the moment. The reactions shown on Fig. 8 represent reversible binding of PLP to the receptor in its various states. This is based on the well-known fact that Schiff's base formation between PLP and proteins is a reversible reaction. Furthermore, we have shown that dithiothreitol and L-lysine reverse the action of PLP on the estrogen receptor by transschiffization. The reaction of PLP with the activated receptor modifies R$_a$E$_2$ thereby preventing either translocation or nuclear retention. It is likely that PLP formed a Schiff base with R$_a$E$_2$ amino acid residues; these may be either directly involved in nuclear binding and retention, or be distal to the receptor–acceptor binding site but crucial to the maintenance of a conformational state which, if slightly altered, decreases the R$_a$E$_2$ affinity

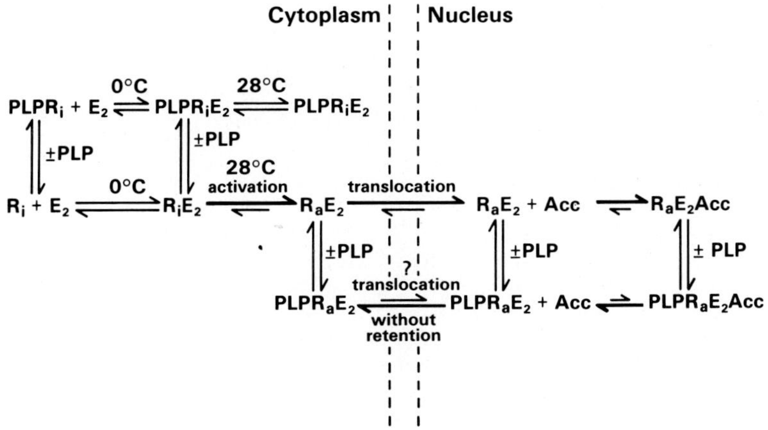

FIG. 8. The multiple points of action of pyridoxal 5′-phosphate leading to reduced nuclear binding of receptor–estrogen complex. R$_i$, inactive unbound receptor; R$_i$E$_2$, untransformed inactive RE$_2$; R$_a$E$_2$, transformed activated RE$_2$; Acc, specific and nonspecific acceptor sites for translocated RE$_2$.

for nuclear binding sites. The finding that PLP extracts intact nuclear RE$_2$ complexes, as judged by hydroxylapatite adsorption and SDG analysis (Müller et al., *unpublished observation*), suggests that it reacts with intranuclear R$_a$E$_2$ in a similar fashion as with the above cytosol R$_a$E$_2$, i.e., by decreasing its affinity for nuclear sites. This effect is not comparable to that of high salt buffers, since the latter must contain at least 0.4 M NaCl or KCl.

The finding that in the presence of PLP 10 to 20% of RE$_2$ became activated and bound to nuclei is explained by the reversibility of the reactions involving PLP.

In conclusion, PLP sensitivity appears to be a general feature of steroid receptors or of cytoplasmic components involved in their activation and nuclear binding. In the case of the uterine estrogen receptor, PLP inhibits activation of R$_i$E$_2$, as well as nuclear binding of R$_a$E$_2$. This effect is reversible and is not only observed in cell-free system, but also in the intact uterine tissue (see also ref. 10). We are currently investigating whether PLP has a similar inhibitory activity *in vivo*.

REFERENCES

1. Brecher, P. I., Vigersky, R., Wotiz, H. S., and Wotiz, H. H. (1967): *Steroids,* 10:635–651.
2. Burton, K. (1956): *Biochem. J.,* 62:315–323.
3. Cake, M. H., DiSorbo, D. M., and Litwack, G. (1978): *J. Biol. Chem.,* 253:4886–4891.
4. Chamness, G. C., Jennings, A. W., and McGuire, W. L. (1974): *Biochemistry,* 13:327–331.
5. Cidlowski, J. A., and Thanassi, J. W. (1978): *Biochem. Biophys. Res. Commun.,* 82:1140–1146.
6. Lowry, O. H., Rosebrough, J., Farr, A. L., and Randall, R. J. (1951): *J. Biol. Chem.,* 193:265–275.
7. Milgrom, E., Atger, M., and Baulieu, E.-E. (1973): *Biochemistry,* 12:5198–5205.
8. Milgrom, E., Atger, M., and Baulieu, E.-E. (1973): *Biochim. Biophys. Acta,* 320:267–283.
9. Mohla, S., DeSombre, E. R., and Jensen, E. V. (1972): *Biochem. Biophys. Res. Commun.,* 46:661–667.
10. Müller, R. E., Traish, A. M., and Wotiz, H. H. (1980): *J. Biol. Chem.,* 255:4062–4067.
11. Müller, R. E., and Wotiz, H. H. (1979): *Endocrinology,* 100:513–519.
12. Notides, A. C., Hamillton, D. E., and Auer, H. E. (1975): *J. Biol. Chem.,* 250:3945–3950.
13. Sato, B., Nishizawa, Y., Noma, K., Matsumoto, K., and Yamamura, Y. V. (1979): *Endocrinology,* 104:1474–1479.
14. Toft, D., Roberts, P. E., Nishigori, H., and Moudgil, V. K. (1979): In *Steroid Hormone Receptor Systems,* edited by W. W. Leavitt and J. C. Clark, pp. 329–341. Plenum, New York.
15. Traish, A. M., Müller, R. E., and Wotiz, H. H. (1977): *J. Biol. Chem.,* 252:6823–6830.
16. Traish, A. M., Müller, R. E., and Wotiz, H. H. (1979): *J. Biol. Chem.,* 254:6560–6563.
17. Weichman, B. M., and Notides, A. C. (1977): *J. Biol. Chem.,* 252:8856–8862.
18. Williams, D., and Gorski, J. (1974): *Biochemistry,* 13:5537–5542.

Cell Biology of Cancer

Hormones and Cancer, edited by S. Iacobelli et al.
Raven Press, New York © 1980.

Growth and Differentiation of Cultured Rat Mammary Epithelial Cells

P. S. Rudland, *D. C. Bennett, and M. J. Warburton

*The Ludwig Institute for Cancer Research, Royal Marsden Hospital,
Sutton, Surrey, England*

The mammary gland consists of two cellular structures, epithelium and mesenchyme. The epithelial components of the mammary gland, which are embedded in a fatty stroma or mesenchyme, comprise a branching system of ducts which, if fully developed, terminate in clusters of alveoli that secrete lipid and milk specific proteins, notably caseins, during lactation. Three main types of mammary epithelial cell are distinguishable; those lining the alveoli, those lining the ducts, and the myoepithelial cells which form a layer around both ducts and alveoli (15). Growth and development of these epithelial structures occurs both by a process of cell multiplication and of differentiation (9). A number of mammotropic hormones affecting these processes in normal glands and in carcinogen-induced tumors have been identified in rodents by means of a series of endocrine gland-ablation and hormone-replacement experiments, and they include prolactin, growth hormone, estrogens, glucocorticoids, and progesterone (12,18,20,35).

However, the relationships between the different cell types, including any program of cellular interconversions, and the primary targets (whether epithelial or mesenchymal) for the mammotropic hormones in mammary development are largely unknown. To tackle the problem of mammary development in a more controlled way we have initially developed a system for obtaining short-term cell cultures of relatively pure stromal and epithelial cells from rat mammary glands and dimethylbenz[a]anthracene(DMBA)-induced mammary adenocarcinomas (11,26) and then separated epithelial cell populations physically or by developing clonal cell lines (3,25).

MAMMARY CELL TYPES PRESENT IN PRIMARY CULTURES

So far we have identified three clearly morphologically distinct types of cells which attach to the Petri dish and grow in primary cultures of mammary tissue from mature rats and from DMBA-induced tumors (26): (a) stromal cells of fibroblastic appearance ("fibroblastoid"), most of which adhere to the plastic

---

* Present address: The Salk Institute, San Diego, California 92138.

surface within 2 hr of plating; (b) the first cells to migrate from the organoids, which attach 3 to 24 hours after plating; these form a layer of flat eosinophilic, usually elongated cells; and (c) tightly packed, basophilic, cuboidal cells that spread last as a sheet, often on top of the flat cells (Fig. 1). A "presticking" step was subsequently used as a method to produce cultures enriched in either stromal (type 1) or epithelial (types 2 and 3) cells. A fourth "type" of cell has been tentatively identified recently—a cell morphologically intermediate between the cuboidal and elongated cell type (P. S. Rudland and R. Thompson, *unpublished results*).

Preliminary characterization of the cells in primary cultures has been attempted, although more detailed studies have been performed on the representative cell lines. Three classes of clonal cell lines, which are thought to originate from the three types of cell in primary cultures, are compared below and in Table 3; we indicate where differences between the primary populations are known and comparable to differences between the cell lines. Many of the cells in the early plating or stromal fraction formed lipocytes on extended culture.

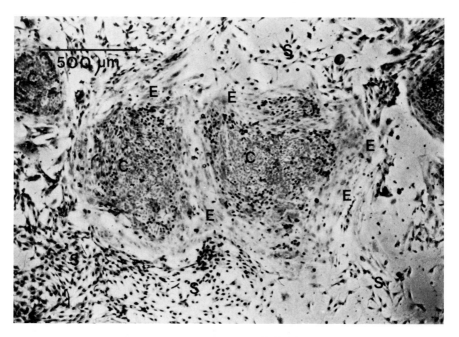

FIG. 1. Primary culture of rat mammary cells from a DMBA-induced tumor. Primary cultures from DMBA-induced tumors were kept in serum-free medium containing 50 ng/ml insulin, 500 ng/ml hydrocortisone for 48 hr, after the original plating. Fetal calf serum (20%) + 50 ng/ml insulin + hydrocortisone were added and the cultures exposed to [³H]thymidine for 48 hr. Cultures were fixed and stained. The three readily identifiable cell types shown are: cuboidal epithelial (C), elongated or "bottom" (E), and stromal (S) cells. The cells that were synthesizing DNA in the previous 48 hr have radioactively labeled nuclei. (From Rudland et al., ref. 25, with permission.)

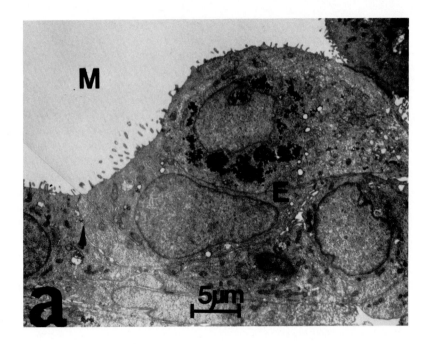

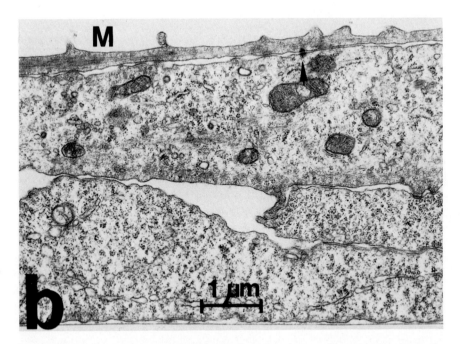

FIG. 2. Electron micrographs of primary epithelium from tumors. Electron micrograph of a vertical section through the region of the cell contacts of epithelium from DMBA-induced tumors. **a:** The surface of the microexplant (E) is covered with microvilli, and a junctional complex *(arrowhead)* is present between the cells spreading to form the colony. M, medium. **b:** Higher magnification showing a desmosome-like structure *(arrowhead)* between the two upper cells in the periphery of the colony, and the lower "mesenchymal-like" cells adjacent to the plastic. (From Rudland et al., ref. 26, with permission.)

When implanted into cleared mammary fat pads of syngeneic rats, this fraction formed only fatty outgrowths, consistent with a mesenchymal origin. Cells in the epithelial fraction from normal tissue, on the other hand, formed fully developed mammary outgrowths (P. S. Rudland and H. Durbin, *unpublished results*) when implanted into the same regions and the rats were subsequently mated, consistent with their epithelial source. When examined in the electron microscope, the colonial cells from both normal and tumorous glands were stacked several layers thick in the central areas (Fig. 2a). The upper layer was usually of cuboidal cells covered with numerous microvilli (Fig. 2a) and linked by specific cell junctional complexes (25), together indicating an absorptive or secretory epithelium. Some of the lower cells failed to exhibit these characteristics but contained bundles of fibers (Fig. 2b). These results suggest that the bottom type 2 cells seen by light microscopy were myoepithelial cells, although their ultrastructure was not sufficiently well differentiated to make an absolute distinction between myoepithelial and mesenchymal cells. A partial separation of these two cell layers could be achieved by preferentially detaching the upper cuboidal cells with EDTA-containing solutions (2). Final proof of the mammary and epithelial nature of the late plating cells was their ability to synthesize casein (26).

MITOGENIC ACTIVITY OF KNOWN HORMONE AND GROWTH FACTORS ON CULTURED CELLS

The growth rate of secondary cultures of stromal or epithelial cell fractions was reduced by lowering the serum concentration to 0.5% for 4 to 5 days before testing for the ability of different hormones and growth factors to increase the rate of initiation of DNA synthesis (Table 1). Large sample sizes were necessary because of marked variation in rates of DNA synthesis between epithelial colonies (or parts of a colony) in the same culture. The most active hormones in stimulating DNA synthesis in the epithelial cells lining the ducts and alveoli (26) were bovine prolactin and growth hormone, although the maximum response with prolactin was only achieved at relatively high concentrations (500 ng/ml). This response was increased still further when hydrocortisone and insulin were included in the medium, but these hormones had little effect alone in the above conditions (synergistic effect; for discussion see ref. 27). Similar effects were seen in the number of cells subsequently dividing. This additional increment was more marked in epithelial cultures from normal than from tumorous glands (26). Prolactin and growth hormone with or without insulin and hydrocortisone had little effect on DNA synthetic rates of cultured stromal cells. Bovine pituitary fibroblast growth factor, on the other hand, stimulated DNA synthetic rates in stromal but not in epithelial cell fractions, and this stimulation was usually augmented with insulin and hydrocortisone as previously reported for mouse fibroblastic cells (28). Epidermal growth factor [also in mouse (39) and human (34) cultures] and prostaglandin $F_{2\alpha}$, but not prostaglandin E_1, were also active

TABLE 1. *Effect of pituitary-related hormones on DNA synthesis in secondary cultures from tumors[a]*

Addition to basal medium containing hydrocortisone and insulin (ng/ml)	Cell fraction	DNA synthesis (1% labeled nuclei ± SEM)
None		4.3 ± 0.1
Epidermal growth factor (10)		13.1 ± 0.7
Fibroblast growth factor (50)		6.4 ± 1.0
Growth hormone (50)		13.9 ± 0.2
Pituitary factor (50)		10.5 ± 1.5
Prolactin (500)	Epithelial	15.1 ± 2.8
Prolactin + pituitary factor		9.4 ± 0.6
Prolactin-hydrocortisone-insulin		11.0 ± 1.4
Rat serum (10%)		33 ± 4
Serum from hypoxed rats (10%)		8.3 ± 1.6
Serum from hypoxed rats (10%) + prolactin + growth hormone[b]		16.2 ± 2.8
None		1.6 ± 0.8
Fibroblast growth factor (50)		17.0 ± 2.5
Fibroblast growth factor-hydrocortisone-insulin	Stromal	8.3 ± 2.5
Pituitary factor (50)		2.5 ± 1.2
Prolactin (500)		2.1 ± 1.0

[a] Triplicate secondary epithelial or stromal cultures from two matched and pooled DMBA-induced tumors remained for 6 days in medium containing 0.5% fetal calf serum, then 500 ng/ml hydrocortisone, 50 ng/ml insulin were added (basal medium) together with various agents. The percentage of cells with [³H]thymidine radioactively labeled nuclei in 40 hr ± SEM was recorded. Serum from hypophysectomized (hypoxed) and normal rats of the same age contained approximately the same amount of protein per milliliter.

[b] The same results were obtained if progesterone (5 ng/ml), estradiol (5 ng/ml), triiodothyronine (5 ng/ml) were also included. The hormones and growth factors used were originally isolated from cows except epidermal growth factor from mice.

Data from Rudland et al., ref. 26, with permission.

in increasing rates of DNA synthesis in the epithelial cell fraction (Table 1). The effects of other hormones reported to have mammotropic activity *in vivo* are shown in Table 2. Glucocorticoids, insulin, and progesterone augmented the response to prolactin at near physiological concentrations, while thyroid hormones inhibited the response, but were themselves stimulatory in its absence. The differential mitogenic effects of thyroid hormones depending on the presence or absence of prolactin may in part explain contradictory reports on the mammotropic effect of thyroid hormones in rodents (1). The stimulatory effect of prolactin on epithelial DNA synthesis mimicked somewhat its effects on tumor growth *in vivo,* since those tumors which could grow in the absence of appreciable levels of circulating prolactin or estrogen also showed little response to prolactin in secondary epithelial cultures (11).

DISCOVERY OF POTENTIALLY NOVEL GROWTH FACTORS

However, the effects on increasing rates of DNA synthesis with the pituitary hormones growth hormone and prolactin, in combination with hydrocortisone

TABLE 2. *Agents that induce changes in DNA synthesis in epithelial cultures from normal and tumorous glands[a]*

Agent	Type	Conc. range (ng/ml)	Effect
Epidermal growth factor	} Growth factors	1–10	+
Pituitary factor		10–100	+
Growth hormone		10–100	+
Prolactin	} Polypeptide hormones	50–500	+
Insulin		5–50	+
Estradiol		50–500	−[b]
Corticosterone		50–500	+
Hydrocortisone		5–50	+
Progesterone	} Steroids	5–50	+
Prednisone		5–50	+
Testosterone		5–50	−
Triiodothyronine	} Thyroid hormones	1–10	±[c]
Thyroxine		5–50	±[c]
Prostaglandin E_1	} Prostaglandins	100–1,000	−
Prostaglandin $F_{2\alpha}$		100–1,000	+
Serum		10% (vol/vol)	+
Conditioned medium	Rat fibroblasts	—	+
Conditioned medium	Rat myoepithelial cells	—	+

[a] Agents were tested for their effects on DNA synthesis in secondary cultures of epithelial cells from normal or tumorous glands in 0.5% fetal calf serum with or without prolactin, hydrocortisone, and insulin. The approximate range of concentrations for the observable effects is shown.

[b] Estradiol below 5 ng/ml failed to show any effect in our system.

[c] Thyroid hormones showed negative effects with prolactin at 500 ng/ml but positive effects in its absence. Polypeptides tested which had little or no effect were fibroblast growth factor, luteinizing hormone, follicle stimulating hormone, thyroid stimulating hormone.

Data from Rudland et al., ref. 26, with permission.

and insulin, were still appreciably smaller than with 10% serum in the above conditions (Table 1). Similarly, serum from hypophysectomized rats yielded lower stimulatory activity than normal rat serum, and this could be only partially restored with prolactin and growth hormone (Table 1) or all the known mammotropic hormones (P. S. Rudland et al., *unpublished results*). This suggested that another pituitary-derived (or at least pituitary-controlled) component that was responsible for increasing rates of DNA synthesis was present in rat serum. Certain fractions of bovine pituitaries from a carboxylmethylcellulose column were tested for their capability to increase rates of DNA synthesis, and one fraction, which also contained ovarian growth factor (7) showed stimulatory activity. This was termed pituitary mammary growth factor (PMGF). Since this fraction contained several components when analyzed by electrophoresis through SDS-polyacrylamide gels, none of which corresponded to bovine prolac-

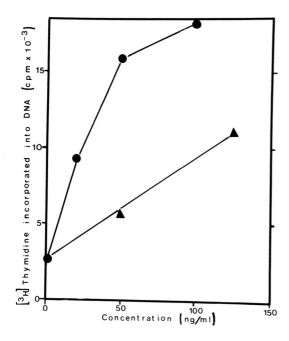

FIG. 3. Relative effects of different concentrations of pituitary factor and prolactin on incorporation of [³H]thymidine into normal secondary epithelial cultures. Secondary epithelial mammary cultures from perphenazine-treated female rats were prepared. After 2 days the medium was changed to one containing 0.5% fetal calf serum + 50 ng/ml insulin + 500 ng/ml hydrocortisone. Then after a further 5 days either varying concentrations (ng/ml) of bovine pituitary factor *(circles)* or bovine prolactin *(triangles)* were added and the cultures exposed to [³H]thymidine for 40 hr. The counts per minute (cpm) incorporated into DNA per culture were recorded. (From Rudland et al., ref. 26, with permission.)

tin, it is unknown if ovarian growth factor or the mammary growth factor of Kano-Sueoka et al. (13) was responsible for this activity. However, this semipurified component was at least 10 times as active on a per weight basis as pure prolactin (Fig. 3). Medium "conditioned" by exposure to rat fibroblasts [also human (37)] or a myoepithelial-like cell line (also human; M. Stampfer, *unpublished results*), Rama 29 (see below), was also a most potent stimulator of DNA synthesis of primary and secondary epithelial cultures. The active components in conditioned medium were termed fibroblast cell mammary growth factor (FMGF) and myoepithelial cell mammary growth factor (MMGF). Their nature, cell specificity, and relationship to each other, to PMGF, and to other pure growth factors is as yet unknown. The possible complexity of the system involving interacting cells in the mammary gland can be seen when rat mammary stromal or "fibroblastoid" cells can be stimulated to grow by pituitary fibroblast growth factor. The stromal cells can in turn produce components that stimulate epithelial cells *in vitro*. Stromal cell-induced stimulation of the growth of epithelial cells *in vitro* is also consistent with the fact that stromal cells form the fat pad *in vivo*, which in turn is required for mammary epithelial cell growth and development (4). Similarly, since the myoepithelial-like cells produce a most potent mitogen for what are probably "lining" epithelial cells, then myoepithelial cells *in vivo* can possibly influence the proliferation of "lining" epithelial cells in close proximity. The physiological significance of all these growth factors is as yet unknown.

ISOLATION OF MAMMARY STEM CELL LINES

All the above results were obtained in cultures composed of at least two epithelial cell types, although labeling indices were only scored in the "cuboidal" one. Further analysis of the epithelial response depended on the isolation of populations of a single cell class, which was achieved by "cloning." However, the resulting cell lines differed from the primary epithelial cells in having generally higher proliferation rates and lower death rates.

The cell line Rama 25 was obtained from the "upper" cell fraction (as described above) of epithelial cultures from a DMBA-induced adenocarcinoma (3). Similar cell lines were obtained from normal rudimentary glands, Rama 75, etc. (P. S. Rudland et al., *unpublished*). Some cells in this fraction proliferated when plated in conditioned medium to form single-layered colonies of cells resembling low, cuboidal epithelium as seen in Fig. 4a. Cells of this appearance were termed "cuboidal." Cell strains derived from colonies of cuboidal cells from this tumor and from normal glands gave rise to a mixture of cuboidal cells and another cell type, somewhat like fibroblasts, but more like cells in the bottom layer of primary epithelial cultures. These cells were termed "elongated" and are shown in Fig. 4c. Cuboidal cells were cloned repeatedly and gave rise to both cuboidal and elongated cells unless the cultures were kept sparse by frequent passage. The tumor-derived cell line Rama 25 is an essentially pure clonal line of cuboidal cells maintained by frequent passage, while Rama 29 is a clonal line of elongated cells derived from a Rama 25 culture which was permitted to become confluent. Dense cultures of cuboidal cells from Rama 25, and from the equivalent cell from normal glands formed not only elongated cells, but also groups of cells with a third morphology: dark and polygonal, with many vacuoles or "droplets" at their peripheries. These cells were termed "droplet" cells (Fig. 4b). Unlike the cuboidal cells, the patches of droplet cells often formed hemispherical blisters or "domes" in the cell-monolayer (19) (Fig. 4b). The rate of droplet cell and dome formation could be rapidly accelerated with agents that induced Friend erythroleukemic cells to differentiate (6,23) notably dimethyl sulfoxide in the presence of insulin, hydrocortisone, and prolactin (25). Clonal cell lines from this tumor, and many of those from other rat mammary tumors and from normal mammary tissue could be classified morphologically as one of cuboidal, elongated, or "fibroblastoid." An example of the last class is Rama 27 (Fig. 4d) which was derived from the stromal fraction of a culture of normal mammary tissue, and was almost certainly a stromal cell since some lipocytes were formed shortly after cloning, although this property was later lost. Properties of the cuboidal, elongated, and fibroblastoid classes of cell line are shown in Table 3, where comparisons are made with the three cell types in primary cultures. Recently we have also isolated cells with morphologies intermediate between the cuboidal and elongated cell (intermediate cells), but these cells are relatively unstable converting to elongated cells at fairly high frequencies (P. S. Rudland and R. Thompson, *unpublished results*).

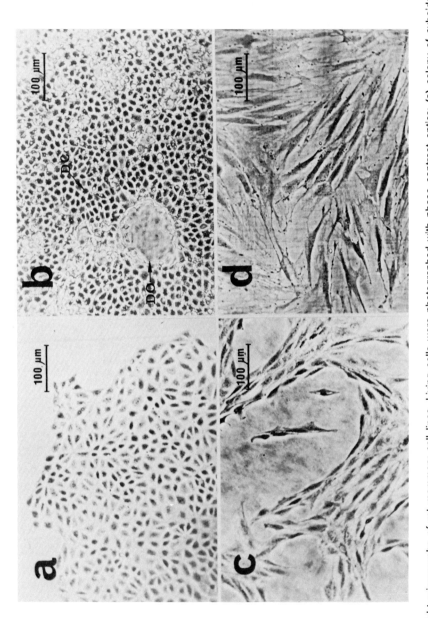

FIG. 4. Light micrographs of rat mammary cell lines. Living cells were photographed with phase contrast optics: **(a)** colony of cuboidal cells, Rama 25; **(b)** droplet cells (DC) in a culture of cuboidal cells at saturation density, with dome (DO); **(c)** elongated cells, Rama 29; **(d)** mammary fibroblastoid cells, Rama 27. (From Rudland et al., ref. 25, with permission.)

TABLE 3. *Cell biological properties of three classes of clones derived from mammary cells*[a]

Properties	Cuboidal (Rama 25)	Elongated (Rama 29)	Fibroblastoid (Rama 27)
Typical cell shape in colony	*Isometric*	*Elongated*	*Elongated*
Typical cell orientation in colony	*None*	*Often parallel*	*Usually spiral*
Saturation cell density (mm^{-2})	3,000	2,000	800
Minimum population doubling time	10 hr	14 hr	nd
Cell cohesion	+++	++(+)	+
Adhesion to plastic	++(+)	++(+)	+
Growth of cuboidal cells on monolayers	0	+	0
Growth on collagen gels	No single cells penetrate into gel	Some single cells penetrate into gel	Eventually destroy gel
Reimplantation into rodents (No. of occurrences/no. of animals)	Carcinoma[b] (10/10)	No structures[b] (19/19)	Fatty outgrowth[c] (8/8)
Ultrastructural features	*Junctional complexes and microvilli*	Basal lamina hemisomes and pinocytotic vesicles	nd

[a] Properties of the three classes of cloned cell lines, Rama 25, Rama 27, and Rama 29 are shown. Properties in *italics* indicate that similar features have been observed in the corresponding cell type seen in primary cultures. nd, not determined. Cell cohesion is an arbitrary estimate of close-alignment of cells, while cell adhesion is a relative estimate of resistance to cell removal from the substrate after treatment with trypsin or pronase.

[b] Tumor-derived material was inserted s.c. into nude mice.

[c] Early passaged uncloned fibroblastoid cultures from normal animals were inserted into the cleared mammary fat pad of synergeneic female rats. Some lipocytes were formed in such cultures and in Rama 27, although this clone later lost this capacity in culture.

Data from Rudland et al., ref. 25, with permission.

CHARACTERIZATION OF MAMMARY CELL LINES

The cultured cells were characterized by a variety of approaches which included electron microscopy, histology, histochemistry, immunology, and biochemistry. On the whole, Rama 29 cells differed from Rama 25 cells and more closely resembled Rama 27 cells in many respects. Thus the ultrastructure (2); the histochemical stains for the Na^+/K^+ adenosine triphosphatase (ATPase) (30) (Table 4); the serological stains for actin (16) myosin found in muscle and fibroblastoid cells (41); the fibroblastoid extracellular matrix glycoprotein, LETS (8); the thymocyte differentiation antigen Thy-1.1 (17,24), which is also found on fibroblasts (33); and the cell surface components that are accessible to lactoperoxidase-catalyzed iodination (Warburton and Head, *unpublished results*) (Table 5) were similar for Rama 27 and 29 but unlike those for Rama 25 cells. The third and fourth results with our cell lines were also obtained

TABLE 4. *Histological and histochemical differences between three classes of clones derived from mammary cells[a]*

Stain	Cuboidal (Rama 25)	Elongated (Rama 29 or fresh converts)	Fibroblastoid (Rama 27)
Fat (oil red 0)	± (Vesicles), DMSO & H ++	± (Vesicles)	± (Vesicles) but +++ in uncloned cultures
Na^+/K^+-ATPase	± (Cell border), DMSO & H ++	+ (Cell periphery), but subpopulation +++, fresh converts ++	++ (Cell periphery)
Mg^{2+}-ATPase	+ (Cell border), DMSO & H ++	+ (Cell periphery), but subpopulation +++, fresh converts ++	++ (Cell periphery)

[a] The relative amounts of stain are shown and the site of intracellular stain is indicated in parentheses. Newly formed elongated cells were observed in cultures of Rama 25 (fresh converts). DMSO & H represents the addition of 250 mM DMSO, 50 ng/ml insulin, hydrocortisone, and 500 ng/ml prolactin to the medium for 48 hr before the cultures were tested. "Vesicles" denotes speckled or granular stains within the cytoplasm; "cell border" denotes a much narrower strip of stain at the edge of a cell than "cell periphery," −, no change, ±, small increase, + increase, etc. The differences in the degree of histochemical staining for the different cell types were independent of the cell density, although confluent cultures of all cell types showed increased staining over sparse cultures.

Data from Rudland et al., ref. 25, with permission.

TABLE 5. Serological and biochemical properties of three classes of mammary cell clones[a]

Reagent		Cuboidal (Rama 25)	Elongated (Rama 29)	Fibroblastoid (Rama 27)
Actin antiserum Myosin antiserum		± (Cell periphery only)	++ (Intracellular fibers)	++ (Intracellular fibers)
LETS antiserum		± (Very faint and patchy)	++ (Patches of filaments)	++ (Intra- and extracellular filaments)
Anti-Thy-1 serum		−	++ (Cell periphery)	± (Cell periphery)
Peanut lectin		± (Cell periphery only)	−	−
+ DMSO + hormones		++	ND	ND
Rat casein antiserum		± (Cytoplasm)	−	−
+ DMSO + hormones		++	−	−
Lactoperoxidase catalyzed	Major MW bands	110,000	200,000 118,000	200,000 118,000
Iodination of cell surface	Minor MW bands		134,000 55,000–90,000	134,000 50,000–90,000
Analysis of collagen type		Probably type IV?	Probably type IV	Type I

[a]Serological tests were performed using immunofluorescent techniques. The relative fluorescent intensity minus its background for nonimmune serum is recorded, and the cellular location is shown in parentheses. Anti-Thy-1 serum was either alloantiserum from AKR mice (Thy-1.1) or antiserum raised against rat brain Thy-1. Alloantiserum from C3H mice (Thy-1.2) was inactive with all our cells. Two tests were performed after confluent cultures were exposed to 250 mm DMSO, 50 ng/ml insulin, hydrocortisone, 500 ng/ml prolactin (DMSO treatment) to yield "droplet" cells. The apparent molecular weight of the iodinated cell surface components after lactoperoxidase-catalyzed iodination of whole cells is shown, there are approximately three indistinct bands in the 55,000–90,000 MW region for Rama 27 and Rama 29. Analysis of collagen type depended on the ratio of chains $\alpha 1[1]/\alpha 2$. For Rama 25, Rama 29, and fresh elongated cell converts harvested from the culture medium of confluent Rama 25 cells, this ratio was greater than 2, and for Rama 27 the ratio was equal to 2. A ratio of more than 2 suggested the presence of collagen consisting of $\alpha 1$ chains only, i.e., type IV collagen. ±, Small increase, +, larger increase, etc., −, no change, ND, not determined.
Data from Rudland et al., ref. 25, with permission.

by R. Dulbecco of the Salk Institute. However, Rama 29 cells contained a few extra features compared with normal fibroblasts, notably extracellular material resembling basal lamina often connected to cells by hemisome-like junctions, pinocytotic vesicles, and evidence consistent with the production of basement membrane specific type IV collagen (38) (M. Warburton and L. Head, *unpublished results*) (Table 5). These results suggested that the Rama 29 cell and the fresh elongated cell converts were myoepithelial-like cells (10) showing both mesenchymal and epithelial properties. Antiserum against casein (42) and peanut lectin (14), on the other hand, reacted with only secreting epithelial cells in the mammary gland and not with myoepithelial or mesenchymal cells, and in culture reacted weakly with cuboidal cells, or more strongly with droplet cells but not with Rama 29 or Rama 27 cells (Table 5) (3,21,40).

POSSIBLE SIGNIFICANCE OF STEM CELLS

We have isolated and characterized types of "lining" epithelial stem cell lines from tumorous glands which can give rise to some myoepithelial-like and secretory, alveolar-like cells in culture (Fig. 5) and, for Rama 25, in tumors formed in rodents, (3; P. S. Rudland et al. *unpublished results*). Morphologically similar cells are obtained from normal glands, but their precise identification awaits biochemical analysis. Differentiation to alveolar-like cells can be regulated in culture by certain mammotropic hormones and dimethyl sulfoxide (DMSO) (25). However, our scheme for two single step conversions of cuboidal cells to alveolar-like or myoepithelial-like cells in culture (Fig. 5) is almost certainly an oversimplification for the following reasons. (a) Two markers for alveolar differentiation, "doming," and casein secretion can be differentially regulated by different hormone and DMSO combinations (25). (b) Strictly only a premyoepithelial-like cell can be produced in culture, an additional change has to occur before mature myoepithelial cells are produced as in the Rama 25-induced tumors (3). (c) Cells of morphology intermediate between that of myoepithelial and cuboidal epithelial cells have been isolated which may represent a true intermediate cell type (P. S. Rudland and R. Thompson, *unpublished results*) similar to the ultrastructurally "indeterminate" cells seen in the human breast (22,36).

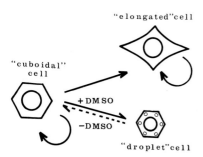

FIG. 5. Summary of interconversions of Rama 25 cells. The cuboidal, droplet, and elongated cells with their possible conversion "pathways" are shown by *arrows*. The *broken line* signifies that reversion of droplet cells to cuboidal cells can be seen under certain conditions, although they cannot be cloned, unlike cuboidal and elongated cells *(circular arrows)*. The presence of DMSO accelerates the conversion to droplet cells. (From Rudland et al., ref. 25, with permission.)

Stem cells that can be converted into myoepithelial cells in the normal gland should be required during two developmental stages. Firstly, early in development, since myoepithelial cells can be found in the mammary rudiment before birth (31,32); and secondly, when terminal end buds form alveolar buds and then mature alveoli containing myoepithelial and secretory epithelial cells (29). Myoepithelial cells in alveoli presumably arise by conversion from myoepithelial cells in the duct, since they are not detected at the tips of terminal end buds which are the precursors of alveolar buds and mature alveoli (29). In support of an early role in development, Rama 25 cells, when grown on floating collagen gells, produce tubular structures with the epithelial cells organized around a central lumen, and also three-dimensional structures reminiscent of rudimentary mammary glands (25). However, the fact that they can be induced to synthesize casein culture supports a role for Rama 25-like cells at the later stages in development. These conclusions raise the possibility that one stem cell could perform both developmental functions.

The testing of the effects of hormones and growth factors on the proliferation, interconversion, and differentiation of our different epithelial cell lines, coupled with the ability to locate cells of these classes in the mammary gland using immunological techniques may lead to a clearer understanding of the role of such agents in the growth and development of the normal mammary gland.

ACKNOWLEDGMENTS

We are indebted to Helga Durbin, Linda Peachey, Linda Head, and Ruth Thompson for excellent technical assistance, and Drs. R. C. Hallowes, S. Franks, N. Mittra, and M. Greaves for useful advice. D.C.B. was a recipient of an I.C.R.F. bursarship during the course of this work.

REFERENCES

1. Banerjee, M. R. (1976): *Int. Rev. Cytol.,* 47:1–97.
2. Bennett, D. C. (1979): Ph.D. thesis. University of London, England.
3. Bennett, D. C., Peachey, L. A., Durbin, H., and Rudland, P. S. (1978): *Cell,* 15:283–298.
4. DeOme, K. B., Faulkin, L. J., Bern, H. A., and Blair, P. B. (1959): *Cancer Res.,* 19:515–520.
5. Franks, L. M., and Wilson, P. D. (1977): *Int. Rev. Cytol.,* 48:55–139.
6. Friend, C., Scher, W., Holland, J. G., and Sato, T. (1971): *Proc. Natl. Acad. Sci. USA,* 68:378–382.
7. Gospodarowicz, D., Jones, K., and Sato, G. (1974): *Proc. Natl. Acad. Sci. USA,* 71:2295–2299.
8. Graham, J. M., Hynes, R. O, Davidson, E. A., and Bainton, D. F. (1975): *Cell,* 4:353–365.
9. Gros, R. J. (1967): In: *Control of Cellular Growth in Adult Organisms,* edited by H. Teir and T. Rytoma, pp. 3–27. Academic Press, New York.
10. Hackett, A. J., Smith, H. S., Springer, E. L., Owens, R. B., Nelson-Rees, W. A., Riggs, J. L., and Gardner, M. B. (1977): *J. Natl. Cancer Inst.,* 58:1795–1806.
11. Hallowes, R. C., Rudland, P. S., Hawkins, R. A., Lewis, D. J., Bennett, D., and Durbin, H. (1977): *Cancer Res.,* 37:2492–2504.
12. Huggins, C., Briziarelli, G., and Sutton, H. (1959): *J. Exp. Med.,* 109:25–42.
13. Kano-Sueoka, T., Campbell, G. R., and Gerber, M. (1978): *J. Cell. Physiol.,* 93:417–424.

14. Klein, P. J., Newman, R. A., Muller, P., Uhlenbruck, G., Schaeffer, H. E., Lennartz, K. J., and Fisher, R. (1978): *Klin. Wochenschr.,* 56:761–765.
15. Kon, S. K., and Cowie, A. T. (1961): *Milk, The Mammary Gland, and Its Secretions.* Academic Press, New York.
16. Lazarides, E., and Weber, K. (1974): *Proc. Natl. Acad. Sci. USA,* 71:2268–2272.
17. Letarte-Muirhead, M., Barclay, A. N., and Williams, A. F. (1975): *Biochem. J.,* 151:685–697.
18. Lyons, R. W., Li, C. H., and Johnson, R. E. (1958): *Recent Prog. Horm. Res.,* 14:219–254.
19. McGrath, C. M. (1975): *Am. Zool.,* 15:231–236.
20. Nandi, S. J. (1958): *J. Natl. Cancer Inst.,* 21:1039–1055.
21. Newman, R. A., Klein, P. J., and Rudland, P. S. (1979): *J. Natl. Cancer Inst.,* 63:1339–1346.
22. Ozzello, L. (1971): *Pathol. Annu.,* 6:1–59.
23. Palfrey, C., Kimhi, Y., Littauer, U. Z., Reuben, R. C., and Marks, P. A. (1977): *Biochem. Biophys. Res. Commun.,* 76:937–942.
24. Reif, A. E., and Allen, J. M. V. (1964): *J. Exp. Med.,* 120:413–433.
25. Rudland, P. S., Bennett, D. C., and Warburton, M. (1979): *Cold Spring Harbor Symposium Conference on Cell Proliferation, Vol. 6: Hormones and Cell Culture,* pp. 677–699. Cold Spring Harbor, New York.
26. Rudland, P. S., Hallowes, R. C., Durbin, H., and Lewis, D. (1977): *J. Cell Biol.,* 73:561–577.
27. Rudland, P. S., and Jimenez de Asua, L. (1979): *Biochim. Biophys. Acta Cancer Res. Rev.,* 560:91–133.
28. Rudland, P. S., Seifert, W., and Gospodarowicz, D. (1974): *Proc. Natl. Acad. Sci. USA,* 71:2600–2604.
29. Russo, J., Saby, J., Isenburg, W. M., and Russo, I. H. (1977): *J. Natl. Cancer Inst.,* 59:435–445.
30. Russo, J., Wells, P. A., and Russo, I. H. A. (1977): *Cancer Res.,* 37:1088–1098.
31. Salazar, H., and Tobon, H. (1974): In: *Lactogenic Hormones, Fetal Nutrition and Lactation,* edited by J. B. Josimovitch, M. Reynolds, and E. Cobo, pp. 221–227. Wiley, London.
32. Schlotke, B. (1976): *Zentralbl. Veterinaermed. [A],* 23:661–669.
33. Stern, P. L. (1973): *Nature (New Biol.),* 246:76–78.
34. Stoker, M. G. P., Piggot, D., and Taylor-Papadimitriou, J. (1976): *Nature,* 264:764–767.
35. Talwalker, P. K., and Meites, J. (1961): *Proc. Soc. Exp. Biol. Med.,* 107:880–883.
36. Tannenbaum, M., Weiss, M., and Marx, A. J. (1969): *Cancer,* 23:958–978.
37. Taylor-Papadimitriou, J., Shearer, M., and Stoker, M. G. P. (1977): *Int. J. Cancer,* 20:903–908.
38. Trelstad, R. L., and Slavkin, H. C. (1974): *Biochem. Biophys. Res. Commun.,* 59:443–449.
39. Turkington, R. R. (1971): *Exp. Cell Res.,* 57:79–85.
40. Warburton, M., Head, L., and Rudland, P. S. (1978): *Biochem. Soc. Trans.,* 7:115–116.
41. Weber, K., and Groeschel-Stewart, U. (1974): *Proc. Natl. Acad. Sci. USA,* 71:4561–4564.
42. Young, S., and Nelstrop, A. E. (1970): *Br. J. Exp. Pathol.,* 51:28–33.

Hormones and Cancer, edited by S. Iacobelli et al.
Raven Press, New York © 1980.

The Regression Process in Hormone-Dependent Mammary Carcinomas

Pietro M. Gullino

Laboratory of Pathophysiology, National Cancer Institute, National Institutes of Health, Bethesda, Maryland 20205

Almost a century ago Beatson (1) observed that growth arrest and regression of some human mammary carcinomas could be obtained by ovariectomy. Since then much work has been oriented toward an understanding of the effect of hormones on modulating the growth of mammary epithelium. A much smaller effort has been devoted to the understanding of events occurring within the neoplastic tissue during hormone-induced regression. The objective of this presentation is to summarize data obtained in our laboratory concerning this last point.

MORPHOLOGIC CHARACTERISTICS OF REGRESSING MAMMARY CARCINOMAS

Structural and cytologic changes in the neoplastic tissue can be classified into two major categories: coagulative necrosis, and apoptosis or shrinkage necrosis. Coagulative necrosis occurs mainly in the center of subcutaneously transplanted tumors and is usually the consequence of an inefficient blood supply. The term apoptosis was coined by Kerr et al. (39) to emphasize cell fragmentation. This event may be the predominant one in a sequence starting with "loosening" of the cytoplasm from the surrounding cells, followed by cytoplasmic shrinkage, disruption of the endoplasmic reticulum and mitochondria, clumping of chromatin, and cell fragmentation. Three features usually characterize the apoptotic process: limitation to single cells, persistence of an intact cytoplasmic membrane, and appearance of many phagosomes within the cytoplasm. Cell atrophy and hydropic degeneration also occur, particularly in tumors with adenomatous structures. Atrophy is most often seen in cells of papillary structures and hydropic degeneration is usually confined to cells of solid cords. Coagulative necrosis occurs in all neoplastic tissues and hormonal deprivation is not considered to be a contributing factor. Apoptosis or shrinkage necrosis is a common event in hormone-dependent regression, not only of mammary tumors but of hormone-dependent tumors in general, e.g., the prostate (32). It is important to realize, however, that no morphologic picture of tissue necrosis is peculiar to hormone-dependent regression. Moreover, cells undergoing regression, i.e., those full of phagosomes and fragmenting, can also be seen in actively growing tumors. The morphologic alterations are, therefore, one aspect of the turnover of a neoplastic cell population which is enhanced during hormone-induced regression. Digestion of cell components within the cytoplasm is usually very rapid as suggested by observations made under different conditions of regression, such as in hepatocytes after occlusion of the portal system (18), or in the lymphatic tissue after glucocorticosteroid treatment (21,42), or in the MTW9 mammary carcinoma model (29). This suggests that the number of cells with morphologic signs of regression is a rather unreliable indicator of the extent of cell destruction during hormone-induced regression.

TURNOVER OF NEOPLASTIC CELL POPULATIONS

Cell growth fraction, rate of cell loss, and cell cycle time are the three most important factors controlling the turnover of neoplastic cell populations. During the life span of a tumor none of them is constant. As soon as hormones are removed the cell growth fraction rapidly declines. In the MTW9 mammary carcinoma model, incorporation of labeled precursors into DNA was about one-third of the control at the end of 24 hr following hormone removal, one-fifth at the end of 48 hr, and practically nil at the end of the third day (30). In the dimethylbenz[a]anthracene (DMBA)-induced mammary tumor model, the rapid decline of the thymidine labeling index was followed by a prolongation of the S phase and the intermitotic time of the few dividing cells (52). The rate of cell loss by the tumor is an approximate value estimated from the discrepancy between the calculated and the observed growth rates *in vivo.* For most tumors, human and experimental, the cell loss has been estimated to be between 54 and 99% of cell production (35,47,53–56). Lysis by digestion appears to be the main route of cell loss. Loss of neoplastic cells by the regressing tumor has been measured in the MTW9 mammary model and found to be on the order of 3 to 4 $\times$ 10^6 cells/24 hr/g tissue, not different from the growing tumor (2). Consequently, cell loss by migration outside the tumor has been interpreted to be a negligible factor in hormone-induced regression.

The relationship between onset of cell lysis and hormonal deprivation of the host has been studied by several approaches. An obvious one was to ascertain whether metabolic deficiencies occurred. The blood supply was found to be as good in regressing as in growing tumors. In growing MTW9 mammary carcinomas, for instance, the blood flow was 6.5 $\pm$ 1.2 ml/hr/g compared with 6.7 $\pm$ 0.4 ml/hr/g in regressing tumors (29). The size of the vascular network, measured as the amount of blood present in the vessels, using high molecular weight dextran as a marker, was also found to be similar in tumors growing or regressed to one-half their original size. For MTW9, the vascular space was about 5% of tumor size and for primary DMBA-induced mammary carcinomas, 10%. The interstitial compartment of MTW9 and DMBA tumors, measured as ^{24}Na space minus the vascular space, was found to be 43 and 59%, respectively, of the total tumor water, again with no substantial change in the tumor regressed to about one-half the original size (29). This indicates that the relationship among physiologic compartments is maintained during regression and tissue destruction occurs in a coordinated fashion.

The global metabolic activity of the regressing tumor was evaluated *in vivo* by measuring the removal of oxygen and glucose from the blood. Transplanted MTW9 or primary DMBA mammary carcinomas, regressed to about one-half the original size, were able to remove about 50% of the oxygen brought by the afferent blood, about the same as the growing counterpart (30). If the blood supply was reduced and thus oxygen input diminished, the regressing tumor increased the capacity to remove oxygen up to 85% of the supply. On the contrary, if the blood supply was enhanced and thus oxygen availability increased, the oxygen removal ratio decreased to 25% of the input. Therefore, the regressing tumor was able to regulate total oxygen consumption to maintain approximately the same utilization despite large variations in availability (26, 29,30).

Glucose utilization by a tumor is related to the plasma concentration (27,28). In acute hyperglycemia, tumors can utilize for the first one-half hour up to 10-fold the glucose consumed during normoglycemia. In chronic hyperglycemia (diabetes), glucose consumption in our models was about 40% greater than during normoglycemia. Tumors regressed to about one-half the original size consumed as much glucose as the growing ones on a wet weight basis and were able to sharply increase the utilization during hyperglycemia (30). The data derived from these experiments indicated that *in vivo* the overall metabolic activity was, per gram of tissue, as high in the regressing as in the growing tumor. Moreover, the efficiency of the regressing tumor in regulating basic metabolic activities such as oxygen and glucose utilization was as good as in the growing counterpart. We concluded that gross metabolic deficiencies were absent during hormone-induced regression of mammary tumors.

TISSUE LYSIS

Another approach to study the turnover of neoplastic cell populations in mammary carcinomas was pursued via a comparison of the gross chemical composition of growing and regressing tumors. Lysis of collagen and DNA was found to be slower than that of other cell components. Carcinomas regressed to about one-half the original size had 20 to 40% more collagen and DNA than growing tumors, while the water content, RNA, and proteins remained proportionally constant on a per wet weight basis. Regressing DMBA tumors accumulated triglycerides to about twice the rate measured in growing tumors, whereas regressing MTW9 had about 30% less triglycerides than the growing counterpart; we have no explanation for this discrepancy (29). The magnitude of the lytic process was expressed by the increment of the free amino acid level in the efferent blood. An increase of 40 to 60% was observed in the plasma leaving regressing as compared with growing tumors (31). When this was compared with the reduction in tumor diameter and blood flow, it became clear that most of the tumor proteins had to be hydrolyzed up to the amino acid or small polypeptide level within the tumor itself.

Lysosomes are known to be involved in tissue digestion (20,57) and the frequency of cells full of phagosomes in our models, particularly MTW9, confirms previous observations. In whole homogenates the activities of lysosomal enzymes, such as acid phosphatase, β-glucuronidase, arylsulfatase, β-galactosidase, cathepsin, and acid ribonuclease were found to be increased during regression (17,43,44,51), and we observed that the increments corresponded to an increase of the number of enzyme molecules per gram of tumor (12,40,41).

An important question to answer was whether lysis occurred as an endocellular process or as the consequence of enzymes spilling into the interstitial space. In the first case, the cell could regulate its own digestion; in the second case, cell lysis should result from an enzymatic attack from the extracellular compartment. When tumor interstitial fluid was sampled by micropore chambers, according to a method previously described (25), lysosomal enzyme activity was found only in the homogenate, not in the interstitial fluid, regardless of whether the tumor was growing or regressing (40). If this result is accepted as a demonstration that lysis is essentially an endocellular process, then the elevation of lysosomol enzyme activity could be the result of either a direct activation or an expansion of a physiologic function of the lysosomes that must digest an increased amount of cell debris. There is no direct evidence in favor of either hypothesis. As an approach to clarify this point, experiments in our laboratory showed that within 24 hr of hormone withdrawal, cytosol proteins of MTW9 became more rapidly degraded by trypsin, α-chymotrypsin and subtilisin BPN. This labilization occurred much earlier than any change in both the level of protein synthesis and the activities of most of the lysosomal enzymes. The increased susceptibility to proteolysis could not be justified by the presence of endogenous proteases, or by destruction of the test enzymes or by the presence of protease inhibitors in the homogenates, nor could it be modified by preincubation with dithiothreitol, prolactin, estradiol-17β, progesterone, or hydrocortisone (48).

The observations of (a) increased susceptibility to degradation of regressing cytosol, (b) preservation of the plasma membrane during digestion of cells or cell fragments (38,39), (c) lack of enzyme "spilling" into the interstitial fluid (40), and (d) increased activity of most lysosomol enzymes only after more than 48 hr from hormone removal suggest that the increment in number and activity of lysosomes may be the effect, not the cause, of regression. Irreversible damage of major consequence to cell survival can be obtained through alteration of a few key proteins. For instance, the 12 liver proteins with the shortest reported half-lives catalyze either the first or the rate-limiting step of metabolic pathways (23,24). A rapid reduction in the concentration of these short-lived proteins can impair a large sector of cell structures that may be rapidly disposed of. Whether something similar occurs in regressing mammary epithelium has not been demonstrated. However, within a few hours after hormone removal, the half-life of acid ribonuclease, for instance, decreased from 7.8 to 2.6 days and enzyme production increased 15-fold (11,12). Although the consequences of this event are unknown, the observation suggests the possibility that a few crucial changes produced by a lack of the appropriate hormones may trigger a massive modification or destruction of cellular components sufficient to kill the cell. In this case, lysosomes could increase in number because the volume of substrate to digest is larger, not because lysosomes aggressively dispose of cell components.

ROLE OF CYCLIC AMP IN TUMOR REGRESSION

Hormone-dependent mammary tumors are known to regress not only after the host is deprived of estradiol but also after an excess of estradiol-17β is given (34). This suggests that an equilibrium in the turnover of the cell population can be altered by hormonal treatment and that cell destruction may prevail over cell multiplication. Since growth inhibition of a lymphosarcoma and Walker 256 carcinoma was obtained by cyclic adenosine monophosphate (AMP) treatment (22,36), Cho-Chung and co-workers in our laboratory initiated an extensive analysis of cyclic AMP participation in hormone-induced regression.

In the hormone-independent Walker 256 mammary carcinoma, injections of dibutyryl cyclic AMP (10 mg/day/200-g rat) were found to cause growth arrest or regression in about 30% of transplants (3,13,14). This treatment induced an increase of cyclic AMP levels in all tumors. However, regressing tumors showed the highest cyclic AMP-binding capacity at pH 6.5 and their binding sites were stable to heat denaturation (50°C), whereas the cyclic AMP-unresponsive tumors showed the highest binding capacity at pH 4.5 and their binding sites were heat labile (8).

Dibutyryl cyclic AMP treatment also caused growth arrest and partial regression of primary DMBA-induced or MTW9 transplanted mammary carcinomas as observed in hosts deprived of hormones. However, the hormone-independent DMBA #1 transplanted mammary carcinoma continued to grow after dibutyryl cyclic AMP treatment, as it did after ovariectomy. The interdependence between ovariectomy and the dibutyryl cyclic AMP effect was reinforced by the observation that in primary DMBA-induced tumors, cyclic AMP-binding activity increased sharply (four- to five-fold) after ovariectomy in both the nuclei and cytosol as compared with the growing counterpart. Under the same conditions, the pattern for estrogen-binding protein changed in the opposite direction. As tumor regression progressed in the ovariectomized rat, the estrogen binding activity decreased in both the cytosol and nuclei (50–80%), while cyclic AMP binding increased. When tumor regrowth was produced by injections of estradiol-17β in the castrated rat, the trend was reversed: cyclic AMP binding decreased and estrogen binding increased (6,7).

The relationship between increment of cyclic AMP-binding protein and tumor regression was assessed (5) by the photoaffinity crosslinking method using 8-azido[^{32}P]cyclic AMP as label (45). The cytosol of a growing DMBA-induced tumor contained 39,000-, 48,000-, and 56,000-dalton proteins binding to the 8-azido[^{32}P]cyclic AMP. The 48,000-dalton species is the cyclic AMP-dependent protein kinase type I. The 39,000- and 56,000-dalton receptors correspond to the kinase type II (33,49), and the first is a proteolytic derivative of the second (19). After ovariectomy or dibutyryl cyclic AMP treatment, the 56,000-dalton protein increased in the cytosol whereas the concentration of the 39,000-dalton protein remained almost constant. Moreover, the 56,000-dalton protein started to accumulate in the nuclei to form a large peak by the third day after ovariectomy. Simultaneously with the transfer of the 56,000-dalton protein into the nuclei, a newly phosphorylated protein (76,000 daltons) also appeared in the nuclei in large amounts (15,16). Nuclear accumulation of both the 76,000- and 56,000-dalton proteins was sharply reduced by injections of estradiol-17β that stimulated the tumor to regrow in the castrated rat.

The increase of the 56,000-dalton protein in the cytosol following endogenous phosphorylation was also demonstrated *in vitro* by incubation of DMBA-tumor slices with cyclic AMP and benzamidine. This increase was blocked when estradiol-17β was added to the incubation medium simultaneously with cyclic AMP (5). These experiments also revealed that phosphorylation of the 56,000-dalton cyclic AMP receptor protein was optimal at cyclic AMP concentrations close to the physiologic level ($\sim 10^{-8}$ M), while concentrations above or below this level had inhibitory effects.

Hormone-independent DMBA-induced tumors that did not regress after ovariectomy incorporated 8-azido[^{32}P]cyclic AMP into the 56,000-dalton cytosol protein; however, neither castration nor dibutyryl cyclic AMP treatment provided an increase of the cytosol binding nor did the bound complex appear in the nuclei (4). Walker 256 carcinomas that are unresponsive to both ovariectomy and dibutyryl cyclic AMP treatment behaved similarly (9,10).

The inability to induce regression in mammary tumors unresponsive to ovariectomy or dibutyryl cyclic AMP treatment correlates with the absence of nuclear translocation and nuclear protein phosphorylation of the cyclic AMP–receptor complex. Experiments were carried out with growing hormone-dependent and -independent DMBA-induced tumors in a cell-free system using activated cytosols (prepared by incubating tumor slices with cyclic AMP, benzamidine, and arginine) and isolated nuclei from untreated tumors. The nuclei were first incubated with activated cytosols in the presence of cyclic AMP, then washed and incubated with [γ^{33}P]-ATP. Results showed nuclear uptake of 56,000-dalton cyclic AMP receptor and phosphorylation of 76,000-dalton protein. However, incorporation of ^{33}P was greatly reduced when the activated cytosol of slices derived from hormone-independent tumors was incubated with nuclei of either hormone-dependent or -independent tumors. Controlled experiments excluded the presence of inhibitors of phosphorylation, and the data were interpreted to indicate that lack of penetration and phosphorylation depends not on the nuclei but on the cyclic AMP + receptor complex of the cytosol (5).

The possibility that an increased "lability" of the cyclic AMP + receptor complex is responsible for the lack of nuclear penetration and phosphorylation was suggested by the observation that arginine potentiates the inhibitory effect of dibutyryl cyclic AMP. Adding arginine (50 mg/200-kg rat s.c.) to daily injections of one-tenth the regression-inducing dose of dibutyryl cyclic AMP resulted in regression of DMBA tumors to 50% the initial size. Arginine also enhanced *in vitro* both the cyclic AMP-induced increase in the 56,000-dalton receptor protein of DMBA-tumor slices and the penetration of the cyclic AMP + receptor complex into the tumor nuclei in a cell-free system. The effect on hormone-independent tumors was nil (4,5).

On the assumption that cyclic AMP action represents a crucial step in the growth arrest and regression of neoplastic cells, Cho-Chung hypothesizes (4) that penetration into the nuclei requires that the catalytic subunit of protein kinase type II remains attached to the regulatory subunit after cyclic AMP binding and phosphorylation of the subunit has occurred. Since phosphorus binds to the serine residue of the regulatory subunit (37) near an arginine residue (19), increased concentrations of arginine may prevent rapid separation of the catalytic from the regulatory subunit, thus keeping the concentration of the phosphorylated cyclic AMP + protein kinase complex at an optimal level for penetration into the nucleus and phosphorylation of the 76,000-dalton nuclear protein.

CONCLUSION

The regression of mammary carcinomas after hormonal deprivation of the host has been approached in our work as resulting from an amplification of the still mysterious signals that control the catabolism of the neoplastic cell population. The shrinkage of the tissue appears to occur as a coordinated sequence of events in the absence of obviously toxic stimuli or a sudden deprivation of metabolites. The regressing tumor utilizes as much energy as the growing one and synthesizes lytic enzymes on a large scale. This process appears as an autodigestion, mostly cell-limited and rather extensive since the level of free amino acids in the efferent blood accounts for an almost complete hydrolysis of proteins. Cyclic AMP plays an important role in triggering regression in the sense that lack of cyclic AMP binding to a cytosol receptor and failure of the cyclic AMP + receptor complex to penetrate into the nuclei is equivalent to absence of regression. Recently Shafie and co-workers (50) in our laboratory observed that this is also true when DMBA-induced mammary tumors regress in streptozotocin-diabetic rats. Consequently, the binding of cyclic AMP to a receptor protein and the transfer of this complex from the cytoplasm into the nuclei appears to be an event influenced by a variety of conditions impinging upon tissue catabolism. Failure to penetrate the nuclei seems to be a distinguishing characteristic between hormone-dependent and -independent tumors. An explanation of the reasons underlying this failure may have important consequences on the possibility of influencing growth of hormone-independent tumors.

As the cyclic AMP + receptor protein complex penetrates the nuclei, a 76,000-dalton protein is phosphorylated (5), acid ribonuclease synthesis is sharply increased (11,12), and α-lactalbumin disappears from the cytosol (46). At this time none of these observations can be projected into a rational picture that offers an explanation of tissue digestion. Ongoing work in our laboratory by Qasba et al. *(unpublished observations)* suggests that mRNA for α-lactalbumin, caseins, and a group of nonsecretory proteins disappear from the tumor tissue as soon as the cyclic AMP + receptor protein has penetrated the nuclei. The onset of autodigestion that follows may result from failure to synthesize correctly or in sufficient quantity key proteins. The consequence could be either obsolescence of large sectors of cell constituents, which invites lysosomal digestion, or an aggressive attack by lysosomol enzymes actively synthesized by the regressing cells. Observations in support of both hypotheses have been reported but no clear picture has yet emerged.

REFERENCES

1. Beatson, G. T. (1896): *Lancet,* 2:104–107; 162–165.
2. Butler, T. P., and Gullino, P. M. (1974): *Cancer Res.,* 35:512–516.
3. Cho-Chung, Y. S. (1974): *Cancer Res.,* 34:3492–3496.
4. Cho-Chung, Y. S. (1980): *Cell. Mol. Biol. (in press).*
5. Cho-Chung, Y. S., Archibald, D., and Clair, T. (1979): *Science,* 205:1390–1392.
6. Cho-Chung, Y. S., Bodwin, J. S., and Clair, T. (1978): *J. Natl. Cancer Inst.,* 60:1175–1178.
7. Cho-Chung, Y. S., Bodwin, J. S., and Clair, T. (1978): *Eur. J. Biochem.,* 86:51–60.
8. Cho-Chung, Y. S., and Clair, T. (1977): *Nature,* 265:452–454.
9. Cho-Chung, Y. S., Clair, T., and Porper, R. (1977): *J. Biol. Chem.,* 252:6342–6348.
10. Cho-Chung, Y. S., Clair, T., and Huffman, P. (1977): *J. Biol. Chem.,* 252:6349–6355.
11. Cho-Chung, Y. S., and Gullino, P. M. (1973): *J. Biol. Chem.,* 248:4743–4749.
12. Cho-Chung, Y. S., and Gullino, P. M. (1973): *J. Biol. Chem.,* 248:4750–4755.
13. Cho-Chung, Y. S., and Gullino, P. M. (1974): *J. Natl. Cancer Inst.,* 52:995–996.
14. Cho-Chung, Y. S., and Gullino, P. M. (1974): *Science,* 183:87–88.
15. Cho-Chung, Y. S., and Redler, B. H. (1977): *Science,* 197:272–275.
16. Cho-Chung, Y. S., Redler, B. H., and Lewallen, R. P. (1978): *Cancer Res.,* 38:3405–3409.
17. Clarke, C., and Wills, E. D. (1976): *Radiat. Res.,* 67:435–446.
18. Cole, S., Matter, A., and Karnovsky, M. J. (1971): *Exp. Mol. Pathol.,* 14:158–175.
19. Corbin, J. D., Sugden, P. H., West, L., Flockhart, D. A., Lincoln, T. M., and McCarthy, D. (1978): *J. Biol. Chem.,* 253:3997–4003.
20. De Duve, C. (1969): In: *Lysosomes in Biology and Pathology, Vol. 1,* edited by J. T. Dingle and H. B. Fell, p. 3. North-Holland, Amsterdam.
21. Dougherty, T. F., Berliner, M. E., Schneebeli, G. I., and Berliner, D. L. (1964): *Ann. NY Acad. Sci.,* 113:825–843.
22. Gericke, D., and Chandra, P. (1969): *Hoppe Seylers Z. Physiol. Chem.,* 350:1469–1471.
23. Goldberg, A. L., and Dice, J. F. (1974): *Annu. Rev. Biochem.,* 43:835–869.
24. Goldberg, A. L., and St. John, A. C. (1976): *Annu. Rev. Biochem.,* 45:747–803.
25. Gullino, P. M. (1970): In: *Methods in Cancer Research, Vol. 5,* edited by H. Busch, pp. 45–91. Academic Press, New York.
26. Gullino, P. M., Grantham, F. H., and Courtney, A. H. (1967): *Cancer Res.,* 27:1020–1030.
27. Gullino, P. M., Grantham, F. H., and Courtney, A. H. (1967): *Cancer Res.,* 27:1031–1040.

28. Gullino, P. M., Grantham, F. H., Courtney, A., and Losonczy, I. (1967): *Cancer Res.,* 27:1041–1052.
29. Gullino, P. M., Grantham, F. H., Losonczy, I., and Berghoffer, B. (1972): *J. Natl. Cancer Inst.,* 49:1333–1348.
30. Gullino, P. M., Grantham, F. H., Losonczy, I., and Berghoffer, B. (1972): *J. Natl. Cancer Inst.,* 49:1675–1684.
31. Gullino, P. M., and Lanzerotti, R. H. (1972): *J. Natl. Cancer Inst.,* 49:1349–1356.
32. Helminen, H. J., and Ericsson, J. L. E. (1971): *J. Ultrastruct. Res.,* 36:708–724.
33. Hoffmann, F., Beavo, J. A., Bechtel, P. J., and Krebs, E. G. (1975): *J. Biol. Chem.,* 250:7795–7801.
34. Huggins, C., Moon, R. C., and Morii, S. (1962): *Proc. Natl. Acad. Sci. USA,* 48:379–386.
35. Iverson, O. H. (1967): *Eur. J. Cancer,* 3:389–394.
36. Keller, R. (1972): *Life Sci.,* 11(Part II):485–491.
37. Kemp, B. E., Bylund, D. B., Huang, T. S., and Krebs, E. G. (1975): *Proc. Natl. Acad. Sci. USA,* 72:3448–3452.
38. Kerr, J. F. R., and Searle, J. (1972): *J. Pathol.,* 108:55–58.
39. Kerr, J. F. R., Wyllie, A. H., and Currie, A. R. (1972): *Br. J. Cancer,* 26:239–257.
40. Lanzerotti, R. H., and Gullino, P. M. (1972): *Cancer Res.,* 32:2679–2685.
41. Lanzerotti, R. H., and Gullino, P. M. (1972): *Anal. Biochem.,* 50:344–353.
42. LaPushin, R. W., and DeHarven, E. (1971): *J. Cell Biol.,* 50:583–597.
43. Paris, J. E., and Brandes, D. (1971): *Cancer Res.,* 31:392–401.
44. Paris, J. E., Brandes, D., and Anton, E. (1969): *J. Natl. Cancer Inst.,* 42:383–398.
45. Pomerantz, A. H., Rudolph, S. A., Haley, B. E., and Greengard, P. (1975): *Biochemistry,* 14:3858–3862.
46. Qasba, P. K., and Gullino, P. M. (1977): *Cancer Res.,* 37:3792–3795.
47. Refsum, S. B., and Berdal, P. (1967): *Eur. J. Cancer,* 3:235–236.
48. Rouleau, M., and Gullino, P. M. (1977): *Cancer Res.,* 37:670–677.
49. Rubin, C. S., and Rosen, O. M. (1975): *Annu. Rev. Biochem.,* 44:831–887.
50. Shafie, S. M., Cho-Chung, Y. S., and Gullino, P. M. (1979): *Cancer Res.,* 39:2501–2504.
51. Shamberger, R. J. (1969): *Biochem. J.,* 111:375–383.
52. Simpson-Herren, L., and Griswold, D. P., Jr. (1973): *Cancer Res.,* 33:2415–2424.
53. Simpson-Herren, L., and Lloyd, H. H. (1970): *Cancer Chemother. Rep.,* 54(Part I):143–174.
54. Steel, G. G. (1967): *Eur. J. Cancer,* 3:381–387.
55. Steel, G. G. (1968): *Cell Tissue Kinet.,* 1:193–207.
56. Steel, G. G. (1972): *Cell Tissue Kinet.,* 5:87–100.
57. Woessner, J. F., Jr. (1969): In: *Lysosomes in Biology and Pathology, Vol. 1,* edited by J. T. Dingle and H. B. Fell, pp. 299–329. North-Holland, Amsterdam.

Hormones and Cancer, edited by S. Iacobelli et al.
Raven Press, New York © 1980.

Towards an Endocrine Physiology of Human Cancer*

Gordon H. Sato

Biology Department, University of California, San Diego, La Jolla, California 92093

When one surveys the available information on cancer, it is difficult to find any body of facts on which to base a general strategy for therapy. In fact, the only consistent rationale for choosing possible therapeutic agents is that they might be selectively toxic to rapidly proliferating cells. There are, of course, isolated exceptions to this rule but they seem to offer no hope for generalization. How is it that we can do no better than this in an era when new marvels of molecular biology are unfolding at a rate too rapid for most of us to assimilate? I believe it is because we lack very basic information on the physiology of tumors, and I would like to describe a possible method for obtaining this information and speculate on how this information may find practical application.

The most obvious approach for studying human cancer is to establish the cancer cells in culture. At the outset a problem exists. It is that it is difficult to culture human tumors. A long lag period usually precedes the phase of active proliferation of the tumor cells and fibroblasts tend to overgrow the cultures in the early stages. This lag period strongly suggests that selection is occurring for a variant cell type, and that the ultimate culture population is not representative of the original tumor cell population. This would, of course, severely limit the use of such cultures.

Our hypothesis is that the main function of serum in cell culture is to provide the cells with complexes of hormones (16). In addition, serum provides growth factors (new hormones), transferrin, and attachment factors (2). If this is true, serum is a poor means for supplying the needs of cells. Serum is toxic to cells at a concentration of 100% vol/vol and so is usually diluted to a concentration of 10% vol/vol. Serum contains many substances which do not leave the vascular spaces to come in direct contact with cells. It is reasonable to surmise that many of these are potentially cytotoxic. Also, many cells are only driven to proliferate by hormone concentrations higher than that usually found in 100% serum. For instance, thyroid follicle cells do not proliferate unless the concentration of thyroid-stimulating hormone (TSH) is much higher than that normally

---

*This chapter is dedicated to the memory of Jacob Furth, a good friend and a great pioneering scientist.

found in blood. Another consideration is that many cell types exist in a highly specialized hormonal environment. Anterior pituitary cells see a high concentration of hypothalamic hormones because of the special vasculature connecting the hypothalmus and the pituitary. Adrenal medullary cells see a much higher concentration of glucocorticoids than other tissues of the body and the same is true of seminiferous tubule cells and androgenic steroids. The specialized environments of these cell types cannot be approximated by diluting serum in standard synthetic culture media.

According to our hypothesis, it is for this reason that long lag periods are observed in primary culture and that many cell types have never been established in cell culture. We attribute the long lag period in primary culture to a selection of variants with reduced hormonal requirements that can be met by diluted serum, and with increased resistance to toxic substances in serum.

Experimental evidence already exists that defined media are suitable for primary culture and, in some cases, superior to serum-based media. S. Ambesi and H. Coon of the National Cancer Institute have established normal rat thyroid cells in the culture using a medium in which the serum was essentially replaced with mixtures of hormones *(personal communication)*. These cultures produce thyroid hormones and iodinated thyroglobulin and require TSH for growth. Such cells had never been established in culture, despite strenuous efforts to do so over the past 70 years, until the new technique of replacing serum with hormones was applied. If normal thyroid cells are placed in conventional serum-based medium, fibroblasts tend to overgrow the cultures, and if epithelial cells are isolated by dint of painstaking care (the green thumb method), they are nonfunctional.

Yossi Orly in our laboratory has shown that functional rat ovarian granulosa cells can be grown in a medium in which serum is replaced with insulin, transferrin, fibronectin, FSH, and androgens. The cultures produce estrogens from androgens and give a hypertrophic response to androgens and FSH. If the cells are initially plated in serum containing medium, they neither produce estrogens nor respond to androgens or FSH. Since only a brief period (a few days) in serum results in the loss of these physiological properties, it appears that serum distorts the physiology of the cells by a mechanism other than selection (15).

Murakami and Masui, from our laboratory, have devised a defined media for the growth of human colonic cancer which grows these cells faster (three times) and to a higher saturation density (three times) than does serum-based medium. This medium can also be used to establish human colonic cancer cells in primary culture (13).

Mary Taub, in our laboratory, has devised a defined media for the growth in primary culture of kidney epithelial cells from a variety of species. From preliminary evidence from microdissection experiments, it appears that the medium supports the growth of cells from Henle's loop and, to a limited extent, of cells from the distal tubule. It should be possible to develop variations of this media to specifically support the growth of cells from other regions such as proximal or collecting tubules (17). Other media developed in our laboratory can be used for the primary culture of neuroblasts and melanomas (4).

The evidence cited in this section strongly supports the notion that conventional serum-based media are inadequate for the primary culture of human tumors. Hormone and factor-supplemented defined media can be expected to allow for the following:

1. The establishment of cells in culture which have not been possible to grow in culture before;

2. The immediate initiation of growth of tumor cells without the usual lag and selection of variants seen using conventional culture techniques;

3. The growth of tumor cells without the usual contamination by fibroblasts because the factors required by fibroblasts are not provided;

4. The continued expression in culture of the specialized functions of the original tumor.

The ultimate aim of this work is to develop a new subdiscipline that I will refer to as the endocrine physiology of tumors. The development of this idea comes from the data on the requirements (mostly hormonal) of tumors for growth in serum-free media. Listed below are the requirements of some tumor cells (2).

GH_3 *(rat pituitary):* Insulin, 5 µg/ml; transferrin, 5µg/ml; fibroblast growth factor (FGF), 1 ng/ml; thyrotropin releasing hormone (TRH), 1 ng/ml; PTH, 0.5 ng/ml; somatomedin C, 1 ng/ml.

HeLa (human cervical carcinoma): Insulin, 5 µg/ml; transferrin, 5 µg/ml; epidermal growth factor (EGF), 10 ng/ml; FGF, 50 ng/ml; hydrocortisone, 50 nM.

M2R (Cloudman mouse melanoma): Insulin, 5 µg/ml; transferrin, 5 µg/ml; testosterone, 10 nM; FSH, 0.4 µg/ml; LHRH, 10 ng/ml; nerve growth factor (NGF), 3 ng/ml. Supports other melanomas and melanomas in primary culture.

MCF-7 (human mammary carcinoma): Insulin, 0.1 µg/ml; transferrin, 25 µg/ml; EGF, 100 ng/ml; cold insoluble globulin (CIg), 7.5 µg/ml; prostaglandin $F_{2\alpha}$, 100 ng/ml; α-1 spreading protein, 1 µg/ml. Medium also supports growth of BT20 human mammary cells.

T84 (human colonic adenocarcinoma): Insulin, 2 µg/ml; transferrin, 2 µg/ ml; EGF, 1 ng/ml; hydrocortisone, 50 nM; glucagon, 0.2 µg/ml; ascorbic acid, 10 µg/ml.

Pituitary tumor, GH_3 cells, require insulin (pancreas), transferrin (liver), T3 (thyroid), PTH (parathyroid), FGF (pituitary), TRH (brain), and somatomedin C (liver). Serum is a complex mixture of substances containing approximately a thousand different species of proteins. For this reason, it is quite surprising that the serum can be replaced by such a small number of defined substances. On the other hand, it is surprising that these tumor cells give a positive growth response to so many hormones. This must mean that the hormonal regulation of tumor cells must be quite complex and may approach the complexity of normal organ systems.

Removing serum from cells in culture is equivalent to a total endocrine ablation. When this is done, wholly unexpected hormonal requirements and responses are revealed. To demonstrate the hormonal requirements of GH_3 cells by classic means, one would have to perform pancreatectomy, hepatectomy, thyroidectomy, parathyroidectomy, and hypothalectomy. I am suggesting that the determination of hormonal requirements by culture techniques can be done for every type of human tumor and the results can be useful in a number of ways.

If human tumors can be plated from biopsy material into a defined media which are optimal for that particular tumor type, screening of therapeutic agents can be initiated immediately to obtain drug sensitivity data that could be clinically useful.

It would be extremely useful to know if the hormones required by tumor cells for growth in serum-free media can affect the growth of tumors in animal hosts or patients. This is fundamental data which is sorely lacking at the present time. Certainly, growth control in the whole animal is more involved than it is in the artificial conditions of tissue culture. Nevertheless, it is entirely conceivable that hormones that are required for serum-free growth in culture can affect the growth of tumors *in vivo*. If so, the possibilities are endless. One can imagine administering complexes of hormones to patients to render their tumor cells maximally proliferative at a precise later time that could be predicted. Drugs could be administered at this period of maximal sensitivity for short times to minimize side effects. It is also conceivable that quiescent tumor cells which normally escape chemotherapy can be incited by hormones into a state of active proliferation and vulnerability to drugs. It is also conceivable that hormones could be used to slow down the proliferation of stem cells in the marrow and gut during periods of chemotherapy to minimize damage to those tissues. Advances of this type represent short-term goals. It seems to me that the best hope for long-term success in cancer therapy lies in the accrual of basic information about the metabolic responses of tumors to hormones. The first step is to discover which hormones are required by these tumors for growth in serum-free medium. The second step is to find out, in a detailed way, how these hormones affect the metabolism of the tumors. I cannot imagine how such a detailed body of basic information could not yield numerous opportunities for therapeutic intervention.

These ideas are not entirely new. They are an extension of the pioneering studies on hormonal induction and dependence of tumors by A. Lacassagne (11), W. S. Murray (14), J. Furth (5), Kim et al. (9), H. Kirkman (10), W. V. Gardner (6), A. Lipschutz and R. Iglesias (12), C. Huggins and C. V. Hodges (8), M. S. Biskind and G. R. Biskind (3), C. W. Hooker (7), and E. Allen (1). In fact, these people laid the foundation on which this entire volume is based.

ACKNOWLEDGMENTS

This work was supported in part by a grant from USPHS (CA 23052) and from the National Science Foundation (NSF-PCM 76-80785).

REFERENCES

1. Allen, E., and Gardner, W. V. (1941): *Cancer Res.,* 1:359–366.
2. Barnes, D., and Sato, G. (1980): *Anal. Biochem.,* 102:255–270.
3. Biskind, M. S., and Biskind, G. R. (1944): *Proc. Soc. Exp. Biol. Med.,* 55:176.
4. Bottenstein, J. E., Sato, G. H., and Mather, J. P. (1979): In: *Hormones and Cell Culture,* edited by G. Sato and R. Ross, pp. 531–534. Cold Spring Harbor Laboratory, Cold Spring Harbor, New York.
5. Furth, J. (1955): *Recent Prog. Horm. Res.,* 2:221–225.
6. Gardner, W. V., Kirschbaum, A., and Strong, C. C. (1940): *Arch. Pathol.,* 29:1–7.
7. Hooker, C. W., and Pfeiffer, C. A. (1942): *Canc. Res.,* 2:759.
8. Huggins, C., and Hodges, C. V. (1941): *Cancer Res.,* 1:293.
9. Kim, U., Furth, J., and Yannopoulos, K. (1964): *J. Natl. Cancer Inst.,* 31:233.
10. Kirkman, H. (1959): *Natl. Cancer Inst. Monogr.,* 1:1–139.
11. Lacassagne, A. (1932): *Compt. Rend. Soc. Biol.,* 129:641–643.
12. Lipschutz, A., and Iglesias, R. (1938): *C. R. Soc. Biol.,* 129:159.
13. Murakami, H., and Masui, H. (1980): *Proc. Natl. Acad. Sci. USA (submitted).*
14. Murray, W. S. (1928): *Cancer Res.,* 12:18–25.
15. Orly, Y., Erickson, G. and Sato, G. (1980): *Cell (submitted).*
16. Sato, G. H. (1975): In: *Biochemical Action of Hormones, Vol. 3,* edited by G. Litwack, pp. 391–396.
17. Taub, M., and Sato, G. (1979): *Proc. Natl. Acad. Sci. USA,* 76:3338–3342.

Hormones and Cancer, edited by S. Iacobelli et al.
Raven Press, New York © 1980.

Cyclic Adenosine Monophosphate Action in Mouse Lymphoma Cells: Somatic–Genetic and Biochemical Analysis

Philip Coffino

Departments of Medicine and Microbiology and Immunology, University of California, San Francisco, California 94143

Mutants have begun to contribute to our understanding of how cyclic adenosine monophosphate (cAMP) acts in animal cells. Cells with mutations affecting discrete and identifiable steps in a regulatory system are valuable tools, because they help us to determine the role of the affected process in more normal (in genetic terms, wild type) cells. Systems of regulation that involve cAMP are ubiquitous, complex, and sometimes poorly understood. Therefore, this approach may prove especially useful here.

Cells with mutations in cAMP-related functions have now been isolated from several sources, including Chinese hamster ovary (5), macrophage-like (16), adrenal (17), and neuroblastoma (19) cell lines. Success was first reported, however, using the S49 mouse T cell lymphoma tissue culture line (2,4). These cells commit suicide when cAMP levels rise, so it is easy to select mutant survivors with a variety of defects in the killing process. While the developmental or physiologic significance of the suicide is unclear, the phenomenon is not unique to S49 cells; three other mouse T cell lymphoma lines we examined all responded similarly (Coffino et al., *unpublished*).

S49 cell mutants were selected for their ability to survive treatments that raised endogenous cAMP levels (1) or treatment with exogenously added congeners of cAMP, such as dibutyryl cAMP (2). The conventional wisdom on how cAMP is made and works can be broadly sketched as follows: Hormones or other effectors bind to receptors displayed on the external cell membrane. A coupling process activates adenyl cyclase within the membrane, leading to the generation of cAMP from adenosine triphosphate (ATP). Binding of cAMP to the regulatory subunit of a protein kinase results in the activation of that enzyme's catalytic subunit, with consequent phosphorylation of specific substrates. These phosphorylations alter the biochemical properties of the proteins on which they occur. This scheme proved an exasperatingly accurate guide in our analysis of the properties of the mutants, here enumerated:

1. Beta-adrenergic receptor-deficient cells are diminished in receptor number, as much as 90% compared with wild type cells (12). The response of their

adenyl cyclase to beta-adrenergic agonists, but not to other effectors of cyclase activity, is similarly diminished.

2. Adenyl cyclase mutants have normal beta-receptors, but are deficient in a function that is required for cyclase activation (1). In some cases, the defect specifically affects the response to hormones, such as beta-adrenergic agonists and prostaglandins; in other cases, the defect is more general and abolishes response to other effectors, such as cholera toxin, as well.

3. Kinase mutants have absent, reduced, or structurally altered cAMP-dependent protein kinase (10).

4. Deathless mutants are not killed by elevation of cAMP, but are otherwise normal in their response to cAMP and have intact cyclase and kinase systems (15).

Cells are thus available with specific lesions in many of the components involved in the cascade leading from occupancy of receptor by hormone, receptor–adenyl cyclase coupling, cAMP generation, protein kinase activation, substrate phosphorylation, and consequent alteration of biologic behavior. The availability of these mutants has facilitated the study of regulation by cAMP of such phenomena as growth control, enzyme induction and deinduction, and programmed cell death. Of course, the usefulness of the mutants is highly dependent on the degree to which we understand the genetic and biochemical basis of their altered phenotypes. Some are relatively well understood.

S49 cyclase mutants have been studied independently by the laboratories of Johnson et al. (13) and Howlett et al. (9). It is likely that hormone-responsive, membrane-associated cyclase consists of at least three components: hormone receptor, catalytic cyclase, and a coupling factor with guanosine triphosphatase (GTPase) activity. The last of these activities is deficient in one type of cyclase mutant, cyc⁻. This same factor is also the substrate for cholera enterotoxin; the toxin promotes adenosine diphosphate (ADP) ribosylation of the factor (7). Consequently, cyc⁻, in contrast to wild type S49, cannot be stimulated to produce cAMP by beta-adrenergic hormones or by cholera toxin. Another class of mutant, termed UNC, does not respond to beta-adrenergic hormones, despite the presence of receptors and catalytic cyclase, but their cyclase does respond to stimulation by cholera toxin. As might be expected, UNC mutants do contain the protein that cholera toxin ADP-ribosylates.

Independently isolated clones of cells with defects of cAMP-dependent protein kinase are also found to exhibit distinct subtypes (10). One class (kin⁻) has no detectable cAMP-stimulated kinase activity. This was initially determined by measuring the phosphotransferase activity of cell extracts in the presence and absence of cAMP, with histone H_{2b} as substrate. More recently, we have been examining the cAMP-stimulated phosphorylation of endogenous substrates, using two-dimensional polyacrylamide gel analysis of extracts from metabolically labeled cells (20). None of the cAMP-stimulated phosphorylations found to occur in wild type cells were seen in kin⁻. A second class of kinase mutants

CYCLIC AMP BINDING

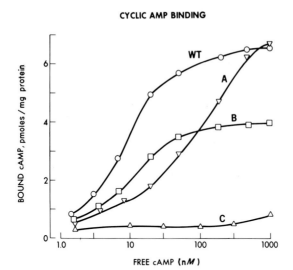

PROTEIN KINASE

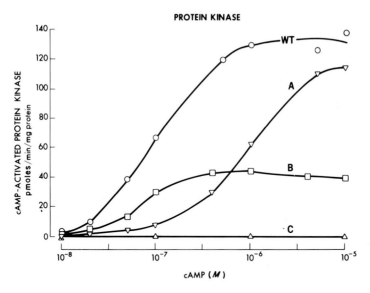

FIG. 1. Cyclic AMP binding **(top)** and cAMP-stimulated phosphotransferase activity **(bottom)** in extracts of wild type and mutant S49 cells. WT designates wild type and A, B, and C designate K_a, V_{max}, and kin⁻ respectively. (From Insel et al., ref. 10, with permission.)

(K_a) have a structural change in their regulatory subunit that reduces its apparent affinity for cAMP. The phosphotransferase activity of these cells extracts can be stimulated to levels approximating that of wild type, but only by relatively high concentrations of cAMP. A third class of mutants (V_{max}) has reduced activity, but the remaining enzyme has apparently normal sensitivity to cAMP. Figure 1 shows the dependence on cAMP concentration of the phosphotransferase activity in extracts of wild type cells and kin$^-$, K_a and V_{max} mutants.

Still another class of mutant, termed cAMP deathless (D$^-$), is defective in cAMP-mediated killing, but preserves the other responses to cAMP that characterizes S49 cells (15). These include growth arrest in the G$_1$ phase of the cycle; induction of cAMP phosphodiesterase; extinction of ornithine decarboxylase and S-adenosylmethionine decarboxylase (11,14); and cAMP-dependent phosphorylation of an apparently full array of endogenous kinase substrates. D$^-$ mutants seem to have intact cyclase and kinase systems. The biochemical basis of the highly specific alteration in their phenotype remains to be determined.

These S49 lymphoma cell mutants have proven efficient tools for investigating problems in biological regulation. They can be used to validate, reject, or generate hypotheses.

HYPOTHESIS VALIDATION

Multiple lines of evidence suggest that cAMP acts in animal cells by activating a protein kinase (8). The kinase mutants can provide formal confirmation of this view. If it is to hold, then alterations in the biochemical properties of cAMP-dependent kinase should be reflected in corresponding alterations in the biological responses of intact cells to cAMP. The dose-dependent effect of dibutyryl cAMP on three such responses—cell death, growth inhibition, and induction of phosphodiesterase—are shown in Fig. 2 (10). In each case, comparison is made among wild type cells and the same kinase mutants whose phosphotransferase activity was illustrated in Fig. 1. All of the biological responses of each mutant are altered in a manner that closely parallels the change in response of its kinase: no response occurs in kin$^-$, maximal response requires more stimulation in K_a and a reduced maximal response is elicited in V_{max} mutants. Besides confirming the central role of kinase in the response to cAMP, two further conclusions are evident. Firstly, the absence of cAMP dependent kinase is compatible with cellular life, despite the loss of certain regulatory opportunities. Secondly, the amount of kinase activity in wild type S49 cells is not in excess of that required to produce a maximal biological response.

HYPOTHESIS REJECTION

The intracellular level of cAMP has been found to vary regularly during the course of cell cycle progression (reviewed by Friedman et al., ref. 6). Consequently, it has been postulated that the cAMP system is a component of a metabolic clock that entrains the orderly progression of events in the cell cycle. But cyclase-deficient, kinase-deficient, and even doubly deficient (cyclase and kinase) mutants progress through the cycle in a normal manner. Therefore,

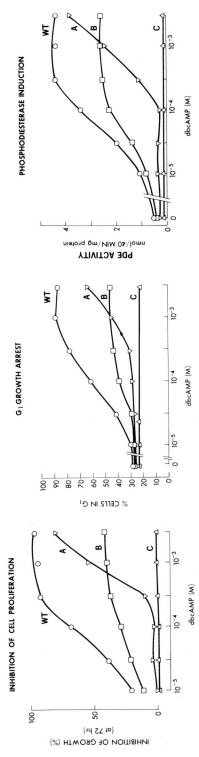

FIG. 2. Biological effects of dibutyryl cAMP and wild type and mutant S49 cells. Cells were treated with the indicated concentrations of dibutyryl cAMP and viable cell number, fraction of cells in G_1 and induction of cAMP phosphodiesterase assessed. Clones are designated as in Fig. 1. (From Insel et al., ref. 10, with permission.)

cAMP-dependent regulation cannot be a prerequisite for exponential cell growth. Shown in Fig. 3 are DNA histograms generated by flow cytometry of wild type, cyc⁻ and kin⁻ cells that have been treated with an inhibitor of cAMP phosphodiesterase alone or with the inhibitor plus cholera toxin or dibutyryl cAMP. In each case, the prominent peak on the left represents the fraction of the cell population in the G_1 phase of the growth cycle. Wild type cells are arrested in G_1, to a minor degree by the inhibitor alone, but profoundly by cAMP generated endogenously through stimulation of cyclase by cholera toxin or by exogenously added dibutyryl cAMP. The cyc⁻ cells arrest in response to dibutyryl cAMP, but not cholera toxin. The kin⁻ are not perturbed at all by either agent, despite the fact that cholera toxin generates even higher levels of cAMP than in wild type (18). One must conclude that cAMP can play no necessary role in the exponential growth of S49 cells. Growth can, however, be modulated by cAMP; wild type (and deathless) cells are reversibly arrested in the G_1 phase of the cell cycle by cAMP elevation.

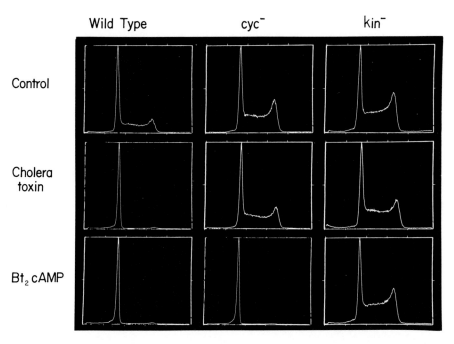

FIG. 3. Effect of cholera toxin and dibutyryl cAMP on the cell cycle distribution of wild type, cyc⁻, and kin⁻ S49 cells. Cultures in exponential growth were untreated or treated with cholera toxin (100 ng/ml) or dibutyryl cAMP (0.5 mM). All cultures contained the phosphodiesterase inhibitor RO 20–1724 (30 μM). After 24 hr the cultures were analyzed by flow cytometry to determine their distribution in the cell cycle. Data are displayed as histograms showing DNA content per cell on the abscissa and cell number on the ordinate, both in arbitrary units. From Coffino and Gray, ref. 3, with permission.)

HYPOTHESIS GENERATION

The deathless mutants were selected to have the phenotype described above, but have an additional property not directly selected for: chemical mutagens are more effective in generating mutations but are not more toxic in these cells. In addition to cAMP-related mutations, a series of other mutant cell types can be isolated in S49 cells. These include cells deficient in hypoxanthine-guanine phosphoribosyltransferase, selected for resistance to 6-thioguanine, and cells with altered Na^+/K^+ ATPase, selected for their resistance to ouabain. The frequency of each of these classes of mutants is greatly increased by treatment with chemical mutagens, such as the alkylating agents ethylmethane sulfonate or N-methyl-N'-nitro-N-nitrosoguanidine. Both these agents produce about three times as many 6-thioguanine- and ouabain-resistant mutants in D⁻ as in wild type cells. It is unlikely that a difference in transport or in the degree of primary damage could account for this, because the toxicity of each agent is similar or identical in the two cell types. This finding suggests the involvement of DNA repair mechanisms in the response of S49 cells to cAMP. Further investigation will be necessary to elucidate the relationship.

ACKNOWLEDGMENTS

This work was supported by National Science Foundation Grant PCM 07382, National Institutes of Health Grant RO1 CA23218, and a Research Career Development Award from the National Institutes of Health.

REFERENCES

1. Bourne, H. R., Coffino, P., and Tomkins, G. M. (1975): *Science,* 187:750–752.
2. Coffino, P., Bourne, H. R., and Tomkins, G. M. (1975): *J. Cell. Physiol.,* 85:603–610.
3. Coffino, P., and Gray, J. W. (1978): *Cancer Res.,* 38:4285–4288.
4. Daniel, V., Litwack, G., and Tomkins, G. M. (1973): *Proc. Natl. Acad. Sci. USA,* 70:76–79.
5. Evain, D., Gottesman, M., Pastan, I., and Anderson, W. B. (1979): *J. Biol. Chem.,* 254:6931–6937.
6. Friedman, D. L., Johnson, R. A., and Zeilig, C. E. (1976): In: *Advances in Cyclic Nucleotide Research, Vol. 7,* edited by P. Greengard and G. A. Robison, pp. 68–114. Raven Press, New York.
7. Gill, D. M., and Meren, R. (1978): *Proc. Natl. Acad. Sci. USA,* 75:3050–3054.
8. Greengard, P. (1978): *Science,* 199:146–152.
9. Howlett, A. C., Sternweiss, Y. C., Macik, B. A., Van Arsdale, P. M., and Gilman, A. G. (1979): *J. Biol. Chem.,* 254:2287–2295.
10. Insel, P. A., Bourne, H. R., Coffino, P., and Tomkins, G. M. (1975): *Science,* 190:896–897.
11. Insel, P. A., and Fenno, J. (1978): *Proc. Natl. Acad. Sci. USA,* 75:862–865.
12. Johnson, G. L., Bourne, H. R., Gleason, M. K., Coffino, P., Insel, P. A., and Melmon, K. L. (1979): *Mol. Pharmacol.,* 15:16–27.
13. Johnson, G. L., Kaslow, H. R., Farfel, Z., and Bourne, H. R. (1980): *Advances in Cyclic Nucleotide Research, Vol. 13,* edited by G. A. Robison and P. Greengard. Raven Press, New York.
14. Kaiser, N., Bourne, H. R., Insel, P. A., and Coffino, P. (1979): *J. Cell. Physiol.,* 101:369–374.
15. Lemaire, I., and Coffino, P. (1977): *Cell,* 11:149–155.

16. Rosen, N., Piscitello, J., Schneck, J., Muschel, R. J., Bloom, B. R., and Rosen, O. M. (1979): *J. Cell. Physiol.,* 98(1):125–136.
17. Schimmer, B. P., Tsao, J., and Knapp, M. (1977): *Mol. Cell. Endocrinol.,* 8:135–145.
18. Shear, M., Insel, P. A., Melmon, K. L., and Coffino, P. (1976): *J. Biol. Chem.,* 251:7572–7576.
19. Simantov, R., and Sachs, L. (1975): *J. Biol. Chem.,* 250(9):3236–3242.
20. Steinberg, R. A., and Coffino, P. (1979): *Cell,* 18:719–733.

Steroid Antagonists

Hormones and Cancer, edited by S. Iacobelli et al.
Raven Press, New York © 1980.

Effect of Clomiphene and Other Triphenylethylene Derivatives on the Reproductive Tract in the Rat and Baboon

J. H. Clark, S. A. McCormack, R. Kling, D. Hodges, and J. W. Hardin

Department of Cell Biology, Baylor College of Medicine, Houston, Texas 77030

Although it has been known for many years that triphenylethylene derivatives, such as nafoxidine and clomiphene (Clomid®) are drugs with both estrogenic and antiestrogenic properties (15), most investigators have been concerned primarily with their antiestrogenic properties. Our laboratory, in contrast, has been interested in the estrogenic capacities of these drugs. Nafoxidine and clomiphene cause long-term retention of the estrogen receptor in the nucleus of uterine cells and this is accompanied by a sustained stimulation of uterotropic activity (5,6,9,11,16,19,27). This stimulation is primarily due to the ability of these drugs to stimulate the epithelium of the uterine lumen, whereas estradiol, a physiological estrogen, causes all tissues of the uterus to grow (8,9,16,32). Therefore, even though these drugs are decidedly antiestrogenic in some tissues, they are long-acting estrogens in others. Since chronic exposure to estrogens is known to result in preneoplastic and neoplastic changes in the reproductive tract (21), we considered the possibility that nafoxidine and clomiphene might cause such changes in the fetal and neonatal rat (10,28). In addition, since clomiphene is used routinely for the induction of ovulation in women, it became of importance to determine whether a similar phenomenon occurs in a primate species.

NEONATAL STUDIES

Uterine Stimulation

Female rat pups of the Sprague-Dawley strain were injected subcutaneously in the nape of the neck on day 7 of life with one of the following estrogens and triphenylethylene derivatives in 0.1 ml oil: 10 μg estradiol, 10 μg diethylstilbestrol (DES), 100 μg tamoxifen, 100 μg nafoxidine, or 500 μg clomiphene. They were killed by cervical dislocation 48 hr later. An additional group of clomiphene-injected animals were killed at 96 hr. Controls consisted of uninjected and oil-injected rats killed at comparable times. The uteri were removed, trimmed to remove fat and mesentery, and weighed. They were immediately placed in Bouin's fixative for histological preparation after weighing.

The relative weight of the reproductive tract was increased significantly by estradiol, DES, and all triphenylethylene derivatives (Table 1). The real weight of the reproductive tract was also increased by hormone treatment in all groups except those animals treated with DES and nafoxidine. However even in these animals estrogenic stimulation was evident upon histological examination (see below).

The body weights of the injected pups were not significantly different from the oil-injected controls except for those receiving DES and clomiphene. Body weights of pups in these two groups were significantly lower than the controls at 48 or 96 hr.

Histological examination revealed that the most striking effects were on the luminal epithelium of the uteri. The luminal epithelial cells of control rats, whether uninjected or oil injected, were cuboidal with spherical nuclei 48 or 96 hr post-injection; the cell height was just adequate to accomodate the nuclei (Fig. 1, top). The luminal epithelial cells of the uteri of all the experimental groups was columnar with ovoid nuclei. The cell height was two to four times that of the nuclear long axis. Tamoxifen or nafoxidine increased luminal epithelial cell height only minimally, often with long, dark cells arranged parallel to the basement membrane with a tendency toward heterogeneity in nuclear arrangement, shape, and cell height. Estradiol- and DES-treated rats had uterine epithelium almost uniformly stimulated to about twice the nuclear long axis. At 48 hr postinjection clomiphene-injected rats showed an increase in luminal epithelial cell height two to three times the nuclear long axis with plump ovoid nuclei. By 96 hr, clomiphene treatment resulted in strikingly tall epithelial cells four to five times the nuclear long axis. These epithelial cells had large apical vacuoles

TABLE 1. *Effects of estradiol, diethylstilbestrol, tamoxifen, nafoxidine, and chlomiphene on body and reproductive tract weights of neonatal rats*

N	Treatment	Body wt (g) $\pm$ SEM	Reproductive tract wt (mg) $\pm$ SEM	Relative reproductive tract wt (mg/100 g body wt) $\pm$ SEM
8	None	14.7 ± 0.6	7.2 ± 0.6	53.8 ± 3.3
4	Oil_{48}	15.5 ± 0.8	6.4 ± 0.8	41.3 ± 3.7
5	Oil_{96}	18.0 ± 0.7	7.4 ± 0.8	41.1 ± 3.3
6	10 μg $E_{2_{48}}$	12.3 ± 0.7	9.5 ± 0.7^a	78.8 ± 3.0
5	10 μg DES_{48}	8.2 ± 0.7^b	6.4 ± 0.8	77.3 ± 3.3^b
8	100 μg TAM_{48}	15.0 ± 0.6	10.9 ± 0.6^a	65.0 ± 3.0^b
7	100 μg NAF_{48}	13.0 ± 0.6	7.9 ± 0.6	61.4 ± 3.0^b
6	500 μg $CLOM_{48}$	12.7 ± 0.7^a	9.4 ± 0.7^a	74.7 ± 3.0^b
6	500 μg $CLOM_{96}$	12.5 ± 0.7^b	11.5 ± 0.7^b	91.8 ± 3.0^b

[a] $p < 0.05$; significantly different from comparable oil-injected control.
[b] $p < 0.01$; significantly different from comparable oil-injected control.

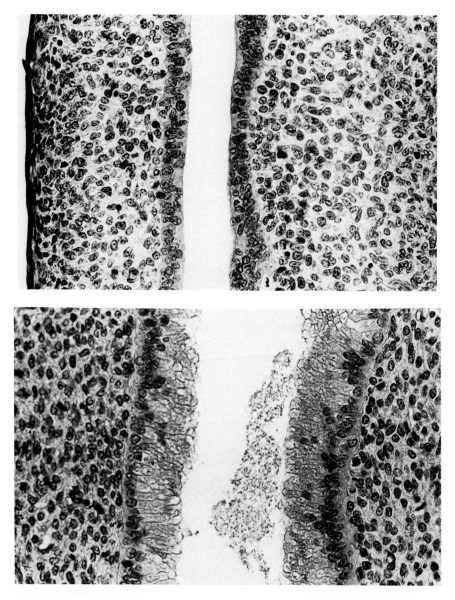

FIG. 1. Effect of clomiphene on the growth of the uterine epithelium in the neonatal rat. Five-day old animals were injected with either oil **(top)** or 500 µg clomiphene **(bottom)** and the uteri were removed 96 hr later.

which gave them a "foamy" appearance. These vacuoles seemed to contribute a stainable material to the uterine lumen (Fig. 1, bottom).

Estrogen Receptor Measurement

Animals were injected with 100 μg nafoxidine on day 5 and the cytosol and nuclear levels of the estrogen receptor were measured on day 10 by the [³H-]estradiol exchange assay as previously described (2).

The cellular distribution of cytosol and nuclear estrogen receptor in the untreated day 5 rat is similar to that which is observed in the immature and adult animal (Fig. 2). An injection of nafoxidine (100 μg) on day 5 causes the majority of the receptor to be localized in the nuclear fraction 5 days later. Oil-injected animals maintain the usual high levels of cytosol receptor and low levels of nuclear receptors 5 days later.

Long-Term Effects

Neonatal female rats were injected on day 1 of life with either nafoxidine (1–100 μg/rat) or clomiphene (10–500 μg/rat). Each compound was dissolved in absolute ethanol, stirred into warmed (~ 45°C) sesame oil until the ethanol had evaporated, and injected subcutaneously in the nape of the neck. Clomiphene is a mixture of *cis* and *trans* isomers and was used as such because this is the form that is administered to women. The animals were weaned at 21 days of age and the time of vaginal opening was noted. Vaginal smears were examined for 3 to 4 weeks before autopsy. The ovaries, oviducts, and uteri were removed between days 60 and 100 of life and were prepared for routine histological analysis.

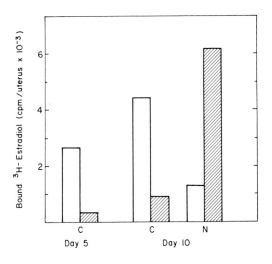

FIG. 2. Effect of nafoxidine on estrogen receptor compartmentalization in the neonatal rat uterus. Animals were injected with 100 μg nafoxidine on day 5 and the levels of cytosol *(open bars)* and nuclear *(hatched bars)* estrogen receptor were determined on day 10. C, control; N, nafoxidine treated.

Vaginal opening occurred in 86% of the rats injected with 100 μg nafoxidine or 500 μg clomiphene between days 26 and 34. Control rats have vaginal opening between days 35 and 50. The vaginal smears of treated rats did not show normal cyclic changes, and a high incidence of estrus smears was noted. Therefore, these animals are probably acyclic and in a state which outwardly resembles persistant estrus. These responses are typical of masculinized female rats; however, a more extensive evaluation of these animals is required before this can be stated with certainty.

Abnormalities of the reproductive tract involved a complicated array of anomalies. These included atrophic ovaries with accompanying atrophic uteri in some animals, while others showed cystic ovaries and enlarged uteri. Hypertrophy of the oviducts was a common observation. An examination of the histology of the uterine tissue revealed various stages of uterine hyperplasia and squamous metaplasia. Tumors of the uterus were also observed in rats that received clomiphene or nafoxidine. Uterine tumors were observed in only a few animals; however, no animals older than 100 days were used in this study. The incidence of uterine tumors may increase considerably in older rats. Other abnormalities include hypertrophied and hyperplastic oviducts; ovarian, oviductal, and uterine inflammation accompanied by pyometra; atrophic ovaries which contained few follicles, a condition that was usually accompanied by atrophic uteri; liquid-filled periovarian sacs with small atrophic ovaries; and hilus cell tumors of the ovary. Control animals that received oil injections did not manifest any reproductive tract abnormalities and were cyclic. The types and frequency of abnormalities varied widely among the various treatment groups. The high doses of either clomiphene (500 μg) or nafoxidine (100 μg) produced some form of abnormality in 80 to 100% of the animals. Although intermediate and lower doses have not been completely evaluated, our results indicate that 10 to 50% of the animals will be adversely affected.

FETAL AND PREGNANCY STUDIES

Rats were mated and the morning that copulatory plugs were found was designated as day 0 of pregnancy. Clomiphene (2.0 mg/kg body weight) was injected on days 0, 5, and 12 of pregnancy in either water or oil. Both injection methods were equally effective. At birth the number of pups was adjusted to eight per mother rat. The pups remained with the mother rat until the day of weaning (day 21) without further handling except for weekly determinations of body weight. At weaning males and females were separated and caged in groups of four and checked daily for preputial separation or vaginal opening. Once this was determined, rats were kept undisturbed until the termination of the experiment at 15 weeks. The rat mothers were also sacrificed at this time. Vaginal smears were obtained on the day of sacrifice and the ovaries, oviducts, uterus, and vagina were removed. These were placed in Bouin's fixative for subsequent sectioning and staining by routine hematoxylin and eosin procedures.

Rats that were injected on day 0 did not become pregnant. This is in agreement with the observations of others (12,30,33); however, when the rats were autopsied 6, 8, and 15 weeks later, the uteri showed extreme stromal and glandular development with hyalinization and small angular nuclei, an almost obliterated lumen, and severely metaplastic and disorganized luminal epithelium. Two of the five animals had follicular cysts while three had many very large corpora lutea showing a peculiar fatty degeneration or vacuolization. Oviducts of these rats showed fluid distension with destruction of the epithelium in some areas. The incidence of atypical or abnormal epithelial tissues in these animals is shown in Table 2.

Three of the rats treated on day 5 became pregnant and delivered normal litters on day 21. When the rats were killed 15 weeks later, the reproductive tracts of both offspring and mothers showed a remarkable array of abnormal or atypical conditions (Table 2). The incidence of disorganized and vacuolated epithelium in the vagina and cervix of the offspring is reminiscent of the vaginal adenosis which has been observed in young girls whose mothers had received DES during pregnancy. These abnormalities of the epithelium were also observed in the uterus and oviduct of both offspring and mother rats. Disorganized hyperplastic epithelium which appeared to be invasive was observed in the uterus and vagina of offspring and mothers. The high incidence of sloughing of noncornified cell cysts (both uterine and ovarian), degenerating epithelium, extensive metaplasia, and hyperplastic vacuolated epithelium indicate the extent of the abnormalities which can be produced by clomiphene. In addition, leukocytic infiltration of the intercellular spaces and glands of the stroma and epithelium of the uterus was observed. This was occasionally seen in the follicles and corpora lutea of the ovaries of both offspring and mothers.

In addition to the abnormalities shown in Table 1, the uteri of the two rats that did not have litters contained extremely wide glandular stroma with a few glandular cysts and low atrophic luminal epithelium.

Of the six females injected on day 12, only four had litters successfully. One mother bore only three pups, two of which were stillborn and one of which died 2 days later. A second female went 9 days beyond normal delivery date, at which time a laparotomy revealed one uterine horn, ovary, and oviduct grossly normal and containing no conceptuses, while the other side had a very large ovarian tumor with adhesions to the oviduct, uterus, intestine, and body wall. This tumor measured $7 \times 10 \times 6$ cm and contained the necrotic remains of at least three pups. Histological examination of the other uterine horn revealed disorganized and possibly invasive epithelium with nests of degenerating stromal cells. The uterine luminal epithelium was metaplastic and cornified throughout the lower half of the uterus. The female pups of these mothers appeared normal at 3 weeks of age, but by 7 weeks areas of luminal epithelial metaplasia had appeared in the uterus. At 15 weeks, the epithelial metaplasia and general extensive stromal development with glandular hyperplasia was marked. In two females the cervical epithelium showed proliferation, downgrowth, and glandular inva-

TABLE 2. *Incidence of epithelial abnormalities in rats treated with clomiphene during pregnancy*[a]

Organ	Experimental group	Abnormality					
		Highly disorganized epithelium	Extensive hyper-plastic vacuolated atypical epithelium	Extensive metaplastic epithelium	Degenerating epithelium	Cysts	Sloughing of noncornified epithelium
Vagina	Control	—	—	—	—	—	—
	Mothers	0	10	0	10	24	31
	Offspring	0	0	0	0	8	21
Cervix	Control	0	0	0	0	4	8
	Mothers	12	35	35	12	0	12
	Offspring	14	21	18	0	0	14
Uterus	Control	0	0	0	0	8	0
	Mothers	12	47	47	0	12	12
	Offspring	14	46	68	0	25	14
Oviduct	Control	0	0	0	0	0	0
	Mothers	0	6	0	47	18	18
	Offspring	0	11	0	14	0	0

[a] Rats were injected with clomiphene (2.0 mg/kg body wt) on day 1, 5, or 12 of pregnancy. Rat mothers ($N = 12$) and offspring ($N = 28$) were autopsied 100 days post-partum. Control females either received no treatment or 0.1 ml of oil. Results are expressed as percentage.

sion of the stroma. The ovaries seemed normal, but the oviducts were distended with fluid and contained cysts without epithelium. One of nine male pups had testicular tubules in which spermatogenesis did not proceed beyond secondary spermatocytes. Interstitial cells were abundant. The epididymis was filled only with fluid and cell fragments and showed local cysts with inflammatory reaction. The remaining male offspring appeared normal.

EFFECTS IN THE BABOON

Two adult, cycling female baboons *(Papio cynocephalus)* with histories of normal gestations were selected from the breeding colony maintained by the Department of Gynecology and Obstetrics at Oklahoma University Health Sciences Center. A bilateral oophorectomy was performed on each animal and serum estrone and estradiol levels were determined 2 weeks post surgery to verify that complete oophorectomy had been accomplished. The estrogen levels in both animals were less than 20 pg/ml, a value in line with postmenopausal humans and remarkably lower than cycling baboons (26).

Clomiphene (100 mg) was given in a banana between 8:00 and 9:00 A.M. for 5 days. Each animal was observed to be certain they consumed the total amount of the drug. Twenty-four hours after the last administration of clomiphene an endometrial biopsy was taken. Pretreatment endometrial biopsies were also taken. Cycling animals received clomiphene (100 mg) on cycle days 6 through 10, and endometrial biopsies were taken on cycle days 5 and 11. Animals were anesthetized with ketamine hydrochloride (10 mg/kg). Following cervical dilatation, an endometrial biopsy was obtained using a sharp endometrial curette. The tissue was either fixed in 10% buffered formalin and stained with hematoxylin-eosin for histological analysis or fixed for 2 hr at room temperature in two aldehydic mixtures: (a) 2% glutaraldehyde, 2% formaldehyde and picric acid or (b) 4% glutaraldehyde and 1% formaldehyde. After rinsing in cacodylate-sucrose buffer (0.1 M sodium cacodylate, 0.25 M sucrose, pH 7.4), they were treated with 1% OsO_4 in veronal acetate buffer, dehydrated, and embedded in Epon 812. Ultrathin sections were stained with uranyl acetate and lead citrates and examined in a Siemens 102A electron microscope.

The endometrium of the oophorectomized baboon before clomiphene treatment was atrophic with low cubodial epithelium. Following 100 mg of clomiphene for 5 days, the endometrium was proliferative with columnar glandular epithelium (Fig. 3). Even more extensive epithelial hypertrophy was observed in the adult intact animals after clomiphene treatment (not shown). In addition to the above evidence for estrogenicity, we also examined endometrial cells for nuclear bodies. Nuclear bodies are found in uterine nuclei of the rat following estrogenic stimulation either by estradiol or triphenylethylene derivatives and their presence is closely correlated with cellular growth (9). Epithelial and stromal cells from the clomiphene-treated oophorectomized baboons contained nuclear bodies, while nontreated controls did not (Fig. 4).

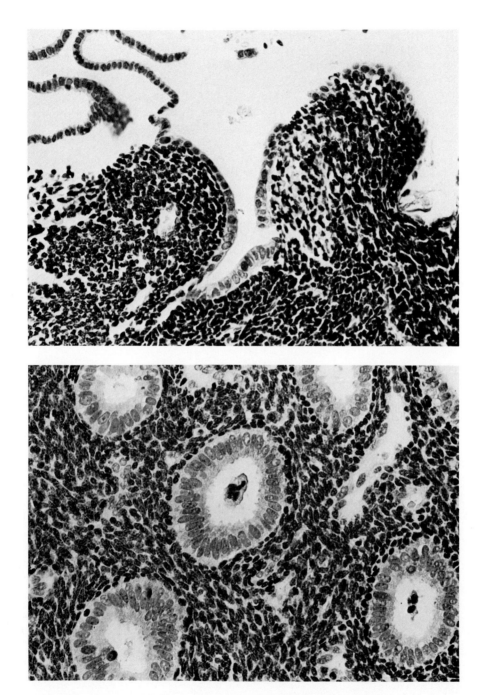

FIG. 3. Effect of clomiphene on the endometrium in the oophorectomized baboon. Endometrium before clomiphene treatment **(top)** and after 5 days of 100 mg/day **(bottom).**

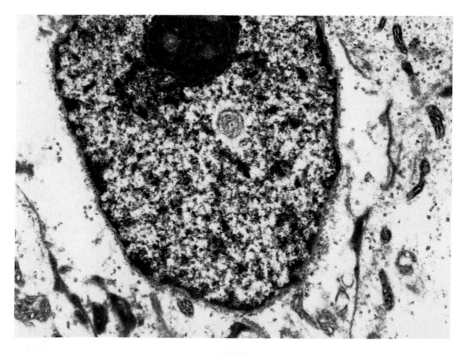

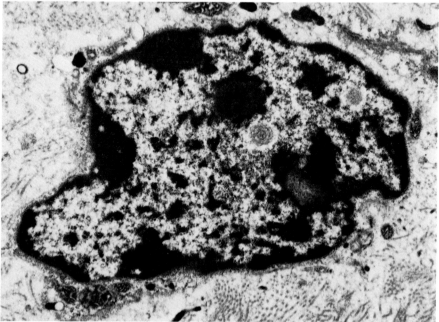

FIG. 4. Nuclear bodies in endometrial nuclei of the baboon following clomiphene treatment. Epithelial cell **(top)** and stromal cell **(bottom).**

DISCUSSION AND CONCLUSIONS

These results indicate that a single injection of clomiphene or nafoxidine during fetal or neonatal life of the rat will cause a wide number of abnormalities of the reproductive tract. These abnormalities may arise from the intense and sustained estrogenic stimulation of the epithelial lining of these organs (Fig. 1). Continuous exposure to high levels of estrogen during fetal and/or neonatal life is known to increase the incidence of preneoplastic and neoplastic changes in the reproductive tract (17,18,20,34). The abnormalities that were observed in the maternal tissues may also result from a similar hyperestrogenization. We have observed extensive epithelial cell stimulation in adult cycling rats *(unpublished results)* and we assume that this also takes place in the pregnant rat.

The variation in the kinds of abnormalities probably relates to both the dose of the compound and the age of the animal to which it is administered. The ability of the reproductive organs to respond to estrogenic compounds depends, in part, on the presence of estrogen receptors, and the concentration of these receptors is known to increase with time in the neonatal rat (7). Therefore, the effectiveness of the compound, as well as its mode of action, may vary with time.

Although we have not ruled out the possibility of indirect effects of nafoxidine and clomiphene, it seems likely that these drugs are acting directly on the various target tissues. We have observed previously that nafoxidine causes long-term retention of the estrogen receptor by uterine nuclei by a sustained stimulation of uterine growth up to 19 days after a single injection (5). This effect also occurs in the neonatal rat (Fig. 2), and therefore, it is likely that the abnormalities which we have observed are due to long-term estrogenic stimulation during critical periods of reproductive tract development.

These results also demonstrate that clomiphene is estrogenic in the uterine endometrium of the baboon. This estrogenicity is evident not only from the cellular hypertrophy shown in Fig. 3, but also from the stimulation of nuclear bodies in epithelial and stromal cells (Fig. 4). Nuclear bodies are of unknown function, however, they are associated with intense transcriptional activity and estrogen receptor binding in uterine nuclei (8,9). Such nuclear bodies have often been identified in neoplastic cells (4,13).

These observations in the baboon imply that similar estrogenic responses to clomiphene may occur in the human. A survey of the literature indicates that similar responses do occur in humans; however, they have been overlooked or deemphasized. This is understandable since these studies were designed to determine the effects of clomiphene on ovulation. Ovulation was judged by endometrial biopsy and the desired endpoint was a secretory endometrium (1,29). Simple endometrial proliferation was taken as evidence that no ovulation had occurred and was assumed to be due to endogenous estrogens. The alternative explanation that endometrial proliferation was due to the inherent estrogenicity of clomiphene was not considered. This, too, is understandable, since the evidence in existence at that time for the antiestrogenic function of clomiphene was substantial. Clomiphene caused decreased vaginal cornification, as judged by decreased pyknotic index; increased the incidence of hot flushes in some women; and decreased the fern pattern in cervical mucous (23,29,31). As discussed in the introduction, these divergent effects may result from the ability of clomiphene to act as a cell-specific agonist/antagonist. Therefore, it may function as an antiestrogen in the vaginal mucosa while acting as an estrogen in the uterine endometrium, thus explaining the results discussed above.

The effect of clomiphene on epithelial cells of the uterus is similar to that observed by the unopposed action of estradiol (hyperestrogenization). Since hyperestrogenization is correlated with the development of endometrial carcinoma (21), the possibility that this may occur in women must be considered. However, it seems unlikely that clomiphene would result in the development of cancer in women who exhibit ovulation and menstruation as a result of clomiphene treatment. Indeed, it has been shown that clomiphene can be used to treat endometrial hyperplasia and presumably reduce the risk of cancer (25,35). However, in women who do not develop a luteal phase, and hence do not benefit from the modifying influences of progesterone, caution should be used. The endometrial epithelium in these women could become hyperestrogenized and thus provide an environment favorable for the development of cancer.

The estrogenic effects of clomiphene in cell types other than those of the reproductive tract also bear consideration. Clomiphene is known to bind estrogen receptors in the hypothalamus and pituitary where it is generally considered to have an inhibitory effect on the estrogenic control of gonadotropin secretion (14,24). Boyer (3) suggested that low doses of clomiphene stimulated gonadotropin secretion because it antagonized the negative feedback of endogenous estrogens. He also suggested that high doses inhibit gonadotropin secretion by virtue of their ability to act as estrogens. This differential response may also be due to cell specific agonist/antagonist effects, i.e., clomiphene may have a positive effect on some hypothalamic or pituitary cells while having negative (antagonistic) effects in others. Hsueh et al. (22) have shown that clomiphene increases the sensitivity of pituitary cells to LH-RH in a fashion similar to that observed with estradiol.

Triphenylethylene derivatives, especially tamoxifen, are used in the treatment of estrogen-dependent breast cancer. Here again the rationale is based on the assumption that these drugs are antiestrogens and this appears to be the case most of the time. However, it is predictable from our findings that some mammary cancers will respond to tamoxifen as though it were an estrogen. We have observed a hormone-dependent transplantable mammary tumor line in the mouse which does have this positive response to nafoxidine (a drug similar to tamoxifen; Watson et al., *unpublished observation*). Therefore, it appears that, although the antiestrogenicity of these drugs is clearly established in the treatment of many breast cancers, clinicians should be cautious of prolonged estrogenic stimulation in certain patients.

ACKNOWLEDGMENT

This work was supported by National Institutes of Health Grants CA-20605 and HD-08436.

REFERENCES

1. Ancla, M., and De Brux, J. (1967): *Am. J. Obstet. Gynecol.,* 98:1043–1049.
2. Anderson, J. N., Clark, J. H., and Peck, E. J., Jr. (1972): *Biochem. J.,* 126:561–567.
3. Boyer, R. M. (1970): *Endocrinology,* 86:629–633.
4. Bouteille, M., Kalifat, S. R., and Delarue, J. (1967): *J. Ultrastruc. Res.,* 19:474–486.
5. Clark, J. H., Anderson, J. N., and Peck, E. F., Jr. (1973): *Steroids,* 22:707–718.
6. Clark, J. H., Anderson, J. N., and Peck, E. J., Jr. (1974): *Nature,* 251:446–448.
7. Clark, J. H., and Gorski, J. (1979): *Science,* 169:76–78.
8. Clark, J. H., Hardin, J. W., McCormack, S. A., and Padykula, H. A. (1978): In: *Hormones, Receptors, and Breast Cancer, (Progress in Cancer Research and Therapy, Vol. 10),* edited by W. L. McGuire, pp. 107–133. Raven Press, New York.
9. Clark, J. H., Hardin, J. W., Padykula, H. A., and Cardasis, C. A. (1978): *Proc. Natl. Acad. Sci. USA,* 75:2781–2784.
10. Clark, J. H., and McCormack, S. A. (1977): *Science,* 197:164–165.
11. Clark, J. H., Paszko, Z., and Peck, E. J., Jr. (1977): *Endocrinology,* 100:91–96.
12. Davidson, O. W., Wada, K., and Schuchner, E. B. (1965): *Fertil. Steril.,* 16:495–501.
13. Dupuy-Coin, A. M., Kalifat, S. R., and Bouteille, M. (1972): *J. Ultrastruct. Res.,* 38:174–183.
14. Eisenfeld, A. J. (1970): *Endocrinology,* 86:1313–1318.
15. Emmens, C. W. (1970): *Annu. Rev. Pharmacol.,* 4:237–254.
16. Ferguson, E. R., and Katzenellenbogen, B. S. (1977): *Endocrinology,* 100:1242–1251.
17. Forsberg, J. G. (1975): *Am. J. Obstet. Gynecol.,* 121:101–104.
18. Furth, J., Ueda, G., and Clifton, K. H. (1973): In: *Methods in Cancer Research, Vol. 10,* edited by H. Busch, pp. 201–277. Academic Press, New York.
19. Hardin, J. W., Clark, J. H., Glasser, S. R., and Peck, E. J., Jr. (1976): *Biochemistry,* 15:1370–1374.
20. Herbst, A. L., Ulfelder, H., and Poskanzer, D. C. (1971): *N. Engl. J. Med.,* 284:878–881.
21. Hertz, R. (1974): *Cancer,* 38:534–540.
22. Hsueh, A. J. W., Erickson, G. F., and Yen, S. S. C. (1978): *Nature,* 273:57–59.
23. Jones, G. S., and de Morales-Ruehsen, M. (1965): *Fertil. Steril.,* 16:461–484.
24. Kistner, R. W. (1975): In: *Progress in Infertility,* edited by S. J. Behrman and R. W. Kistner, pp. 509–536, Little, Brown, Boston.
25. Kistner, R. W., Gore, H., and Hertig, A. T. (1966): *Am. J. Obstet. Gynecol.,* 95:1011–1024.
26. Kling, O. R., and Westfahl, P. K. (1978): *Biol. Reprod.,* 18:392–400.
27. Markaverich, B. M., Clark, J. H., and Hardin, J. W. (1978): *Biochemistry,* 17:3146–3152.
28. McCormack, S. A., and Clark, J. H. (1979): *Science,* 204:629–631.
29. Pildes, R. B. (1965): *Am. J. Obstet. Gynecol.,* 91:466–478.
30. Prasad, M. R. N., Segal, S. J., and Kalra, S. P. (1965): *Fertil. Steril.,* 16:101–105.
31. Riley, G. M., and Evans, T. M. (1964): *Am. J. Obstet. Gynecol.,* 89:97–109.
32. Ruh, T. S., and Baudendistel, L. H. (1977): *Endocrinology,* 100:420–426.
33. Staples, P. E. (1966): *Endocrinology,* 78:82–86.
34. Takasugi, N., and Bern, H. A. (1964): *J. Natl. Cancer Inst.,* 33:855–865.
35. Whitelaw, M. J. (1963): *Fertil. Steril.,* 14:540–546.

Hormones and Cancer, edited by S. Iacobelli et al.
Raven Press, New York © 1980.

Antiestrogen Action in Estrogen Target Tissues: Receptor Interactions and Antiestrogen Metabolism

Benita S. Katzenellenbogen, *John A. Katzenellenbogen, Richard L. Eckert, James R. Hayes, *David W. Robertson, *Tochiro Tatee, and Ten-lin S. Tsai

*Departments of Physiology and Biophysics and *Chemistry, University of Illinois, and School of Basic Medical Sciences, University of Illinois College of Medicine, Urbana, Illinois 61801*

There has long been an interest in the development of compounds capable of interfering with the actions of estrogens. Antiestrogens are compounds that prevent estrogens from expressing their full effects on estrogen target tissues and, as such, they antagonize a variety of estrogen-dependent processes, including uterine growth and the growth of hormone-dependent mammary tumors. They also act to stimulate pituitary gonadotropin output and subsequent ovulation in certain women by antagonism of estrogen feedback at the level of the hypothalamus and pituitary. It should be noted, however, that these compounds are not pure antagonists in some species and tissues, and they usually show some estrogenicity themselves (2,4,7,9). The compounds that we have used in some of our studies, CI-628, U-11,100A, and U-23,469 have a characteristic triphenylethylene structure.[1] They are structurally related to the better-known antiestrogens clomiphene and tamoxifen and to the potent estrogen diethylstilbestrol.

Our main interest in these compounds has been the elucidation of some of the molecular aspects of their mode of action. Our studies have endeavored to analyze both the cellular (target tissue) interaction of these compounds, as well as their pharmacokinetic behavior and metabolism which may markedly modulate their efficacy *in vivo*.

Conceivably, the antagonistic action of an antiestrogen could take place at any of the stages of estrogen interaction with the receptor mechanism of target cells or at hypothetical control points postreceptor. An antiestrogen might (a) interfere with the cellular uptake of estradiol, (b) compete for cytoplasmic complex formation, (c) interfere with the transformation of the estrogen receptor

---

[1] CI-628 = α-[4-pyrrolidinoethoxy]phenyl-4-methoxy-α'-nitrostilbene; U-11,100A = 1-(2-[p-(3,4-dihydro-6-methoxy-2-phenyl-1-naphthyl)phenoxy]ethyl) pyrrolidine hydrochloride; U-23,469 = *cis*(3-[p-(1,2,3,4,-tetrahydro-6-methoxy-2-phenyl-1-naphthyl)-phenoxy]-1,2-propanediol).

to an active form, (d) interfere with the transfer of the receptor complex to the nucleus or with its proper association with nuclear sites, (e) interfere with nuclear turnover or release of receptor and regeneration of cytoplasmic receptor, and/or (f) exert a postreceptor block (such as at the level of transcription).

There is evidence from the studies to be described here and from the studies of other laboratories (reviewed in part in refs. 4,7, and 9; see below) indicating that antiestrogens have some effects at levels 2, 4, and 5. That is, they compete for cytoplasmic complex formation; they appear to alter the association of the receptor complex and the nuclear binding sites; and under some conditions, particularly at high doses, they alter the regeneration of the cytoplasmic receptor.

EFFECTS OF ANTIESTROGENS IN UTERUS AND MAMMARY TUMOR SYSTEMS

In some early studies (3,10), we examined the effects of antiestrogens on the subcellular distribution of estrogen receptors in the immature (day 20–23) rat uterus. We found that, like estradiol, a variety of antiestrogens moved cytoplasmic receptor sites into the nucleus. However, while the estradiol–receptor complex was lost from the nucleus rather rapidly, and cytoplasmic receptor levels were replenished soon thereafter, the antiestrogens retained some receptor in the nucleus for a prolonged period of time and cytoplasmic receptor levels remain depleted for a long period. These findings confirmed the earlier reports of Clark et al. (2) and Rochefort and Capony (16) demonstrating prolonged nuclear retention and cytoplasmic depletion of receptor following administration of high doses of U-11,100A.

We wanted to explore what the state of the uterus was in terms of its responsiveness to estrogen, during this period when antiestrogen had depleted the cytoplasmic receptor. Further studies (10) showed that during the period in which antiestrogen had depleted the cytoplasmic receptor, the uterus was incapable of responding to estradiol as monitored by the synthesis of the estrogen-induced protein or by uterine weight gain. However, after estradiol, the more rapid return of uterine responsiveness to estrogen parallelled the return of cytoplasmic receptor.

Nuclear maintenance and cytoplasmic depletion of estrogen receptors are dose-related events and there is evidence (8,14) that antiestrogens can antagonize estrogen-stimulated uterine growth at lower doses than cause only partial cytoplasmic receptor depletion. Hence, even low doses of antiestrogen may interfere in a more direct way with estrogen sensitivity beyond that attributable to cytoplasmic receptor depletion.

Since antiestrogens are able to antagonize the actions of estrogens, these compounds hold the potential of being noninvasive, nonsurgical agents capable of controlling the growth of hormone-dependent tumors. Hence, we (22) analyzed the effectiveness of the antiestrogen U-23,469, previously shown to be potent in antagonizing estrogen-induced uterine growth (3), in preventing the development of 7,12-dimethylbenz[a]anthracene (DMBA)-induced rat mammary tumors and in eliciting the regression of established tumors. We have attempted to elucidate the mechanisms of U-23,469's tumor antagonism. In addition to finding U-23,469 to be highly effective in preventing the development of mammary tumors, antiestrogen treatment was able to elicit the regression of established tumors. The time course of tumor regression (3 months after DMBA) by U-23,469 or ovariectomy was found to be similar with 50% regression by about 2 weeks and both procedures elicited regression of almost all tumors (22).

In an attempt to understand the mechanism by which this antiestrogen might be eliciting tumor regression, we examined its effects on tumor estrogen, progesterone, and prolactin receptors. In control mature cycling rats, approximately half of the estrogen receptor was found in the nucleus and high levels of progesterone cytosol receptor were found. Following ovariectomy, as would be expected in the absence of ovarian estrogen, very little estrogen receptor was present in nuclei of regressing tumors, and likewise, progesterone receptor levels were low. Following antiestrogen treatment, as tumors regressed, approximately 90% of the total tumor estrogen receptor was found in the nucleus, and progesterone receptor was similar to that of control rats and much higher than in mammary tumors regressing due to ovariectomy (22). This latter finding may reflect some estrogen-like action of this compound U-23,469.

Antiestrogens also influence the level of prolactin binding in DMBA-induced mammary tumors (Table 1). Tumor prolactin receptor content is greatly reduced in tumors regressing during treatment with a variety of antiestrogens, or with high doses of estrogen. Ovariectomy results in an even more marked reduction in tumor prolactin receptor.

Hence, as was seen in the uterus earlier, high doses of antiestrogen perturb the normal distribution of estrogen receptor such that much of the receptor is found in the nucleus with low levels of cytoplasmic receptor; this situation may render the mammary tumor incapable of responding to the animal's own endogenous estrogens and hence unable to grow. In addition, antiestrogens may also influence mammary tumor growth in this system by reducing the tumor content of prolactin receptors (13) (Table 1).

Antiestrogen treatment also markedly depresses the growth of the ovarian autonomous but estrogen-sensitive R3230AC rat mammary tumor (12,23). Administration of the antiestrogen U-23,469 and two related antiestrogens, U11,100A and CI-628, beginning at the time of tumor transplantation into Fischer 344 host rats, results in a two-to fourfold depression in tumor growth rate, and the degree of growth reduction is related to the dose of antiestrogen. Estradiol-17β (15 μg) also depresses R3230AC tumor growth, while growth is at or slightly above the control rate in ovariectomized hosts. These findings suggest that antiestrogens may provide palliative benefit in the case of some ovarian-unresponsive but estrogen-sensitive breast cancers, in addition to being highly beneficial in the treatment of ovarian-dependent breast cancers.

TABLE 1. *Prolactin receptor in DMBA-induced mammary tumors*

Group[a]	% Specific binding[b]
Control	8.0 ± 0.8 (31)
U23,469 (250 μg/day)	4.5 ± 0.8[c] (16)
U11,100A (250 μg/day)	4.9 ± 0.6[c] (7)
CI-628 (200 μg/day)	5.4 ± 0.9[c] (18)
Estradiol-17β (50 μg/day)	3.7 ± 0.9[c] (19)
Estradiol-benzoate (50 μg/day)	2.8 ± 0.3[c] (11)
Ovariectomy	1.3 ± 0.4[c] (8)

[a] Each rat bearing tumors (ca. 60–80 days after DMBA) received s.c. injections of antiestrogen or estrogen in 0.5 ml 0.15 M NaCl daily for 2–4 weeks. Controls received 0.15 M NaCl alone and rats that were ovariectomized received no injections. The tumors were assayed 19–23 hr after the last injection, or approximately 2 weeks after ovariectomy.

[b] The difference in bound [125I]prolactin with or without excess cold prolactin expressed as the percentage of total radioactivity added in each tube. Values are expressed as mean ± SEM. Numbers in parentheses are number of tumors assayed.

[c] $p < 0.05$ versus control value.

RECEPTOR INTERACTIONS AND METABOLISM STUDIES WITH RADIOLABELED ANTIESTROGENS

With the hope of looking directly at the interaction of antiestrogens with receptor, and at possible antiestrogen metabolism, we have tritiated two of the antiestrogens (CI-628 and U-23,469) to high specific activity. In studies presented below, we have found that the interaction of radiolabeled antiestrogen with the estrogen receptor parallels that of estradiol in many respects. Both of the antiestrogens are metabolized *in vivo* to more polar forms that have a higher affinity for receptor than the parent compound. These antiestrogen metabolites are found to be associated with the nuclear estrogen receptor and we believe that they may be the true agents active *in vivo*.

Studies revealed high affinity estrogen specific binding of [3H]CI-628 in uterine cytosol, $K_D = 1.7 \times 10^{-9}$ M, corresponding to an affinity approximately 6% that of estradiol (11). Sucrose density gradient analyses of antiestrogen cytoplasmic receptor complexes on low salt gradients indicated that over 90% of the antiestrogen–receptor complexes sedimented at 8 S, as did estradiol–receptor complexes (9).

After administration of tritiated CI-628 *in vivo,* radioactivity can be found associated with specific estrogen receptor sites in uterine nuclei, and salt-extracted nuclear receptor antiestrogen complexes sediment at 5.4 S on high salt-containing sucrose gradients as do [³H]estradiol nuclear receptor complexes (Fig. 1). In DMBA-induced mammary tumors, nuclear antiestrogen–receptor complexes and estradiol–receptor complexes are likewise indistinguishable by sucrose density gradient analysis (T. L. Tsai and B. S. Katzenellenbogen, *unpublished*).

Studies with a series of structurally modified antiestrogens (3) suggested that some antiestrogens, such as CI-628, possessing a methyl ether group might undergo metabolism to form a compound with a higher affinity for receptor and a faster onset of action. Therefore, we investigated the chemical nature of the antiestrogen associated with the nuclear receptor (11). Analyses of ethyl acetate extracts of the nuclear receptor peak fractions from sucrose gradients showed that a polar metabolite of CI-628 was selectively bound to the 5-S nuclear receptor (11).

This polar metabolite cochromatographs with the demethylated form of CI-628 in a variety of solvent systems. Further confirmation of its identity with demethylated CI-628 was indicated by experiments employing diazomethane. Treatment of the metabolite with diazomethane, a reagent that selectively methylates phenolic hydroxyl groups, completely converts the metabolite back to CI-628 (D. W. Robertson and J. A. Katzenellenbogen, *unpublished*).

Pharmacokinetic studies (11) have also revealed that high levels of antiestrogen persist in serum and uterus for long periods of time (half cleared in 18–24 hr), whereas estradiol is much more rapidly cleared (half cleared in 30 min). Hence, it is likely that the prolonged *in vivo* activity of this antiestrogen derives, at least in part, from its slow rate of clearance, and that the agent active *in vivo* may be a metabolite of CI-628.

Studies with another antiestrogen, U-23,469, indicate that it also is rapidly converted to a more polar metabolite that selectively accumulates in the target cell nucleus (Fig. 2). By 1 hr after the *in vivo* administration of [³H]U-23,469, there is already some metabolite present in the nucleus, and by 13 hr it accounts for almost all of the nuclear radioactivity. In DMBA-induced mammary tumors, a similar situation is seen (B. S. Katzenellenbogen and T. L. Tsai, *unpublished*).

U-23,469 itself has a low affinity for the cytoplasmic estrogen receptor (approximately 0.1% that of estradiol; ref. 3). Preliminary characterization indicates that the metabolite is the demethylated material which has an affinity for receptor more than 100 times that of the parent compound (21). In addition, specific nuclear antiestrogen–receptor complexes can be detected after administration of [³H]U-23,469 *in vivo* (Fig. 3). Salt-extractable nuclear receptor complexes sediment at 5 S on high salt sucrose gradients as do estradiol–receptor complexes (Fig. 3A), and chromatographic analysis (Fig. 3B) reveals that it is only the metabolite that accumulates in the nuclear receptor fraction.

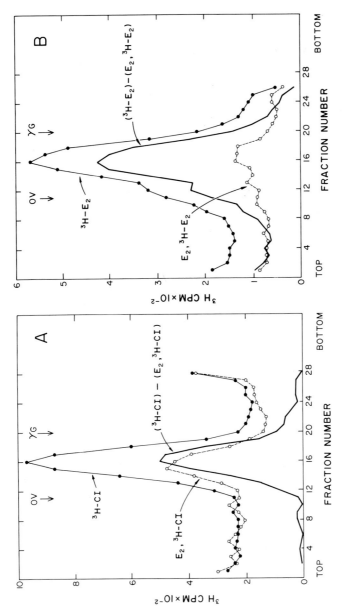

FIG. 1. High salt sucrose density gradient centrifugation profiles of salt-extracted nuclear receptor complexes after exposure to [^{3}H]CI-628 **(A)** or [^{3}H]estradiol ([^{3}H]E$_2$) **(B)** *in vivo*. Groups of rats were pretreated for 1 hr *in vivo* with 5 µg unlabeled estradiol or with vehicle saline alone and then received an s.c. injection of 50 µg [^{3}H]CI or 3 µg [^{3}H]E$_2$ (containing 0.9 µg [^{3}H]E$_2$ plus 2.1 µg E$_2$). At 1 hr after injection, uteri were excised and the three-times washed 800 × *g* nuclear pellet was extracted with buffer containing 0.4 M KCl for 1 hr at 0°C. Extracts were treated with 10% charcoal-dextran prior to addition of ^{14}C-labeled marker proteins, and 300-µl aliquots (containing 1.6 uterine equivalents, **A**; 1.0 uterine equivalents, **B**) were layered onto gradients. Centrifugation was for 17 hr at 4°C at 270,000 × *g*. (From Katzenellenbogen et al., ref. 11, with permission.)

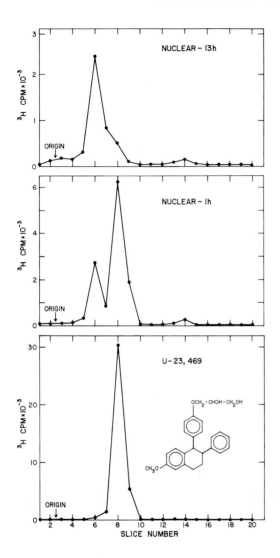

FIG. 2. Thin-layer chromatographic profiles of authentic [³H]U-23,469 *(lower panel)* and of uterine nuclear radioactivity after *in vivo* injection of [³H]U-23, 469. Immature rats were injected with [³H]U-23,469 (25 μg s.c./rat), and at 1 and 13 hr after injection, uteri were excised and homogenized and the three-times washed nuclear pellet was then ethanol extracted. Ethanol extracts were analyzed on thin-layer silica gel plates developed in anesthetic ether:ethanol (98:2 vol/vol). (From Katzenellenbogen et al., ref. 9, with permission.)

We have now synthesized the presumed antiestrogen metabolites and we are beginning to examine their interactions with estrogen receptors. Figure 4 shows competitive binding assays using rat uterine cytosol receptor. It is seen that the metabolites have a much higher affinity for estrogen receptor than do the parent compounds. In the case of U-23,469, the demethylated form has an affinity for receptor approximately 300 times that of the parent compound, while there is a 10-fold increased affinity of the CI-628 metabolite, resulting in an affinity for receptor greater than that of estradiol.

In MCF-7 human breast cancer cells, the metabolite forms of these two anties-

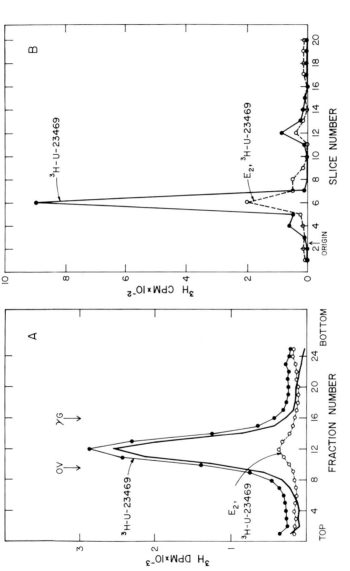

FIG. 3. High salt sucrose density gradient analysis of salt-extracted nuclear receptor complexes after exposure to [³H]U-23,469 *in vivo* (**A**) and thin layer chromatographic analysis of 5-S estrogen receptor complex purified on sucrose gradients (**B**). Groups of rats were pretreated for 1 hr *in vivo* with 5 μg unlabeled estradiol or with vehicle saline alone, and each then received an s.c. injection of 25 μg [³H]U-23,469. At 2 hr after injection, uteri were excised and the three-times washed 800 × *g* nuclear pellet was extracted with buffer containing 0.4 M KCl for 1 hr at 0°C. **A:** Extracts were treated with charcoal-dextran prior to addition of ¹⁴C-labeled marker proteins (ovalbumin, OV; gamma globulin, γG), and a 350 μl-aliquot (containing 1.2 uterine equivalents) was layered onto gradients. Centrifugation was for 17 hr at 4°C at 270,000 × *g*. **B:** The peak region of the gradient (fractions 9–15, **A**) was extracted with ethyl acetate and analyzed by thin-layer chromatography. The profile of material from animals treated with [³H]U-23,469 alone is indicated by the *solid curve* and that of [³H]U-23,469 after unlabeled estradiol pretreatment is indicated by the *broken curve*. The difference between these two profiles represents radioactivity associated with estrogen-specific nuclear binding sites. Authentic [³H]U-23,469 chromatographs at slice 8. (From Tatee et al., ref. 21, with permission.)

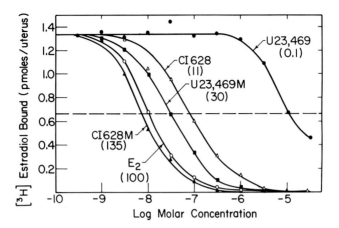

FIG. 4. Competitive binding assay of the parent antiestrogens and antiestrogen metabolites with rat uterine cytosol. Cytosol from immature rat uteri was incubated for 6 hr at 0°C with 10^{-8} M [^{3}H]estradiol and the indicated concentrations of unlabeled competitor. Bound [^{3}H]estradiol was then determined by charcoal-dextran adsorption. Numbers in parentheses indicate the binding affinity of the compounds relative to estradiol, which is set at 100.

trogens also show a greatly increased affinity for nuclear or cytosol estrogen receptor (Fig. 5).

Since biological potency obviously depends upon many factors in addition to receptor affinity, our present studies are focused on assessing whether these *in vivo* metabolites have enhanced biological effectiveness as estrogen antagonists. In addition, their high affinity for receptors should enable detailed analyses of the receptor interactions that may serve to characterize their agonist and antagonist activities. Of interest here are related studies that have documented *in vivo* metabolism of tamoxifen and the enhanced activity of monohydroxytamoxifen (1,6,7).

CONCLUSION

We do not yet have sufficient information to propose a definitive model to explain the molecular mechanism of antiestrogen action, but Fig. 6 may serve to summarize some of the experiments discussed.

The top portion of Fig. 6 presents the standard picture of estrogen action. After exposure to estrogen, the steroid binds to the cytoplasmic receptor present in the target cell. The cytoplasmic receptor becomes localized in the nucleus and the nuclear receptor interacts with chromatin in a manner such that a spectrum of biochemical and physiological responses are elicited including replenishment of cytoplasmic receptor (15,19).

When an antiestrogen or a more active metabolite of the antiestrogen enters the target cell, it also binds to the cytoplasmic receptor. By the criteria we

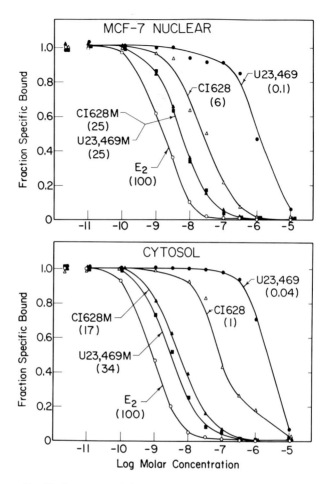

FIG. 5. Competitive binding assay of the parent antiestrogens and antiestrogen metabolites with nuclear or cytosol estrogen receptor from MCF-7 human breast cancer cells. Receptor preparations were incubated for 16 hr at 0°C with 2×10^{-9} M [³H]estradiol (nuclear) or 1×10^{-9} M [³H]estradiol (cytosol) and the indicated concentrations of unlabeled competitor. Bound [³H]estradiol was then determined and values are expressed as the fraction of specific estradiol counts bound. Numbers in parentheses indicate the binding affinity of the compounds relative to estradiol, which is set at 100.

have used thus far, the interaction of antiestrogen with cytoplasmic receptor does not appear to be different from the interaction of estrogen with this receptor, but we have indicated R_C as R_C' here to indicate that the receptor complex with antiestrogen may be different, as suggested by some binding studies of Rochefort and Capony (17). The antiestrogen–receptor complex does move into the nucleus and binds to chromatin, but its nuclear interaction must be different because it initiates only some responses; in tissues such as the chick oviduct,

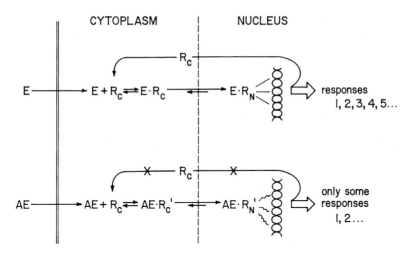

FIG. 6. Model for antiestrogen action, indicating our present state of knowledge about how estrogens (E) and antiestrogens (AE) interact with the estrogen receptor system in target cells. R_C, cytoplasmic receptor; R_N, nuclear receptor. (From Katzenellenbogen et al., ref. 9, with permission.)

it does not appear to evoke any estrogen-like responses (20), although receptor does localize in the nucleus. Differences in the salt extractability of nuclear receptor–estrogen complexes versus nuclear receptor–antiestrogen complexes (11,18) and in the processing of such nuclear receptor complexes (5) may be manifestations of genuine differences in the chromatin interaction of these compounds.

At high doses, antiestrogens alter cytoplasmic receptor replenishment resulting in depletion of cytoplasmic receptor levels. This may account for the antagonistic effects of antiestrogens in terms of certain responses (9). However, antiestrogens can be antagonists of responses such as uterine growth under conditions where there is only partial depletion of cytoplasmic receptor (8,14), suggesting a more direct or active role of the antiestrogen–receptor complex. Additional studies are required to provide further refinement of a molecular model of antiestrogen action.

ACKNOWLEDGMENTS

Research from our laboratories discussed in this chapter was supported in part by National Institutes of Health Research Grants CA 18119 and HD 06726 (to B. S. Katzenellenbogen); and United States Public Health Service Grant AM 15556, American Cancer Society Grant BC-223, a Camille and Henry Dreyfus Foundation award (to J. A. Katzenellenbogen) and Ford Foundation Grant 700–0333. We are grateful to the Parke-Davis and Upjohn Companies for providing us with antiestrogens, to the NIAMDD Hormone Distribution

Program for providing us with ovine prolactin, and to Dr. Charles McGrath for providing MCF-7 cells. We thank Robyn Luke for excellent secretarial assistance.

REFERENCES

1. Capony, F., and Rochefort, H. (1978): *Mol. Cell. Endocrinol.,* 78:71–81.
2. Clark, J. H., Anderson, J. N., and Peck, E. J., Jr. (1973): *Steroids,* 22:707–718.
3. Ferguson, E. R., and Katzenellenbogen, B. S. (1977): *Endocrinology,* 100:1242–1251.
4. Horwitz, K. B., and McGuire, W. L. (1978): In: *Breast Cancer, Vol. 2,* edited by W. L. McGuire, pp. 155–204. Plenum Press, New York.
5. Horwitz, K. B., and McGuire, W. L. (1978): *J. Biol. Chem.,* 253:8185–8191.
6. Jordan, V. C., Collins, M. M., Rowsby, L., and Prestwich, G. (1977): *J. Endocrinol.,* 75:305–316.
7. Jordan, V. C., Dix, C. J., Naylor, K. E., Prestwich, G., and Rowsby, L. (1978): *J. Toxicol. Environ. Health,* 4:363–390.
8. Jordan, V. C., Rowsby, L., Dix, C. J., and Prestwich, G. (1978): *J. Endocrinol.,* 78:71–81.
9. Katzenellenbogen, B. S., Bhakoo, H. S., Ferguson, E. R., Lan, N. C., Tatee, T., and Katzenellenbogen, J. A. (1979): *Recent Prog. Horm. Res.,* 35:259–300.
10. Katzenellenbogen, B. S., and Ferguson, E. R. (1975): *Endocrinology,* 97:1–12.
11. Katzenellenbogen, B. S., Katzenellenbogen, J. A., Ferguson, E. R., and Krauthammer, N. (1978): *J. Biol. Chem.,* 253:697–707.
12. Katzenellenbogen, B. S., Tsai, T. L., Rorke, E., and Rutledge, S. (1979): *Proceedings 61st Annual Endocrine Society Meeting,* Abstr. 296, p. 146.
13. Kelley, P. A., Asselin, J., Caron, M. G., Labrie, F., and Raynaud, J. P. (1977): *J. Natl. Cancer Inst.,* 58:623–628.
14. Koseki, Y., Zava, D. T., Chamness, G. C., and McGuire, W. L. (1977): *Endocrinology,* 101:1104–1109.
15. Mester, J., and Baulieu, E. E. (1975): *Biochem. J.,* 146:617–623.
16. Rochefort, H., and Capony, F. (1973): *C.R. Acad. Sci. Paris,* 276:2321–2325.
17. Rochefort, H., and Capony, F. (1977): *Biochem. Biophys. Res. Commun.,* 75:277–285.
18. Ruh, T. S., and Baudendistel, L. J. (1977): *Endocrinology,* 100:420–426.
19. Sarff, M., and Gorski, J. (1971): *Biochemistry,* 10:2557–2563.
20. Sutherland, R., Mester, J., and Baulieu, E. E. (1977): *Nature,* 267:434–435.
21. Tatee, T., Carlson, K. E., Katzenellenbogen, J. A., Robertson, D. W., and Katzenellenbogen, B. S. (1979): *J. Med. Chem.,* 22:1509–1517.
22. Tsai, T. L., and Katzenellenbogen, B. S. (1977): *Cancer Res.,* 37:1537–1543.
23. Tsai, T. L., Rutledge, S., and Katzenellenbogen, B. S. (1979): *Cancer Res.,* 39:5043–5050.

Hormones and Cancer, edited by S. Iacobelli et al.
Raven Press, New York © 1980.

Influence of Sex Steroids and Steroid Antagonists on Hormone-Dependent Tumors in Experimental Animals

M. F. El Etreby and F. Neumann

Research Laboratories, Schering AG, D-1000 Berlin 65, West Germany

Ever since steroid hormones were introduced into human medicine and particularly since the widespread use of contraceptive steroids, the question of their influence on the development of hormone-dependent tumors has been controversial. There is no clear evidence to date that steroids cause any form of human cancer. However, sex steroids may influence the development of breast, endometrial, cervical, and prostatic cancer (8,10,41,42,46,50). For that reason, these steroids (estrogens, progestagens, androgens) or steroid antagonists (antiandrogens, antiestrogens) appear to be beneficial in the prophylaxis and/or treatment of some types of human tumors (20,46,50).

The object of this chapter is to evaluate and summarize knowledge of the influence of sex steroids or steroid antagonists on tumor development in mice, rats, dogs, and monkeys. The interpretation of such an effect in experimental animals and the predictive value of different animal models for detecting a prophylactic or therapeutic potential of these biologically active compounds on hormone-dependent tumors will be discussed in the light of available human data.

SEX STEROIDS

Long-term systemic tolerance and carcinogenicity studies of sex steroids suggest that high doses of certain estrogens, progestagens, and progestagen–estrogen combinations may stimulate development of tumors in different organs, particularly the pituitary, mammary gland, uterus, gonads, and/or liver of experimental animals (4,7–14,16,18,23,28,40–42,44,45). The influence of sex steroids on tumor developments will be summarized separately for the different organs of experimental animals and man.

Pituitary Gland

In mice and rats, the specific neuroendocrine regulatory mechanisms of prolactin (PRL) secretion appear to be involved in pathogenesis of both spontaneous and steroid-related PRL cell tumors ("prolactinomas") of the pituitary gland. These biologically benign growth processes are observed in long-term studies of some sex steroids (certain estrogens, progestagens, and progestagen-estrogen combinations) which are shown to be potent PRL stimulatory agents as a result of their estrogenic activity in these species (Tables 1–4). Mice were more susceptible than rats (7,10,12,13,18,23).

In the dog, monkey, and man contraceptive steroids stimulate PRL and/or growth hormone (GH) (11–13,30). However, in the dog and monkey, steroid-related pituitary tumors are not observed, even after long-term treatment with high doses of estrogens, progestagens, and their combinations (10,12,13,16, 40,41). On the other hand, a high dose of estrogens may, in special cases and in certain individuals, stimulate growth of PRL cell adenomas in man (5,10, 12,13,27).

These findings indicate that with regard to the influence of sex steroids on development of pituitary tumors, not only the species-specific neuroendocrine

TABLE 1. *Contraceptive steroids that have caused an increased incidence of pituitary tumors in carcinogenicity tests in CF-LP strain of mice[a]*

		Pituitary tumors (%)			
		Males		Females	
Compound	Ratio of HCD	Control	Dose range (2–400 × HCD)	Control	Dose range (2–400 × HCD)
Ethinylestradiol		2 (0–5)	22	5 (0–12)	27
Norethisterone acetate + ethinylestradiol	50 + 1		21		27
Norethynodrel			28		25
Norethynodrel + mestranol	25 + 1		35		32
	66 + 1		39		35
Mestranol			10		14
Norethisterone			7		19
Norethisterone + mestranol	20 + 1		12		26
Ethynodiol diacetate	2 + 1		34		40
+ ethinylestradiol	20 + 1		25		41
Ethynodiol diacetate	1 + 1		25		22
+ mestranol	10 + 1		31		29
	20 + 1		19		27
Mestranol			20		—
Chlormadinone acetate + mestranol	25 + 1		17		33

[a] 3 × 40 mice/group/sex. Numbers in parentheses indicate range in 6 × 40 control animals. Compounds were administered daily in the diet for 80 weeks. HCD, human contraceptive dose.
Data from the Committee on Safety of Medicines, ref. 7.

TABLE 2. *Effect of norethynodrel on tumor incidence (%) in pituitary gland, mammary gland, and liver in a carcinogenicity test in male rats[a]*

Norethynodrel (dose range × HCD)[b]	Pituitary gland	Mammary gland		Liver
		Benign	Malignant	
Control	6	0	0	2
2–5	12	2	0	7
50–150	27	12	5	32
200–400	87	12	40	32

[a] The female rats used in this study did not show significant treatment-related effects on tumor incidence.
[b] 40 rats/treated group, 120 control rats. Compound was administered daily in the diet for 104 weeks. HCD, human contraceptive dose (0.05 mg/kg/day p.o.).
Data from the Committee on Safety of Medicines, ref. 7.

TABLE 3. *Effect of norethisterone and norethisterone + mestranol on tumor incidence (%) in pituitary gland, mammary gland, and liver in a carcinogenicity test in male rats[a]*

Compound[b]	Dose range × HCD	Pituitary gland	Mammary gland		Liver
			Benign	Malignant	
Control (40)	—	22	0	0	4
Norethisterone (120)	2–400	27	4	4	12
Norethisterone + mestranol 20 + 1 (120)	2–400	33	4	12	23

[a] The female rats used in this study did not show significant treatment-related effects on tumor incidence.
[b] Number of rats indicated in parentheses. Compounds were administered daily in the diet for 104 weeks. Norethisterone HCD = 0.02 mg/kg/day p.o., mestranol HCD = 0.001 mg/kg/day p.o.
Data from the Committee on Safety of Medicines, ref. 7.

system but also an unexplained susceptibility of certain species, strains, or individuals are of decisive importance (10,12,13).

The available human data suggest that women taking sex steroids should be watched for amenorrhea, galactorrhea, or other indications of hypothalamic–pituitary dysfunction, which could be considered as common symptoms of pituitary tumors (prolactinomas). Moreover, careful documentation, investigation, and follow-up of the relationship between sex steroids and pituitary tumors in humans are still required and full prospective and retrospective studies should be undertaken (5,10,12,13,27,41,42).

Mammary Gland

Long-term treatment of mice and rats with high doses of certain sex steroids, mainly those with estrogenic activity in these species, may stimulate development

TABLE 4. *Effect of norethisterone enanthate on tumor incidence (%) in pituitary gland, mammary gland, and liver in a carcinogenicity test in rats[a]*

| Norethisterone enanthate (dose × HCD) | Pituitary gland | | Mammary gland | | | | | | Liver | |
| | | | Benign | | Malignant | | | | | |
	M	F	M	F	M	F	M	F	M	F
Control	10	42	0	55	0	7			5	10
20	25	40	55	42	0	5			37	45
60	43	17	61	60	20	27			56	67
200	59	27	33	43	43	76			61	78

[a] Test conducted by Schering AG; 40 rats/group/sex. Compound was administered once weekly i.m. for 104 weeks. HCD = 0.5 mg/kg/week i.m. M, males; F, females.

TABLE 5. *Effects of chronic 2-Br-α-ergocryptine (CB-154) and estradiol-17β treatment of young nulliparous C3H/HeJ mice on number of mammary hyperplastic nodules and mammary tumor incidence[a]*

Treatment	No. mice beginning of study	No. hyperplastic nodules in inguinal mammary gland	No. mice with mammary tumors
Controls	100	3.1 ± 1.0	11
Estradiol-17β	100	4.8 ± 1.2	27
Estradiol-17β + CB-154	100	2.8 ± 0.6	9

[a] Compounds were administered daily (CB-154, 0.1 mg/animal s.c.; estradiol-17β 0.5 mg/liter drinking water) for 20 months. The potent PRL inhibitor CB-154 was able to antagonize the stimulatory effect of estradiol-17β on mammary hyperplasia and neoplasia.
Data from Welsh, ref. 53.

of mammary carcinoma in male and/or female animals (Tables 2–4). In treated rats, this is usually accompanied by higher (male animals) or lower (female animals) incidences of benign mammary tumors (Table 4), as compared with the corresponding controls (7,10,18,23,28). The species-specific neuroendocrine system, i.e., estrogen-dependent stimulation of pituitary hormone secretions, mainly PRL, appear to be of great importance in the pathogenesis of mammary tumors in mice (Table 5) and rats (10,28). However, a close correlation between the incidence of pituitary and mammary tumors in both control and treated animals is not usually evident, which probably reflects a different strain susceptibility to the various tumors (Table 6).

On the other hand, stimulation of mammary tumors in dogs by certain proges-

TABLE 6. *Percentage incidences of pituitary, mammary and adrenal tumors in different control groups in carcinogenicity tests in female rats of five different strains[a]*

Group	No. rats	Pituitary	Mammary	Adrenal
1	120	7	27	1
2	35	2	23	0
3	60	—	15	2
4	40	30	37	0
5	40	27	35	0
6	40	35	25	2
7	100	0	90	26
8	50	30	41	2
9	25	4	24	0
10	114	1	2	0
11	80	41	54	1
12	25	12	12	0
Incidence range		0–40	2–90	0–26

[a] The rat strains used in these studies are Charles River (USA), Charles River (France), Wistar, Sprague Dawley, and the Holtzmann Albino.
Data from the Committee on Safety of Medicines, ref. 7.

tagens or progestagen–estrogen combinations seems to be related to high hormonal potency (progestational activity) of these compounds in the dog (endometrium and mammary gland) and their stimulatory effect on highly mammotropic canine GH (4,10–13,16,28,40). In total contrast to the situation in mice and rats, long-term treatment with high doses of estrogens and weak progestagens with possible inherent estrogenic activity does not stimulate mammary tumor development in the beagle bitch, in spite of their ability to stimulate PRL secretion in this species (11–13). Similarly, in the monkey and man certain sex steroids (high doses) may stimulate PRL secretion (12,30). However, in the monkey steroid-related mammary tumors are not observed, even after long-term treatment with high doses of estrogens, progestagens, and their combinations (16,28). Moreover, use of contraceptive steroids appears to decrease the risk of benign breast tumors in women, and this apparently protective effect seems to be related to the dose of progestagen and duration of use (10,41,42).

Pituitary and gonadal hormones, e.g., certain estrogen metabolites, androgens, progesterone, and PRL, have all been suspected of playing a role in breast cancer development, but none has been confirmed. Further studies, several of which are now in progress, are still required to define and establish the possible relationship between steroids and development of breast cancer in women (41,42).

Gonads

In a few long-term studies, an excess of gonadal tumors was observed in male mice of certain strains treated with high doses of estrogens or other steroids with estrogenic activity (7,8,10).

Estrogens may also stimulate mesothelial proliferations of the serous membranes surrounding the gonads and other genital organs of the dog (10,38,39).

There is no evidence that prolonged treatment with different sex steroids is associated with higher incidences of gonadal tumors in the monkey and man (10,41,42). Oral contraceptives may even have a protective effect against the incidence of ovarian cysts, which are the most common benign ovarian neoplasm of women (41,42).

Uterus

A small and uncertain excess of endometrial and cervical carcinoma was observed in mice as a result of long-term treatment with high doses of a few estrogens and estrogen–progestagen combinations. The estrogenic activity may be important in the promotion of these tumors. However, a strain difference in response seems to be present (7,8,10,18,23).

In rats, with the exception of one study, endometrial carcinomas were almost equally distributed among the control and treated animals. This exception probably reflects strain susceptibility (Table 7). In the dog, steroid-related uterine

TABLE 7. *Effect of norethisterone acetate and ethinylestradiol on proliferative changes of the uterus in a carcinogenicity test in rats[a]*

Treatment group	Dose × HCD[b]	No. animals examined	Endometrium hyperplasia (%)	Carcinoma (%)
Control	—	20	30	0
Norethisterone acetate +	10 ×	19	21	26
ethinylestradiol	30 ×	21	48	33
20 + 1	100 ×	18	72	22
Norethisterone acetate	100 ×	20	10	5
Ethinylestradiol	100 ×	19	79	11

[a] Test conducted by Schering AG. Compounds were administered daily in the diet for 104 weeks.
[b] × Multiples of 0.02 + 0.001 mg/kg/day p.o.

tumors have not been observed (10,16). In the monkey, cancer of the endometrium was found in two animals which had been given extremely high doses of medroxyprogesterone acetate for 10 years (14).

There is some evidence that prolonged treatment of women with high doses of estrogens may enhance development of endometrial carcinoma. On the other hand, progestagens and progestagen–estrogen combinations may have a protective effect against this type of cancer. Further studies are still required to define and establish the relationship between use of sex steroids and development of cervical cancer in women (8,10,41,42).

Liver

The results of available carcinogenicity studies of sex steroids in mice show slight but uncertain evidence of an increased incidence of steroid-related liver-cell tumors. In rats, only some studies have yielded evidence that a few progestagens and estrogens, separately and in combination, stimulated dose-dependent liver tumor development (Tables 2–4). However, some of the same compounds (e.g., ethinylestradiol) had no effect on tumorigenesis in the liver of rats in further studies (7,10,44,45).

In the dog and monkey, there is no clear evidence so far that sex steroids are associated with increased incidences of liver tumors (10,44,45). However, adenoma-like lesions were found in the liver of a few Beagle bitches treated parenterally with progesterone and medroxyprogesterone acetate for 20 months (10).

A possible association of long-term use of contraceptive steroids with a (dose-dependent) higher risk of benign liver tumorigenesis in older women should be borne in mind. However, the increase in incidence attributable to oral contraceptives was estimated to be no more than 3 per 100,000 women per year for those under age 30 (10,41,42).

ANTIESTROGENS AND ANTIANDROGENS

Results of long-term systemic and carcinogenicity studies of antiestrogens and antiandrogens in different experimental animals are not available. The antiandrogen cyproterone acetate was tested in rats for 78 weeks. The classical antiandrogenic effects of this drug (reduction in prostate, seminal vesicle, and testicular weight) were observed in treated rats. With regard to the influence on tumor development, cyproterone acetate showed an increase in the incidence of hepatomas (probably benign liver cell tumors) in both male and female rats (10,44,45). This effect of cyproterone acetate is only evident at extremely high doses (Table 8), in contrast to some other sex steroids (see Tables 2–4).

Since antiestrogens are able to antagonize the actions of estrogens, these compounds have been used to control the growth of estrogen-dependent tumors. Antiestrogens are effective in preventing the development of 7,12-dimethylbenz-[a]anthracene (DMBA)-induced rat mammary tumors, and in eliciting the regression of established tumors (20). The regression is almost similar to that observed after ovariectomy. Mammary tumors which regress by ovariectomy or antiestrogen treatment begin regrowth soon after the administration of estradiol (20).

The mechanism of action of these antiestrogens has been shown to be through competitive binding to the estrogen receptor in the target organ (47). In addition, these drugs may also block the resynthesis of the cytosol estrogen binding protein (6). This presents an advantage over endocrine ablative procedures which do not completely eliminate circulating estrogens.

Receptor studies suggest that the effectiveness of the antiestrogens in antagonizing mammary tumor development and growth may reside in the ability of the antiestrogen to lower markedly the levels of cytoplasmic estrogen receptor. This renders the mammary tissue incapable of responding to the animal's own endogenous estrogens and hence unable to grow (20). Antiestrogens may also reduce the level of prolactin binding in mammary tumors (20,21).

The effectiveness of antiestrogens as antitumor agents in women with breast

TABLE 8. *Effect of cyproterone acetate on the incidence of liver-cell tumors in a carcinogenicity test in rats[a]*

Compound	Type of treatment	Dose × HCD	Liver-cell tumors (%)	
			M	F
Control	Daily p.o.	—	0	0
Cyproterone acetate	78 weeks	250	0	0
		1250	3	17
		6250	17	40

[a] Test conducted by Schering AG; 40 rats/group/sex. HCD = 0.04 mg/kg/day p.o. M, males; F, females.

and endometrium cancer has been well documented (20,21). Preliminary results further suggest that pituitary hormones may also play a role in stimulating the growth of some human breast cancers (10). Effective PRL-inhibiting drugs are now available. A combination of antiestrogen and anti-PRL drugs might yield an effective therapy of hormone-dependent breast cancer (20,21).

Hyperplasia of the prostate is due to a proliferation of the epithelial and fibromuscular compartments whereby one of the two components can be involved more intensely in this process than the other (2,31). Generally, hyperplasia of the stromal elements dominate in man and the clinical symptoms of obstruction can also be attributed to this. It is assumed that changes in the androgen∶estrogen ratio in favor of the estrogen are responsible for the formation of hyperplasia of the prostate (31).

In old dogs with spontaneous hyperplasia of the prostate, effective antiandrogens such as cyproterone acetate and flutamide can lead to atrophy (33,34). Spontaneous hyperplasia of the prostate in dogs concern the whole prostate, however, in contrast to that in man. Furthermore in dogs, in contrast to man, no increase of the fibromuscular stroma is present. The age-dependent hyperplasia of the prostate in dogs is therefore not a very good model for experimental research (3,37).

Walsh and Wilson (52) were the first to succeed in inducing hyperplasia of the canine prostate by treatment with dihydrotestosterone alone or in combination with estradiol. The antiandrogen cyproterone acetate prevents development of prostatic epithelial hyperplasia, induced in castrated dogs as a result of 6 months' treatment with 5α-androstane-3α, 17β-diol (49).

On the basis of these investigations it can be concluded that in hyperplasia of the prostate in man, treatment with antiandrogens will lead to a certain amount of regression in the epithelial compartment, but the stromal hyperplasia and especially the activated smooth muscle will hardly react. Some clinical observations confirm this assumption (46,50). Hyperplasia of the stroma is primarily estrogen dependent. Thus, it would seem appropriate to administer antiestrogens or a combination of antiestrogens and antiandrogens in order to influence all compartments involved in hyperplasia. Investigations of this kind were conducted in the dog using the antiestrogen tamoxifen. First results indicate that this hypothesis could be correct.

Regarding the value of antiandrogens in the therapy of prostate carcinoma, we are essentially dependent on clinical observations because we have no suitable models. In a series of clinical but uncontrolled studies, therapy with cyproterone acetate was at least as effective as surgical castration or treatment with estrogens (46).

The experimental induction and prevention of prostatic hyperplasia in the castrated dog seem to be associated with an endocrine imbalance in hypothalamic–pituitary–adrenal function of a complex nature. Treatment with sex steroids seems to influence and modify the PRL target sites in the canine prostate gland. This may provide an insight into understanding the, as yet, undefined role of steroids and pituitary hormones in prostatic function. A combination of antiandrogen, antiestrogen, and prolactin-inhibiting drugs might yield an effective therapy of hormone-dependent prostatic tumors in man.

THE ALDOSTERONE ANTAGONIST SPIRONOLACTONE

Long-term tolerance and carcinogenicity studies of spironolactone were only performed in rats. The available toxicity studies in dogs (13 weeks) and monkeys (26 and 52 weeks) are too short, and thus do not allow the detection of potential tumorigenic effects of spironolactone in these species (26). In the long-term (78 and 104 weeks) systemic tolerance (and carcinogenicity) studies of spironolactone in rats, changes were observed in the pituitary, mammary gland, thyroid, gonads, and liver. Only significant findings will be discussed, especially with regard to the influence of spironolactone on tumor developments.

Pituitary and Mammary Gland

There was the usual incidence of chromophobe hyperplasias and adenomas of the pituitary gland, scattered randomly among control and test groups. Similarly, there was no significant increase in mammary tumor incidence in treated animals as compared with the corresponding controls (26). An inhibitory effect of spironolactone on development of pituitary and mammary tumors could even be assumed in female animals (Table 9). However, this may reflect a variation in the spontaneous incidence of these tumors (7,10,18,23). There is also evidence that spironolactone significantly delays the development of experimentally induced mammary tumors in rats (22).

Diffuse acinar hyperplasia (adenosis) of the mammary gland was observed as a function of dose in male monkeys treated for 52 weeks with spironolactone. This may be related to the antiandrogenic effects of this drug (reduction in prostate, seminal vesicle, and testicular weights) observed in these treated male monkeys (26).

Gynecomastia is known as a side effect in human males given spironolactone (24,36,43). Breast cancer was also reported in five women during or after prolonged administration of spironolactone. However, this association may be purely coincidental (25). On the other hand, a further five cases of breast carcinoma in men were observed after prolonged spironolactone treatment (17). Since the incidence of breast cancer in men is extremely low, a possible association between long-term use of spironolactone and a higher risk of mammary tumors in humans should be borne in mind.

Thyroid Gland

Relative thyroid weights were increased as a function of dose in both sexes at 78 and 104 weeks. A marked increase of functional nodular hyperplasia or

TABLE 9. Effect of spironolactone on the incidence of different tumors (%) in carcinogenicity tests in rats[a]

Duration	Dose levels (mg/kg/day × HD)		Pituitary gland		Mammary gland				Thyroid gland		Gonads	Malignant tumors	
					Benign		Malignant						
			M	F	M	F	M	F	M	F	M	M	F
78 weeks	0	0	29	50	0	15	0	0	0	0	0	3	6
	50	25	26	26	3	22	0	3	12	3	0	11	8
	150	75	8	23	3	8	3	8	48	35	14	14	11
	500	250	28	3	0	3	0	0	64	38	33	14	6
104 weeks	0	0	24	76	0	25	0	38	10	0	0	10	47
	10	5	22	90	3	29	0	11	17	7	7	7	20
	30	15	34	68	0	33	0	10	14	14	0	10	17
	100	50	11	43	0	23	0	4	0	18	0	13	10

[a]M, males; F, females. Compound was administered daily in the diet. HD = recommended human dose (2 mg/kg/day p.o.). Data from Lumb et al., ref. 26.

adenomas (simple or papillary) of the thyroid gland was observed in both sexes at the 150 and 500 mg/kg/day levels (26). Three papillary cystadenocarcinomas with no evidence of invasiveness or metastases were also detected in different treated groups (Table 9). The adaptive dose-related increase in mass of the thyroid gland presumably created a hormonal environment of hyperthyroidism. This may explain the decreased incidence of mammary tumors in spironolactone-treated rats, since mammary tumors in different animal species (rats, dogs) and in women seem to develop more frequently in a modified hormonal environment with reduced thyroxine (9).

There are no reports of thyroid gland abnormalities in other experimental animals and in man associated with spironolactone administration. For that reason, the thyroid response to spironolactone in rats may be a species-specific endocrine aberration, which is difficult to explain.

Gonads (Testis)

The diffuse interstitial cell hyperplasias, frequently observed in populations of old rats, were less common in the treated animals than in the controls. However, nodular microscopic hyperplastic lesions of normal-appearing interstitial cells (adenomas) were frequently observed at the 150 and 500 mg/kg/day levels (Table 8). Again, these lesions may be related to the antiandrogenic effects of spironolactone (1,24,29,36,43,48).

Testicular tumors also developed in rats during the chronic toxicity study of flutamide, a nonsteroidal antiandrogen (32). The development of this compensatory hyperplasia of interstitial cells of the testis as a result of long-term treatment with these antiandrogens (flutamide, spironolactone) may be explained by the fact that these drugs stimulate luteinizing hormone secretion via inhibition of the negative androgen feedback and/or androgen biosynthesis (35).

In other experimental animals and/or in man, with the exception of typical antiandrogenic effects (maturation arrest of spermiogenesis, semen abnormalities, atrophy of prostate and seminal vesicle), no proliferative lesions were observed in male genital organs (26). This steroid has even been found effective in the treatment of patients with hyperplasia or carcinoma of the prostate (51).

Liver

There was a dose-related increase of liver weight. Liver nodules were observed on gross examination in some animals of all groups at 78 and 104 weeks. These nodules were more frequent at 150 and 500 mg/kg dose levels and occurred in males rather than in females. Most of these nodules were areas of nonspecific inflammation associated with focal necrosis. Cellular hypertrophy was observed after 78 weeks in animals receiving 150 and 500 mg/kg/day. On the other hand, there were no significant differences in the incidence of microscopic nodular hyperplasia between control and test animals (26). The increased liver mass in rats after prolonged spironolactone administration is a species-specific effect, which is expected since the drug induces a marked increase in liver microsomal enzyme in the rat (15). This is also related to the species-specific pharmacokinetic and metabolic pattern of spironolactone. The rat readily metabolizes this drug and most of the metabolites are excreted via the bile. This is in contrast to the situation in man and monkeys, where the major excretory route for metabolites is the urine (19).

Hepatocellular carcinomas with no evidence of invasiveness and metastases were also observed in single treated male rats. However, the numbers are very small and none are statistically significant when compared with controls (26).

Malignant Tumors in General

Tumors diagnosed as malignant on the basis of morphology alone including a few with metastases are listed in Table 9. These figures may suggest a possible slight carcinogenic effect of spironolactone in males in the 78-week rat study. However, a more marked, dose-related anticarcinogenic effect of spironolactone in females of the 104-week rat study could also be assumed. The biological significance of all these findings is not convincing. They may only reflect a variation in the spontaneous incidence of malignant tumors in an aging rat population (26).

SUMMARY

Long-term studies of sex steroids suggests that high doses of certain estrogens, progestagens, and progestagen–estrogen combinations may stimulate development of tumors in different organs, particularly the pituitary, mammary gland, uterus, gonads and/or liver of mice and/or rats. However, treatment with some of the same or similar compounds (estrogens, progestagens and their combinations) may result in no effect on tumor incidence or even in suppression of tumorigenesis in further studies. Therefore, the results of these studies in mice and rats are so conflicting that definitive general statements are not possible.

In the dog, with the exception of stimulation of development of mammary tumors by long-term treatment with certain progestagens and progestagen–estrogen combinations, no other tumorigenic effect of sex steroids has been seen in this species. These steroid-related canine mammary tumors must be considered as being a species-specific effect, depending on the high proliferative effect of these compounds on the mammary gland of the dog. This may be a direct and/or indirect effect via stimulation of pituitary canine GH secretion.

In the monkey, cancer of the endometrium was found in two animals given extremely high doses of medroxyprogesterone acetate for 10 years. However, no definite conclusion can be made until ongoing long-term studies with other steroids are completed.

In man, long-term use of contraceptive steroids seems to be associated with a lower incidence of benign breast tumors and ovarian cysts as well as with a higher risk of benign liver tumors. Sex steroids may also affect the occurrence of breast, endometrial, cervical, and prostatic cancer.

Antiestrogens control the growth of the estrogen-dependent tumors. They cause regression of experimentally induced mammary tumors in rats. The effectiveness of antiestrogens as antitumor agent in women with breast and endometrium cancer has also been well documented.

Recent results suggested the effectiveness of antiandrogens alone or in combination with antiestrogens in the prophylaxis and treatment of hyperplasia and neoplasia of the human prostate. Cyproterone acetate, an antiandrogen, prevents the development of androgen-induced epithelial hyperplasia of the canine prostate. The estrogen-related fibromuscular proliferation and epithelial metaplasia in the prostate of the dog seem to be prevented by the treatment with the antiestrogen tamoxifen.

Spironolactone, an aldosterone antagonist with antiandrogenic effects, has been studied by long-term (78 and 104 weeks) administration to rats, with daily dose levels up to 250 times the recommended human dose. There tends to be a reduction in the number of pituitary and mammary tumors in female rats as exposure to spironolactone is increased. The drug was also shown to cause a dose-related increase in thyroid follicular hyperplasia, hepatocellular hypertrophy, and interstitial cell adenoma of the testis. However, these lesions occur in the form of adaptive processes, as aberrations due to specific endocrine and/or metabolic activity, rather than as a true neoplasm.

In conclusion, there is no evidence to suggest that sex steroids or steroid antagonists are carcinogenic in experimental animals or in man. However, depending on timing, dosage, and experimental design, susceptibility of the species and strain, age and sex of the animals, and diet and housing conditions, administration of these hormonally active compounds can enhance or delay the development of tumors in different target organs, particularly in the pituitary, mammary gland, uterus, thyroid, gonads, and/or liver of experimental animals. The species-specific differences in biological activity, pharmacokinetics, and metabolism of steroids and steroid antagonists must be considered when attempting to extrapolate these results to man. Eventually, however, further clinical data should be collected and evaluated to confirm or refute the assumption of a potential tumorigenic or antitumor effect of these compounds in man.

ACKNOWLEDGMENT

The authors are indebted to Mrs. B. Schilk for her highly qualified assistance and to Dr. P. Günzel for his advice and encouragement.

REFERENCES

1. Baba, S., Murei, M., Jitsukawa, S., Hata, M., and Tazaki, H. (1978): *J. Urol.,* 199:375–380.
2. Bartsch, G., and Rohr, H. P. (1979): *Aktuel Urol.,* 10:137–143.

3. Berg, O. A. (1958): *Acta Endocrinol. (Kbh.),* 27:140–154.
4. Briggs, M. H. (1977): *Life Sci.,* 21:175–284.
5. Campenhout, J., van, Blanchet, P., Beauregard, H., and Papas, S. (1977): *Fertil. Steril.,* 28:728–732.
6. Clark, J. H., Peck, E. J., and Anderson, J. N. (1974): *Nature,* 251:446–448.
7. Committee on Safety of Medicines (1972): *Carcinogenicity Tests of Oral Contraceptives,* Her Majesty's Stationary Office, London.
8. Drill, V. A. (1979): *Arch. Toxicol. [Suppl.],* 2:59–84.
9. El Etreby, M. F. (1979): *Pharmacol. Ther.,* 5:403–405.
10. El Etreby, M. F. (1980): In: *Pharmacological Modulation of Steroid Action,* edited by E. Genazzani, F. Di Carlo, and W. I. P. Mainwaring, pp. 239–260. Raven Press, New York.
11. El Etreby, M. F., and Gräf, K.-J. (1978): *Pharmacol. Ther.,* 5:369–402.
12. El Etreby, M. F., Gräf, K.-J., Günzel, P., and Neumann, F. (1979): *Arch. Toxicol.,* Suppl. 2:11–39.
13. El Etreby, M. F., and Günzel, P. (1973): *Arzneim. Forsch.,* 23:1768–1790.
14. *Family Planning Perspectives* (1979):11:47.
15. Feller, D. R., and Gerald, M. C. (1970): *Proc. Soc. Exp. Biol. Med.,* 136:1347–1350.
16. Geil, R. G., and Lamar, J. K. (1977): *J. Toxicol. Environ. Health,* 3:179–193.
17. Hammerstein, J. (1977): *Endokrinol. Inform.,* 5:162.
18. IARC Monographs on the Evaluation of Carcinogenic Risk of Chemicals to Man (1974): In: *Sex Hormones, Vol. 6,* International Agency for Research on Cancer, Lyon.
19. Karim, A., Kook, C., Zitzewitz, D. J., Zagarella, J., Doherty, M., and Campion, J. (1976): *Drug Metab. Dispos.,* 4:547–555.
20. Katzenellenbogen, B. S., Bhakoo, H. S., Ferguson, E. R., Lan, N. C., Tatee, T., Tsai, T. S., and Katzenellenbogen, J. A. (1979): In: *Recent Progress in Hormone Research, Vol. 35,* edited by R. O. Greep, pp. 259–300. Academic Press, New York.
21. Kelly, P. A., Asselin, J., Caron, M. G., Labrie, F., and Raynaud, J. P. (1977): *J. Natl. Cancer Inst.,* 58:623.
22. Kovacs, K., and Somogyi, A. (1970): *Eur. J. Cancer,* 6:195–201.
23. Leonard, B. J. (1974): In: *Pharmacological Models in Contraceptive Development,* edited by M. H. Briggs and E. Diczfalusy, pp. 34–73. WHO Research and Training Centre on Human Reproduction, Karolinska Institutet, Stockholm.
24. Loriaux, D. L., Menard, R., Taylor, A., Pita, J. C., and Santen, R. (1976): *Ann. Intern. Med.,* 85:630–636.
25. Loube, A. D., and Quirk, R. A. (1975): *Lancet,* 1:1428–1429.
26. Lumb, G., Newberne, P., Rust, R. R., and Wagner, B. (1978): *J. Environ. Pathol. Toxicol.,* 1:641–660.
27. March, C. M., Kleitzky, O. A., Israel, R., Davajan, V., and Mishell, D. R. (1977): *Fertil. Steril.,* 28:346.
28. Meites, J. (1979): *Arch. Toxicol.,* Suppl. 2:47–58.
29. Menard, R. H., Loriaux, D. L., Bartter, F. C., and Gillette, J. R. (1978): *Steroids,* 31:771–782.
30. Mishell, D. R., Jr., Kletzky, O. A., Brenner, P. F., Roy, S., and Nicoloff, J. (1977): *Am. J. Obstet. Gynecol.,* 128:60–74.
31. Mostofi, F. K. (1970): In: *Urology,* edited by M. F. Campbell and J. H. Harrison, pp. 1065–1129. Saunders, Philadelphia.
32. Neri, R. O. (1977): In: *Androgens and Antiandrogens,* edited by L. Martini and M. Motta, pp. 179–189. Raven Press, New York.
33. Neri, R. O., Casmer, Ch., Zeman, W. V., Fielder, F., and Tabachnick, I. I. A. (1968): *Endocrinology,* 82:311.
34. Neri, R. O., and Monahan, M. (1972): *Invest. Urol.,* 10:123.
35. Neumann, F., and Gräf, K.-J. (1979): *Pharmacol. Ther.,* 5:271–286.
36. Ochs, H. R., Greenblatt, D. J., Bodem, G., and Smith, T. W. (1978): *Am. Heart J.,* 96:369–400.
37. O'Shea, J. D. (1962): *J. Comp. Pathol. Ther.,* 72:321–331.
38. O'Shea, J. D., and Jabara, A. G. (1967): *Pathol. Vet.,* 4:137–148.
39. O'Shea, J. D., and Jabara, A. G. (1971): *Vet. Pathol.,* 8:81–90.
40. Owen, L. N., and Briggs, M. H. (1976): *Curr. Med. Res. Opin.,* 4:309–329.
41. Population Reports (1977): Series A, No. 4. George Washington University Medical Center, Department of Medical and Public Affairs, Washington, D.C.

42. Population Reports (1979): Series A, No. 5. George Washington University Medical Center, Department of Medical and Public Affairs, Washington, D.C.
43. Rose, L. I., Underwood, R. H., Newmark, S. R., Kisch, E. S., and Williams, G. H. (1977): *Ann. Intern. Med.,* 87:398–403.
44. Schuppler, J., and Günzel, P. (1978): *Arch. Toxicol.,* Suppl. 2:181–195.
45. Schuppler, J., Günzel, P., and El Etreby, M. F. (1977): *J. Toxicol. Environ. Health,* 3:370–371.
46. Scott, W. W. (1971): In: *Life Science Monographs, Vol. 1: International Symposium on the Treatment of Carcinoma of the Prostate,* edited by G. Raspé and W. Brosing, pp. 161–163, 173–180. Pergamon, Oxford.
47. Terenius, L. (1971): *Eur. J. Cancer,* 7:57–64.
48. Tidd, M. J., Horth, C. E., Ramsay, I. E., Shelton, J. R., and Palmer, R. F. (1978): *Clin. Endocrinol. (Oxf.)* 9:389–399.
49. Tunn, U., Senge, Th., Schenck, B., and Neumann, F. (1979): *Acta Endocrinol. (Kbh.),* 91:373–384.
50. Vahlensieck, W., and Gödde, S. (1968): *Munch. Med. Wochenschr.,* 110:1573–1577.
51. Walsh, P. C., and Siiteri, P. K. (1975): *J. Urol.,* 114:254–256.
52. Walsh, P. C., and Wilson, J. D. (1976): *J. Clin. Invest.,* 57:1093–1097.
53. Welsch, C. W. (1976): *J. Toxicol. Environ. Health,* 1:161–175.

Clinical Use of Receptor Assay

Hormones and Cancer, edited by S. Iacobelli et al.
Raven Press, New York © 1980.

An Update on Estrogen and Progesterone Receptors in Prognosis for Primary and Advanced Breast Cancer

William L. McGuire

Department of Medicine/Oncology, University of Texas Health Science Center, San Antonio, Texas 78284

Considerable progress has been made in the last decade in our approach to patients with breast cancer. Endocrine therapy for advanced disease has now progressed to the point where physicians can confidently select patients who are likely to respond. New information is emerging regarding the use of estrogen receptor (ER) assays to predict which patients will have an early recurrence. It is the purpose of this brief review to present data from my own laboratory on the use of ER and progesterone receptor (PgR) assays in the management of both primary and advanced breast cancer.

ESTROGEN RECEPTOR IN THE PRIMARY BREAST CANCER

It is widely accepted that only about one-half of breast cancer patients are cured by surgical and/or radiation therapy of the primary tumor. The majority of these patients have tumors confined to the breast without extension to the axillary lymph nodes (4). Those patients with regional lymph node involvement will usually present with metastatic disease at some later date. Until the past few years, axillary node positive patients were simply observed following surgery with the hope, albeit slim, of cure. Upon recurrence, palliative endocrine and cytotoxic therapies provided prolongation of life, but eventually all patients died of the disease. More recently, the concept of adjuvant therapy with the goal of cure has emerged, particularly in the case of axillary node positive patients. The reasoning is that extension of tumor to regional lymph nodes is operationally equivalent to finding distant microscopic tumor metastases. Rather than waiting until these foci are clinically evident, systemic antitumor therapy begun soon after surgery might be very successful, since tumor burden is relatively low. There is considerable experimental animal tumor data to support this concept and now many large clinical trials are underway with some preliminary reports showing early success (3,5,11). The question is not whether to use adjuvant therapy, but rather which drugs to use, which patients, and for how long. Since there are considerable arrays of systemic agents available and undoubtedly many subsets of patients with varying degrees of risk of recurrence and potential response to these agents, a method to select patients at risk and the proper adjuvant therapy for particular subsets of these patients is needed.

In San Antonio, we had begun to measure ER in primary breast tumors in hopes of eventually correlating these data with the response to endocrine therapy at some later date. In many of these patients we had follow-up data including time to recurrence and survival. So we decided to look at the natural history of our patient population to see if the ER status was correlated with any particular outcome. To our surprise, we found that regardless of axillary node status, age, size of the primary tumor, or location of the tumor in the breast, those patients with ER − tumors recurred earlier than ER + patients (12). Approximately a year later we reanalyzed our data with the addition of more patients and the elimination of patients who had received any systemic endocrine or cytotoxic therapy. Our earlier conclusions were confirmed and extended to show that ER − patients not only recurred earlier but had worse survival than ER + patients (13). These data are illustrated in Table 1. Subsequently, similar data have recently been reported from other centers around the world which substantiates the results of our pilot study (1,6,14,16). The implications of these findings are considerable. First, we now can identify a subset of axillary node positive patients who have an extremely poor prognosis if left untreated. Second, the ER assay results indicate that the latter group should receive intensive combination chemotherapy and that the ER + axillary node positive patients should receive an endocrine therapy as part of the adjuvant therapy. In fact, this approach is now being tested. In collaboration with Hubay, Pearson, and

TABLE 1. *Estrogen receptor and recurrence*

Characteristic	Recurrence at 20 months		
	ER − (%)	vs	ER + (%)
Age			
< 50	32		0
> 50	36		16
Nodes			
Negative	19		6
Positive	59		26
1–3	36		25
> 4	72		27
Primary size			
< 2 cm	40		5
> 2 cm	37		16
Primary location			
Outer	31		9
Inner and central	50		19

Adapted from Knight et al., ref. 12.

TABLE 2. *ER and response to endocrine therapy*

	Primary biopsy	Metastatic biopsy
ER−	1/6 = 17%	4/47 = 8%
ER+	22/44 = 50%	48/101 = 48%

colleagues in Cleveland, we have been assaying ER in primary breast tumors of patients randomized to receive combination chemotherapy with or without antiestrogen therapy. The preliminary data are very encouraging (11). ER + patients are recurring less frequently if they receive a combination of chemo–endocrine therapy compared with chemotherapy alone. ER − patients recur at the same rate whether or not antiestrogens are added to the chemotherapy. Independent trials from other centers are needed to confirm these data, but the approach is based on sound physiological principles and the use of ER assays in the primary tumor for prognostic information as well as therapeutic strategy seems assured.

As will be discussed later, the presence or absence of ER in a biopsy of metastatic breast cancer correlates well with the response of that cancer to endocrine therapy. The question remains, however, whether ER assay results at the time of primary surgery are valuable, perhaps years later, if the patient develops metastatic disease. This is of considerable importance since less than 50% of patients presenting with advanced disease have readily accessible lesions for biopsy and assay—whereas practically all patients undergoing primary breast surgery have tissue available for this purpose. The theoretical objection to this approach is that the ER status of a tumor could change between the time of primary surgery and the clinical presentation of advanced disease. This has been examined by various investigators and in the great majority of cases, the ER status is unchanged when comparing primary and metastatic biopsies in the same patient. The most direct test, of course, is to measure ER in the primary tumor and correlate the results with subsequent endocrine therapy for metastatic disease; data from Jensen's laboratory clearly suspects such a correlation (2). Our own data are illustrated in Table 2. We find approximately the same response rate to endocrine therapy of advanced disease in ER + tumors regardless of whether ER determination was made on the original primary tumor or a subsequent metastatic lesion.

THE VALUE OF QUANTITATIVE ESTROGEN RECEPTOR ASSAYS

In the early days of ER correlations, few laboratories reported quantitative data. It seemed sufficient to merely indicate whether the receptor was present or absent. Our earliest analysis, however, though based on a limited number of patients, indicated that the response rate was the highest in those patients with the highest quantitative tumor ER content (15). As we examine in Table 3

TABLE 3. *Quantitative ER values in primary and metastatic breast cancer*

ER value	< 50 Years		> 50 Years	
	1° Biopsy	2° Biopsy	1° Biopsy	2° Biopsy
< 3	162 (37%)	49 (52%)	279 (23%)	75 (31%)
3–10	90 (20%)	13 (14%)	176 (15%)	39 (16%)
11–100	183 (41%)	28 (29%)	432 (35%)	67 (27%)
100–2,000	10 (2%)	5 (5%)	312 (26%)	63 (26%)
Total	445	95	1199	244

TABLE 4. *Quantitative ER and the response to endocrine therapy*

ER (fmoles/mg)	Response	
	1° Biopsy	2° Biopsy
< 3	1/6 = 17%	4/47 = 8%
3–10	3/7 = 42%	11/24 = 45%
11–100	14/31 = 45%	15/41 = 36%
> 100	5/6 = 83%	22/36 = 61%

the actual values in primary versus metastatic biopsies and younger versus older patients, certain features stand out. First, metastatic biopsies are more often ER − than primary biopsies, regardless of age. Second, the older patient is much more likely to have a high receptor content than the younger patient, regardless of whether the biopsy is from a primary or metastatic lesion. This might be expected since the older patient is more likely to have a favorable response to endocrine therapy. Our actual clinical correlations are shown in Table 4. In almost 200 endocrine trials we find that the response rate is proportional to the absolute receptor content.

PROGESTERONE RECEPTOR AND RESPONSE TO ENDOCRINE THERAPY

Despite the success of ER assays for prediction, a large number of ER + patients fail to respond to endocrine therapy. Several years ago we reasoned that since cytoplasmic binding to estrogen to receptor was only the first step in a complex biochemical pathway leading to growth and specific protein synthesis in a breast tumor cell, perhaps certain ER + tumors failed to respond because of defects distal to the binding step. We hypothesized that PgR might be an ideal marker of estrogen action in breast tumor cells as it had been shown to be estrogen dependent in normal reproductive tissue (7). We developed an assay for PgR which was quite specific and sensitive in breast cancer tissue (8) and

TABLE 5. *Distribution of ER and PgR in 1,366 breast cancer patients*

	Premenopausal (%)	Postmenopausal (%)
ER−, PgR−	30	19
ER−, PgR+	9	3
ER+, PgR−	12	23
ER+, PgR+	49	55

demonstrated that PgR synthesis was strictly controlled by estrogen in both experimental (9) and human breast cancer cells (10). The distribution of PgR in a large number of human breast cancer biopsies is shown in Table 5. As anticipated, PgR is rarely found in those tumors lacking ER. Conversely, the likelihood of finding PgR in a tumor was proportional to the absolute amount of ER in the tumor. Thus it was likely that PgR would correlate with a favorable response to endocrine therapy. Our own data on clinical response are illustrated in Table 6. As anticipated, those tumors without ER and PgR are unlikely to respond. Tumors containing only PgR are rare and not enough information is available to reach any conclusions. Those patients with both ER and PgR have a remarkably high response rate. The interesting group is that with ER but without PgR. We would have anticipated that few if any of these patients would have responded. Yet the response rate is appreciable even though far below those patients with both receptors. We have considered several possibilities to explain the behavior of this group. First, the assays for PgR are imperfect and it is possible that a few patients in this group are false negative. However, it is doubtful that this could explain the whole result. Second, we must consider the influence of endogenous progesterone in premenopausal women. Saez and colleagues (17) have reported that PgR cannot be found in breast tumor cytosols of women with high circulating levels of progesterone during the luteal phase of the menstrual cycle. Presumably all of the cytoplasmic PgR sites have been translocated to nuclei. A nuclear exchange assay might solve this problem. Finally, since PgR synthesis is estrogen dependent, could some postmenopausal women have insufficient circulating estrogen to stimulate PgR in the tumor even when the appropriate biochemical pathways are present? Degenshein and

TABLE 6. *Objective remission of metastatic breast cancer as a function of ER and PgR*

	Objective response
ER−, PgR−	3/20 = 15%
ER−, PgR+	—
ER+, PgR−	14/45 = 31%
ER+, PgR+	16/20 = 80%

associates *(personal communications)* have, in fact, biopsied patients before and after a few days of estrogen therapy and found several women who converted to PgR+. So it appears that many of the ER+, PgR− cases who respond to endocrine therapy can be explained.

QUANTITATIVE ESTROGEN RECEPTOR ASSAYS VERSUS PROGESTERONE RECEPTOR ASSAYS

Although the merits of PgR assays are now well documented, one could take the position that since the likelihood of finding PgR in a tumor is correlated with the amount of ER in the tumor, and since the likelihood of favorable response is proportional to the amount of ER in the tumor, then perhaps PgR is just a signal that a high level of ER is present. If so, PgR measurements would be redundant. Fortunately, the matter can be resolved by direct analysis of the data. We have studied 65 ER + patients where we have quantitative ER and PgR data as well as objective response to endocrine therapy. The data are illustrated in Table 7. If we use quantitative ER alone to discriminate between

TABLE 7. *Quantitative ER vs PgR*

		Objective response rate
PgR	+	16/20 = 80%
	−	14/45 = 31%
ER	> 100	17/27 = 63%
	3–100	13/38 = 34%

low and high response rates in ER + patients, we find that the best separation obtained is 34 versus 63%. If we use the presence of PgR, the discrimination becomes 31 versus 80%. So we must conclude from our own data that the measurement of ER and PgR is superior to just quantitating ER alone.

The implications for therapy are just emerging. In those patients with both ER and PgR, endocrine therapy is the therapy of choice. The group ER+, PgR− is a little more difficult in that about 30% of these patients will still have a good response. Perhaps many of these responders could be reclassified as ER+, PgR+ if nuclear exchange assays are employed or estrogen stimulation were used. At present, we would not recommend withholding endocrine therapy from this group but would suggest that only those therapies with low morbidity be used (e.g., antiestrogens); this group might be ideal candidates for combined chemo–endocrine therapies.

ACKNOWLEDGMENTS

This work was partially supported by the National Cancer Institute (CA 11378, CB 23682) and The American Cancer Society.

REFERENCES

1. Allegra, J. C., Lippman, M. E., Simon, R., Thompson, E. G., Barlock, A., Green, L., Huff, K., Do, H. M. T., Aitken, S. C., and Warren, R. (1979): *Cancer Treat. Rep.,* 63:1271–1278.
2. Block, G. E., Ellis, R. S., DeSombre, E., and Jensen, E. (1978): *Ann. Surg.,* 188:372.
3. Bonadonna, G., Rossi, A., Valaqussa, P., Banfi, A., and Veronesi, U. (1977): *Cancer,* 39:2904.
4. Fisher, B. (1977): In: *Breast Cancer: Advances in Research and Treatment,* edited by W. L. McGuire, p. 1. Plenum Press, New York.
5. Fisher, B., and Wolmark, N. (1977): In: *Breast Cancer: Advances in Research and Treatment,* edited by W. L. McGuire, p. 25. Plenum Press, New York.
6. Hahnel, R., Woodings, T., and Vivian, A. B. (1979): *Cancer,* 44:325.
7. Horwitz, K. B., and McGuire, W. L. (1975): *Science,* 189:726–727.
8. Horwitz, K. B., and McGuire, W. L. (1975): *Steroids,* 25:497–505.
9. Horwitz, K. B., and McGuire, W. L. (1977): *Cancer Res.,* 37:1733–1738.
10. Horwitz, K. B., and McGuire, W. L. (1978): *J. Biol. Chem.,* 253:2223–2228.
11. Hubay, C. A., Pearson, O. H., Marshall, J. S., Rhodes, R. S., DeBanne, S. M., Mansour, E. G., Herman, R. E., Jones, J. C., Flynn, W. J., Eckert, C., and McGuire, W. L. (1980): *Surgery (in press).*
12. Knight, W. A., Livingston, R. B., Gregory, E. J., and McGuire, W. L. (1977): *Cancer Res.,* 37:3667–4671.
13. Knight, W. A., Livingston, R. B., Gregory, E. J., Walder, A. I., and McGuire, W. L. (1978): *Proc. Am. Soc. Clin. Oncol.,* 19:392.
14. Maynard, P. V., Davies, C. J., Blamey, R. W., Elston, C. W., Johnson, J., and Griffiths, K. (1978): *Br. J. Cancer,* 38:745.
15. McGuire, W. L., Carbone, P. P., and Vollmer, E. P., eds. (1975): *Estrogen Receptors in Human Breast Cancer.* Raven Press, New York.
16. Rich, M. A., Furmonski, P., and Brooks, S. C. (1978): *Cancer Res.,* 38:4296.
17. Saez, S., Martin, P., and Chouvet, C. (1978): *Cancer Res.,* 38:3468.

Hormones and Cancer, edited by S. Iacobelli et al.
Raven Press, New York © 1980.

The Therapeutic Utility of Glucocorticoid Receptor Studies in Non-Hodgkin's Malignant Lymphoma

Clara D. Bloomfield, *Kendall A. Smith, *Laurie Hildebrandt,
JoAnn Zaleskas, **Kazimiera J. Gajl-Peczalska, **Glauco
Frizzera, Bruce A. Peterson, *John H. Kersey,
†Gerald R. Crabtree, and †Allan Munck

*Section of Medical Oncology, Department of Medicine, and **Department of Laboratory
Medicine and Pathology, University of Minnesota Health Sciences Center, Minneapolis,
Minnesota 55455; and Departments of *Medicine and †Physiology, Dartmouth Medical
School, Hanover, New Hampshire 03755, U.S.A.*

Glucocorticoids are included in almost all combination chemotherapy regimens currently used for the treatment of adult non-Hodgkin's malignant lymphoma (NHML) (1,6,7,10,24). However, a number of studies suggest that many patients have lymphomas which are not sensitive to glucocorticoids and that steroids are frequently toxic in elderly patients (12,13,15,18). Consequently, *in vitro* tests that would rapidly identify before treatment those lymphoma patients likely to benefit from steroids would be of considerable therapeutic utility.

Glucocorticoid receptor complexes appear to be required for hormone action in all glucocorticoid-sensitive tissues (21). In addition, *in vitro* studies show that the uptakes of leucine, uridine, and thymidine are inhibited by glucocorticoids in sensitive lymphocytes (21). Consequently, to see if we could identify those patients likely to respond to glucocorticoids, we have studied malignant cells from adults with NHML for glucocorticoid receptors and *in vitro* sensitivity to glucocorticoids (4). These *in vitro* parameters have been correlated with antitumor response to therapy with glucocorticoid as a single agent (5). Our data suggest that *in vitro* glucocorticoid studies may allow us to select, before treatment, those patients with lymphoma who should receive glucocorticoids in their chemotherapy regimens (2,5).

PATIENTS AND METHODS

Patients

Between February 1978 and September 1979 we studied 42 adults (≥ 18 years of age) consecutively admitted with a diagnosis of NHML and with sufficient accessible lymphomatous tissue. Informed consent was obtained in writing from each patient. There were 26 males and 16 females. They ranged in age from 18 to 84 years (median age 60 years). Twenty-three patients were first studied at diagnosis, nineteen at relapse. Relapse patients had been off all chemotherapy for a minimum of 1 week and off glucocorticoids for at least 10 days.

Glucocorticoid therapy as a single agent was administered to 22 of the 42 patients. In this group were 11 males and 11 females, ranging in age from 19 to 84 years (median age 59 years). Fourteen patients were newly diagnosed; eight had received prior treatment, including glucocorticoids in five. Following biopsy for *in vitro* studies, patients were treated with 4 mg dexamethasone every 6 hr. Single-agent glucocorticoid therapy was administered for a minimum of 5 days, since that is the duration of glucocorticoid treatment in most combination chemotherapy regimens for lymphoma (1,6,7). In patients who did not have progressive disease and who would consent, glucocorticoid alone was continued for at least 2 weeks. In three patients with rapidly progressive disease on glucocorticoid therapy, combination chemotherapy was initiated after only 3 to 4 days of glucocorticoids alone.

Antitumor response to dexamethasone was measured by a single investigator who had no knowledge of the results of the *in vitro* glucocorticoid studies. At the end of single-agent glucocorticoid therapy, patients were classified as responders or nonresponders. They were scored as responders if they had at least a 50% decrease in size of all tumor masses and had developed no new lesions. In addition, when peripheral blood involvement was present, it was required that the absolute lymphoma cell count (percent lymphoma cells × leukocyte count) had decreased by at least 50%. Patients who did not meet these requirements were scored as nonresponders.

Histologic and Immunologic Classification

Neoplastic lymphoid tissue was obtained from all patients, usually by biopsy of involved lymph nodes. Different portions of the same tissue were used to obtain sections for histologic diagnosis, cryostat sections for immunologic analysis, and single cell suspensions. Part of the cell suspension was utilized for glucocorticoid studies and part for lymphocyte surface marker analysis.

Lymph node sections were classified histologically according to the Rappaport classification (16,22,23). The biopsy specimens were classified without knowledge of the *in vitro* glucocorticoid data. Both lymph node cryostat sections and cell suspensions were assayed for lymphocyte surface markers. Immunologic analyses for surface immunoglobulin, complement receptors, sheep erythrocyte receptors, and Fc receptors were performed utilizing techniques previously described in detail (3).

Lymphomas were classified as B cell, T cell, or "Null" cell using previously defined criteria (3). In brief, lymphomas were classified as B cell when they represented a monoclonal proliferation of surface immunoglobulin-bearing cells. Lymphomas were identified as T cell when more than 50% of the cells formed erythrocyte rosettes and at least 20% of these cells were identified in cytocentrifuge preparations as malignant. A tumor was defined as "Null" cell if studies of suspensions of living cells and cryostat sections showed neither surface immunoglobulin nor sheep erythrocyte, complement, or Fc receptors.

Glucocorticoid Receptors and *In Vitro* Glucocorticoid Sensitivity

In single cell suspensions prepared from neoplastic lymphoid tissue, the percent of malignant cells was first determined by lymphocyte surface marker analysis. When the single cell suspension demonstrated at least 50% malignant cells, the tissue was studied for glucocorticoid receptors and *in vitro* sensitivity. In 35 patients (83%), the specimen studied contained at least 75% malignant cells, and in 24 cases more than 80% malignant cells. Single cell suspensions from normal, nonmalignant lymph nodes from 11 adults were studied as controls.

Cytoplasmic and nuclear receptors were measured utilizing a whole cell assay as previously described (8). Briefly, cells were incubated for 30 min at 37°C as follows: A: with approximately 40 nM [^{3}H]1,4-pregnadien-9-fluoro-16α-methyl-11β,17α,21-triol-3,20-dione (dexamethasone); or B: with 40 nM [^{3}H]dexamethasone with approximately 2 μM unlabeled dexamethasone. For assay of nuclear receptors, cells were broken by adding an aliquot of the cell suspension to 60 volumes of 1.5 mM $MgCl_2$ at 3°C, the broken cell suspension was centrifuged, and the resulting nuclear pellet was counted. For assay of cytoplasmic receptors, cells were broken by adding an aliquot of the cell suspension to 5 volumes of 1.5 mM $MgCl_2$ containing dextran-coated charcoal at 3°C, the charcoal (which adsorbs free steroid) was sedimented along with the nuclei and cell particulates by centrifugation, and an aliquot of the supernatant (containing bound steroid) was counted.

For both nuclear and cytoplasmic binding, receptor binding in counts per minute (cpm) was calculated by subtracting the bound cpm obtained from incubation B (which estimates nonsaturable binding) from the cpm obtained from incubation A, appropriately corrected for differences in the radioactive steroid concentrations in the two incubations (20). These cpm were converted to bound steroid molecules per cell. Receptor sites per cell were then calculated from these values by extrapolating to infinite steroid concentration (20), assuming dexamethasone has a dissociation constant for glucocorticoid receptors of 10 nM (9).

Total receptor sites per cell (R_T) were calculated as the sum of the cytoplasmic (R_C) and nuclear (R_N) receptor sites per cell. In cases in which the single cell suspensions contained only 50 to 80% malignant cells, the R_T was corrected (R_{T*}) based on the average R_T for the nonmalignant control lymph nodes. Most of our glucocorticoid receptor data are reported in terms of total receptors (R_{TC}). These data consist of R_T for patients for whom the cell suspension studied contained $\geq$ 80% malignant cells and the R_{T*} for patients for whom the cell suspension contained 50 to 80% neoplastic cells.

In vitro sensitivity to glucocorticoids was measured by studying the incorporation of leucine, uridine, and thymidine and cell viability using methods previously described (8). Briefly, for assays of isotope incorporation, cells (1×10^6/ml) were incubated in quadruplicate with and without 100 nM dexamethasone for 20 hr at 37°C. Radiolabeled leucine, uridine, and thymidine were then added and the incubation continued for 4 hr. The cells were then harvested on glass fiber filter paper and the isotope incorporation determined by liquid scintillation counting. For assay of cell survival, cells (5×10^5/ml) were incubated in quadruplicate in the absence and presence of dexamethasone (400 nM) at 37°C. At 96 hr samples were removed for cell counts and viabilities by Trypan blue dye exclusion. Results for *in vitro* sensitivity studies have been expressed as percent change from the values obtained when cells were incubated without dexamethasone.

Statistical Methods

Differences among groups were evaluated for significance at the $p = 0.05$ level or less. Differences in percentage for discrete variables were tested using the Pearson chi-square statistic correcting for continuity in 2×2 tables. Differences in continuous variables between groups were tested using the Mann-Whitney test.

RESULTS

Glucocorticoid Receptors

The 11 normal lymph nodes studied as controls had median receptor numbers of 661 for R_C, 1,481 for R_N, and 2,082 for R_T (Table 1). The 42 malignant lymphomas studied had median receptor numbers of 1,031 for R_C, 2,880 for R_N, and 4,110 for R_T. The values from lymphomas are significantly higher than those from the control lymph nodes (Table 1). The differences are even greater when the number of total receptor sites per cell for the lymphomas is corrected for contamination by normal lymphocytes. R_{TC} for the lymphomas ranged from 0 to 17,218 (median = 4,254). Only one case had no detectable glucocorticoid receptors.

The numbers of receptors were similar in patients studied at diagnosis, prior to any treatment, and in patients studied at relapse (Table 1). However, in all four patients studied sequentially (at diagnosis and relapse), the receptor number fell (Fig. 1).

The median receptor numbers by Rappaport histologic class were determined (Table 2). Only classes in which a minimum of six patients were studied are shown in the table. There were no significant differences in receptor numbers

TABLE 1. In vitro glucocorticoid characteristics of malignant lymphomas and normal lymph nodes

	Malignant lymphoma		Normal lymph nodes		
	N = 42		N = 11		
	Glucocorticoid receptors (sites/cell)				
	Median	Range	Median	Range	p
Cytoplasmic (R_C)	1,031	230–10,627	661	0–1,099	< 0.05
Nuclear (R_N)	2,880	421– 7,491	1,481	0–3,086	< 0.01
Total (R_T)	4,110	671–17,218	2,082	0–3,996	< 0.01
Total corrected (R_{TC})[a]	4,254	0–17,218	—	—	—
Diagnosis (N = 23)	4,107	1,718–16,336	—	—	—
Relapse (N = 19)	4,865	0–17,218	—	—	—

| | Malignant lymphoma | | Normal lymph nodes | | |
| | In vitro glucocorticoid sensitivity | | | | |
	Median (%)	No. pts	Median (%)	No. pts	
Inhibition of isotope incorporation					
Leucine	19	27	21	5	ns[b]
Uridine	33	30	28	5	ns
Thymidine	21	25	21	5	ns
Cell survival decreased	48	28	20	8	< 0.05

[a] See text.
[b] ns, not significant.

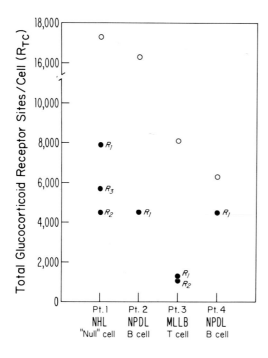

FIG. 1. Total glucocorticoid receptors (R_{TC}) in lymphomas from four patients whose tumors were studied sequentially. The histologic and immunologic diagnoses are indicated for each patient (see text and tables for explanations of abbreviations). R_{TC} from the pretreatment lymphomas are indicated by *open circles*. R_{TC} from tumors obtained at each relapse are indicated by R_n *(closed circles)*.

among the histologic classes. Within classes, no significant differences were found between lymphomas sampled at diagnosis and those studied at relapse, but the numbers of patients in each category are still small.

The median numbers of receptors by immunologic class are also shown in Table 2. The median numbers of total receptors were 7,552 for "Null" cell lymphomas, 3,411 for T cell lymphomas, and 4,251 for B cell lymphomas. Only a small number of cases of T cell and "Null" cell lymphoma were studied, but the "Null" cell lymphomas appear to have more receptors than the T cell lymphomas ($p < 0.05$).

In Vitro Glucocorticoid Sensitivity

The effects of glucocorticoids on isotope incorporation were studied in 5 normal lymph nodes. Similar results were obtained for leucine, uridine, and thymidine (Table 1). Compared with cultures not containing dexamethasone, isotope incorporation was decreased by a median of 21% for leucine, 28% for uridine, and 21% for thymidine.

The effects of glucocorticoids on isotope incorporation, for the total group of malignant lymphomas, were similar to the effects on nonmalignant lymph nodes (Table 1). Median inhibitions were 19% for leucine, 33% for uridine, and 21% for thymidine. However, the range of inhibition by glucocorticoid was much greater in the lymphomas (Fig. 2). Among the controls, the largest

TABLE 2. In vitro glucocorticoid characteristics according to histologic and immunologic classes

| Classes[a] | No. pts. | Total glucocorticoid receptors (R_TC) Sites/cell | | Inhibition of isotope incorporation | | | | | | | | Cell survival decreased | |
| | | Median | Range | Leucine | | Uridine | | Thymidine | | | | | |
				Median (%)	No. pts.	Median (%)	No. pts.	Median (%)	No. pts.			Median (%)	No. pts.
Histologic													
Nodular-PDL	12	4,327	0–16,336	19	5	32	7	7	6			23	7
Diffuse-WDL	6	4,223	2,560– 8,413	3	5	27	4	4	4			64	4
Diffuse-IDL	9	3,067	1,908– 6,624	29	6	32	8	32	5			65	6
Lymphoblastic	6	3,507	695– 8,150	0	3	19	3	11	3			49	4
Immunologic													
B cell (SIg+)	32	4,251	0–16,336	19	19	32	23	19	18			31	19
μκ	19	4,952	1,718–13,638	18	11	24	12	24	9			55	10
μλ	10	3,264	1,908– 9,254	30	6	43	8	19	6			30	7
T cell (E+)	6	3,411	695– 8,150	0	3	20	3	11	3			60	4
"Null" cell	4	7,552	4,112–17,218	36	3	50	3	47	3			63	4

[a] PDL, poorly differentiated lymphocytic lymphoma; WDL, well-differentiated lymphocytic lymphoma; IDL, intermediately differentiated lymphocytic lymphoma.

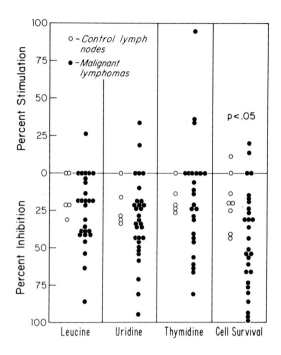

FIG. 2. Effects of dexamethasone on the incorporation of leucine, uridine, and thymidine and on the *in vitro* survival of lymphocytes obtained from normal lymph nodes *(open circles)* and of neoplastic cells obtained from malignant lymphoma *(closed circles)*.

glucocorticoid inhibition of leucine incorporation was 31%; among the lymphomas, leucine incorporation was inhibited more than this in 11 of 27 cases studied. Similarly, the greatest inhibition of uridine incorporation was 34% among the controls; 13 of 30 lymphomas had more inhibition than this. For thymidine, among controls the greatest inhibition was 27%; 10 of 25 lymphomas studied had more inhibition.

In a given lymphoma, when the neoplastic cells were taking up the isotope, the percent inhibition of incorporation was usually similar for leucine, uridine, and thymidine (correlation coefficients $r = 0.57-0.81$). There were no apparent differences in isotope incorporation between those patients studied at diagnosis and those studied at relapse.

The effect of glucocorticoid on *in vitro* cell survival was studied in eight normal lymph nodes. Cell survival was inhibited by a median of 20% (Table 1). In the 28 lymphomas studied, cell survival was inhibited by a median of 48%. The effect of glucocorticoids on cell survival was significantly greater in the lymphomas than in the nonmalignant lymph nodes ($p < 0.05$). In half of the lymphomas, glucocorticoids caused at least a 50% decrease in cell survival.

We examined *in vitro* glucocorticoid sensitivity according to histologic and immunologic classes. No significant differences between either histologic or immunologic classes were observed, but the numbers studied in most groups are very small (Table 2).

In Vitro Glucocorticoid Studies and Response to Glucocorticoid Therapy

Of the 22 patients who received single agent glucocorticoid therapy, 10 responded and 12 did not. Clinical characteristics of the two patient groups are shown in Table 3. Responders and nonresponders did not differ significantly in gender, age, diagnosis, or prior treatment status. All patients had disseminated disease at the time glucocorticoid was started (Ann Arbor stage IV disease).

Responders and nonresponders received single-agent glucocorticoid therapy for comparable periods of time (median 10 and 9 days, respectively). Among the responders, seven achieved a partial remission (50% decrease in measurable tumor) after 5 days of therapy. Three patients did not meet response criteria after 5 days, but responded after 2 weeks of therapy. Following 14 days of glucocorticoid therapy, two patients achieved clinical complete remissions defined as disappearance of all palpable lymphoma; one of these patients also demonstrated disappearance of lymphoma from the bone marrow, thus achieving a pathologically documented complete remission.

Among the nonresponders at the end of single agent glucocorticoid therapy,

TABLE 3. *Clinical characteristics of responders and nonresponders*

Characteristic[a]	Responders	Nonresponders
No. patients	10	12
Gender (M:F)	4:6	8:4
Age (years)		
Median	54	59
Range	20–84	18–79
Diagnosis		
Histologic (Rappaport)		
Nodular-PDL	4	5
Nodular-HL	3	0
Diffuse-IDL	2	3
Lymphoblastic (MLLB)	1	1
Undifferentiated	0	2
Diffuse-PDL	0	1
Immunologic		
B cell (SIg+)	7	10
$\mu\kappa$	5	6
$\mu\lambda$	1	4
$\mu\gamma$	1	0
T cell (E+)	1	1
"Null" cell	2	1
Prior treatment	3	5
Prior glucocorticoid	1	4
Stage IV at treatment	10	12
Blood involvement	4	6

[a] HL, histiocytic lymphoma; PDL, poorly differentiated lymphocytic lymphoma; WDL, well-differentiated lymphocytic lymphoma; IDL, intermediately differentiated lymphocytic lymphoma.

TABLE 4. *Correlation of* In Vitro *glucocorticoid studies with response to glucocorticoid therapy*

| | Median value | | |
In vitro test	Responders	Nonresponders	*p*
Glucocorticoid receptor number (sites/cell)			
Total receptors (R_{TC})	5,617	3,321	0.01
Inhibition of isotope incorporation			
Leucine	36%	7%	0.02
Uridine	44%	19%	<0.05
Thymidine	35%	24%	ns[a]
Cell survival decreased	43%	18%	ns

[a] ns, not significant.

six patients demonstrated stable disease ($< 25\%$ decrease in measurable tumor). All of these patients received glucocorticoid therapy alone for at least 1 week and four of them for 2 weeks or more. Six patients had progressive disease on glucocorticoid therapy. In three of these patients, because of rapidly progressive disease, single agent glucocorticoid administration was terminated after only 3 to 4 days. The remaining three patients received glucocorticoids alone for 6, 9, and 11 days, respectively.

Toxicity was generally not severe, but occurred more frequently in the respon-

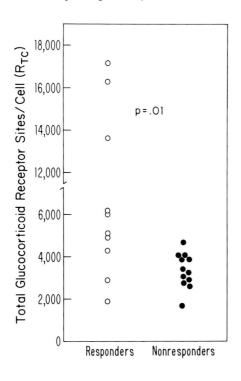

FIG. 3. Total glucocorticoid receptors (R_{TC}) in lymphomas from 10 patients whose tumors clinically decreased at least 50% on glucocorticoid therapy (Responders: *open circles*) and 12 patients whose lymphomas did not respond to treatment with glucocorticoids (Nonresponders: *closed circles*).

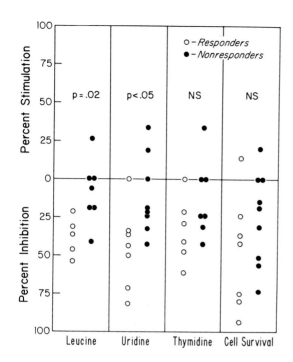

FIG. 4. Effects of dexamethasone on the incorporation of leucine, uridine, and thymidine and on the *in vitro* survival of lymphoma cells from patients who clinically responded to glucocorticoid therapy (Responders: *open circles*) and patients who did not respond (Nonresponders: *closed circles*).

ders than the nonresponders. Among the responders there was one *Escherichia coli* septicemia (on day 18 of glucocorticoid therapy), one episode of mild disseminated intravascular coagulation due to rapid tumor lysis, two instances of mild fluid retention, two instances of steroid-induced acne, four instances of psychologic changes (increased sleeplessness or nervousness), two instances of joint pain, and one of hiccups. In comparison, among the 12 nonresponders, gastrointestinal bleeding, mild fluid retention, mild sleeplessness, hiccups, and mild sweating were seen in one case each.

The results of the *in vitro* glucocorticoid studies for the responders and the nonresponders are summarized in Table 4 and Figs. 3 and 4. Although there were no significant differences in pretreatment clinical characteristics, total glucocorticoid receptors were significantly higher in the responders than the nonresponders (median 5,617 versus 3,321, $p = 0.01$) (Fig. 3). The inhibition of leucine and uridine incorporation were also significantly greater in the responders than the nonresponders (Fig. 4). Significant differences between responders and nonresponders were not seen in dexamethasone inhibition of thymidine incorporation or cell survival, though the number of patients studied in each group is still small.

DISCUSSION

These data (4) confirm and extend our preliminary results (2) which suggested that almost all cases of malignant lymphoma in adults have measurable numbers of glucocorticoid receptors. Of 42 cases, only 1 appeared to have no detectable receptors; the remaining cases had 1,781 to 17,218 total glucocorticoid receptor sites per cell. We know of no other systematic study of glucocorticoid receptors in adult lymphoma, although reports of receptors in occasional patients have appeared (8,14).

The number of receptor sites varied markedly among lymphomas; the range was similar to that reported in acute lymphocytic leukemia (ALL) (17). Attempts to relate the variability in receptor number to histologic or immunologic classification of the lymphoma were not successful. Wide ranges in receptor number were found in all subtypes of lymphoma. However, "Null" cell lymphomas usually had higher receptor levels than T cell lymphomas similar to what has been reported in childhood ALL (17). Since in this series the number of cases studied in many histologic subtypes was very small, it can not be excluded that in larger series significant differences among histologic classes may also be demonstrated.

Variability in receptor number occurred both in cases studied at diagnosis (range 1,718–16,336) and at relapse (range 0–17,218). However, since receptor levels fell in all four cases that we studied repeatedly during the course of their disease, it is possible that in individual patients glucocorticoid therapy results in the selection of neoplastic cells with fewer glucocorticoid receptors. The only lymphoma we found with no receptors was from a patient who had previously received intensive combination chemotherapy including glucocorticoids. However, some lymphomas at diagnosis may have no receptors.

All patients studied at relapse had been off glucocorticoids at least 10 days to avoid the apparent down-regulation of receptors that occurs following treatment with glucocorticoids (26). In the few normals we have studied, glucocorticoid receptor levels have returned to pretreatment levels within 1 week of stopping glucocorticoids, but longer preiods may be required in lymphomas. The effects of other chemotherapy on receptor levels in lymphoma are unknown.

Although almost all lymphomas had fairly large numbers of glucocorticoid receptors, *in vitro* glucocorticoid sensitivity as measured by inhibition of radiolabeled isotope incorporation and cell survival varied widely. Many cases showed marked sensitivity, while proliferation appeared to be stimulated in others. There was not a strong correlation ($r < 0.5$) between glucocorticoid receptor levels and *in vitro* sensitivity. Too few cases have been studied to correlate *in vitro* sensitivity with histologic or immunologic subtypes.

Involved lymph nodes were the source of neoplastic cells in most of our patients (73%). Adults with lymphoma rarely have sufficient blood or marrow involvement for these sites to provide enough lymphoma cells for *in vitro* glucocorticoid studies. In order to compare the results from *in vitro* glucocorticoid assays in lymphoma with comparable results in normal tissue, we studied lymphocytes from 11 normal lymph nodes. These demonstrated significantly lower numbers of glucocorticoid receptors than did the neoplastic cells and also a narrower range in receptor number. Similarly, although on average dexamethasone-induced inhibition of isotope incorporation was compa-rable in nonmalignant and malignant lymphocytes, the range was quite narrow in the normal lymphocytes and much greater among lymphomas. The effect of dexamethasone on inhibition of *in vitro* cell survival was significantly greater in the malignant cells. These differences between neoplastic and normal lympho-cytes are of considerable interest, especially in light of the fact that human lymphocytes are felt to be relatively corticoresistent (11), while lymphomas frequently appear quite sensitive. Although glucocorticoids may exert their anti-tumor effect via mechanisms other than direct cell lysis (Smith et al., *this volume*), our *in vitro* studies in lymphomas (4) provide possible explanations for the clinically apparent direct lytic activity in lymphoma. Obviously, these differences between cells from normal and malignant lymph nodes require further study.

No studies like ours (4) with lymphocytes from normal lymph nodes appear to have been reported previously. There are, however, *in vitro* glucocorticoid studies with human circulating lymphocytes (9,11,17). Although *in vitro* glucocorticoid sensitivity appears similar in lymphocytes from blood and nodes, the number of receptors is significantly lower in lymph nodes (in this series R_T mean $\pm$ SEM were 4,190 $\pm$ 337 and 2,110 $\pm$ 396, respectively, $p < 0.01$). Our results for circulating lymphocytes are similar to those reported by others (11). Whether the lower receptor levels in lymphocytes from nodes are related to monocyte contamination in preparations from the blood (29) or the degree of lymphocyte stimulation (17,27) is unknown.

The wide range in glucocorticoid receptor levels and *in vitro* glucocorticoid sensitivity among lymphomas suggested that these tests might be useful in pre-dicting the antitumor effect of glucocorticoids in individual patients. To test this hypothesis, adults with lymphoma were treated with glucocorticoids alone and antitumor response assessed. Lymphomas from patients who had at least a 50% decrease in measurable tumor after short-term glucocorticoid therapy had higher numbers of glucocorticoid receptors and greater *in vitro* gluco-corticoid sensitivity as measured by inhibition of leucine and uridine incor-poration (5). These data suggest that *in vitro* glucocorticoid studies may allow us to select before treatment those patients with lymphoma who should receive glucocorticoids in their chemotherapy regimens and those patients for whom the antitumor benefit may not be worth the potential toxicity.

Our results in lymphoma with regard to glucocorticoid receptors and antitu-mor response to glucocorticoids are similar to those reported in breast cancer with regard to estrogen receptors and response to estrogen (19). Glucocorticoid receptors and response to single agent glucocorticoid therapy have not been extensively studied in other lymphoproliferative disorders. However, the numbers of glucocorticoid receptors have been reported to be useful in predicting clinical response to glucocorticoids in a small series of patients with advanced chronic lymphocytic leukemia (28). Similar anecdotal results have been reported in Sézary syndrome (25). The correlation between glucocorticoid receptor levels and response to glucocorticoids has not been studied in ALL, but the duration of remission induced with regimens including glucocorticoids has been positively correlated with receptor levels (17).

The need to study lymph nodes to obtain sufficient malignant cells for *in vitro* glucocorticoid assays in patients with lymphoma is associated with two major problems. The first is the relative inaccessibility of nodal tissue as a source of malignant cells. The second and more important problem relates to the purity of the malignant cell population obtained from lymph nodes. The major contaminating cells are nonmalignant lymphocytes. No satisfactory rapid method, such as exists for removing contaminating granulocytes from blood, is available for the elimination of nonmalignant lymphocytes. A practical approach is to assess the degree of contamination by lymphocyte surface marker analysis and discard specimens with less than 50% malignant cells and correct for lesser degrees of contamination. Since the degree of contamination can vary markedly within a node, especially in nodular lymphomas, surface marker analysis must be performed on the same cell suspension from which cells are taken for *in vitro* glucocorticoid assays. In the present series, even among cases where adequate numbers of cells were obtained from biopsied lymph nodes and more than 50% malignant cells were present in the cell suspension, only half of the cases had more than 80% malignant cells in the cell suspension; the remaining cases were mathematically corrected for contamination. Obviously the availability of rapid and reliable methods for separation of contaminating nonmalignant lymphocytes that would not waste large numbers of cells or alter them in any way would be preferable.

Even though difficulties exist in assaying glucocorticoid receptors and *in vitro* sensitivity in adults with lymphomas, our data (5) suggest that such studies may be useful and allow the selection of the 50% or less of adults who will significantly benefit from glucocorticoid therapy. If our results are confirmed by further studies, glucocorticoid receptor determinations may become a necessary part of the evaluation of lymphoma in the same way in which estrogen receptor analysis is required in breast cancer (19).

ACKNOWLEDGMENTS

This research was supported in part by National Institutes of Health Grants CA-26273, CA-17323, AM-03535, the Masonic Hospital Fund, Inc., the Norris Cotton Cancer Center, and the Minnesota Medical Foundation.

REFERENCES

1. Bagley, C. M., Jr., DeVita, V. T., Jr., Berard, C. W., and Canellos, G. P. (1972): *Ann. Intern. Med.,* 76:227–234.
2. Bloomfield, C. D., Crabtree, G., Smith, K. A., Gibbs, G., Peterson, B. A., Jeffries, M., Gajl-Peczalska, K., Kersey, J., McKenna, R., Frizzera, G., and Munck, A. (1978): *Blood,* 52(Suppl. 1):240.
3. Bloomfield, C. D., Gajl-Peczalska, K. J., Frizzera, G., Kersey, J. H., and Goldman, A. I. (1979): *N. Engl. J. Med.,* 301:512–518.

4. Bloomfield, C. D., Smith, K. A., Hildebrandt, L., Zaleskas, J., Gajl-Peczalska, K. J., Frizzera, G., Peterson, B. A., Kersey, J. H., Crabtree, G. R., and Munck, A. (1979): *Submitted for publication.*

5. Bloomfield, C. D., Smith, K. A., Peterson, B. A., Hildebrandt, L., Zaleskas, J., Gajl-Peczalska, K. J., Frizzera, G., and Munck, A. (1980): *Lancet,* 1:952–956.

6. Canellos, G. P., Lister, T. A., and Skarin, A. T. (1978): *Cancer,* 42:932–940.

7. Coltman, C. A., Luce, J. K., McKelvey, E. M., Jones, S. E., and Moon, T. E., (1977): *Cancer Treat. Rep.,* 61:1067–1078.

8. Crabtree, G. R., Smith, K. A., and Munck, A. (1978): *Cancer Res.,* 38:4268–4272.

9. Crabtree, G. R., Smith, K. A., and Munck, A. (1978): In: *Seventh Tenovus Workshop. Glucocorticoid Action and Leukemia,* edited by P. A. Bell and N. M. Borthwick, pp. 191–204. Alpha Omega, Cardiff.

10. DeVita, V. T., Jr., Canellos, G. P., Chabner, B., Schein, P., Hubbard, S., and Young, R. C. (1975): *Lancet,* 1:248–250.

11. Duval, D., Homo, F., and Thierry, C. (1978): In: *Seventh Tenovus Workshop. Glucocorticoid Action and Leukemia,* edited by P. A. Bell and N. M. Borthwick, pp. 143–154. Alpha Omega, Cardiff.

12. Ezdinli, E. Z., Stutzman, L., Aungst, C. W., and Firat, D. (1969): *Cancer,* 23:900–909.

13. Fortuny, I. E., Theologides, A., and Kennedy, B. J. (1972): *Minn. Med.,* 55:715–716.

14. Gailani, S., Minowada, J., Silvernail, P., Nussbaum, A., Kaiser, N., Rosen, F., and Shimaoka, K. (1973): *Cancer Res.,* 33:2653–2657.

15. Jones, S. E., Rosenberg, S. A., Kaplan, H. S., Kadin, M. E., and Dorfman, R. F. (1972): *Cancer,* 30:31–38.

16. Kim, H., Heller, P., Rappaport, H. (1973): *Am. J. Clin. Pathol.,* 59:282–294.

17. Lippman, M. E., Yarbro, G. S. K., and Leventhal, B. G. (1978): In: *Seventh Tenovus Workshop. Glucocorticoid Action and Leukemia,* edited by P. A. Bell and N. M. Borthwick, pp. 175–190. Alpha Omega, Cardiff.

18. Livingston, R. B., and Carter, S. K. (1970): In: *Single Agents in Cancer Chemotherapy,* pp. 337–358. Plenum Press, New York.

19. McGuire, W. L. (1978): *Cancer Res.,* 38:4289–4291.

20. Munck, A. (1976): In: *Receptors and Mechanism of Action of Steroid Hormones. Part I,* edited by J. R. Pasqualini, pp. 1–40. Marcel Dekker, New York.

21. Munck, A., and Leung, K. (1977): In: *Receptors and Mechanism of Action of Steroid Hormones. Part II,* edited by J. R. Pasqualini, pp. 311–397. Marcel Dekker, New York.

22. Nathwani, B. N., Kim, H., and Rappaport, H. (1976): *Cancer,* 38:964–983.

23. Rappaport, H. (1966): In: *Atlas of Tumor Pathology, Sect. 3, Fasc. 8.* Armed Forces Institute of Pathology, Washington, D.C.

24. Schein, P. S., DeVita, V. T., Jr., Hubbard, S., Chabner, B. A., Canellos, G. P., Berard, C., and Young, R. C. (1976): *Ann. Intern. Med.,* 85:417–422.

25. Schmidt, T. J., and Thompson, E. B. (1979): *Cancer Res.,* 39:376–382.

26. Shipman, G. F., Bloomfield, C. D., Smith, K. A., Peterson, B. A., and Munck, A. (1979): *Blood,* 54(Suppl.1):209a.

27. Smith, K. A., Crabtree, G. R., Kennedy, S. J., and Munck, A. U. (1977): *Nature,* 267:523–526.

28. Terenius, L., Simonsson, B., and Nilsson, K. (1978): In: *Seventh Tenovus Workshop. Glucocorticoid Action and Leukemia,* edited by P. A. Bell, and N. M. Borthwick, pp. 155–160. Alpha Omega, Cardiff.

29. Werb, Z., Foley, R., and Munck, A. (1978): *J. Exp. Med.,* 147:1684–1694.

Hormones and Cancer, edited by S. Iacobelli et al.
Raven Press, New York © 1980.

Present and Future Clinical Value of Steroid Receptor Assays in Human Prostatic Carcinoma

Peter Ekman, *Erik Dahlberg, *Jan-Åke Gustafsson, **Bertil Högberg, *Åke Pousette, and †Marek Snochowski

*Department of Urology, Karolinska Hospital; Departments of *Chemistry and Medical Nutrition and **Pharmacology, Karolinska Institutet, S-104 01 Stockholm, Sweden*

The prostate is a target organ for androgens. The gland atrophies after castration but regains its normal size and characteristics after androgen supply (33). The prostate also seems to be influenced by other hormones, e.g., estrogens (23) and prolactin (39,40). The possible direct effects of these hormones on the human prostate cells are less well investigated. Ever since the pioneering work of Charles Huggins in the early 1940s (35,36), endocrine manipulations, either by castration or administration of estrogens, have been useful tools in controlling the growth of prostatic carcinoma for various periods of time. The mechanism of action of estrogens has not been fully clarified. Some authors have reported a direct effect of estrogens on prostatic cancer cells (18,28). However, the main effect seems to be indirect and mediated via the hypothalamo–pituitary–testicular axis. Luteinizing hormone (LH) production and, hence, testicular androgen production is decreased following estrogen administration (2).

Progestins (23,39) and progestational antiandrogens such as cyproterone acetate (7,24) have also been of value in the treatment of prostatic carcinoma. Corticosteroids have been used mainly in advanced stages of the disease (44).

Prostatic carcinoma is common in elderly men, with a reported incidence of 50% in males over 80 years of age (32). Still little is known concerning the mechanisms of tumor development in the gland. A continuous androgen supply seems to be of importance, since neither cancer nor hyperplasia develop in the prostate of males castrated before the age of 40 (46). To date, however, data on hormone concentrations in serum have been controversial and have offered only a minor contribution to our knowledge of these pathological processes (29,48,53). Studies on steroid receptor profiles in normal and pathological prostatic tissue might increase our knowledge concerning the etiology of prostatic carcinoma. Because of the slow development of prostatic tumors, progressing in intervals over several years, it is difficult to know in which phase the investigations should be performed. Another difficulty is finding adequate age-matched controls.

---

†Visiting scientist from the Polish Academy of Sciences.

Endocrine therapy is effective in 75 to 80% of all cases of prostatic carcinoma (19). Poorly differentiated tumors are often resistant to endocrine manipulations (15), but histology and cytology offer only a very crude screening for choice of therapy. In fact, today there are still no reliable methods for the selection of which patients should be given hormonal treatment and which patients should preferably be given alternative therapy such as irradiation or cytotoxic drugs.

In view of the promising results from clinical use of steroid receptor assays for prediction of tumor response to endocrine therapy in human breast cancer (37), a disease with some characteristics in common with prostatic carcinoma, it seems reasonable to propose that steroid receptor assays should also be investigated in prostatic carcinoma for use as a screening test for hormone sensitivity.

Receptor studies on the human prostate have long been hampered for many reasons. One major problem has been contamination of the tissue specimen with a plasma protein, testosterone-binding globulin (TeBG), which binds testosterone and 5α-dihydrotestosterone (DHT) with an affinity similar to that of the androgen receptor (45). A variety of techniques have been tried to overcome this obstacle, including precipitation with ammonium or protamine sulfate (17,25,43), fractionation on Sephadex G-100 or G-200 columns (27,41), cold agar gel electrophoresis (56,57), sucrose density gradient centrifugation (27, 41,43), and ion exchange chromatography (17). Although these techniques have provided evidence for the existence of an androgen binding species in human prostatic tissue, they have failed to demonstrate reproducibly the presence of an androgen receptor in the cytosol.

The human prostate contains large amounts of endogenous DHT; therefore, many receptor sites may be saturated (1). "Exchange" assays are complicated by slow dissociation of the steroid from its receptor at low temperature and instability of the receptor at higher temperature (16,54). Natural ligands are often rapidly metabolized even at low temperature, a fact that also makes them less suitable for receptor research (3,54). Hence, the introduction of radiolabeled synthetic steroids has been of great importance for research on steroid receptors in the human prostate. Methyltrienolone, a synthetic androgen, has the advantage of binding to the intracellular receptor but not to TeBG (6,54). Furthermore, it is resistant to metabolic conversion and exchanges with receptor-bound endogenous steroid to about 70% during incubation overnight at 0°C (12,42,54). Methyl trienolone has the disadvantage of crossreacting with progestin receptors, which seem to be present in significant amounts in human benign prostatic hyperplasia (6,9,12,26,52). Recent findings, however, indicate that this obstacle may be overcome by adding an excess of unlabeled triamcinolone acetonide to the incubation medium (3,31,58), thereby blocking the progestin receptor without interfering with the binding of methyltrienolone to the androgen receptor.

The purpose of this chapter is to review briefly recent results from steroid receptor assays in human prostatic tissue and also to speculate on future possible methodological improvements.

MATERIALS

Human hyperplastic prostates may easily be obtained at routine operations. However, electroresected material is definitely unsuitable for receptor studies, since varying amounts of protein denatured by this procedure (13,26,54). Homogeneous human cancer tissue may be obtained by removal of soft tissue metastases (11). In biopsies from the primary tumor, significant amounts of stroma cells have always been found to contaminate the specimen (13). Moreover, the prostatic carcinoma is sometimes heterogeneous with a mixture of cancer cells of different degrees of differentiation. It is therefore not certain that the most malignant part of the tumor is represented in the biopsy.

For biopsies of primary tumors we have used the punch needle instrument designed by Veenema in 1953 (55). Other authors have used the TRU-CUT needle (31,56). The biopsies usually yield a total specimen weight of less than 0.2 g. Material obtained at radical prostatectomies can also be used for receptor studies, but in such cases comparison between receptor content and response to endocrine therapy can seldom be carried out, as prostatectomized cancer patients are usually not given further therapy.

Normal prostatic tissue is difficult to obtain and is also difficult to classify. Normal human prostates are probably only found in males aged 15 to 35. The normal sized prostate of elderly men usually displays many alterations characteristic of senescence, such as atrophic parts, sclerosis, and cyst formations (21). When attempting to find possible differences in prostatic cell properties and serum hormone levels among patients with or without prostatic disease, however, it seems reasonable to use age-matched controls even though their prostate glands may no longer be truly normal. Another problem is that the histology of early benign hyperplasia is often indistinguishable from that of the normal prostate; therefore, all comparisons of assay results of normal versus hyperplastic and cancerous prostatic tissue must be made with caution. "Normal" prostates have usually been obtained in connection with cystectomy operations for bladder carcinoma. the gland is then routinely removed. Minor parts of the peripheral prostate may also be removed in connection with adenoma enucleations for benign prostatic hyperplasia.

METHODS

Evaluation of Clinical Response to Therapy

To study the value of steroid receptor assays for prediction of tumor response to endocrine treatment, the assay results have been compared with the outcome of the patients. However, tumor regression is not always easy to evaluate in the individual patient with prostatic carcinoma. No generally accepted criteria exist. The most reliable parameters seem to be as follows:

1. Decrease of elevated acid phosphatase levels by at least 50%;
2. Shrinking of the primary tumor as estimated by rectal palpation and/or computerized tomography or ultrasound;
3. Squamous cell metaplasia and cell necrosis, as disclosed by needle biopsy (20);
4. Regression of metastases.

A remission may also be supported by improved micturition as estimated by a uroflow meter or removal of an indwelling catheter and/or relief of skeletal pains for at least 3 months. Also improvement of the general condition, decreased sedimentation rate, increased hemoglobin count, and other routine laboratory tests have been used for evaluation of response. Improvement usually occurs within 3 months of therapy. It is our opinion that the therapy should be regarded as unsuccessful if no improvement occurs.

Storage of Tissue

The strict use of fresh material would be impractical; therefore, it seems reasonable to use frozen tissue specimens in all cases to make the handling of the material as uniform as possible. According to our experience, no significant loss of receptors occurred when tissue had been kept for about 2 hr at room temperature before freezing to $-70°C$. The androgen receptors seem to be relatively stable when larger pieces of tissue are stored at $-70°C$ (12). On the other hand, the receptors are unstable in frozen cytosol preparations (12,35). Also, repeated freezing and thawing decreases the receptor content of the specimen (12).

Incubation Temperature

The temperature at which the incubation should be performed is a matter of debate. Many authors use 0 to $4°C$ (3,12,31,42,54); others prefer $15°C$ (51,52), since this leads to a more efficient exchange of endogenous steroid and radiolabeled ligand. It has also been suggested that incubation at $15°C$ exclusively destroys the progestin receptor so that an incubation with SH-MT at $15°C$ only measures the androgen receptor (51). However, according to our results, not only the progestin but also the androgen receptor is lost to some extent at $15°C$ *(unpublished data)*. Also other recent investigations demonstrate lower maximal binding levels at $15°C$ as compared with $0°C$ (3,31). Furthermore, the cross-reactivity of MT to the progestin receptor seems to be avoided by saturating the incubation medium with triamcinolone acetonide as previously mentioned.

Methods Used in Our Laboratory

Our own data are based on assays using a dextran-coated charcoal technique (54). For reasons given above, androgen receptor measurements have been performed using [³H]methyltrienolone (MT) (17β-hydroxy-17α-methyl-4,9,11-estratrien-3-one) as ligand (6). For similar reasons, estrogen receptors were measured with [³H]R 2858 (17α-ethynyl-11β-methoxy-17β-estradiol) (49) and progestin receptors with [³H]R 5020 (17α-21-dimethyl-19-nor-4,9-pregnadiene-3,20-dione) (47). For glucocorticoid receptor assays [³H]dexamethasone was used (9α-fluoro-11β,17α,21-trihydroxy-16α-methyl-1,4-pregnadiene-3,20-dione) (5).

For receptor quantitation incubations were carried out overnight at 4°C with ³H-labeled ligands in the presence or absence of a 100-fold excess of unlabeled ligand. The apparent maximum number of binding sites (B_{max}) and the dissociation constant (K_D) were calculated according to Scatchard from data corrected for nonspecific binding according to Chamness and McGuire (8). A program was developed for a Nord computer for calculations of relevant statistical data. Nondetectable levels of binding were said to exist when the slope of the Scatchard plot was not significantly different ($p < 0.05$) from zero. Binding was related to wet weight of tissue, to DNA, and to protein content.

Calculation of Binding Data

When comparing data from different laboratories it is of importance to observe how the calculations have been performed. Calculation of binding data by Scatchard analysis seems to have gained the widest acceptance. More simple assays for clinical use may be of value, but such estimations must be compared with those obtained with Scatchard plots to assess the reliability of such assays (31).

RESULTS

Literature data on receptor amounts in the human prostate vary, due in part to the use of different assay methods, procedures for calculation, and choice of reference parameters. This makes comparison of results from different laboratories difficult.

"Normal" and Hyperplastic Tissue

The presence of androgen receptors in the cytosol of all specimens of "normal" and hyperplastic human prostates seems to be well accepted by most groups. When MT is used as ligand for androgen receptor measurement the mean value for binding data (B_{max}) varies between 25 and 50 fmoles/mg of protein or 500 to 1,000 fmoles/mg DNA (12,31,42,51,52). When a 1,000-fold excess of triamcinolone acetonide is added to the incubation medium the maximum number of binding sites is reduced by approximately 50% (31). Progestin receptors are also found in some "normal" and most hyperplastic human prostates (3,9,12,26). Although some groups have found estrogen receptors in the cytosol of benign prostatic hyperplasia (4,30), we and others have failed to demonstrate estrogen receptors in cytosol (12,14) or in cell nuclei (14) of benign prostatic hyperplastic

TABLE 1. *Cytosolic receptor contents in metastases of human prostatic carcinoma*

Pat no.	Previously treated with	MT^a	R 5020[a]	R 2858[a]	Dexamethasone[a]
I	Estramustine phosphate	8,150	402	nd	1,350
II	—	3,440	92	nd	2,270
III	Estrogens/estramustine phosphate	2,870	nd	nd	nd
IV	Orchiectomy	1,790	nd	nd	254
V	—	1,319	54	nd	401
VI	Estrogens	674	nd	nd	942
VII	—	21	nd	nd	nd
VIII	Estrogens/estramustine phosphate	nd	nd	nd	nd
No. of receptor positive cases		7/8	3/8	0/8	5/8
Mean value for K_D (nM)		0.3	0.8	—	3.6

[a] B_{max} = Maximum number of binding sites (fmoles/mg DNA). nd, not detectable, i.e., slope of Scatchard plot not significantly ($p < 0.05$) different from zero.

TABLE 2. *Relationship between receptor content and response to endocrine therapy*

Content of specific MT binding sites	No. patients responding to endocrine therapy	Total no. patients given endocrine therapy	% Responders
51–318 fmoles/mg DNA	18	21	86
Not detectable	3	8	38

tissue. On the other hand, we have been able to demonstrate estrogen receptors in a few "normal" prostates (12). Glucocorticoid receptors seem to be absent in "normal" as well as hyperplastic prostates (12).

Prostatic Carcinoma

Our own receptor data on human prostate cancer metastases are given in Table 1. The receptor profile of prostatic carcinoma seems to be quite heterogeneous. An interesting finding is the presence of glucocorticoid receptors in metastases of prostatic carcinoma (11), which may indicate the possibility of a direct effect of corticosteroids on the cancer cells of advanced prostatic carcinoma. Progestin "receptor-positive" cases may be sensitive to treatment with progestational agents. In no metastases were cytosolic receptors for estrogens detected, which may support the opinion that the main effect of estrogen therapy is indirect and mediated via the hypothalamo–pituitary–testicular axis. (10,11).

Biopsies from primary prostatic carcinoma were also analyzed with regard to the cytosol content of MT binding. Eighteen of the 21 patients (86%) with tumors containing binding sites for MT had tumor regression following endocrine therapy, whereas 5 of the 8 patients (63%) without demonstrated MT binding in their cancer biopsies failed to respond to endocrine manipulations (Table 2) (13). The lower relationship for the MT "receptor-negative" cases may be explained to some extent by the small amount of tissue; when the specimen weight is as low as 0.05 to 0.10 g it may fall below the level of sensitivity of the assay used.

GENERAL DISCUSSION

Endocrine therapy has been a dominant form of treatment for prostatic carcinoma for almost 40 years. However, the exact mechanism of action of different types of hormones used for treatment is still not known. Moreover, we still have no reliable diagnostic aids for the selection of individual cases for endocrine versus nonendocrine therapy. Steroid receptor quantitation constitutes one possible tool to increase our knowledge of the processes responsible for the development of tumors in the human prostate.

Preliminary studies indicate that receptor assays in prostatic carcinoma, as in breast cancer, may become of value to optimize and individualize the therapy. The figures on the relationship between receptor content and tumor response to endocrine therapy are encouraging and should stimulate future research. Improved assay techniques, and also nuclear receptor studies (31), may increase the predictive value of such measurements.

However, the small amount of tissue obtained by needle biopsy may lead to results below the sensitivity of the assay. Another important factor when evaluating the results of the assays is the possible heterogeneity of prostatic carcinoma. Areas of well-differentiated prostatic carcinoma may occur together with components of poorly differentiated carcinoma. A biopsy estimated as receptor positive may in fact also contain considerable amounts of receptor negative cell populations of great importance for the prognosis. It seems to be more difficult to find a correspondence between clinical interpretation and the results from receptor assays of tumors in relapsing cases.

The use of steroid receptor assays as a predictive test in the treatment of prostatic carcinoma may become more general once the receptors have been purified. If it becomes possible to obtain monoclonal antibodies against the receptors, immunoassay methods may be introduced. Considerably smaller amounts of tissue will then be needed for each assay, and material obtained by fine needle aspiration biopsy (22) should be sufficient. Furthermore, an adequate estimation of the receptor content may be performed whether endogenous steroid is bound to the receptor or not.

An advantage with aspiration biopsies as source of tissue for receptor assays is that the technique is rapidly and easily performed; it is used routinely in northern Europe for the diagnosis and follow-up of prostatic carcinoma. Another advantage is that the aspirate may be suspended in an aqueous solution, part of which can be used for cytological examination. It will then be ascertained that the cytological smear will be representative of the material used for the receptor assay. The relative proportion of receptor positive cells as estimated by immunofluorescence techniques may predict the value of endocrine therapy and possibly also which type of endocrine therapy will be the most effective.

In the future it is possible that a multimodality regimen will be introduced in the treatment of prostatic carcinoma, as has been the case for many other types of cancer. Improved survival rates may perhaps be achieved by a combination of radiotherapy, cytotoxic drugs, and/or endocrine manipulations. An adequate screening of the relative number of different cell types with regard to sensitivity to different types of therapy will then be of great importance.

ACKNOWLEDGMENTS

This work was supported by grants from Riksföreningen mot Cancer, AB LEO Research Foundation, and the Swedish Society of Medical Sciences.

REFERENCES

1. Albert, J., Geller, J., Geller, S., and Lopez, D. (1976): *J. Steroid Biochem.,* 7:301–307.
2. Alder, A., Burger, H., Davis, J., Dalmanis, A., Hudson, P. B., Sarfaty, G., and Straffon, W. (1968): *Br. Med. J.,* 1:28–30.
3. Asselin, J., Melancon, R., Gourdeau, Y., Labrie, F., Bonne, C., and Raynaud, J.-P. (1979): *J. Steroid Biochem.,* 10:483–486.
4. Bashirelahi, N., O'Toole, J. H., and Young, J. D. (1976): *Biochem. Med.,* 15:254–261.
5. Baxter, J. D., and Tomkins, G. M. (1970): *Proc. Natl. Acad. Sci. U.S.A.,* 65:709–715.
6. Bonne, C., and Raynaud, J.-P. (1976): *Steroids,* 27:497–507.
7. Bracci, U. (1979): *Eur. Urol.,* 5:303–306.
8. Chamness, G. C., and McGuire, W. L. (1975): *Steroids,* 26:538–542.
9. Cowan, R. A., Cowan, S. K., and Grant, J. K. (1977): *J. Endocrinol.,* 74:281–289.
10. Ekman, P. (1980): In: *Prostatic Cancer Workshop,* edited by H. DeVoogt. Excerpta Medica, Amsterdam (*in press*).
11. Ekman, P., Snochowski, M., Dahlberg, E., and Gustafsson, J.-Å. (1979): *Eur. J. Cancer,* 15:257–262.
12. Ekman, P., Snochowski, M., Dahlberg, E., Bression, D., Högberg, B., and Gustafsson, J.-Å. (1979): *J. Clin. Endocrinol. Metab.,* 49:205–215.
13. Ekman, P., Snochowski, M., Zetterberg, A., Högberg, B., and Gustafsson, J.-Å. (1979): *Cancer,* 44:1173–1181.
14. Emmott, R. C., Murphy, J. B., Hicks, L. L., and Walsh, P. C. (1979): 74th Meeting, American Urological Association, New York, Abst. 56.
15. Esposti, P. L. (1971): *Scand. J. Urol. Nephrol.,* 5:199–209.
16. Fang, S., and Liao, S. (1971): *J. Biol. Chem.,* 246:16–23.
17. Fang, S., and Hsu, R. S. (1975): *Fed. Proc.,* 34:348 *(abstr.).*
18. Farnsworth, W. E. (1969): *Invest. Urol.,* 6:423–427.
19. Fergusson, J. D. (1972): In: *Endocrine Therapy of Malignant Disease,* edited by B. A. Stoll, pp. 247–262. Saunders, London.
20. Fergusson, J. D., and Franks, L. M. (1953): *Br. J. Surg.,* 40:422–428.
21. Franks, L. M. (1954): *J. Pathol.,* 68:617–621.
22. Franzén, S., Giertz, G., and Zajicek, J. (1960): *Br. J. Urol.,* 32:193–196.
23. Geller, J. (1974): In: *The Treatment of Prostatic Hypertrophy and Neoplasia,* edited by J. E. Castro, pp. 27–54. MTP, Lancaster, England.
24. Geller, J., Vazakas, G., Fruchtman, B., Newman, H., Nakao, L., and Loh, A. (1968): *Surg. Gynecol. Obstet.,* 127:748–758.
25. Geller, J., and Worthman, C. (1973): *Acta Endocrinol. [Suppl.] (Copenh.),* 177:Abstr. 4.
26. Gustafsson, J.-Å., Ekman, P., Pousette, Å., Snochowski, M., and Högberg, B. (1978): *Invest. Urol.,* 15:361–366.
27. Hansson, V., Tveter, K. J., Unhjem, O., and Djøseland, O. (1972): *J. Steroid Biochem.,* 3:427–439.
28. Harper, M. E., Fahmy, A. R., Pierrepoint, C. G., and Griffiths, K. (1970): *Steroids,* 15:89–103.
29. Harper, M. E., Peeling, W. B., Cowley, T., Brownsey, B. G., Phillips, M. E. A., Groom, G., Fahmy, D. R., and Griffiths, K. (1976): *Acta Endocrinol. (Kbh.),* 81:409–426.
30. Hawkins, E. F., Nijs, M., Brassinne, C., and Tagnon, H. J. (1975): *Steroids,* 26:458–469.
31. Hicks, L. L., and Walsh, P. C. (1979): *Steroids,* 33:389–406.
32. Hirst, A. E., Jr., and Bergman, R. T. (1954): *Cancer,* 7:136–142.
33. Holland, J. B., and Grayhack, J. T. (1976): In: *Scientific Foundations of Urology, Vol. 2,* edited by D. I. Williams and G. D. Chisholm, pp. 338–347. Heinemann, London.
34. Høisaeter, P. Å. (1973): *Biochim. Biophys. Acta,* 317:492–499.
35. Huggins, C., and Hodges, C. V. (1941): *Cancer Res.,* 1:293–297.
36. Huggins, C., Stevens, R. A., and Hodges, C. V. (1941): *Arch. Surg.,* 43:209–213.
37. Jensen, E. V., Block, B. E., Smith, S., Kyser, K., and De Sombre, E. R. (1971): *Natl. Cancer Inst. Monogr.,* 34:55–61.
38. Johnson, D. E., Kaesler, K. E., and Ayala, A. G. (1975): *J. Surg. Oncol.,* 7:9–15.

39. Keenan, E. J., Kemp, E. D., Ramsey, E. E., Garrison, L. B., Pearse, H. D., and Hodges, C. V. (1979): *J. Urol.,* 122:43–46.
40. Kledzik, G. S., Marshall, S., Campbell, G. A., Gelato, M., and Meites, J. (1976): *Endocrinology,* 98:373–379.
41. Mainwaring, W. I. P., and Milroy, E. J. G. (1973): *J. Endocrinol.,* 57:371–384.
42. Menon, M., Taninis, C. E., Hicks, L., Hawkins, E. F., McLoughlin, M. G., and Walsh, P. C. (1978): *J. Clin. Invest.,* 61:150–162.
43. Menon, M., Taninis, C. E., McLoughlin, M. G., Lippman, M. E., and Walsh, P. C. (1977): *J. Urol.,* 117:309–312.
44. Miller, G. M., and Hinman, F. (1954): *J. Urol.,* 72:483–496.
45. Mobbs, B. G., Johnson, I. E., and Connolly, J. G. (1975): *J. Steroid. Biochem.,* 6:453–458.
46. Moore, R. A. (1944): *Surgery,* 16:152–168.
47. Philibert, D., and Raynaud, J.-P. (1973): *Steroids,* 22:89–98.
48. Pirke, K. M., and Doerr, P. (1973): *Acta Endocrinol. (Copenh.),* 74:792–800.
49. Raynaud, J.-P., Bouton, M. M., Ballet-Bourquin, D., Philibert, D., Tournemine, C., and Azadien-Boulanger, G. (1973): *Mol. Pharmacol.,* 9:520–533.
50. Scatchard, G. (1949): *Ann. N. Y. Acad. Sci.,* 51:660–672.
51. Shain, S. A., Boesel, R. W., Lamm, D. L., and Radwin, H. M. (1978): *Steroids,* 31:541–556.
52. Sirett, D. A. N., and Grant, J. K. (1978): *J. Endocrinol.,* 77:101–110.
53. Sköldefors, H., Blomstedt, B., and Carlström, K. (1978): *Scand. J. Urol. Nephrol.,* 12:111–117.
54. Snochowski, M., Pousette, Å., Ekman, P., Bression, D., Andersson, L., Högberg, B., and Gustafsson, J.-Å. (1977): *J. Clin. Endocrinol. Metab.,* 45:920–930.
55. Veenema, R. K. (1953): *J. Urol.,* 69:320–322.
56. de Voogt, H. J., and Dingjan, P. (1978): *Urol. Res.,* 6:151–158.
57. Wagner, R. K. (1972): *Hoppe Seylers Z. Physiol. Chem.,* 353:1235–1245.
58. Zava, D. T., Landrum, B., Horwitz, K. B., and McGuire, W. L. (1979): *Endocrinology,* 104:1007–1012.

Hormones and Cancer, edited by S. Iacobelli et al.
Raven Press, New York © 1980.

Glucocorticoid Receptors and Steroid Sensitivity of Acute Lymphoblastic Leukemia and Thymoma

Stefano Iacobelli, Paola Longo, *Renato Mastrangelo, *Raffaella Malandrino, and **Franco O. Ranelletti

*Laboratory of Molecular Endocrinology and Institutes of *Clinical Pediatrics and **Histology and Endocrinology, Catholic University, 00168 Rome, Italy*

Glucocorticoid hormones have a wide range of tissue specificity, intracellular receptor proteins having been demonstrated in various tissues and cultured cells (27). The manifold effects produced by glucocorticoids reflect the variety of ways in which the different cell types respond to the hormonal signal. For example, in liver cells glucocorticoids have been shown to induce the synthesis of several enzymes (18,41), while in fibroblasts and lymphoid cells they inhibit cell growth and eventually induce cell death (1,4,32,38,39). The magnitude of the response to glucocorticoids can also vary as a function of mutational events (2,43) or as a result of modifications produced during ontogenesis (17,26,29).

The relationship between cell differentiation and response to the hormonal signal is particularly interesting in the case of tumor cells. Thus, if response to hormone is attributable to cell differentiation, it may be inferred that the content of cell receptors may represent an indicator of differentiation and malignancy.

Over the last 10 years several studies have demonstrated that the analysis of hormone receptor content in breast cancer can provide useful information regarding the management of choice (25). It has also been demonstrated that patients with tumors containing high levels of receptors survive longer—independently of treatment—than patients with tumors containing low levels of receptors (19). These studies suggest that the presence of hormone receptors in tumor cells is an important biochemical marker with prognostic significance. Whether this important function of the receptor is entirely related to the degree of cell differentiation has not yet been elucidated.

The aim of the present investigation was to clarify this relationship. Two different models were studied: (a) acute lymphoblastic leukemia (ALL) for the relationship between glucocorticoid receptors (GR) and response to therapy, and (b) human thymus for the relationship between GR and differentiation of lymphatic cells.

METHODOLOGICAL ASPECTS

Acute Lymphoblastic Leukemia

Studies were carried out on 19 children (age 2–15 years). In each of the patients diagnosis of ALL was confirmed by cytological and cytochemical examination of blood and bone marrow smears. The percentage of lymphoblasts in the smears was never less than 80%. Leukocytes were isolated from defibrinated venous blood by spontaneous sedimentation through dextran mixtures (46). The contaminating red blood cells were lysed by hypotonic shock with 0.2 M NaCl. Cell viability was always greater than 85%.

Thymus and Thymoma

Normal thymus and thymoma tissues were collected from children undergoing cardiac surgery (normal thymus) or from patients with myasthenia gravis subjected to removal of the tumor. Diagnosis of thymoma was verified histologically.

Glucocorticoid Receptor Assay

GR analysis on ALL cells was carried out by a whole cell assay. Cells were suspended ($1–3 \times 10^7$ cells/ml) in Dulbecco modified Eagle medium (DME) supplemented with 25 mM Hepes, penicillin, and streptomycin and incubated with increasing concentrations of [^{3}H]triamcinolone acetonide [^{3}H]TA; (25 Ci/mM, The Radiochemical Center, Amersham) in the absence or presence of an excess of unlabeled triamcinolone acetonide at 37°C for 60 min. Following incubation, 1 ml of ice-cold phosphate-buffered saline (PBS) was quickly added and cells were sedimented by centrifugation at $160 \times g$ for 6 min. After two additional washes, the cell pellets were extracted with 1 ml ethanol; the extracts were counted with 8 ml scintillation fluid.

GR analysis on thymus and thymoma was carried out using a cytosol assay according to the procedure previously detailed (30).

Binding sites and equilibrium dissociation constant were calculated by Scatchard analysis (40) with the aid of a desk computer (Olivetti P6060).

In Vitro Steroid Sensitivity

Aliquots of cell suspensions in DME ($2–5 \times 10^6$ cells/ml) were incubated at 37°C for 22 hr in the presence of dexamethasone ($1–100 \times 10^{-9}$M). Cells were radioactively labeled for 60 min with [^{3}H]thymidine (The Radiochemical Center, Amersham) at the final concentration of 1×10^{-6}M. Cultures were terminated by adding 1 ml ice-cold PBS and centrifuged at $200 \times g$ for 6 min. Cell pellets were washed with PBS (twice) and extracted with 10% trichloroacetic acid (twice), ethanol/ethyl ether (1:1, vol/vol) and ethyl ether. The dried residues were dissolved with 0.3 ml formic acid and counted with 10 ml scintillation fluid.

In Vivo Sensitivity to Glucocorticoids

To all 19 ALL patients a short-term (3–10 days) trial of prednisone (60 mg/m²) was given before the start of combination polychemotherapy (24). Response was evaluated at the end of the third day of treatment, on the basis of changes (when present) in the percentage of peripheral blast cells, size of the spleen, lymph nodes, and mediastinal mass.

STUDIES ON ALL

Nosologically, ALL is a hetereogenous disease and attempts are currently being made to identify new parameters for use in prognostic evaluation. Lippman et al. (23) recently demonstrated a positive correlation between the levels of GR in lymphoblasts of patients with ALL and remission duration and survival independent of other factors such as age, sex, white blood count, and presence of surface markers. It was not evident from this study if the more favorable prognosis of patients with high receptor levels is a consequence of greater sensitivity to glucocorticoids included in the combination polychemotherapy. According to others, the extent of glucocorticoid effects *in vitro* on leukemic cells is not correlated with the levels of cellular GR (5,12,44). These observations suggest that the prognostic significance of GR in ALL is not related to the functional capacity of the receptor molecule and emphasizes that receptors are necessary for hormonal effects, but are not the sole regulators of sensitivity.

In the present study the following parameters were taken into consideration: (a) GR levels and steroid sensitivity of leukemic lymphoblasts, (b) remission following polychemotherapy, and (c) response to short-term glucocorticoid treatment.

An example of the results obtained following the above parameters is given in Fig. 1. In this particular case the cells contain approximately 5,000 receptor sites of high affinity ($K_D = 8.3 \times 10^{-9}$ M; upper right panel) and are sensitive to dexamethasone *in vitro* with $\sim 40\%$ reduction of thymidine incorporation at a steroid concentration in the range 1–10×10^{-9} M (lower left panel). Conversely, cell uptake of the nucleoside was not affected by steroid concentrations up to 1×10^{-7} M (lower left panel). Finally, prednisone treatment (60 mg/m² for 4 days) causes a decrease in the percentage of circulating blast cells (lower right panel) and subsequent polychemotherapy induces complete remission.

GR levels, inducibility of remission, and response to glucocorticoid treatment in 19 patients with ALL are reported in Table 1. The most significant results can be summarized as follows: (a) GR are present in all patients (mean receptor sites per cell = 6,909; median = 5,576); receptor concentration varies considerably from one patient to another (range = 688–20,791 sites per cell). (b) Approxi-

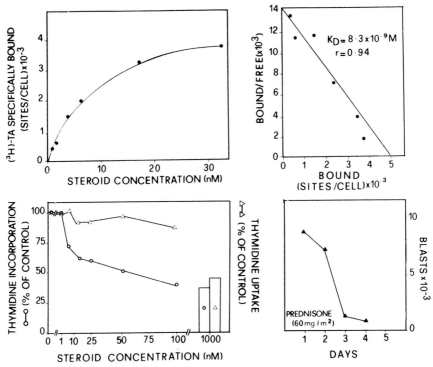

FIG. 1. GR, cell sensitivity to steroid and response to glucocorticoid treatment in one patient with ALL. **Upper left:** [³H]TA specifically bound as a function of free steroid concentration. **Upper right:** Specific binding data are plotted according to Scatchard's transformation. **Lower left:** Effects of increasing dexamethasone concentrations on thymidine uptake and incorporation into leukemic cells. **Lower right:** Decrease in the number of circulating lymphoblasts during prednisone treatment.

mately half the patients respond to glucocorticoid treatment with a reduction of more than 50% in the number of circulating lymphoblasts. (c) In patients responding to glucocorticoids, cells contain more than 4,000 GR sites while in nonresponders, the number of cases with more than 4,000 sites per cell is similar to that of patients with less than 4,000 sites per cell (5 versus 6). On the basis of receptor site number (more or less than 4,000), a highly significant difference is observed between responders and nonresponders ($p < 0.005$, Table 2A). (d) The difference between the two categories of patients is no longer significant when remission induction is used as the response parameter. From a comparison of results in Table 2A and B it appears that the increase in the rate of response to polychemotherapy refers exclusively to patients with less than 4,000 sites per cell, these patients being insensitive to glucocorticoid treatment. Thus a low number of GR would appear to reflect greater malignancy of cells, since the other drugs included in the combination polychemotherapy, the action of which are presumably not mediated by GR, were also poorly

TABLE 1. *GR levels in leukemic lymphoblasts isolated from patients with ALL in relation to* in vivo *response to glucocorticoids and inducibility of complete remission*

Case	Age (yr)	Sex	GR (sites/cell)	Response to glucocorticoids[a]	CR[b]
1	7	M	688	−	−
2	6	F	980	−	−
3	9	M	1,430	−	+
4	8	F	2,027	−	−
5	4	M	2,994	−	+
6	15	M	3,260	−	−
7	5	M	4,134	+	−
8	12	M	4,476	+	+
9	2	M	5,289	−	−
10	12	M	5,433	−	−
11	10	M	5,566	−	−
12	5	M	5,757	+	+
13	8	M	7,072	+	+
14	9	M	7,150	+	+
15	7	M	10,769	−	+
16	3	M	11,576	+	+
17	9	M	15,000	+	+
18	4	M	17,684	+	+
19	7	F	20,791	−	−

[a] The response was considered positive if the number of circulating lymphoblasts and/or the size of the measurable lesions decreased by more than 50%.
[b] CR, complete remission.

effective. This hypothesis is in keeping with the good correlation between responsiveness to glucocorticoids and inducibility of complete remission (15 versus 19; Table 1).

The difference in the response rate according to the cell content of GR induced us to see whether the affinity, besides the density of receptor sites in these

TABLE 2. *Distribution of responders and nonresponders to (A) glucocorticoids and (B) polychemotherapy on the basis of GR number in leukemic lymphoblasts*

	GR (sites/cell)	
	< 4,000	> 4,000
A. Glucocorticoids[a]		
Responders	0	8
Nonresponders	6	5
B. Polychemotherapy[b]		
Responders	2	8
Nonresponders	4	5

[a] $\chi^2 = 6.37$ ($p < 0.005$).
[b] $\chi^2 = 1.3$ (ns).

leukemic lymphoblasts, could give some indication of the degree of cell malignancy. As illustrated in Fig. 2, the dissociation constant (K_D) values in the nonresponders group varied from one patient to another (median $= 5.58 \times 10^{-9}$ M; range $= 1.34$–14.4×10^{-9} M) and show an inverse correlation with the number of GR sites. Conversely, the K_D values of the responders were distributed within a narrow interval (median $= 4.8 \times 10^{-9}$ M; range $= 2.53$–7.6×10^{-9} M), independently of cell content of GR.

Steroid Sensitivity of Leukemic Lymphoblasts

To establish whether or not the number of GR and the affinity of GR in the leukemic lymphoblasts were correlated with sensitivity to glucocorticoids, the effects elicited by dexamethasone on thymidine uptake and incorporation were investigated. These studies were prompted by the assumption that the interaction of steroids with receptors is only an early event in hormone action and that the presence of receptors in the cell does not guarantee per se the cell response to hormone. The results obtained revealed that the sensitivity of cells to dexamethasone varied markedly from one patient to another and also in the same patient depending on steroid concentration. Some examples are given in Fig. 3. In one case (Fig. 3A), maximal inhibition of cell uptake of thymidine occurred at 1×10^{-9} M dexamethasone, while higher steroid concentrations produced a fivefold increase in control levels. In another case (Fig. 3B), cell uptake and incorporation were not affected by dexamethasone concentrations up to 1×10^{-7} M. In other cases (Fig. 3C), thymidine incorporation displayed a biphasic pattern similar to that seen in the case reported in Fig. 3A. Finally, both cell uptake and incorporation can be paradoxically stimulated by dexamethasone (Fig. 3D).

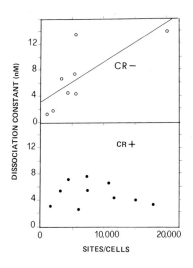

FIG. 2. The apparent equilibrium dissociation constant (K_D) of receptor–hormone complex as a function of the number of GR sites per cell of patients achieving (CR+) or not achieving (CR−) complete remission. CR+, $r = 0.19$ (ns); $N = 10$. CR−, $r = 0.79$; $p < 0.005$; $N = 8$.

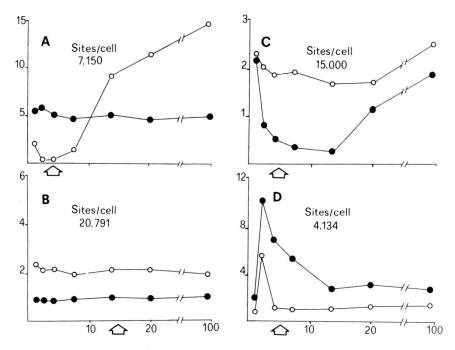

FIG. 3. Effects of increasing concentrations of dexamethasone on thymidine uptake (open circles) and incorporation (closed circles) in cells of four patients with ALL. Values of K_D relative to each case are indicated by *arrows. Abscissa,* concentrations of dexamethasone ($\times 10^{-9}$ M); *Ordinate,* [³H]thymidine (cpm $\times 10^{-2}$)/10^6 cells.

The fact that in a same population of leukemic lymphoblasts the effects induced by glucocorticoids can be either inhibitory or stimulatory, depending on steroid concentration, made it impossible for us to evaluate the overall sign of cell response to steroids. For example, in the case illustrated in Fig. 3C, if we had chosen a concentration of dexamethasone of 1×10^{-8} M, would the effect of steroid on these cells have been inhibitory? If the concentration selected had been only 10-fold higher than the previous concentration, would the cells have been insensitive to steroid? From the results in Fig. 3, neither the number nor the affinities of GR sites appear to correlate with cell sensitivity to dexamethasone, even assuming the K_D value as the concentration of steroid to which the hormonal effect refers. Evaluation of cell sensitivity to glucocorticoids at a fixed steroid concentration would therefore lead to contradictory results.

Following the correlation found by others in many animal and cell culture models (10,21,22,31) it is difficult to offer an explanation for the lack of correlation between the number of cellular GR and cell sensitivity to steroid. It should be emphasized, however, that factors other than number of receptors may regu-

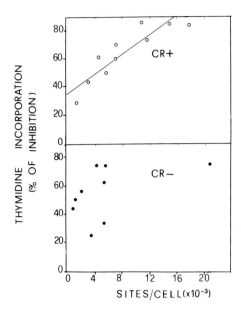

FIG. 4. Percentage inhibition of thymidine incorporation in leukemic cells in the presence of 1×10^{-6} M dexamethasone as a function of the number of GR sites per cell in patients achieving (CR+) or not achieving (CR−) complete remission. CR+, $r = 0.88$; $p < 0.001$; $N = 10$. CR−, $r = 0.45$ (ns); $N = 9$.

late the cellular response to hormone, for example, possible defects in the receptor mechanism due to neoplastic transformation (35,42,43). Furthermore, steroid receptor levels vary independently of the extent of hormone action, depending on the proliferative stage of the cells (3,15,28,45). Recent observations have also indicated that response to glucocorticoids may vary from inhibitory to stimulatory according to the metabolic state of the cell (16). Finally, some of the effects observed on whole cell population might be the result of combined effects on single cell components (11).

Cell Sensitivity to Pharmacological Concentrations of Glucocorticoids

In ALL, the lack of any evident correlation between the density of GR and the cell sensitivity to glucocorticoids *in vitro* is not in agreement with the high response rate to steroid observed in this disease (33,34). Since antileukemic treatment includes potent synthetic glucocorticoids reaching elevated blood concentrations, the sensitivity of leukemic lymphoblast to pharmacological doses of steroid was determined. The cells in all patients were sensitive to the inhibitory effect of 1×10^{-6} M dexamethasone on thymidine incorporation (mean decrease = 46%; range = 24–90%). Moreover, if the patients are divided into two groups according to remission induction by polychemotherapy, it can be seen (Fig. 5) that the extent of steroid-induced inhibition of thymidine incorporation

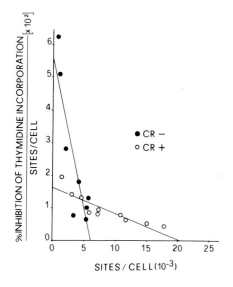

FIG. 5. Linear regression analysis of the number of GR sites per cell on the *in vitro* sensitivity of leukemic cells to 1×10^{-6} M dexamethasone in patients achieving (CR+) or not achieving (CR−) complete remission. CR+, $r = 0.88$; $N = 10$. CR−, $r = 0.88$; $N = 8$. The slopes of regression lines were significantly different ($F = 34$, $p < 0.001$).

correlates with the number of cell GR in the group of responders but not in that of nonresponders. These results are better illustrated by the plot shown in Fig. 6 which correlates the number of GR sites per cell with the ratio of steroid-induced inhibition of thymidine incorporation to the number of GR sites per cell. As can be seen, these two parameters show a linear correlation in both categories of patients and the slopes of regression lines are significantly different ($p < 0.001$).

This uniformity of effects at a pharmacological concentration of glucocorticoids, if compared with the variability observed using physiological concentra-

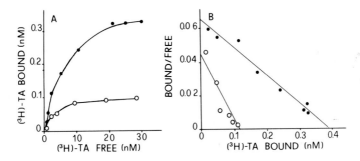

FIG. 6. Concentration dependence of [³H]TA binding to cytosols derived from normal thymus *(open circles)* and lymphoepithelial thymoma *(closed circles)*. **A:** Specific binding calculated as the difference between total binding and nonspecific binding. **B:** Scatchard analysis of the binding data taken from A.

tions, raises the question of whether these effects should still be considered as mediated by a receptor mechanism and not due to a nonspecific cytotoxic action. An answer will only be forthcoming when it is known how receptors work under pharmacological doses of hormone. On the other hand, the correlation between density of GR and sensitivity of the cells to pharmacological concentrations of glucocorticoids found in the group of responders could suggest that the hormone action in these cells is mediated by a receptor mechanism. This possibility, however, seems unlikely, since it does not explain why a similar correlation is not present in the non-responders. It is probable that besides its role of mediating hormone action, receptor in these leukemic cells represents an indicator of cell sensitivity to cytotoxic action of glucocorticoids related to the degree of cell malignancy.

STUDIES ON HUMAN THYMUS

Recent studies from various laboratories have demonstrated that lymphoid cell sensitivity to glucocorticoids depends simultaneously on several factors, i.e., the cell content of GR (6–8,13), metabolic and/or proliferative state of the cell (3,16,28,45), and the degree of cell differentiation (17,26,29,31). Over the last 3 years our studies have focused on the relationship between GR and cell differentiation in human thymic lymphocytes.

In the thymus, the bone marrow stem cell is committed through a sequence of maturation steps and released into the circulation as a mature T lymphocyte. This maturation pathway is regulated, among other factors, by the activity of epithelial cells. In the case of thymoma, the neoplastic transformation of these cells leads to changes in the maturation processes of lymphatic cells. As indicated in Table 3, thymocytes derived from thymoma undergo a more advanced maturative stage as compared with thymocytes from normal thymus. Thus, like the peripheral lymphocytes, a high percentage of cells bear the Fc receptor for IgM and respond to mitogens. The capacity to form heat-stable E rosettes, on

TABLE 3. *Surface markers and mitogen responsiveness in thymocytes from normal thymus and thymoma and in peripheral T lymphocytes*[a]

	Thymus	Thymoma	Peripheral T lymphocytes
SERFC$_S$	70–90%	70–90%	3%
LERFC$_S$	No	No	70%
T$_G$	0–4%	2–5%	5–16%
T$_M$	2–12%	20–53%	36–68%
Con A	NR	NR	R
PHA	NR	NR	R

[a] SERFC$_S$, heat-stable E rosettes forming cells; LERFC$_S$, heat-labile E rosettes forming cells; NR, not responsive; R, responsive.

the other hand, suggests that these cells originate from the thymus where, under the influence of neoplastic epithelial cells, they reach a more advanced degree of immunological maturation (20).

Both normal thymus and thymoma contain specific receptors for glucocorticoids. Binding of [³H]TA to cytosol is saturable at steroid concentrations between 10 and 20×10^{-9} M (Fig. 6A). A Scatchard plot of the binding data (40) indicates that [³H]TA, both in the thymus and thymoma, binds to a single class of high affinity receptor sites (Fig. 6B).

Receptors from thymus and thymoma show a similar specificity (Table 4), and in both tissues the receptor–steroid complexes are readily transported into the nuclei through a temperature-dependent process (Fig. 7) in a manner similar to that observed in rat thymus (48).

As shown in Table 5, GR content in thymoma is approximately three times higher than in normal thymus; other properties such as affinity and sedimentation

TABLE 4. *Steroid specificity of GR sites in human thymus and thymoma*

Competing steroid	Thymus		Thymoma	
	Molar ratio	% Inhibition[a]	Molar ratio	% Inhibition[a]
TA	10^{-1}	60	10^{-1}	46
	10	40	10	32
	10^2	35	10^2	30
Dexamethasone	10^{-1}	62	10^{-1}	45
	10	42	10	30
	10^2	36	10^2	28
Prednisolone	10^{-1}	74	10^{-1}	65
	10	57	10	38
	10^2	42	10^2	32
Cortisol	10^{-1}	77	10^{-1}	77
	10	51	10	44
	10^2	36	10^2	28
Corticosterone	10^{-1}	80	10^{-1}	77
	10	60	10	45
	10^2	35	10^2	28
R 5020[b]	10^{-1}	90	10^{-1}	93
	10	80	10	76
	10^2	50	10^2	40
Aldosterone	10^{-1}	85	10^{-1}	93
	10	70	10	64
	10^2	46	10^2	38
Estradiol-17β	10^{-1}	100	10^{-1}	100
	10	100	10	92
	10^2	84	10^2	90
Testosterone	10^{-1}	100	10^{-1}	100
	10	95	10	92
	10^2	92	10^2	92

[a] Results are expressed as percentage of inhibition of [³H]TA bound in the presence of unlabeled steroid relative to control (no steroid added).
[b] 17,21-Dimethyl-19-nor-4,9-pregnadiene-3,20-dione.

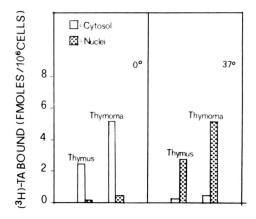

FIG. 7. Effect of temperature on the distribution of receptor–hormone complex between supernatant and nuclei of thymocytes derived from normal thymus and lymphoepithelial thymoma.

TABLE 5. *GR and steroid sensitivity of thymocytes from normal thymus and thymoma*

	GR (fmoles/mg protein) mean ± SD	K_D ($\times 10^{-9}$ M)	S_{20_ω} [a]	Thymidine incorporation[b]
Normal thymus (4)[c]	109 ± 5.3	2.34 ± 3.0	3.6/7.0	65–75
Thymoma (4)	292 ± 83	4.0 ± 5.0	8.0	50–70

[a] S_{20_ω} = sedimentation coefficient of receptor–steroid complex.
[b] Percent of inhibition relative to control.
[c] Number of cases in parentheses.

rate of receptor sites are similar in the two tissues. Despite the greater GR content, the sensitivity of thymoma cells to steroid-induced inhibition of thymidine incorporation is not unlike that observed in normal thymus (Table 5). This lack of correlation between GR content and cell response to steroid emphasizes that the receptor levels alone cannot explain the amplitude of cell sensitivity to hormone. Furthermore it suggests that the density of receptors in the cell may be regulated by the degree of cell differentiation, independently of changes in cell sensitivity to hormone.

CONCLUSIONS AND PERSPECTIVES

The growing interest in hormone receptors in recent years, while providing data in the molecular events of the receptor mechanism, has, on the other hand, masked the more general problem of its integration with other systems regulating cell function. As a result, our present knowledge on hormone action, which is based on a "static" receptor model not taking into account other regulatory factors, is even more inadequate. Some of these factors, e.g., the metabolic and/or proliferative state of the cell, aging, and differentiation, have recently been identified (3,16,17,26,28,29,31,36,37,45). The complexity of the receptor model has increased with the discovery of a variety of receptor defects in the neoplastic cells and the mutants (2,35,42,43). From these studies it becomes apparent that the regulation points in the receptor–steroid interaction sequence are multiple and interrelated with other systems (9,47).

The present study on ALL and human thymus indicates that GR can provide useful information on differentiation of lymphoid cells. Some of this information may be employed for prognostic purposes. However, the apparent lack of correlation in ALL cells between GR content and sensitivity to steroid indicates that the evaluation of hormone actions *in vitro,* even employing dose–response curves, fails to provide any reliable information.

Using a whole cell binding assay, no relationship was found among the levels of steroid receptors in leukemic lymphoblasts of ALL and the *in vitro* actions of glucocorticoids or response to therapy. Similar results have recently been reported by Duval et al. *(this volume).* Among the factors explaining this lack of correlation are the heterogeneity of the leukemic cell population and the artificial subtraction of influences present *in vivo.* These influences may condition the cell response to glucocorticoids, even reversing the sign of response observed *in vitro* (14).

In normal thymus and thymoma the GR content correlates with the immunological maturation of lymphoid cells, but not with cell sensitivity to steroid. This lack of correlation between receptor density and hormone action is, however, not surprising, given that the interaction of steroid with the receptor is an early event in hormone action and at various levels, multiple mechanisms can integrate the receptor with other regulatory systems. The dependence of receptor levels on the functional state of the cell is at present the better understood regulation. Other regulatory mechanisms acting more distally along the sequence of receptor mechanism may eventually be discovered. These data will then lead to a better understanding of the role of hormone receptors in the economy of the cell and will broaden its prognostic significance in neoplasia. The observation that in a high percentage of cases, mutants insensitive to glucocorticoids have altered receptor systems suggests that the receptor is one of the regulatory points more frequently influenced by genetic alteration and also provides a stimulus to pursue receptor studies in an attempt to establish a better management of endocrine-related tumors.

REFERENCES

1. Berliner, D. L., and Ruhmann, A. G. (1966): *Endocrinology,* 78:373–382.
2. Bourgeois, S., and Newby, R. (1977): *Cell,* 11:423–430.
3. Cidlowski, J. A., and Michaels, G. A. (1977): *Nature,* 267:643–645.
4. Claman, H. N., Moorhead, J. W., and Benner, W. H. (1971): *J. Lab. Clin. Med.,* 78:499–507.
5. Crabtree, G. R., Smith, R. A., and Munck, A. (1979): In: *Seventh Tenovus Workshop. Glucocorticoid Action and Leukemia,* edited by P. A. Bell and N. M. Borthwick, pp. 191–204. Alpha Omega, Cardiff.

6. Duval, D., Dausse, J. P., and Dardenne, M. (1976): *Biochim. Biophys. Acta,* 451:82–91.
7. Duval, D., Dardenne, M., Dausse, J. P. and Homo, F. (1977): *Biochim. Biophys. Acta,* 496:312–320.
8. Duval, D., Homo, F., Fournier, C., and Dausse, J. P. (1979): *Cell Immunol.,* 46:1–11.
9. Giddings, S. J., and Young, D. A. (1974): *J. Steroid Biochem.,* 5:587–595.
10. Harmon, J. M., Norman, M. R., Folwlkes, B. J., and Thompson, E. B. (1979): *J. Cell. Physiol.,* 98:267–278.
11. Homo, F., and Duval, D. (1979): *J. Clin. Lab. Immunol.,* 2:329–332.
12. Homo, F., Duval, D., Meyer, P., Belas, F., Debre, P., and Binet, J. L. (1978): *Br. J. Haematol.,* 38:491–499.
13. Homo, F., Harousseau, J. L., and Duval, D. (1979): *Cancer Treat. Rep.,* 63:1198.
14. Iacobelli, S., and Ranelletti, F. O., Longo, P., Riccardi, R., and Mastrangelo, R. (1978): *Cancer Res.,* 38:4257–4262.
15. Iacobelli, S., Ranelletti, F. O., Natoli, C., and Longo, P. (1980): In: *Control Mechanisms in Animal Cells: Specific Growth Factors,* edited by L. Jimenez de Asua, R. Levi-Montalcini, R. Shields, and S. Iacobelli, pp. 121–132. Raven Press, New York.
16. Johonson, K. L., Lan, N. C., and Baxter, J. D. (1979): *J. Biol. Chem.,* 254:7785–7794.
17. Jost, A. (1971): In: *Hormones in Development,* edited by H. Hambrough and E. J. W. Barrington, pp. 1–18. Appleton-Century-Crofts, New York.
18. Kenney, F. T., (1962): *J. Biol. Chem.,* 237:3495–3498.
19. Knight, W. A., III, Livingstone, R. B., Gregory, E. J., and McGuire, W. L. (1977): *Cancer Res.,* 37:4669–4671.
20. Lauriola, L., Piantelli, M., Carbone, X., Dina, M. A., Scoppetta, C., and Musiani, P. (1979): *Clin. Exp. Immunol.,* 37:502–506.
21. Lippman, M. E., and Barr, R. (1977): *J. Immunol.,* 118:1977–1981.
22. Lippman, M. E., Halterman, R. M., Leventhal, B., Perry, S., and Thompson, E. B. (1973): *J. Clin. Invest.,* 52:1715–1725.
23. Lippman, M. E., Konior-Yarbro, G. S., and Leventhal, B. C. (1978): *Cancer Res.,* 38:4251–4256.
24. Mastrangelo, R., Romanini, A., Cellini, N., Parenti, D., De Renzis, C., Riccardi, R., Cimatti, G., and Malandrino, R. (1978): *Tumori,* 64:607–612.
25. McGuire, W. L., editor (1978): *Hormones, Receptors, and Breast Cancer,* Raven Press, New York.
26. Moscona, A. A., and Piddington, R. (1966): *Biochim. Biophys. Acta,* 121:409–411.
27. Munck, A., and Leung, K. (1977): In: *Receptors and Mechanisms of Action of Steroid Hormones, Part II,* edited by J. R. Pasqualini, pp. 311–397, Marcel Dekker, New York.
28. Neifeld, J. P., Lippman, M. E., and Tormey, D. C. (1977): *J. Biol. Chem.,* 254:2972–2977.
29. Platzker, A. C. G., Kitterman, J. A., Mescher, E. J., Clements, J. A., and Tooley, W. H. (1975): *Pediatrics,* 56:554–561.
30. Ranelletti, F. O., Carmignani, M., Iacobelli, S., and Tonali, P. (1978): *Cancer Res.,* 38:516–520.
31. Ranelletti, F. O., Iacobelli, S., Carmignani, M., Sica, G., Natoli, C., and Tonali, P. (1980): *Cancer Res. (in press).*
32. Ranelletti, F. O., Iacobelli, S., Longo, P., Natoli, C., and Carmignani, M. (1979): *Cancer Treat Rep.,* 63:1197.
33. Ranney, H., and Gelhorn, A. (1975): *Am. J. Med.,* 22:405–413.
34. Roath, S., Israels, M., and Wilkinson, J. (1964): *Q. J. Med.,* 33:257–283.
35. Rosenau, W., Baxter, J. D., Rousseau, G. G., and Tomkins, G. M. (1972): *Nature (New Biol.),* 237:20–24.
36. Roth, G. S. (1975): *Biochim. Biophys. Acta,* 399:145–156.
37. Roth, G. S., and Livingston, J. N. (1976): *Endocrinology,* 99:831–839.
38. Ruhmann, A. G., and Berlier, D. L. (1965): *Endocrinology,* 76:916–927.
39. Santisteban, G. A., and Doughterty, T. F. (1954): *Endocrinology,* 66:550–558.
40. Scatchard, G., (1949): *Ann NY Acad. Sci.,* 51:660–672.
41. Schimke, R. T., Sweeney, E. A., and Berlin, C. M. (1965): *J. Biol. Chem.,* 240:322–331.
42. Sibley, C. H., and Tomkins, G. M. (1974): *Cell,* 2:213–220.
43. Sibley, C. H., and Tomkins, G. M. (1974): *Cell,* 2:221–227.

44. Sloman, J. C., and Bell, P. A. (1979): In: *Seventh Tenovus Workshop. Glucocorticoid Action and Leukemia,* edited by P. A. Bell and N. M. Borthwick, pp. 161–169. Alpha Omega, Cardiff.
45. Smith, K. A., Crabtree, G. R., Kennedy, S. G., and Munck, A. (1977): *Nature,* 267:523–525.
46. Thompson, E. B., Granner, D. K., Geleherter, T., Erikson, J., and Hager, G. L. (1979): *Mol. Cell. Endocrinol.,* 15:135–150.
47. Wira, C., and Munck, A. (1974): *J. Biol. Chem.,* 249:5328–5336.

Hormones and Cancer, edited by S. Iacobelli et al.
Raven Press, New York © 1980.

Glucocorticoid Receptors in Normal and Neoplastic Human Lymphoid Cells

F. Homo, D. Duval, *J. L. Harousseau, and **C. Thierry

*Departments of Physiology and Pharmacology, INSERM Unit 7, Necker Hospital, 75015 Paris; *Hematology Service, Saint Louis Hospital, 75475 Paris Cedex 10; and **Department of Tumor Immunopharmacology, Paul Lamarque Center, St. Eloi Hospital, 34059 Montpellier, France*

In all steroid-responsive tissues the initiation of the hormonal response is thought to be mediated by a specific receptor system in the cytoplasm of the target cells (12). The main argument supporting this assumption is the existence of a close correlation between the affinity of various steroids for the cytoplasmic binding sites and their biological activity (2,38). Given the fact that the binding step is an obligatory event in the mechanism of steroid action, attempts have been made to infer the steroid sensitivity of various tissues from the determination of their steroid receptor content. This procedure has been used mainly in neoplastic tissues such as mammary tumors (29), prostatic carcinoma (18), or leukemia (13). Indeed, in lymphoid cells glucocorticoids have been shown to induce several events such as the inhibition of both transport and synthesis of macromolecules (30,32) and, to some extent, nuclear damage and cell lysis (1,15,26). Although this approach has been shown to be useful for predicting the response to hormonal therapy in breast cancer, the situation still remains obscure in leukemic cells despite a considerable amount of investigation.

Lippman et al. (27) first presented evidence in favor of such a correlation between cytosolic receptor content and *in vitro* sensitivity in patients with acute lymphocytic leukemia. However, Sibley and Tomkins (40) and Lippman et al. (28) later described the existence of corticoresistant lymphoma or lymphoblastoid cell lines which contained glucocorticoid receptors. Furthermore, Bird et al. (3), as well as Crabtree et al. (7), Homo et al. (22), and Sloman and Bell (41), failed to demonstrate any significant correlation between the number of steroid receptors and the *in vitro* sensitivity of human lymphoblastoid cell lines or human leukemic cells.

We present evidence for the presence of glucocorticoid receptors in all human lymphoid cells, both normal and malignant. In addition, we report that in leukemia, the extent of glucocorticoid effects *in vitro* does not correlate with the level of cellular glucocorticoid receptors. Finally, we have also studied the short-term *in vivo* response and the level of glucocorticoid receptors in some cases of acute lymphocytic leukemia.

METHODS

The methods used for the measurement of *in vitro* steroid sensitivity by following the inhibitory effects of dexamethasone on uridine and thymidine incorporation or the lytic effect of this drug have been described in detail elsewhere (23). Briefly, the cells were isolated from peripheral blood by centrifugation on Ficoll-Hypaque, washed and adjusted at a concentration of 10^7 cells/ml in minimum essential medium (MEM) supplemented with 2 mM glutamine, 1 mM sodium pyruvate, 100 U/ml penicillin, 100 μg/ml streptomycin, and nonessential amino acids. The cell suspensions were preincubated for 22 hr at 37°C in an atmosphere of 5% CO_2 in air in the absence or presence of 10^{-6}M dexamethasone and then received 1 μCi of either [^{3}H]uridine (25 Ci/mmole) or [^{3}H]thymidine (27 Ci/mmole). After 2 hr additional incubation, the reaction was terminated by addition of ice-cold 5% trichloroacetic acid. The precipitates were filtered on Whatman GF/A filters and washed three times with 10 ml of ice-cold 5% trichloroacetic acid. The radioactivity collected on the filters was counted by liquid scintillation spectrometry.

Cell viability was estimated by the trypan blue exclusion procedure. The methods used for the determination of glucocorticoid receptors have been described in detail elsewhere (8,10,23).

Nevertheless, it should be pointed out that all the measurements of steroid binding sites in this study were performed on freshly isolated lymphocyte suspensions using a whole cell assay at 37°C. In many of the previously published experiments (13,27), the binding studies were conducted on cytosol preparations at 0 to 4°C. It has been shown that this procedure leads to an underestimation of the number of receptors. To illustrate this possibility, we have determined the number of dexamethasone binding sites in mouse thymocytes either by whole cell assay or by the classic cytosol assay (11). As shown in Table 1, the number of glucocorticoid receptors found by the latter assay is significantly lower than that obtained in the whole cell assay. This difference may be attributed either

TABLE 1. *Determination of dexamethasone binding sites in mouse thymocytes*[a]

	Whole cell assay (N = 4)	Cytosol assay (N = 3)
R_n	7,050 ± 822	4,200[b]
K_D	3.04 ± 1.05 × 10^{-8} M	4.8 × 10^{-8} M

[a] R_n, number of binding sites per cell; K_D, dissociation constant of the steroid–receptor complex determined by Scatchard plot analysis.

[b] Calculated on the basis of 3.9 × 10^{-3} mg cytosolic protein/10^6 cells, mean value of 16 experiments.

This experiment was done in collaboration with T. J. Schmidt (May 1978).

to the fact that the whole cell assay ensures the determination of both cytoplasmic and nuclear receptors or to a partial inactivation of the receptors during cytosol preparation (16,24,35,41).

RESULTS

Determination of Glucocorticoid Receptors in Normal and Malignant Human Lymphoid Cells

Human Peripheral Lymphocytes

The level of glucocorticoid receptors was determined in the whole leukocyte population isolated from peripheral blood of normal subjects (25–35 years old) and in lymphocyte subpopulations enriched either in T + "null" cells or in B cells by filtration on an immunoabsorbant column [Anti-F(ab')$_2$]. Figure 1 shows the specific binding of [^{3}H]dexamethasone as a function of the tracer concentration in the unseparated population, after monocyte depletion, and in various lymphocyte subpopulations.

Scatchard analysis of these binding curves gives straight lines consistent with the existence of a single class of binding sites. The number of binding sites and the affinities of the receptors for the tracer do not differ significantly from one population to another. The number of binding sites is in the range of 3,600 to 6,000 sites per cell, and K_D values average 5×10^{-8} M (23).

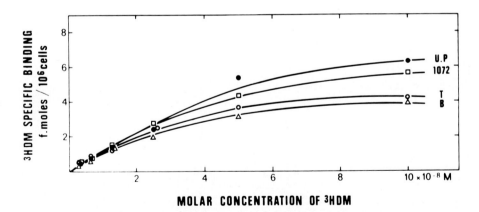

FIG. 1. The specific binding of [^{3}H]dexamethasone ([^{3}H]DM) as a function of tracer concentration in unseparated lymphocyte populations after monocyte depletion (U.P.) in populations isolated from immunoabsorbant column (T + "null" and B cells) and in a T + "null" cell subpopulation obtained by gradient centrifugation (fraction d = 1.072). Cells (10^7/ml) were incubated for 20 min at 37°C in the presence of various concentrations of the tracer, in the range 3×10^{-9} to 10^{-7} M. The results, expressed as fmoles/10^6 cells, represent the average values obtained in five normal male subjects (25–35 years old).

Human Thymus Cells

We have also measured the number of steroid receptors in thymus cells obtained from children (four females, five males, 2–96 months old) during cardiac surgery. Figure 2 shows a binding curve obtained in a typical experiment. The average number of binding sites in nine experiments was 3,100 sites per cell, a value consistently, but not significantly, lower than that measured in circulating lymphocytes (4,700 binding sites per cell, after monocyte depletion). Affinity constants, determined by Scatchard analysis, were similar in both tissues ($\sim 5 \times 10^{-8}$M) (19).

Studies in Chronic Lymphocytic Leukemia

The patients under investigation were classified on the basis of clinical and hematological features according to Rai's modified classification (36) and comprised nine patients in stage 0, nine patients in stage I, four patients in stage III, and five patients in stage IV. This last group is of poor prognosis and is the only one in which corticotherapy is used. The values for specific binding of [³H]dexamethasone in lymphocytes from 21 patients are shown in Fig. 3. For 18 patients (7 stage 0, 5 stage I, 4 stage III, and 2 stage IV) these values fell within the range of normal values regardless of whether or not the patients were under treatment. The only patient with a highly abnormal level of steroid receptors (fivefold normal) was a stage IV patient who, in addition to chronic lymphocytic leukemia, was suffering from Hodgkin's disease.

In all of these patients, the affinity of the receptor for dexamethasone was

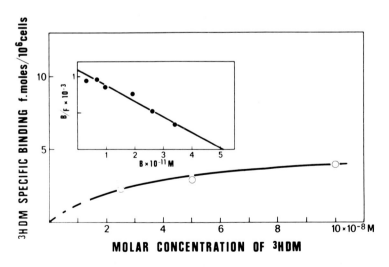

FIG. 2. Specific binding of [³H]dexamethasone [³H]DM) in children's thymocytes from a typical experiment. *Inset* represents Scatchard plot analysis of the binding curve.

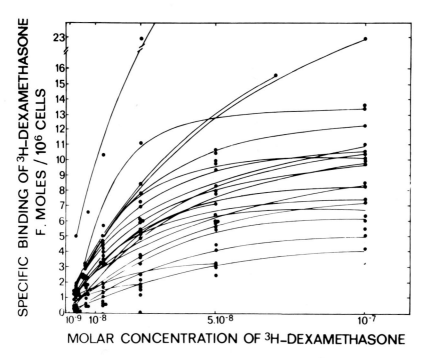

FIG. 3. Specific binding of [³H]dexamethasone in lymphocytes isolated from the blood of 21 patients with chronic lymphatic leukemia. Each line denotes the binding curve obtained for one patient.

close to control values (22). These results are in good agreement with those obtained in another series of 19 patients previously investigated in our laboratory (21).

Acute Lymphocytic Leukemia

Studies were performed in 26 patients with acute leukemia, comprising mostly patients with acute lymphocytic leukemia and 2 patients with chronic myelocytic leukemia in "lymphoid" blast crisis.

In each of the patients studied, cytological examinations were performed. Blood and bone marrow samples were stained by several methods including May-Grünwald-Giemsa, periodic acid/Schiff peroxidase, and, in numerous cases, acid phosphatase reagent. Detection of T cells was performed by the E-rosette test using sheep erythrocytes, and detection of B cells was performed by immunofluorescence of surface immunoglobulins. All the studies were done at the time of diagnosis and none of these patients had received prior chemotherapy.

Figure 4 (right panel) shows the values of glucocorticoid binding sites, determined by Scatchard plot analysis, in 23 patients. The concentration of glucocorti-

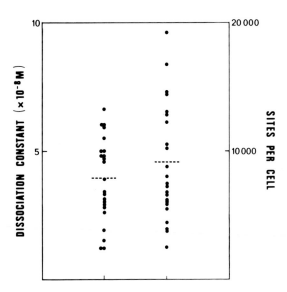

FIG. 4. Specific binding of [³H]dexamethasone ([³H]DM) **(right)** and the apparent dissociation constant of the steroid–receptor interaction (K_D 37°C, **left**) were determined in leukocytes isolated from the blood of 23 patients with acute lymphocytic leukemia. In each case these values were calculated by Scatchard plot analysis. *Dotted lines* represent the means of individual determinations.

coid receptors varied widely from one patient to another, ranging from 2,600 to 19,200 sites per cell. The mean receptor value was about 9,000 sites (9,140 ± 4,390, $N = 23$) per cell. Dissociation constants, determined from the slope of the Scatchard plots, were in the range of 1.2 to 6.7×10^{-8} M (mean value 3.9 ± 1.6×10^{-8} M, $N = 23$) and appeared similar to those determined for dexamethasone receptor interaction in normal human lymphocytes (Fig. 4, left panel).

Attempts have been made to correlate the level of steroid receptors with several parameters including immunological markers, white blood cell (WBC) counts, and patient sex or age. The results presented in Table 2 reveal that the number of glucocorticoid receptors tends to be higher in males than in females. Konior-Yarbro et al. (25) also mentioned some variation in the level of glucocorticoid receptors with sex and age, but their results were not statistically significant. This possible sex difference in receptor level should therefore be confirmed in more extensive studies. Within our group of patients we failed to show any difference in receptor content between T cell and "null" cell acute leukemia in contrast with previously reported results (25). These results also confirm the predominance of acute lymphocytic leukemia of T cell origin in older boys with a high WBC count, whereas leukemia devoid of receptors for sheep erythrocytes was generally found in younger children, with an almost equal distribution between the sexes.

TABLE 2. *Number of glucocorticoid receptors in leukocytes isolated from the blood of patients with acute lymphocytic leukemia or chronic myelocytic leukemia in "lymphoid" blast crisis, in relation to sex and age*

	Acute lymphocytic leukemia						
	"Null" cell leukemia				T cell leukemia		
	Female		Male		Male		
	5,958 ± 2,336	$N=6$	10,128 ± 3,332	$N=6$	10,365 ± 4,990	$N=6$	
< 10 yr							
GR[a]	5,657 ± 2,906	$N=4$	10,087 ± 2,606	$N=4$	5,820[b]	$N=1$	
WBC (× 10³/ mm³)	2.22 ± 15.8		23.5 ± 16.7		18.5		
> 10 yr							
GR[a]	6,560	$N=2$	10,210	$N=2$	11,274 ± 4,993	$N=5$	
WBC (× 10³/ mm³)	60.6		26		95.5 ± 76.9		

	CML in "lymphoid" blasts crisis		
	Female	Male	
GR[a]	7,830 $N=1$	12,240 $N=1$	
WBC (× 10³/ mm³)	334	150	

[a] GR, glucocorticoid receptors.
[b] This patient does not exhibit circulating lymphoblasts.

Absence of Correlation Between the Effects of Glucocorticoid *In Vitro* and the Levels of Glucocorticoid Receptors in Human Lymphoid Cells

Normal Human Lymphoid Tissues

The inhibitory effects of glucocorticoids on uridine and thymidine incorporation were determined *in vitro* in peripheral human lymphocytes and in thymocytes of children, in relation to their glucocorticoid receptors (19,23). Although the number of steroid binding sites was consistently (but not significantly) lower in human thymocytes than in peripheral lymphocytes (average values are 3,100 and 4,700 sites per cell, respectively), thymocytes were far more sensitive to the effects of steroid than circulating lymphocytes. After 24 hr of incubation in the presence of 10^{-6} M dexamethasone, the percentages of inhibition in thymocytes were 70% for uridine incorporation and over 90% for thymidine incorporation, whereas under similar conditions the extent of steroid-induced inhibitions of precursor incorporation into peripheral lymphocytes did not exceed 20 to 30% (Table 3). It should be emphasized that the thymus of children is characterized by a high rate of cell division (5,6) which is reflected in the high level of

TABLE 3. Number of glucocorticoid receptors and the inhibitory effects of dexamethasone on [³H]uridine and [³H]thymidine incorporation in circulating lymphocytes of normal adult subjects and in thymocytes of children

	GR[a] (mean	[³H]Uridine		[³H]Thymidine	
		Incorporation (cpm/10^6 cells)	Inhibition (%)	Incorporation (cpm/10^6 cells)	Inhibition (%)
Circulating lymphocytes (N=5)	4,700	830 ± 203	20.4 ± 12.9	433 ± 178	23.8 ± 19.3
Children's thymocytes (N=9)	3,100	328.9 ± 138.5	70.1 ± 8.1	5,958 ± 6,397	95.9 ± 3.9

[a] GR, glucocorticoid receptors.

spontaneous (i.e., in the absence of steroid) thymidine incorporation *in vitro*. Indeed, this level is almost 10 times higher in child thymocytes than in circulating lymphocytes. Claman (5) postulated that the *in vivo* shrinkage of human thymus in the presence of hydrocortisone is not due to cytolysis but can be explained in terms of growth inhibition. Given the high rate of cell division in infant thymus, any agent which blocks cell proliferation without changing the intrathymic cell death would cause a decrease of the thymus size.

Chronic Lymphocytic Leukemia

Glucocorticoid sensitivity was also studied in lymphoid cell suspensions isolated from patients with chronic lymphocytic leukemia. The results of these experiments are presented in Fig. 5. From this figure it is apparent that the percentage of dexamethasone-induced inhibition of uridine incorporation increases significantly with the evolution of the disease to reach about 70% in the patients at stage III/IV, whether or not they had previously been treated by chemotherapy. No such parallel increase could be observed for the effect of steroid on thymidine incorporation. In each group of patients the percentage of inhibition in the presence of steroid was close to the value determined for normal circulating lymphocytes. It is, however, well known that in chronic lymphocytic leukemia few proliferating cells escape into the circulation, and they are therefore often undetectable by peripheral examination.

Acute Lymphocytic Leukemia

Attempts have been made to establish a correlation between the level of glucocorticoid receptors and the inhibitory effects of steroids on uridine or thymidine incorporation *in vitro*. As shown in Fig. 6, no correlation could be found between

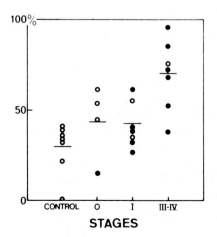

FIG. 5. Percentages of steroid-induced inhibition of uridine incorporation in isolated lymphocytes from control subjects and patients with chronic lymphocytic leukemia at stages 0, I, and III–IV. *Open circles* correspond to untreated patients, and *closed circles* to patients under treatment. The differences between the average values of inhibition of nucleoside incorporation in control subjects and stage III–IV patients were statistically significant: 29.3 and 69.6%, respectively; $p < 0.02$.

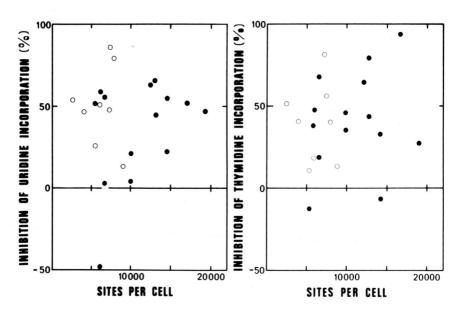

FIG. 6. Percentages of steroid-induced inhibition of uridine incorporation **(left)** and thymidine incorporation **(right)** are plotted as a function of the number of binding sites per cell, in 22 patients with acute lymphocytic leukemia. *Open circles* denote female patients; *closed circles* denote male patients.

the number of steroid binding sites and the percentage of steroid-induced inhibition of both uridine and thymidine incorporations.

Moreover, in some patients we have even noted a stimulation of nucleoside incorporation in the presence of dexamethasone, although the patients possess lymphocyte glucocorticoid receptors. Similarly, the sex difference observed in terms of glucocorticoid receptors is not associated with any sex difference in steroid sensitivity.

Dexamethasone-induced inhibition of uridine (left panel) and thymidine (right panel) incorporation as a function of the spontaneous levels of nucleoside incorporation are plotted in Fig. 7. A significant correlation exists between these parameters ($r = 0.49$, $p < 0.01$, $N = 25$; and $r = 0.51$, $p < 0.01$, $N = 25$ for uridine and thymidine, respectively), suggesting that the effects of the steroid *in vitro* could be linked to the proliferative and metabolic state of the cells.

The effect of dexamethasone on cell viability, which represents the endpoint of the steroid action, was also determined over a 22-hr incubation period *in vitro* in relation to receptor levels. As shown in Fig. 8, in the absence of steroid the cell viability remained greater than 75% in 15 of 23 patients and showed only an appreciable decrease in 8 of 23 patients. Dexamethasone (10^{-6} M) produced a supplementary diminution of cell viability in only 7 of 23 patients. This effect was more frequent in those patients who showed an already high incidence

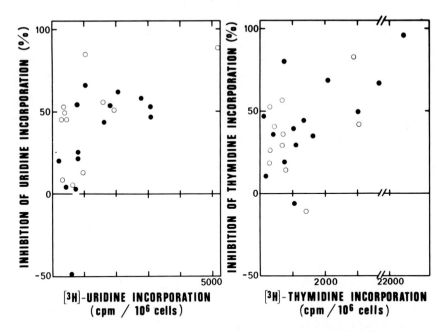

FIG. 7. Percentages of steroid-induced inhibition of uridine incorporation **(left panel)** and thymidine incorporation **(right panel)** are plotted as a function of the spontaneous levels of nucleoside incorporation (i.e., in the absence of steroid) over a 24-hr period in 25 patients with acute lymphocytic leukemia. *Open circles* denote female patients; *closed circles* denote male patients. In each case, there is a significant correlation between the inhibitory effect of the steroid and the level of nucleoside incorporation ($r = 0.49$, $p < 0.01$; and $r = 0.5$, $p < 0.01$, as determined using a linear regression adjustment, for uridine and thymidine, respectively).

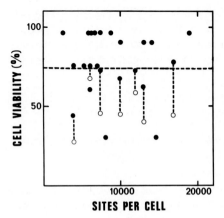

FIG. 8. Percentage of viable cells, after 22-hr incubations *in vitro*, in lymphoid cells isolated from the blood of 23 patients with acute lymphocytic leukemia. *Closed circles:* spontaneous viability (i.e., in the absence of steroid). *Open circles:* percentage of viable cells after 22-hr incubations in the presence of 10^{-6} M dexamethasone.

TABLE 4. *Number of glucocorticoid receptors and the percentage inhibition of thymidine incorporation (in the presence of 10^{-6} M dexamethasone) determined in 11 patients with acute lymphocytic leukemia before the start of corticotherapy*

	Positive response		Negative response	
	Before	After	Before	After
WBC ($\times 10^3$/ mm³)	$39.4 \pm 32{,}7$	9.8 ± 5.6	21.7 ± 16.2	17.7 ± 14.6
Blast (%)	$80.5 \pm 14{,}1$	44.8 ± 20	50.4 ± 30.7	53.2 ± 36.9
GR (sites/cell)	8,275	F 5,565 M 10,080	6,170	F 4,650 M 8,440
Inhibition (%)	41.5 ± 21.8		35.2 ± 31.4	
Sex ratio (M/F)	3/3		2/3	
Age (yr)	6 < 15		5 < 15	
	5N, 1T		3N, 1T, 1(−)	

GR, glucocorticoid receptors.

of spontaneous cell death (5 of 7). Under similar conditions, the viability of normal human peripheral lymphocytes remained virtually unaffected by steroid. Again, no correlation could be found between the lytic effect of steroid *in vitro* and the number of glucocorticoid receptors.

Response to Short-Term Glucocorticoid Therapy

Eleven patients were treated with prednisone (40 mg/m²) for 2 to 4 days before starting combined chemotherapy. Among these patients only six responded to steroids by a marked decrease both in WBC count and in the percentage of circulating blast cells.

The clinical features and the results of *in vitro* determinations in responding and nonresponding patients are compared in Table 4. No significant differences could be found between these two groups in terms of glucocorticoid receptors, or in terms of inhibition of nucleoside incorporation by dexamethasone and steroid-induced cell lysis. Similarly, there were no striking differences in clinical features between the two groups.

DISCUSSION

In these experiments we have reported the results of glucocorticoid receptor determinations in lymphoid cells isolated from approximately 60 subjects, either normal or with various forms of leukemia. The number of steroid receptors expressed on a cellular basis appears to vary greatly from one subject to another. In patients with acute lymphocytic leukemia the number of binding sites ranged from about 2,000 sites per cell to about 20,000 sites per cell, whereas in patients with chronic lymphocytic leukemia or in normal subjects this number was contained within a narrower range.

In no case, however, did we find lymphoid cells devoid of receptors. As previously discussed (9), numerous factors may account for the variability in the receptor content of lymphoid cells. Among these is the possibility of a regulation of the number of binding sites by the level of endogenous hormone. Although this phenomenon has been little investigated for glucocorticoid receptors, where only an increase in receptors following adrenal ablation has been shown in various tissues including lymphoid tissue (11,17,20) such a regulation has been clearly demonstrated in the case of sex steroid receptors (31). In addition, the number of steroid receptors in lymphoid cells has been shown to vary according to the immunological nature of the cell, the degree of maturation or differentiation, and the stage of proliferation. Changes in steroid receptor content have thus been demonstrated during ontogeny or aging over the cell cycle or after mitogen-induced blast transformation (4,10,14,33,37,39,42). In one patient with acute monoblastic leukemia, we determined in parallel the level of glucocorticoid receptors in peripheral leukocytes and in bone marrow cells and found three times more receptors in bone marrow samples than in peripheral cells (26,500 and 9,600 sites per cell, respectively). These physiological factors, together with some methodological problems such as inactivation of the receptors during cytosol preparation (24,41) or in the absence of sulfhydril group protecting agents (16), the inability to measure the binding sites occupied by the endogenous hormone (11), or perhaps the use of frozen cells, all contribute to the unreliability of steroid receptor determination as a clinical index.

Using a whole cell binding assay to minimize technical problems, we failed to show any relationship between the level of steroid receptors in lymphoid cells and either the *in vitro* actions of glucocorticoid or the clinical features of the patients investigated.

In normal subjects, for example, thymocytes which contain slightly fewer receptors than peripheral lymphocytes were strongly sensitive to the inhibitory effects of dexamethasone on RNA and DNA synthesis, whereas circulating lymphocytes were not. Similarly, the moderate sex difference observed among the patients with "null" cell acute leukemia, in terms of steroid receptors, was not associated with a comparable difference in the *in vitro* effects of steroids. These discrepancies confirm the lack of correlation between receptor content and steroid sensitivity observed previously by others in animal or cell culture models (3,7,8,34,40,41).

Attempts made to relate the level of steroid receptors to the short-term response to steroid therapy or the clinical aspects, such as staging in chronic lymphocytic leukemia or immunological features of the acute leukemia, were also unsuccessful. The only significant correlation found with regard to the steroid effects *in vitro* was the relationship between uridine and thymidine incorporation in acute lymphocytic leukemia, and the steroid-induced inhibition of their incorporation. This suggests, as previously reviewed (2,5), that the effects of glucocorticoids on lymphoid cells greatly depend on the state of the cell at the time of drug exposure. We therefore conclude that steroid receptor determinations in human leukemic cells are not sufficient to preclude steroid sensitivity.

REFERENCES

1. Baxter, J. D., and Harris, A. W. (1975): *Transplant. Proc.,* 7:55–65.
2. Baxter, J. D., and Tomkins, G. M. (1970): *Proc. Natl. Acad. Sci. USA,* 65:709–715.
3. Bird, C. C., Waddel, A. W., Robertson, A. M. G., Currie, A. R., Steel, C. M., and Evans, J. (1976): *Br. J. Cancer,* 33:700–707.
4. Cidlowski, J. A., and Michaels, G. A. (1977): *Nature,* 266:643–645.
5. Claman, H. N. (1972): *N. Engl. J. Med.,* 287:388–397.
6. Claman, H. N., Moorhead, J. W., and Benner, W. H. (1971): *J. Lab. Clin. Med.,* 78:499–507.
7. Crabtree, G. R., Smith, K. A., and Munck, A. (1979): In: *Seventh Tenovus Workshop. Glucocorticoid Action and Leukemia,* edited by P. A. Bell and N. M. Borthwick, pp. 191–204. Alpha Omega, Cardiff.
8. Duval, D., Dausse, J. P., and Dardenne, M. (1976): *Biochim. Biophys. Acta,* 451:82–91.
9. Duval, D., and Homo, F. (1978): *Cancer Res.,* 38:4263–4267.
10. Duval, D., Homo, F., Fournier, C., and Dausse, J. P. (1979): *Cell Immunol.,* 46:1–11.
11. Feldman, D. (1974): *Endocrinology,* 95:1219–1227.
12. Feldman, D., Funder, J. W., and Edelman, I. S. (1972): *Am. J. Med.,* 53:545–560.
13. Gailani, S., Minowada, J., Silvernail, P., Nussbaum, A., Kaiser, N., Rosen, F., and Shimaoka, K. (1973): *Cancer Res.,* 33:2653–2657.
14. Giannopoulos, G., Hassan, Z., and Solomon, S. (1974): *J. Biol. Chem.,* 249:2424–2427.
15. Giddings, S. J., and Young, D. A. (1974): *J. Steroid Biochem.,* 5:587–595.
16. Granberg, J. P., and Ballard, P. L. (1977): *Endocrinology,* 100:1160–1168.
17. Gregory, M. C., Duval, D., and Meyer, P. (1976): *Clin. Sci. Mol. Med.,* 51:487–493.
18. Gustafsson, J. A., Ekman, P., Snochowski, M., Zetterberg, A., Pousette, A., and Högberg, B. (1978): *Cancer Res.,* 38:4345–4348.
19. Homo, F., and Duval, D. (1979): *J. Clin. Lab. Immunol.,* 2:329–332.
20. Homo, F., Duval, D., Hatzfeld, J., and Evrard, C. (1980): *J. Steroid Biochem.,* 13:135–143.
21. Homo, F., Duval, D., and Meyer, P. (1975): *C. R. Acad. Sci. Ser. D,* 280:1923–1926.
22. Homo, F., Duval, D., Meyer, P., Belas, F., Debre, P., and Binet, J. L. (1978): *Br. J. Haematol.,* 38:491–499.
23. Homo, F., Duval, D., Thierry, C., and Serrou, B. (1979): *J. Steroid Biochem.,* 10:609–613.
24. Kaine, J. L., Nielsen, C. J., and Pratt, W. B. (1975): *Mol. Pharmacol.,* 11:578–587.
25. Konior-Yarbro, G. S., Lippman, M. E., Johnson, G. E., and Leventhal, B. G. (1977): *Cancer Res.,* 37:2688–2695.
26. Leung, K., and Munck, A. (1975): *Endocrinology,* 97:744–748.
27. Lippman, M. E., Halterman, R., Leventhal, B., Perry, S., and Thompson, E. B. (1973): *J. Clin. Invest.,* 52:1715–1725.
28. Lippman, M. E., Perry, S., and Thompson, E. B. (1974): *Cancer Res.,* 34:1572–1576.
29. MacGuire, W. L., Horwitz, K. B., Pearson, O. H., and Segaloff, A. (1977): *Cancer,* 39:2934–2947.
30. Makman, M. H., Nakagawa, S., Dvorkin, B., and White, A. (1970): *J. Biol. Chem.,* 245:2556–2563.
31. Milgrom, E., Luu Thi, M., and Baulieu, E. E. (1973): In: *Sixth Karolinska Symposia on Research Methods in Reproductive Endocrinology: Protein Synthesis in Reproductive Tissue,* pp. 380–403. Karolinska Institutet, Stockholm.
32. Munck, A., Wira, C., Young, D. A., Mosher, K. M., Hallahan, C., and Bell, P. A. (1972): *J. Steroid Biochem.,* 3:567–578.
33. Neiffeld, J. P., Lippman, M. E., and Tormey, D. C. (1977): *J. Biol. Chem.,* 252:2972–2977.
34. Nicholson, M. L., and Young, D. A. (1978): *Cancer Res.,* 38:3673–3680.
35. Rafestin-Oblin, M. E., Michaud, A., Claire, M., and Corvol, P. (1977): *J. Steroid Biochem.,* 8:19–23.

36. Rai, K. R., Sawitsky, A., Cronkite, E. P., Chanana, A. D., Levy, R. N., Pasternak, B. S. (1975): *Blood,* 46:219–228.
37. Roth, G. S. (1975): *Biochim. Biophys. Acta,* 399:145–156.
38. Rousseau, G. G., and Schmit, J. P. (1977): *J. Steroid Biochem.,* 8:911–919.
39. Schaumburg, B. P., and Crone, M. (1971): *Biochim. Biophys. Acta,* 237:494–501.
40. Sibley, C. H., and Tomkins, G. M. (1974): *Cell,* 2:221–227.
41. Sloman, J. C., and Bell, P. A. (1979): In: *Seventh Tenovus Workshop. Glucocorticoid Action and Leukemia,* edited by P. A. Bell and N. M. Borthwick, pp. 161–169. Alpha Omega, Cardiff.
42. Smith, K. A., Crabtree, G. R., Kennedy, S. J., and Munck, A. (1977): *Nature,* 267:523–525.

Hormones and Cancer, edited by S. Iacobelli et al.
Raven Press, New York © 1980.

Endocrine Treatment and Steroid Receptors in Urological Malignancies

G. Concolino, A. Marocchi, C. Conti, *M. Liberti, *R. Tenaglia, and **F. Di Silverio

*Fifth Institute of General Clinical Medicine and Therapy and *Institute of Clinical Urology, University of Rome, 00100 Rome; and **Institute of Clinical Urology, University of Chieti, Chieti, Italy*

Endocrine treatment of urological malignancies may be hard to accept. Nevertheless, over the last few years much effort has been made to clarify the role played by hormonal factors in the growth of these neoplasias not only in experimental animals, but also in man. Some of the carcinomas developed in the experimental animal may represent suitable models for studying how modifications in the hormonal status might lead to regression or progression of the tumor. In this regard, these neoplasias can thus be considered hormone-dependent, and their hormone dependence has been further supported by the demonstration of hormone receptors within the carcinoma. Since steroid hormones act, in fact, through steroid receptors, and since steroid hormones may induce regression or progression of some neoplasia, steroid receptors are considered the biochemical support of the hormone dependence of the tumor.

Renal and prostatic cancers will be discussed together for several reasons. First, the presence of steroid receptors has been demonstrated in many sites of the urological tract, e.g., kidney, bladder and prostate gland. Second, these receptors have been found in the urological tract both in experimental animals and in humans. Third, experimentally induced tumors of the kidney in the hamster, and of the prostate in the rat, are the best models for investigating the relationship between the steroid receptors and the hormone responsiveness of the neoplasia investigated. Finally, on the basis of correlations found between receptors and cancer in the animal, attempts can also be made to correlate steroid receptors and endocrine treatment of these neoplasias in man.

It is well known that hormones are not primarily involved in tumor induction (87), but may be considered as cofactors in the carcinogenic process (46). Certain similarities have been demonstrated between the effects of hormones and those of promoting agents (139). These considerations led to the conclusion that hormones are of secondary importance in the onset of carcinomas, while they may significantly affect the tumors' progression or regression. In this regard, the role played by hormones in the growth of urological neoplasia in the experimental animal and the importance of hormonal status to the development and clinical history of urological carcinomas in man, need to be extensively examined.

UROLOGICAL NEOPLASIA IN EXPERIMENTAL ANIMALS

Many reports have appeared on the effects of steroid hormones (as well as pituitary hormones) on the development and growth rate of renal and prostatic carcinomas in animals. Data from animal experiments cannot be entirely extrapolated to man. Nevertheless, the knowledge of the effects that hormonal factors and manipulations (such as orchiectomy, adrenalectomy, and hypophysectomy) have on the control of renal and prostatic carcinoma growth in animals may help to understand the way in which the growth of these tumors of the urological tract can be modified or controlled in man as well.

Steroid Hormones and Renal Cancer

The influence of sex hormones on renal structures in laboratory animals has been studied for many years (70,72,86,122), and the morphological and biochemical changes elicited by androgens and estrogens in the kidney have been described (59,69,74,102,111,132–134). These anatomical and enzymatic changes may be followed or accompanied by the induction of renal tumor, particularly after the animals have had long-term treatment with natural or synthetic estrogens. While androgens in fact induce renal hypertrophy, estrogens induce a reduction in kidney weight as well as degenerative changes; estrogen action is antagonized by progesterone, which increases renal mass (121). Renal cell carcinoma (RCC) has been induced with estrogens in 2% of male mice (113) and female guinea pigs. Male dogs are more frequently affected by RCC than females (85).

RCC induced with chemical carcinogens in rats and mice is influenced by sex hormones (103,129). Male Syrian hamsters *(Mesocricetus auratus)* and castrated female animals developed RCC after prolonged treatment with estrogens (56,68,93). RCC of Syrian hamsters are the most extensively investigated tumors, and the effects of ablative or additive endocrine therapy in these animals are most important in understanding the role of sex hormones on tumor growth. In the Syrian hamster, RCC induced with prolonged estrogen administration are often bilateral with multiple tumors arising from the tubular epithelium. These RCC have a high degree of malignancy with metastases in the lymph nodes and lungs. Furthermore, the histological pattern of these tumors resembles adenocarcinomas in humans, with the high content of lipophilic material in the neoplastic cells.

Estrogen-induced RCC of the Syrian hamster is the best model of the hormone dependence of renal tumor. RCC of the hamster may, in fact, be produced in male animals or in females after ovariectomy either before or after reproductive maturity when secretion of progesterone from the ovaries is low or absent (67). Estrogen-induced RCC in the hamster is sensitive to the inhibitory properties of estrogen antagonists, such as progesterone, testosterone propionate, and deoxycorticosterone (67,114). Furthermore, this tumor can be transplanted in other hamsters that have been pretreated with either estrogens (56,67) or androgens (66). Although with serial transplant passages RCCs acquire varying degrees of autonomy, it is important to underline that their growth is still hormone dependent; they are still affected by endogenous estrogens and they remain sensitive to the inhibitory properties of some estrogen antagonists such as testosterone propionate or progesterone (67).

It is important, however, to try to answer several questions: (a) Are neoplastic changes directly or indirectly produced by the sex hormones? (b) Do neoplastic changes occur only in injured cells or also in normal cells? (c) Does high estrogen dosage act through the activation of a latent oncogenic virus preexisting in the normal renal cells of the experimental animal? These questions have only been answered in part. For example, the presence of possible oncogenic viruses in frog renal adenocarcinoma (41) and in renal tumors of leopard frog (84), fowl (23), mouse (25), and Syrian hamster (39) has been reported. It is more difficult to understand the exact role of sex hormones in tumor induction, although the discovery of steroid receptors in the induced neoplasia has thrown further light on this problem and might explain the hormone dependence and hormone responsiveness of RCC (39).

Steroid Hormones and Prostatic Cancer

Regarding the relationship between steroid hormones and prostatic cancer in the experimental animal, it is useful to refer mainly to the Dunning R3327 tumor of the rat. This tumor, transplanted in the same inbred line of rats, fulfills almost all the criteria needed for an animal model to be related to human prostatic cancer. It arises spontaneously in the rat prostate, has histological and biological similarities to human prostatic adenocarcinoma, gives rise to bone and lymph node metastases, and displays an androgen dependence with therapeutic response to castration and estrogen treatment followed by a subsequent relapse when the tumor acquires varying degrees of hormone insensitivity.

Smolev et al. (126) have performed extensive studies on the characteristics of this transplantable rat tumor (Dunning R3327H), with the injection of a tumor cell suspension into the flank of the recipient animal. When a suspension of 1.5×10^6 cells of Dunning R3327H prostatic adenocarcinoma is injected into an intact male rat, a tumor appears at the site of injection and grows at a slow rate increasing more than 400-fold in cell number after 6 months. Histologically, the transplanted tumor is a moderate- to well-differentiated prostatic adenocarcinoma with acinar development, microvilli and secretory granules, and cellular and nuclear pleomorphism. This morphology is similar to that found in a well-differentiated human prostatic adenocarcinoma. From a biochemical point of view, the enzymes found in this tumor confirm its origin from the dorsolateral lobe of the rat prostate (127). The incidence of metastases (in lymph nodes and lungs) is only 5%.

The hormone dependence of this tumor is extremely interesting. The neoplasia, in fact, reaches a large size in the presence of androgens with 93% growing cells, although some growth and a different morphology is also obtained in castrated animals (29% of growing cells). Following administration of testosterone proprionate (2 mg/kg/day) for 6 months to castrated animals, tumor growth was comparable to that in intact animals. Administration of diethylstilbesterol (DES) (100 mg/kg/day) or antiandrogens such as flutamide for 6 months to intact animals prevented the growth of the injected tumor. Growth of the tumor in the castrated animal, i.e., in the absence of androgens, could be due to the presence of hormone-insensitive cells (8–29% of the original inoculated cells). These hormone-insensitive cells have a doubling time of 20 days, equal to that of hormone-sensitive cells, and could explain the subsequent relapse of tumor growth after the partial regression obtained with castration or DES.

In experimentally induced RCC it has been hypothesized that estrogen could act through the activation of a latent oncogenic virus (39). The possibility that hormones, also in prostatic cancer, act through the formation of products coded for by transforming genes of oncogenic viruses has been reported in the hamster (110).

Polypeptide Hormones and Urological Malignancies

Prolactin as well as insulin affect tumor growth and tumor development. This has been demonstrated both *in vitro* and *in vivo*. In Syrian hamsters treated with estrogens to induce RCC, an increase was found in the number of prolactin-secreting cells, with morphological changes of pituitary pars intermedia accompanied by an increase in melanocyte-stimulating hormone (MSH) (51). Prolactin has also been reported to influence androgen metabolism by increasing its accumulation and use in the rat prostate (49,131). However, the effect of prolactin on prostatic cancer is still controversial, since it has been demonstrated that in the rat prostate prolactin reduces the conversion of testosterone to 5α-dihydrotestosterone (DHT), while the inhibition of prolactin secretion by bromocryptine stimulates DHT formation and activates the prostatic glandular cells (5).

HORMONES AND UROLOGICAL MALIGNANCIES IN MAN

A relationship has already been established between hormones and tumor growth rate in many human neoplasias. Furthermore, epidemiological studies as well as differences observed in the incidence of renal malignancy at different ages and in subjects of opposite sex have confirmed the roles of hormones in this neoplasia. More information on the hormones involved in the growth of renal and prostatic carcinomas in man can be derived from tumor regression (or progression) obtained by spontaneous or induced endocrine modifications.

Hormones and Human Renal Cell Carcinoma

The incidence of RCC shows a predominance in males, the ratio of males to females being 3.8:1.0 (92). The peak excess in males corresponds to the childbearing period in females, i.e., when progesterone secretion seems to protect women from the development of RCC (63). With the cessation of gonadal activity, the male-to-female ratio drops to 2:1. Differences in hormonal status could also explain the difference in racial statistics, RCC being found frequently in Caucasians, seldom in Negroes, and almost never in Orientals (7).

Hormonal factors have also been cited for the spontaneous regression of RCC, reported more frequently in men than in women (10). The possibility that hormones of the adrenal cortex have an inhibitory effect on RCC growth rate was proposed, since adrenal tumors have been found in the presence of regressing RCC (4). Therefore, adrenal cortical hormones were used in combination with testosterone propionate and/or progesterone to decrease the size of radiologically proven lung metastases (8,11), or to obtain a long "tumor-free interval" after nephrectomy and decreased incidence of metastases (19). Sex differences have been reported also for the ten-year survival rate, being higher for females than for males (101).

It is possible that hormones act through the activation of a latent oncogenic virus preexisting in the normal kidney. However, attempts thus far to isolate viruses directly from human RCC have failed, while virus particles have been detected under electron microscopy in papillary cancer of the human pelvis and in papillary transitional cell carcinoma of renal pelvis from adult males (42).

Hormones and Human Prostatic Cancer

Prostatic carcinoma, the most frequent tumor occurring in the male urogenital tract, has been known to be responsive to hormonal manipulation since the early work of Huggins and Hodges (60), who introduced endocrine therapy for prostatic cancer in 1941. Androgens have a direct promoting action on the growth of prostatic tissue and on the development of prostatic neoplasia, while pituitary hormones may act indirectly through testicular or adrenal cortical hormones, or by interfering with androgen metabolism in the prostate. Therefore orchiectomy, which abolishes more than 95% of plasma testosterone concentration, may represent one of the best means of decreasing the tumor growth

(119). Administration of estrogen, as well as progestational compounds, has been reported to be effective in the control of this hormone-dependent neoplasia by lowering plasma testosterone levels and displaying a peripheral antiandrogenic activity (32,64,104).

Racial differences have also been reported, the rate of occurrence of prostatic cancer being higher among blacks than among whites in the United States (43). Socioeconomic status and related hormonal differences must also be relevant, since the incidence rate is higher in American blacks than in Africans (61).

Patient hormonal status has been recognized as an important factor, since prostatic carcinoma remains, at least for a time, androgen dependent. Patients can be divided into three groups: (a) those with normal plasma luteinizing hormone (LH) and testosterone levels; (b) those with high plasma LH and normal plasma testosterone levels; and (c) those with high plasma LH and low plasma testosterone levels. The last group has interstitial cell failure and is unlikely to respond to orchiectomy, the tumor having already acquired a degree of androgen independence (20).

The effects of female sex hormones on human prostatic carcinoma have been examined also by means of electron microscopic autoradiographic study with the *in vitro* localization of tritiated estradiol in the tumor. It was thus possible to demonstrate that estrogens have a direct effect on some of the prostatic cancer cells within 2 hr, although the extent of changes at the subcellular level of the tumor cells has not yet been determined (124).

Could steroid hormones in prostatic carcinoma activate a latent oncogenic virus? This question remains unanswered. Nevertheless, a genital strain of cytomegalovirus (CMV) isolated from a human prostate has been shown to transform normal human prostatic tissue into cells with malignant characteristics (118). This finding is extremely important since 50 to 100% of the general population may have been infected with CMV (140). Furthermore, prostatic cancer patients frequently develop a CMV antibody (112). However, the human cells transformed *in vivo* may fail to express viral-specific cell membrane antigens, except under specific conditions. Steroid hormones might act as cocarcinogens in the malignant changes in human prostatic tissue.

STEROID RECEPTORS IN UROLOGICAL MALIGNANCIES

Steroid hormone action in the urological tract requires the presence of steroid receptors and could explain the hormone sensitivity or urological malignancies. Steroid receptors have been demonstrated in the kidney of various experimental animals (21,22,37,47,48,65,75,76,80,83,91,108,109,115) and prostate gland of rats (1,81,88), dogs (24), and baboons (117). Furthermore, steroid receptors have been found in normal and carcinomatous renal tissue in man and in normal and neoplastic human prostate.

As far as the relationship between hormone dependence and steroid receptors is concerned, only the receptor studies on estrogen-induced RCC in Syrian hamsters and on Dunning R3327 rat prostatic carcinoma will be described here, together with the data on receptors found in human RCC and human prostatic cancer.

Steroid Receptors in Renal Cell Carcinoma of Syrian Hamsters

Li and Villee (78) and Li et al. (76,76) demonstrated the presence of estradiol receptor (ER) in the Syrian hamster kidney and in estrogen-induced RCC. This receptor has a sedimentation coefficient of 8 S and a high affinity constant ($K_D = 1.7 \times 10^{-9}$ M). Triphenylethylene derivatives at high concentrations compete effectively for the estrogen receptor complex in renal tumor. These same authors also found the progesterone receptor (PR) in the 7 to 8 S regions of the sucrose gradient of primary tumor cytosol from DES-treated male hamster. Scatchard plot analysis gave a single homogeneous component of high affinity binding sites that can be saturated with 10 nM progesterone (80). In response to estrogen treatment, progesterone binding activity of the kidney increases, and this marked increase (from 17- to 27-fold untreated control levels) represents the earliest consistent change during the induction period. PR concentration in the tumor is much higher (520 times) than that of the untreated control (79).

Androgen receptors (AR) are also present in this tumor (75,77), although in low amounts, and the concentration in the untreated hamster kidney is unaffected by estrogen treatment prior to renal tumorogenesis (73).

Steroid Receptors in Dunning R3327 Rat Prostatic Carcinoma

Markland et al. (90) reported on the characterization of steroid hormone receptors (AR and ER) both in the hormone-responsive R3327 tumor and in a hormone-insensitive line that emerged during transplantation of the established R3327 tumor. The titration curve for AR and Scatchard analysis produced a linear plot which represented a single class of high affinity binding sites: the dissociation constant was 1.6 to 7.0×10^{-9} M. The sedimentation profile and receptor concentration varied with the histological type of the tumors examined. The moderately differentiated hormone-sensitive adenocarcinoma possesses a 7.8 S AR on a sucrose gradient with the number of binding sites ranging between 100 and 300 fmoles/mg of cytosol protein. The mixed tumor, with extensive proliferation of the stromal fibroblastic cells, i.e., carcinosarcoma, possesses a 4.5 to 5 S AR with the number of binding sites ranging between 65 and 70 fmoles/mg of cytosol protein. Fibrosarcoma, the most rapidly growing hormone-insensitive tumor, which consists of pure connective tissue, does not contain detectable AR.

The titration curve and Scatchard analysis for ER also gave a single component of high affinity binding sites ($K_D = 3.1$–8.0×10^{-10} M). The adenocarcinoma possesses an 8.3 S ER with a concentration of 100 to 300 fmoles/mg of cytosol protein; the carcinosarcoma has an 8.3 S ER with a concentration of 35 to 40 fmoles/mg of cytosol protein; while the fibrosarcoma contains no detectable ER.

A high affinity binding component of AR with low capacity (20 fmoles/mg of cytosol protein) was found in the normal prostate gland of Copenhagen rat which was, however, devoid of ER.

Steroid Receptors in Human Renal Cell Carcinoma

Estrogen, progesterone, and aldosterone receptors have been demonstrated in normal renal tissue surrounding carcinomatous area (14,45,94). Microscopic foci of tumor cells in the untransforming tissue may, however, be included in this way. Therefore, in our studies on renal steroid receptors we preferred to use normal renal tissue removed from nonneoplastic patients (i.e., after polar renal resection in patients with kidney stones).

Our studies focused mainly on ER and PR in human RCC using tritiated estradiol-17β and progesterone or promegestone as radioligands. For PR studies cytosols were preincubated with cortisol (1–10×10^{-6} M). Unlabeled steroids were usually added to stabilize the receptors. Exchange assay at 25 and 20°C for 5 and 1 hr, respectively, for ER and PR and agar gel electrophoresis according to Wagner (136) were employed. Some specimens were also analyzed by means of the protamine sulfate precipitation assay (141). The results of our studies correlate with those reported by other authors (12–14,45,107). Saturation analysis and Scatchard plot revealed the presence of high affinity binding both for ER and PR ($K_D{}^{ER} = 0.89$–2.61×10^{-9} M; $K_D{}^{PR} = 0.13$–3.72×10^{-9} M). However, the binding capacity of both receptors was found to be lower than that measured in normal renal tissue. We (28) suggested that this could be related to nuclear translocation of the receptors as reported by other authors (45).

The distribution of ER and PR in the cytosol of the 37 human RCC so far investigated is shown in Table 1. ER was found in 54.1% and PR in 62.1%. Of the tumors 29.7% were positive for both ER and PR and 13.5% were negative for both ER and PR.

TABLE 1. *Distribution of ER and PR in human renal cell carcinoma[a]*

	PR+	PR⁻	Total
ER+	11 (29.7)	9 (24.3)	20 (54.1)
ER⁻	12 (32.4)	5 (13.5)	17 (45.9)
Total	23 (62.1)	14 (37.8)	37 (100)

[a] Numbers in parentheses are percentages.

STEROID RECEPTORS IN HUMAN PROSTATIC CARCINOMA

It is well known that the assay of androgen receptors is complicated by the large amounts of endogenous DHT and sex hormone binding globulin (SHBG), by the metabolism of DHT during incubation time, and by the small amount of tissue usually obtained at biopsy. However, it was possible by means of density gradient centrifugation, Sephadex chromatography, agar gel electrophoresis, and protamine sulfate precipitation to separate putative human prostate cytoplasmic androgen receptors from SHBG (35,52,71,89,96,98). The use of methyltrienolone (R1881), a synthetic steroid that is not metabolized with the temperature of incubation and does not bind to SHBG, has also been successfully employed, but one must be aware of the fact that R1881 is also bound to progestin receptor of human prostate (2,15,33,40,50,95,123,138). Following these technical improvements AR have been demonstrated not only in normal prostate and in benign prostatic hypertrophy (BPH), but also in human prostatic carcinoma (36,97,128,138). The identification of AR in the nuclear fraction of human prostate has also been reported: the concentration of AR was found to be 800 and 1,500 receptor molecules/cell by Davies et al. (36); and 1,000 and 1,900 receptor molecules/cell by Lieskovsky and Bruchovsky (82) in normal and carcinomatous prostatic tissue, respectively.

Recently the presence of estrogen receptor has also been demonstrated in BPH and in human prostatic cancer (6,26,53,128). Furthermore, the occurrence of a progestin receptor in the cytosol from hyperplastic and carcinomatous human prostatic tissue has also been demonstrated (6,30,33,50).

Steroid receptors are the biochemical support of the hormone dependence of BPH and prostatic carcinoma and may be usefully employed in the selection of patients with a tumor growth still influenced by hormonal factors.

We studied AR in 30 prostatic cancers employing exchange assay and agar gel electrophoresis or protamine sulfate precipitation assay using R1881 as radioligand. The presence of ER and PR was sought in the cytosol fraction of 15 tumors. AR was found in 24 of the 30 tumors examined, and ER in 3 and PR in 7 out of the 15 examined. Total receptor concentration was found to be of the order of 17 to 37 fmoles/mg of protein for AR, 14 to 80 fmoles/mg protein for PR, and 100 to 110 fmoles/mg protein for ER (Table 2).

TABLE 2. *Steroid receptors in human prostatic carcinoma*

Receptor	No. +/ no. patients	N (fmoles/mg protein)	K_D (10^{-9} M
ER	3/15	—	—
PR	7/15	14–80	—
AR	24/30	17–37	0.25–1.75

STEROID RECEPTORS AND HORMONE TREATMENT IN EXPERIMENTAL ANIMALS

Studies on the relationship between steroid receptors and hormonal manipulation in suitable animal models should provide comprehensive information on the possible correlation between hormone-dependent tumors and endocrine treatment in humans. Although data on receptors, tumors, and the endocrine treatment of experimental animal cannot be extrapolated to man, the more information available in this field the better the treatment of prostatic cancer patients selected on the basis of putative parameters of hormone dependence of the neoplasia.

Renal Cell Carcinoma In the Hamster

In 1959 Kirkman (67) reported that progestins have an inhibitory effect on estrogen induction of RCC in Syrian hamsters. The inhibitory action of progestins on the induction and growth of breast and endometrial cancers has also been reported (57,120). Li et al. (80) reported a modest reduction (22%) of cytoplasmic ER in renal tumors from estrogen- and progesterone-treated animals, compared with animals treated with estrogens alone. Although the reduction of ER is not as rapid or as marked as that found under similar conditions for the uterus (58), it may be important in contributing to progesterone-induced renal tumor regression in the hamster.

However, can the demonstration of steroid receptors in the epithelium of hamster RCC explain the relation of estrogen to tumor induction or the hormone responsiveness of the neoplasm? The embryonal origin of renal nephron from coelomic epithelial cells and from the urogenital ridge (from which epididymis and ductus deferens also derive) may explain the sensitivity of renal tissue to sex hormones. Perhaps a more detailed study on the presence of steroid receptors in the stromal compartment may lead to a better understanding of the relationship between tumor induction and tumor regression in response to hormonal factors.

Dunning R3327 Rat Prostatic Carcinoma

R3327 rat prostatic tumor possesses both AR and ER, but is devoid of PR. The presence of steroid hormone receptors correlates with the hormone responsiveness. In fact, adenocarcinoma, which contains substantial amounts of both AR and ER, is hormone sensitive. It grows quite slowly and grows better in male than in female rats. The other histological variant, fibrosarcoma, with an excessive amount of stroma, is completely devoid of receptors and is hormone insensitive. It grows quite rapidly and equally well when injected into the female rat or into the intact or castrated male rat. It should not be forgotten that androgen, progesterone, and estrogen receptors might have a different distribution in the prostatic gland (with AR prevalent in the epithelial and PR and ER in the stromal compartment). This different distribution might account for some of the tissue changes in response to endocrine manipulation in man (90).

The endocrine treatment of urological cancers gives rise to several questions: (a) whether hormonal therapy is really effective; (b) if and when hormonal therapy should be started; and (c) which form of hormonal therapy is preferable.

ENDOCRINE TREATMENT OF HUMAN UROLOGICAL MALIGNANCIES

Effectiveness

Hormonal therapy has been shown to be of benefit to some patients with inoperable renal cell carcinoma, and a 20% remission rate has been reported (9–11,18,105,116,135). Androgen has been used when patients failed to respond to progestins (11,62,100,106). Nevertheless, no objective response after either progestagens and/or androgens has been obtained (34,100,130), and the remission rate of 20% obtained with progestins in cases of RCC with metastases was considered to be due to spontaneous regression of the tumor. Montie et al. (99) reported on the incidence of regression of metastases following nephrectomy in nine series and found only 4 cases of regression in a total of 474 patients collected. In view of the rarity of spontaneous regression of metastases in RCC, the objective improvement, observed 2 to 6 weeks after starting endocrine treatment, could not be merely a spontaneous event. As far as the 5-year survival rate is concerned (Fig. 1), a significant statistical difference was found by our group between nephrectomized patients and those submitted to nephrectomy plus endocrine therapy.

Between 60 and 80% of patients with prostatic carcinoma respond to hormonal manipulation (17,125); the lack of responsiveness in the remaining cases is associated with poorly differentiated tumors (54). Besides the histological grade, the age of the tumor is also important. In the early phase the tumor may be constituted almost entirely by clones of hormone-sensitive cells, whereas in a subsequent phase it may be represented by clones of hormone-insensitive cells.

The suppression of the main source of androgens by bilateral orchiectomy induces a decrease in tumor size (119). Indirect suppression of testosterone production with estrogens or inhibition of androgen action on the target organs by means of progestins or antiandrogens have also been reported to be effective (32,64,104). Although many patients with prostatic cancer show an improvement of signs and symptoms with endocrine therapy, there is no evidence that survival

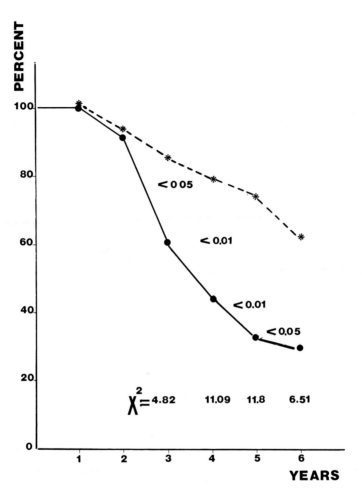

FIG. 1. Survival rate in two groups of patients nephrectomized for RCC, treated *(broken line)* or untreated *(solid line)* with hormonal therapy.

is prolonged (3,31). The type of hormone therapy employed should, however, always be borne in mind. Bracci (16) reported a mean survival rate of 64% 5 years after orchiectomy associated with cyproterone acetate.

Commencement of Endocrine Therapy

The other point of debate is related to the commencement of hormone theapy. Two rules are usually followed by our group: Selection of patients with hormone-responsive tumor, and early commencement of endocrine treatment (soon after surgery).

Estrogens which induce renal cell carcinoma in some experimental animals may also play a role in the onset of human RCC. The identification of ER and PR in the cytosol of human RCC together with the results of ablative or additive endocrine treatment in animals, particularly the Syrian hamster with RCC, led us to hypothesize that progestational treatment may be usefully employed in patients with steroid receptor positive RCC (29). Conflicting results may be due to the different dosages of progestin employed. Li et al. (80) observed a slight reduction in ER after progesterone treatment of RCC in the hamster and suggested that a longer period of progesterone treatment might be necessary to elicit a substantial decrease in ER concentration. The results of our competitive experiments, in fact, favor a weak competitive action of progesterone for ER (Fig. 2). DHT is a strong competitor for ER in some RCC and this could possibly explain the favorable results of androgen therapy obtained in patients who failed to respond to progestational therapy (27). Treatment with pharmacological doses should be started soon after nephrectomy and should never be discontinued, since the appearance of metastases has been reported after withdrawal of treatment in some patients, thus leading to the hypothesis that development of metastases is due to the lack of inhibition of tumor growth by progestins (38). Combined chemo-, endocrine, and radiotherapy is reserved for the hormone-insensitive tumors, i.e., RCC devoid of both ER and PR.

As far as prostatic carcinoma is concerned, the selection of patients with hormone-responsive tumors is based on results obtained with cyproterone acetate on tumor size and tumor growth (16) and, more recently, on the results of receptor studies on specimens of prostatic cancer (30). Endocrine treatment is usually employed when the size of the tumor decreases in response to cyproterone acetate or DES or when AR (or PR and ER) are detected in the biopsy specimen.

We prefer to use orchiectomy in combination with other forms of endocrine therapy, such as DES or cyproterone acetate. Cyproterone acetate is usually employed because of its capacity to block the effect of male hormones on the target organs influencing the intracellular events induced by the action of steroid hormones. Cyproterone acetate, 50 mg/day, should be commenced at the time of diagnosis and administered immediately after orchiectomy. Use of cyproterone acetate, while not inducing untoward and harmful side effects, has been shown in many cases (even in those previously treated with estrogens) to have a favorable effect upon the disease, with marked regression of both tumor mass and symptoms (16). Chemotherapy is preferable in patients with hormone-insensitive tumor, i.e., those in whom the tumor mass does not regress following cyproterone acetate or DES administration and in whom the tumor is devoid of steroid. Recently estramustine phosphate (Estracyt®), a drug composed of an antiblastic substance and estradiol, was employed in the palliative therapy of prostatic carcinoma. Although this association was originally made in order to have a compound acting at receptor level, it is not known whether the main effect is elicited by the antiblastic substance or by the estrogen. Therefore, we reserve

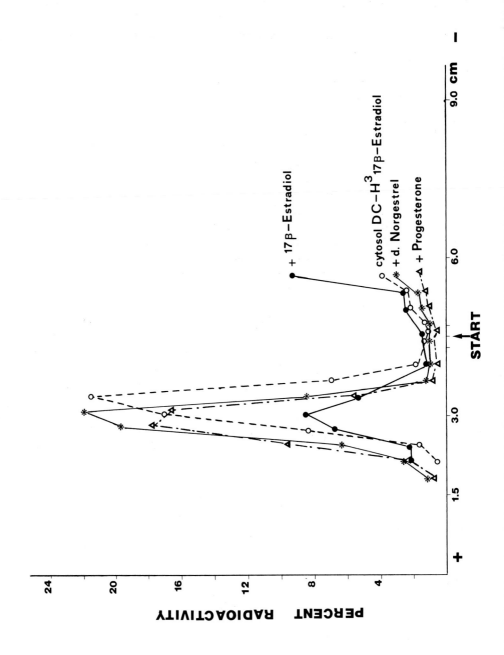

estramustine phosphate for hormone-insensitive tumors since the mean survival rate seems to be increased.

CORRELATION BETWEEN STEROID RECEPTORS AND ENDOCRINE TREATMENT IN UROLOGICAL MALIGNANCIES

We have examined 37 human RCC for the presence of ER and PR and attempted to correlate hormonal treatment and receptor studies in 30 patients in whom follow-up data were available. Of these patients (23 males and 7 females, mean age 44 years), 5 had evidence of metastases. One with bilateral RCC died soon after nephrectomy, one was not treated, three were treated with combined chemo- and radiotherapy, one with tamoxifen (10 mg p.o. twice a day), and twenty-four received medroxyprogesterone acetate at pharmacological doses, as previously reported (28) (Table 3).

TABLE 3. *Distribution of hormone receptors in human RCC and response to endocrine therapy*

Presence of hormone receptors	ER+ PR+	ER+ PR−	ER− PR+	ER− PR−	Total
Incidence	10	8	8	4	30
Response to endocrine therapy	6/6	7/7	6/7	1/4	20/24[a]

[a] Responsive cases/total cases subjected to endocrine therapy.

In order to evaluate the response of patients to endocrine treatment, the following parameters were taken into consideration: return to normal of all laboratory values, stabilization of metastases, and a decrease of more than 50% in the sum of the products of the diameters of all measurable lesions. The parameters studied at follow-up in the patients with no metastatic lesions at time of nephrectomy were: (a) return to normal of laboratory findings, (b) subjective improvements with positive Karnosky index, (c) increase in body weight, and (d) a long "time-free" interval (> 18–24 months). The response to endocrine therapy (Table 3) shows that 6 out of 6 patients with ER+ PR+ tumor, 7 out of 7 patients with ER+ PR− tumor, and 6 out of 7 patients with ER−

FIG. 2. Agar gel electrophoresis of cytosol from human RCC. Presence of a specific estradiol-17β receptor complex. Incubation for 18 hr at 4°C with 1 nM tritiated estradiol-17β (*asterisks and solid line*), or plus 100 nM unlabeled estradiol-17β (*asterisks and dotted line*), or plus 100 nM unlabeled d-norgestrel *(closed circles)*, or plus 100 nM unlabeled progesterone *(closed squares)*. 1% agar gel in 0.05 μm sodium diethyl-barbiturate/acetate buffer, pH 8.2; run 280 V for 3 hr, 50 μl applied for analysis, 30 sections of 3.0 mm.

PR+ tumor responded to medroxyprogesterone acetate treatment. Of the 4 patients with tumor devoid of ER and PR, only one responded to endocrine therapy. The response to endocrine treatment in these patients with RCC, therefore, shows a good correlation with the presence of steroid receptors (20/24).

As far as prostatic cancer patients are concerned we wish to emphasize two points: (a) The different distribution of the receptors in the prostatic gland [AR being localized mainly in the epithelial cells and ER and PR in the stromal compartment of the prostate (6,33,137)], leading to different morphological tissue changes in response to estrogenic, antiandrogenic, or progestational treatment. (b) The possibility that a correlation between endocrine treatment and steroid receptor may exist particularly when the hormonal manipulation is directed to the respective receptor molecule. For these reasons we have estimated not only AR, but also ER and PR as predictive parameters of the hormone responsiveness of human prostatic carcinoma and evaluated the clinical response to orchiectomy and to the administration of cyproterone acetate. The results obtained are summarized in Table 4. For evaluation of the response, subjective

TABLE 4. *Response to different forms of endocrine therapy[a] in patients[b] with prostatic cancer*

	Response after 1–4 yr		Response after 1–2 yr		
Remission	15/30[c]	(50)	2 AR+	3/15[d]	(20)
Partial objective regression	3/30	(10)	3 AR+	3/15	(20)
Objectively stable	6/30	(20)	4 AR+	8/15	(53)
Objective progression	6/30	(20)		1/15	(7)

[a] Orchiectomy; orchiectomy + cyproterone acetate (CPA); CPA + orchiectomy + CPA.
[b] 60–81 years old; TNM: T_2-T_4/M_0-M_1/N_0-N_1.
[c] Hormone dependence evaluated without receptor studies.
[d] Hormone dependence evaluated after TVR with receptor studies.

and clinical criteria were used to define *remission* in those cases in which adequate data for objective evaluation were not available.

Tumor regression and objectively stable tumor were evaluated using objective criteria including changes in bone metastases, tumor mass, and prostatic acid phosphatase. Two groups of patients have been studied. One group of 30 patients was considered to have a hormone responsive tumor if the size of the palpable mass decreased 1 month after cyproterone acetate administration; these patients were then submitted to orchiectomy and further treatment with cyproterone acetate. The second group was comprised of 15 patients in whom hormone responsiveness was evaluated by means of receptor studies; these patients were also submitted to orchiectomy and treatment with cyproterone acetate. The two groups were comparable as to age and TNM classification. The response to endocrine therapy in the first group after 1 to 4 years of treatment demonstrated that 15 patients had a remission, 3 a partial objective regression, and 6 an objectively stable tumor. Six out of thirty patients showed tumor progression. The response to endocrine therapy of the second group after 1 to 2 years demonstrated that 3 patients (2 with AR+ and 1 with PR+) had a remission; 3 patients with AR+ had partial objective regression; 8 patients (4 with AR+ and 4 with PR+) had an objectively stable tumor; 1 patient with PR+ cancer had an objective progression.

Therefore, from these results it can be concluded that a correlation between androgen or progesterone receptors and endocrine treatment (orchiectomy and cyproterone acetate) exists in 93.3% of cases (14/15). Whether cyproterone acetate is active through an inhibitory effect on AR or through a stimulatory effect on PR remains to be elucidated.

CONCLUSIONS

From the data presented it seems that receptor studies are useful parameters to establish hormone dependence of renal cell carcinoma and prostatic carcinoma. However, the measurement of steroid receptors may be useful mainly as a prognostic parameter in neoplastic diseases. This can be stated after longer follow-up.

The commencement of endocrine treatment should be as early as possible, after diganosis or, at least, after orchiectomy.

The presence of different clones of hormone-responsive and hormone-unresponsive cells in urological malignancies suggests that endocrine- and chemotherapy should perhaps be combined in order to avoid possible relapse due to the presence of residual hormone-insensitive cells.

ACKNOWLEDGMENTS

This work was supported in part by a grant from the Italian Research Council (CNR), special project "Control of Neoplastic Growth."

REFERENCES

1. Armstrong, E. G., and Bashirelahi, N. (1978): *J. Steroid Biochem.,* 9:507–513.
2. Asselin, J., Labrie, F., Gourdeau, J., Bonne, C., and Raynaud, J. P. (1976): *Steroids,* 28:449–459.
3. Barnes, R., Hirst, A., and Rosenquist, R. (1976): *J. Urol.,* 115:404–405.
4. Bartley, O., and Hultquist, G. T. (1950): *Acta Pathol. Microbiol. Scand.,* 27:448–460.
5. Bartsch, G., and Roho, H. P. (1979): *Arch. Androl.,* 2(Suppl. 1):80 (Abstr.).
6. Bashirelahi, N., and Sanefugi, H. (1979): In: *Steroid Receptors, Metabolism and Prostatic Cancer.* Workshop of the European Prostatic Cancer Research Group, Amsterdam, April 27–28. Excerpta Medica, Amsterdam *(in press).*
7. Bennington, J. L. (1973): *Cancer,* 32:1017–1029.
8. Bloom, H. J. G. (1964): In: *Tumours of the Kidney and Ureter,* edited by E. Riches, pp. 311–338. Churchill Livingstone, Edinburgh.
9. Bloom, H. J. G. (1971): *Br. J. Cancer,* 25:250–265.
10. Bloom, H. J. G. (1973): *Cancer,* 32:1066–1071.

11. Bloom, H. J. G., and Wallace, D. M. (1964): *Br. Med. J.,* 2:476–480.
12. Bojar, H., Balzer, K., Dreyfurst, R., Staib, W., and Wittliff, J. L. (1976): *J. Clin. Chem. Clin. Biochem.,* 14:515–520.
13. Bojar, H., Dreyfurst, R., Balzer, K., Staib, W., and Wittliff, J. L. (1976): *J. Clin. Chem. Clin. Biochem.,* 14:521–526.
14. Bojar, H., Wittliff, J. L., Balzer, K., Dreyfurst, R., Boeminghans, F., and Staib, W. (1975): *Acta Endocrinol. (Kbh.) [Suppl.],* 193:51.
15. Bonne, C., and Raynaud, J. P. (1976): *Steroids,* 27:497–507.
16. Bracci, U. (1979): *Eur. Urol.,* 5:303–306.
17. Bracci, U., and Di Silverio, F. (1973): *Prog. Med.,* 29:779–785.
18. Bracci, U., and Di Silverio, F. (1976): In: *Atti della Società Italiana di Urologia, Vol. 1,* edited by C. Corbi, pp. 167–189. Tripi De Meria, Roma.
19. Bracci, U., Gagliardi, V., and Di Silverio, F. (1973): In: *Proc. XVI Congr. Int. Soc. Urol. Vol. 2,* edited by C. Doin, pp. 569–572. G. & R. Joly, Paris.
20. Bramble, F. J., and Jacobs, H. S. (1975): *Br. Med. J.,* 3:307.
21. Bullock, L. P., and Bardin, C. W. (1974): *Endocrinology,* 94:746–756.
22. Bullock, L. P., and Bardin, C. W. (1975): *Endocrinology,* 97:1106–1111.
23. Carr, J. G. (1960): *Br. J. Cancer,* 14:77–82.
24. Chasiri, N., Valotaire, Y., Evans, B. A. J., and Pierrepoint, C. G. (1978): *J. Endocrinol.,* 78:131–139.
25. Claude, A. (1962): *J. Ultrastruct. Res.,* 6:1–18.
26. Concolino, G., Di Silverio, F., Marocchi, A., and Tenaglia, R. (1978): *Atti della Soc. Ital. Biochim. Clin.,* 7:512. (abstr.).
27. Concolino, G., Marocchi, A., Concolino, F., Di Silverio, F., Sciarra, F., and Piro, C. (1976): *V Int. Congr. Endocrinology,* Hamberg July 18–24, p. 194 *(abstr.).*
28. Concolino, G., Marocchi, A., Conti, C., Tenaglia, R., Di Silverio, F., and Bracci, U. (1978): *Cancer Res.,* 38:4340–4344.
29. Concolino, G., Marocchi, A., Di Silverio, F., and Conti, C. (1976): *J. Steroid Biochem.,* 7:923–927.
30. Concolino, G., Marocchi, A., Ricci, G., Liberti, M., Di Silverio, F., and Bracci, U. (1979): In: *Steroid Receptors, Metabolism and Prostatic Cancer.* Workshop of The European Prostatic Cancer Group, Amsterdam, April 27–28. Excerpta Medica, Amsterdam *(in press).*
31. Correa, R. J., Jr., Anderson, R. G., Gibbons, R. P., and Mason, J. T. (1974): *J. Urol.,* 111:644–646.
32. Corvol, P., Michaud, A., Menard, J., Freifeld, M., and Mahoudeau, J. (1975): *Endocrinology,* 97:52–58.
33. Cowan, R. A., Cowan, S. K., and Grant, J. K. (1977): *J. Endocrinol.,* 74:281–289.
34. Cronin, R. E., Kaehny, W. D., Miller, P. D., Stables, D. P., Gabow, P. A., Ostroy, P. R., and Schierer, R. W. (1976): *Medicine,* 55:291–331.
35. Davies, P., and Griffiths, K. (1975): *Mol. Cell. Endocrinol.,* 3:143–164.
36. Davies, P., Thomas, P., and Griffith, K. (1977): In: *Interdisciplinary Trends in Surgery,* Proc. X Eur. Congr. Int. College of Surgeons, edited by W. Montorsi. Minerva Medica, Milan *(in press).*
37. De Vries, J. R., Ludens, J. H., and Fanestil, D. D. (1972): *Kidney Int.,* 2:95–100.
38. Di Silverio, F., Liberti, M., and Biacobini, S. (1976): In: *Sillabus, Vol. 1,* edited by P. Periti, pp. 359–364. Giuntini, Florence.
39. Dodge, A. M. (1974): *Lab. Invest.,* 31:250–257.
40. Dubé, J. Y., Chapdelaine, P., Tremblay, R. R., Bonne, C., and Raynaud, J. P. (1976): *Horm. Res. (Basel),* 7:341–347.
41. Duryce, W. R. (1959): *Acta Int. Cancer,* 15:587–594.
42. Elliott, A. Y., Fraley, E. E., Cleveland, P., Castro, A. E., and Stein, N. (1973): *Science,* 179:393–395.
43. Ernster, V. L., Winkelstein, W., Jr., Selvins, S., Brown, S. M., Sacks, S. T., Austin, D. F., Mandel, S. A., and Bertolli, T. A. (1977): *Cancer Treat. Rep.,* 61:187–191.
44. Fanestil, D. D., and Edelman, I. S. (1966): *Proc. Natl. Acad. Sci. USA,* 56:872–879.
45. Fanestil, D. D., Vaughn, D. A., and Ludens, J. H. (1974): *J. Steroid Biochem.,* 5:338 (abstr.).
46. Fialkow, P. J. (1974): *N. Engl. J. Med.,* 4:26–35.
47. Funder, J. W., Feldman, D., and Edelman, I. S. (1973): *Endocrinology,* 92:1005–1013.

48. Ghaleb, H. A. (1964): In: *Tumours of the Kidney and Ureter,* edited by E. Riches. Churchill Livingstone, Edinburgh.
49. Grayhack, J. T. (1963): *Natl. Cancer Inst. Monogr.,* 12:189.
50. Gustaffson, J. A., Ekman, P., Pousette, A., Snochowski, M., and Hogberg, B. (1978): *Invest. Urol.,* 15:361–366.
51. Hamilton, J. M., Saluja, P. G., Thody, A. J., and Flaks, A. (1977): *Eur. J. Cancer,* 13:29–32.
52. Hansson, V., Tveter, K. J., Attramadal, A., and Torgersen, O. (1971): *Acta Endocrinol. (Kbh.),* 68:79–88.
53. Hawkins, E. F., Nijs, M., and Brassinne, C. (1976): *Biochem. Biophys. Res. Commun.,* 70:854.
54. Heaney, J. A., Chang, H. C., Daly, J. J., and Prout, G. R., Jr. (1977): *J. Urol.,* 118:283–287.
55. Horning, E. S. (1956): *Z. Krebsforsch.,* 61:1–21.
56. Horning, E. S., and Whittick, J. W. (1954): *Br. J. Cancer,* 8:451–457.
57. Howard, J. A., Cornes, J. S., Jackson, W. D., and Bye, P. (1974): *J. Obstet. Gynecol. Br. Commonw.,* 81:786–790.
58. Hsuch, A. J. W., Peck, E. J., and Clark, J. H. (1976): *Endocrinology,* 98:438–444.
59. Huang, K. C., and McIntosh, B. J. (1955): *Am. J. Physiol.,* 183:387–390.
60. Huggins, C., and Hodges, C. V. (1941): *Cancer Res.,* 1:293–297.
61. Jackson, M. A., Ahluwalia, B. S., Herson, J., Heshmat, M. Y., Jackson, A. G., Jones, G. W., Kapoor, S. K., Kennedy, J., Kovi, J., Lucas, A. O., Nkposong, E. O., Olisa, E., and Williams, A. O. (1977): *Cancer Treat. Rep.,* 61:167–172.
62. Jenkin, R. D. I. (1967): *Br. Med. J.,* 1:361.
63. Kantor, A. L. F., Meigs, J. M., Heston, J. F., and Flannery, J. T. (1976): *J. Natl. Cancer Inst.,* 57:495–500.
64. Kent, J. R., Bishoff, A. J., Arduino, L. J., Mellinger, G. T., Byar, D. P., Hill, M., and Kozbur, X. (1973): *J. Urol.,* 109:858–860.
65. King, R. J. B. (1967): *Arch. Anat. Micros. Morphol. (Suppl. 3–4),* 56:570–575.
66. Kirkman, H. (1957): *Cancer,* 10:757–764.
67. Kirkman, H. (1959): Parts I and II: *J. Natl. Cancer Inst.,* 13:745–771.
68. Kirkman, H., and Bacon, R. L. (1952): *J. Natl. Cancer Inst.,* 13:745–755.
69. Kochakian, C. D., Tomana, M., and Strickland, B. (1974): *Mol. Cell Endocrinol.,* 1:129–138.
70. Korenchevsky, V. M., and Ross, M. A. (1940): *Br. Med. J.,* 1:645.
71. Krieg, M., Bartsch, W., Herzer, S., Becker, H., and Voigt, K. D. (1977): *Acta Endocrinol.,* 86:200–215.
72. Lattimer, J. K. (1942): *J. Urol.,* 48:778–794.
73. Li, J. J., Cuthbertson, T. L., and Li, S. A. (1977): *Endocrinology,* 101:1006–1015.
74. Li, J. J., Kirkman, H., and Hunter, R. L. (1969): *J. Histochem. Cytochem.,* 17:386–393.
75. Li, J. J., and Li, S. A. (1977): In: *Research on Steroids, Vol. 7,* edited by A. Vermeulen, P. Jungblut, A. Klopper, and F. Sciarra, pp. 325–344. North-Holland, Amsterdam.
76. Li, J. J., Talley, D. J., Li, S. A., and Villee, C. A. (1974): *Endocrinology,* 95:1134–1141.
77. Li, J. J., Talley, D. J., Li, S. A., and Villee, C. A. (1976): *Cancer Res.,* 36:1127–1132.
78. Li, J. J., and Villee, C. A. (1972): *Proc. Fifth Int. Congr. Pharmacol.,* San Francisco, p. 140.
79. Li, S. A., and Li, J. J. (1978): *Endocrinology,* 103:2119–2128.
80. Li, S. A., Li, J. J., and Villee, C. A. (1977): *Ann. NY Acad. Sci.,* 286:369–383.
81. Liao, S., Liang, T., and Tymoczko, J. L. (1971): *J. Steroid Biochem.,* 3:401.
82. Lieskovsky, G., and Bruchovsky, N. (1979): *J. Urol.,* 121:54–58.
83. Lin, Y. C., Talley, D. J., and Villee, C. A. (1978): *Cancer Res.,* 38:1286–1290.
84. Lucke, B. (1934): *Am. J. Cancer,* 20:352–379.
85. Lucke, W. M., and Kelly, D. F. (1976): *Vet. Pathol.,* 13:264–276.
86. Ludden, J. B., Kreuger, E., and Wright, I. S. (1941): *Endocrinology,* 28:619–623.
87. Main, J. H. P. (1972): In: *Developmental Aspects of Oral Biology,* edited by H. G. Slavkin and L. A. Bavetta, pp. 385–405. Academic, New York.
88. Mainwairing, W. I. P. (1969): *J. Endocrinol.,* 45:531–541.
89. Mainwairing, W. I. P., and Milroy, E. J. G. (1973): *J. Endocrinol.,* 57:371–384.
90. Markland, F. S., Chopp, R. T., Cosgrove, M. D., and Hovard, E. B. (1978): *Cancer Res.,* 38:2818–2825.
91. Marver, D., Goodman, D., and Edelman, I. S. (1972): *Kidney Int.,* 1:210–223.

92. Matsuda, M., Osafune, M., Kotake, T., and Sonoda, T. (1976): *Jap. J. Urol.,* 67:635–646.
93. Mattews, V. S., Kirkman, H., and Bacon, R. L. (1947): *Proc. Soc. Exp. Biol. Med.,* 66:195–200.
94. Matulich, D. T., Spindler, B. G., Schambelan, M., and Baxter, J. D. (1976): *J. Clin. Endocrinol. Metab.,* 43:1170–1174.
95. Menon, M., Tananis, C. E., Hicks, L. L., Hawkins, E. F., McLoughlin, M. G., and Walsh, P. G. (1978): *J. Clin. Invest.,* 61:150–162.
96. Menon, M., Tananis, C. E., McLoughlin, M. G., Lippman, M. E., and Walsh, P. C. (1977): *J. Urol.,* 117:309–312.
97. Menon, M., Tananis, C. E., McLoughlin, M. G., and Walsh, P. C. (1977): *Cancer Treat. Rep.,* 61:265–271.
98. Mobbs, B. J., Johnson, I. E., and Connolly, J. G. (1976): *Proc. Am. Assoc. Cancer Res.,* 17:9 (abstr.).
99. Montie, I. E., Stewart, B. H., Straffon, R. A., Bonowsky, L. H., Hevitt, C. B., and Montague, D. K. (1977): *J. Urol.,* 117:272–275.
100. Morales, A., Kiruluta, G., and Lott, S. (1975): *J. Urol.,* 114:692–693.
101. Mostofi, F. K. (1967): In: *Renal Neoplasia,* edited by K. J. Stanten, Jr., pp. 63–75. Churchill, London.
102. Mowszowicz, I., and Bardin, C. W. (1974): *Steroids,* 23:793–807.
103. Noronha, R. F. (1975): *Invest. Urol.,* 13:136–141.
104. Orestano, F., Altwein, J. E., Knapstein, P., and Bandhauer, K. (1975): *J. Steroid Biochem.,* 6:845.
105. Paine, C. H., Wright, F. W., and Ellis, F. (1970): *Br. J. Cancer,* 24:277–282.
106. Papac, R. J. (1970): *Proc. Am. Assoc. Cancer Res.,* 25:26–40.
107. Pasqualini, J. R., Portois, M. C., Kuss, R., Khoury, S., Petit, J., Degennes, J. L., and Dirou, F. (1979): In: *Interdisciplinary Trends in Surgery, Vol. 1,* edited by W. Montorsi, L. Donati, and T. Longo, pp. 393–396. Minerva Medica, Milan.
108. Pasqualini, J. R., Sumida, C., and Gelly, C. (1974): *J. Steroid Biochem.,* 5:977–985.
109. Pasqualini, J. R., Sumida, G., Gelly, C., and Nguyen, B. l. (1973): *C. R. Acad. Sci. (Paris) Ser. D,* 276:3359–3362.
110. Paulson, D. F., Fraley, E. E., Rabson, A. S., Ketcham, A. S. (1968): *Surgery,* 64:241–247.
111. Radev, A. T. (1971): *Probl. Endokrinol. (Mosk.),* 76:96–100.
112. Rapp, F., and Geder, L. (1979): *Archives of Andrology,* 2(Suppl. 1):278 (abstr.).
113. Richardson, F. L. (1957): *J. Natl. Cancer Inst.,* 18:813–815.
114. Riviére, M., Chouroulinkov, I., and Guérin, M. (1961): *Bull. Assoc. Franc. Cancer,* 48:499–524.
115. Rouseeau, J., Baxter, J. D., Funder, J. W., Edelman, J. S., and Tomkins, G. M. (1972): *J. Steroid Biochem.,* 3:219–227.
116. Samuels, M. L., Sullivan, P., and Hove, C. D. (1968): *Cancer,* 22:525–532.
117. Sandberg, A. A., Muntzing, J., Kadohama, N., Karr, J. P., Sufrin, G., Kirdani, R. Y., and Murphy, G. P. (1977): *Cancer Treat. Rep.,* 61:289–295.
118. Sanford, E. J., Geder, L., Laychock, A., Rohner, T. J., Jr., and Rapp, F. (1977): *J. Urol.,* 118:789–792.
119. Sciarra, F., Sorcini, G., Di Silverio, F., and Gagliardi, V. (1973): *Clin. Endocrinol.,* 2:101–109.
120. Segaloff, A. (1973): *Cancer Res.,* 33:1136–1137.
121. Selye, H., (1940): *Can. Med. Assoc.,* 42:188.
122. Selye, H., (1941): *J. Urol.,* 46:110–131.
123. Shain, S. A., Boesel, R. W., Lamm, D. L., and Radwin, H. M. (1978): *Steroids,* 31:541–556.
124. Sinha, A. A., Blackard, C. E., Doe, R. P., and Seal, U. S. (1973): *Cancer,* 31:682–688.
125. Smith, P. H., Robinson, M. R. G., and Cooper, E. H. (1976): *Eur. J. Cancer,* 12:937–944.
126. Smolev, J. K., Coffey, D. S., and Scott, W. W. (1977): *J. Urol.,* 118:216–220.
127. Smolev, J. K., Heston, W. D. W., Scott, W. W., and Coffey, D. S. (1977): *Cancer Treat. Rep.,* 61:273–287.
128. Snochowski, M., Pousette, A., Ekman, P., Bression, D., Andersson, L., Hogberg, B., and Gustaffson, J. A. (1977): *J. Clin. Endocrinol. Metab.,* 45:920–930.
129. Takizawa, S. (1976): *Gann,* 67:33–40.

130. Tazaki, H., Baba, S., Murai, M., and Ohkoshi, M. (1973): *Proc. XVI Congr. Int. Soc. Urol. Vol. 2,* edited by C. Doin, pp. 79–83. Joly, Paris.
131. Thomas, J. A., and Manandhar, M. (1975): *J. Endocr.,* 65:149–150.
132. Venk, K. (1968): *Endokrinologie,* 53:378–389.
133. Verhoven, G., and De Moor, P. (1977): *J. Steroid Biochem.,* 8:113–119.
134. von Deimling, O., Barmeyer, A., Bausch, I., and Rossner, R. (1968): *Histochimie,* 15:348–362.
135. Wagle, D. G., and Murphy, G. P. (1971): *Cancer,* 28:318–321.
136. Wagner, R. K. (1972): *Hoppe Seylers Z. Physiol. Chem.,* 353:831–835.
137. Wagner, R. K., and Jungblut, P. W. (1979): In: *Steroid Receptors, Metabolism and Prostatic Cancer.* Workshop of the European Prostatic Center Research Group, Amsterdam, April 27–28. Excerpta Medica, Amsterdam *(in press).*
138. Wagner, R. K., Schulze, K. H., and Jungblut, P. W. (1975): *Acta Endocrinol. (Kbh.) [Suppl.],* 193:52 *(abstr.).*
139. Weinstein, B. I., and Troll, W. (1977): *Cancer Res.,* 37:3461–3463.
140. Weller, T. H. (1971): *N. Engl. J. Med.,* 285:203–214.
141. Zava, D. T., and McGuire, W. L. (1977): *J. Biol. Chem.,* 252:3703–3708.

Hormones and Cancer, edited by S. Iacobelli et al.
Raven Press, New York © 1980.

Relationship Between Estrogen Receptor Status and Relapse-Free Survival After Adjuvant CMF Chemotherapy

Gianni Bonadonna, Gabriele Tancini, Emilio Bajetta,
and Giovanni di Fronzo

National Tumor Institute, 20133 Milan, Italy

During the past few years, several independent studies have confirmed that the estrogen receptor (ER) status of a tumor biopsy specimen with advanced mammary carcinoma correlates with the response to hormone treatment. Thus, the ER status and the ER concentration represent a useful guideline to improve patient selection for endocrine therapy (16).

In more recent years the ER status has been evaluated to predict survival of primary breast cancer as well as response to chemotherapy. In almost all reported series, women with ER+ tumors were shown to have 3-year relapse-free survival (RFS) and total survival rates following primary surgery which were superior to those of women with ER− tumors (1,2,9,15). However, there has been considerable controversy concerning the relationship of ER status and response to chemotherapy in advanced breast cancer. Lippman et al. (13) have published that the response to combination chemotherapy is more likely to occur in patients whose tumors are characterized as ER− than in those patients whose tumors can be characterized as ER+. Other investigators (12; Carbone, *personal communication*) have reported that the opposite occurs, namely that ER+ tumors are more likely to regress with chemotherapy. All these reports have involved highly disparate differences in patient characteristics (prognostic variables, drug regimens, and response criteria) which could, in large part, explain for the contradictory results (8). In fact, when results were evaluated in a more uniform series of women with advanced breast cancer and previously untreated with chemotherapy and/or endocrine therapy, there was no relationship between ER status and response to chemotherapy (4,7).

The aim of this report is to briefly present our experience between ER status and response to cyclophosphamide, methotrexate, fluorouracil (CMF) combination chemotherapy in the adjuvant setting. The details of this prospective study were reported elsewhere (7,19).

PATIENTS AND METHODS

The series includes 256 women (193 premenopausal, 63 postmenopausal) with primary resectable breast cancer (UICC classification: T_{1a}-T_{2a}-T_{3a}) in whom the axillary lymph nodes were found to be histologically positive after radical or modified radical mastectomy. Adjuvant treatment consisted of the classic CMF chemotherapy (3). Within 4 weeks of surgery, patients were randomized to receive 12- or 6-monthly cycles of adjuvant CMF (6,19). Drug response was measured in terms of RFS at 3 years from mastectomy after performing systematic follow-up studies. Whenever technically feasible, the first treatment failure was also documented through biopsy (19).

The ER content was determined on the primary tumor utilizing the dextran-coated charcoal method (10,11). The binding parameters (ER concentration or fmoles/mg protein and association constant or K_A) were determined through Scatchard analysis. Levels below 5 fmoles/mg cytosol protein and $K_A < 1.5 \times 10^9 \ \text{M}^{-1}$ were regarded as negative (10).

The actuarial life table method has been utilized to summarize relapse-free distributions starting from the date of mastectomy. The statistical significance of differences observed between ER+ and ER− populations was assessed by the Mantel-Haenszel test for survivorship data (14).

ER STATUS AND RFS

Table 1 shows that in the series of patients in whom ER determination could be performed at the time of mastectomy, the 3-year actuarial analysis failed to reveal a significant difference between the subsets who received 12 or 6 cycles of adjuvant CMF. This lack of difference was also observed between pre- and postmenopausal women in both major nodal subgroups (1–3 and > 3 nodes positive).

Due to the lack of difference in therapeutic results and knowing that other prognostic variables (e.g., size of primary tumor, number of involved axillary nodes, and especially ER status) were comparable between the two groups receiving 12 or 6 cycles of adjuvant CMF, patients were grouped in one single series.

TABLE 1. *Three-year relapse-free and total survival rates in 193 premenopausal and in 63 postmenopausal women*

	CMF 12 cycles (%)	CMF 6 cycles (%)	*p*
RFS			
Premenopause	83.9	84.8	0.59
Postmenopause	85.2	75.2	0.39
Survival			
Premenopause	87.8	86.2	0.49
Postmenopause	92.4	84.7	0.44

TABLE 2. *Three-year relapse-free survival after adjuvant CMF related to ER status*

	No. patients	% Relapse-free			
		ER+	ER−	ER±	p^b
Premenopause	193	82.9	78.2	70.6	0.23
Nodes 1–3	104	96.3	81.9	79.0	0.13
>3	89	68.8	61.2	59.6	0.52
CMF amenorrhea[a]	131	87.2	71.3	70.1	0.16
No amenorrhea[a]	37	77.5	62.5	—	0.60
Postmenopause	63	81.9	75.2	100	0.82
Nodes 1–3	42	85.3	83.4	100	0.60
>3	21	74.1	66.7	100	0.90

[a] Patients with last menstrual period prior to mastectomy are excluded.
[b] On time distribution (ER+ versus ER−).
From ref. 7, G. Bonadonna et al., *Cancer Chemother. Pharmacol.* (1980), with permission.

TABLE 3. *ER status and "chemical castration" after adjuvant CMF*

	No. patients	CMF-induced amenorrhea (%)		3-Yr RFS (%)	p
ER+	117	Yes:	75	87.2	0.28
		No:	25	77.5	
ER−	29	Yes:	72	71.3	0.75
		No:	28	62.5	

Furthermore, a detailed analysis failed to reveal that the duration of adjuvant treatment affected the RFS when related to ER status. Table 2 shows that the 3-year RFS was similar between ER+ and ER− tumors, regardless of menopausal status. In particular, for ER+ and ER− tumors the RFS was comparable in the two major nodal subgroups as well as in women with and without CMF-induced amenorrhea. The hypothesis of some investigators that in premenopausal women the therapeutic effect of CMF is largely related to "chemical castration" finds no support from the findings (5) presented in Table 3. It is also important to point out that the results presented in Tables 2 and 3 remained essentially unchanged when the cut-off point between ER+ and ER− was raised to 10 fmoles/mg protein.

CONCLUSION

The present results indicate that in an adjuvant setting utilizing CMF chemotherapy, the 3-year RFS is not influenced by the ER status. Furthermore, the results were not substantially different when two levels of fmoles (> 5 or > 10) were considered. Thus, with the dose schedule of CMF utilized in primary breast cancer having positive axillary nodes, combination chemotherapy was equally effective both in ER+ and ER− tumor cells (7).

While tumor size, location in the breast, and axillary nodal status do not correlate with the presence of ER, preliminary evidence suggests that ER content does correlate with certain histologic features. Breast tumors are more frequently ER− when poorly differentiated, with high nuclear grade and growth fraction (17,18). Published results (1,2,9,15,16) showed that following surgery alone, the 3-year RFS and total survival rates of women with involved axillary nodes are superior in ER+ tumors as compared with ER− tumors. However, the data on the predictive value of ER status for survival is not sufficient to warrant acceptance at this time without further study (Carbone, *personal communication*).

In conclusion, present data confirm that, for the time being, the most important prognostic indicator for adjuvant chemotherapy remains the axillary nodal status. Our results strongly suggest that when effective adjuvant combination chemotherapy is applied, the reported prognostic difference between ER+ and ER− tumors becomes negligible. Since chemotherapy appears effective regardless of ER status, in the presence of ER+ tumors there is no reason to delay the early administration of adjuvant chemotherapy, alone or combined with endocrine therapy, in women with positive axillary nodes.

ACKNOWLEDGMENT

Supported in part by Contract NO1-CM-33714 with DCT, NCI, and NIH.

REFERENCES

1. Allegra, J. C., Simon, R., and Lippman, M. E. (1979): In: *Adjuvant Therapy of Cancer, Vol. 2*, edited by S. E. Salmon and S. E. Jones, pp. 47–54. Grune & Stratton, New York.
2. Bishop, H. M., Blamey, R. W., Elston, C. W., Haybittle, J. L., Nicholson, R. I., and Griffiths, K. (1979): *Lancet*, 2:283–284.
3. Bonadonna, G., Brusamolino, E., Valagussa, P., Rossi, A., Brugnatelli, L., Brambilla, C., De Lena, M., Tancini, G., Bajetta, E., Musumeci, R., and Veronesi, U. (1976): *N. Engl. J. Med.*, 294:405–410.
4. Bonadonna, G., Di Fronzo, G., and Tancini, G. (1979): *Proc. Am. Soc. Clin. Oncol.*, 20:359(*Abstr. C-281*).
5. Bonadonna, G., Valagussa, P., and De Palo, G. (1980): In: *Controversies in Medical Oncology*, edited by M. B. Van Scoy-Mosher. G. K. Hall, Boston (*in press*).
6. Bonadonna, G., Valagussa, P., Rossi, A., Zucali, R., Tancini, G., Bajetta, E., Brambilla, C., De Lena, M., Di Fronzo, G., Banfi, A., Rilke, F., and Veronesi, U. (1978): *Semin. Oncol.*, 5:450–463.
7. Bonadonna, G., Valagussa, P., Tancini, G., and Di Fronzo, G. (1980): *Cancer Chemother. Pharmacol.*, 4:37–41.
8. Carter, S. K. (1979): *Cancer Clin. Trials*, 2:49–53.
9. Cooke, T., George, D., Shields, R., Maynard, P., and Griffiths, K. (1979): *Lancet*, 1:995–997.
10. Di Fronzo, G., Bertuzzi, A., and Ronchi, E. (1978): *Tumori*, 64:259–266.
11. EORTC Breast Cancer Cooperative Group (1973): *Eur. J. Cancer*, 9:379–381.
12. Kiang, O. T., Frenning, D. H., Goldman, A. I., Ascensao, V. F., and Kennedy, B. J. (1978): *N. Engl. J. Med.*, 299:1330–1334.
13. Lippman, M. E., Allegra, J. C., Thompson, E. B., Simon, R., Barlock, A., Green, L., Huff,

K. K., Do, H. M. T., Aitken, S. C., and Warren, R. (1978): *N. Engl. J. Med.,* 298:1223–1228.

14. Mantel, N. (1966): *Cancer Chemother. Rep.,* 50:163–170.
15. Maynard, P. V., Blamey, R. W., Elston, C. W., Haybittle, J. L., and Griffiths, K. (1978): *Cancer Res.,* 38:4292–4295.
16. McGuire, W. L. (1978): *Semin. Oncol.,* 5:428–433.
17. Meyer, J. S., Rao, B. R., Stevens, S. C., and White, W. L. (1977): *Cancer,* 40:2290–2298.
18. Osborne, C. K., and McGuire, L. (1979): *Bull. Cancer,* 66(3):203–210.
19. Tancini, G., Bajetta, E., Marchini, S., Valagussa, P., Bonadonna, G., and Veronesi, U. (1979): *Cancer Clin. Trials,* 2:285–292.

Predisposing Factors

Hormones and Cancer, edited by S. Iacobelli et al.
Raven Press, New York © 1980.

Control of the Metabolism of Testosterone in the Prostate and in Other Androgen-Dependent Structures

F. Celotti, P. Ferraboschi, P. Negri-Cesi, and L. Martini

Department of Endocrinology, University of Milan, 20129 Milan, Italy

It is now well established that the prostate of the rat converts testosterone (T) into 5α-androstan-17β-ol-3-one (dihydrotestosterone, DHT) and 5α-andro-stan-3α,17β-diol(3α-diol) (3,26,33). These conversions occur under the influence of a 5α-reductase-3α-hydroxysteroid dehydrogenase system, and play a signifi-cant role for the expression of the multiple actions T exerts on the gland. The 3β-isomer of 3α-diol, 5α-androstan-3β,17β-diol (3β-diol), which is a regular T metabolite in the human (2,17) and in the dog prostate (16,21), is not formed in significant amounts by the rat prostate (15,33,37,38). A similar metabolic pattern has been shown to be present in other androgen-responding peripheral structures (seminal vesicles, sebaceous glands, etc.) (35,36,42). Evidence obtained in this and other laboratories indicates that the central nervous system (CNS) (mainly the hypothalamus) and the anterior pituitary gland are also able to metabolize T into DHT and 3α-diol both *in vitro* and *in vivo* (5,10,19,28,34,40,41; see also 6 for refs.). As in the case of the prostate, very little 3β-diol seems to be formed by the central structures of the rat (10,18,31,39).

Very little information is available on the endocrine factors which control the activity of the 5α-reductase-3α-hydroxysteroid dehydrogenase system in the peripheral and in the central structures. The experiments to be reported here have been planned (a) to analyze whether androgens and prolactin might modu-late the activity of these enzymatic systems, and (b) to clarify whether these hormonal factors might operate differentially in the various androgen-dependent tissues. In the present experiments, all hormonal treatments have been performed *in vivo,* while the metabolites of T have been quantitated *in vitro* according to procedures previously described by this laboratory (19,25). Depending on the experiment, either T or DHT have been used as substrates. It was not believed essential to separate 3α-diol from 3β-diol, since the amounts of the latter formed by the various androgen-sensitive structures of the rat are very limited. Conse-quently, the term "diols" will appear in the figures and in the text.

ROLE OF ANDROGENS

Effect of Castration

For this experiment, adult male rats were castrated under light ether anesthesia 20 days before sacrifice; at autopsy, the prostates, the seminal vesicles, the anterior pituitaries, and the hypothalami were collected.

Figure 1 shows that, when T is used as the substrate, orchidectomy does not modify the quantities of DHT recovered at the end of the incubation period in the prostate; however, the formation of the "diols" is significantly increased. As a consequence of this increase, the "total" 5α-metabolites formed in the prostate are also higher following the operation. These results, which agree with previous findings of Massa et al. (27), suggest that the 3-hydroxysteroid dehydrogenase system is stimulated in the prostate following orchidectomy; the activity of the 5α-reductase is also increased, possibly as the consequence of a higher utilization of DHT for the conversion into the "diols." Castration does not modify the formation of DHT and of the "diols" in the seminal vesicles (Fig. 2) or in the hypothalamus (Fig. 3), suggesting that endogenous androgens do not intervene in the control of the two enzymatic activities under consideration in these structures. The negative result obtained at hypothalamic level is confirmatory of previous evidence obtained in this laboratory (19,24,28). Orchidectomy is followed by a significant increase in the formation of DHT and of the "diols" at anterior pituitary level (Fig. 4); obviously, also the "total" 5α-reduced metabolites are enhanced in this structure following castration. These findings are similar to those obtained in previous studies performed in this and other laboratories

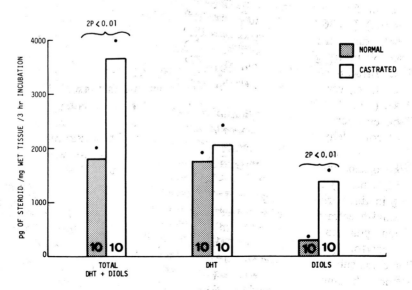

FIG. 1. Effect of castration (20 days) on T metabolism in the ventral prostate of male rats.

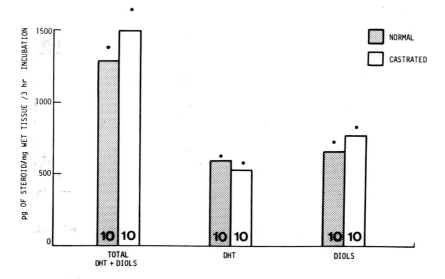

FIG. 2. Effect of castration (20 days) on T metabolism in the seminal vesicles of male rats.

(10,19,28,40), and suggest that both the 5α-reductase and the 3-hydroxysteroid dehydrogenase are hyperactive following castration in the anterior pituitary. However, it is not clear whether the increased formation of DHT and of the "diols" is due to a real stimulation of the activity of the two enzymatic systems, or whether it only reflects the changes in pituitary cell population which is

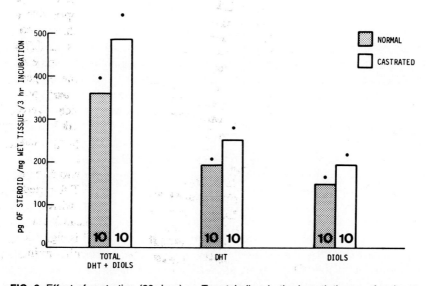

FIG. 3. Effect of castration (20 days) on T metabolism in the hypothalamus of male rats.

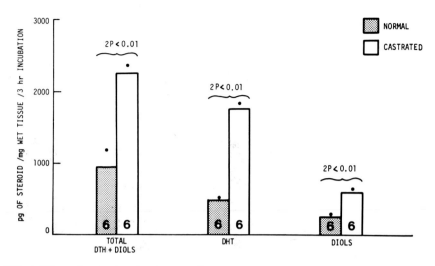

FIG. 4. Effect of castration (20 days) on T metabolism in the anterior pituitary of male rats.

induced by castration. *In vitro* and *in vivo* evidence suggests that the 5α-reductase is particularly concentrated in the gonadotrophs (4,9,23) which augment in number and in size following castration.

Effect of Androgen Administration

It is clear from the results described above that the elimination of endogenous T (and of other androgens of testicular origin) brings about totally different effects in the various organs considered. Because of this observation, it was felt necessary to perform the opposite experiment and to study the effect of treatment of castrated rats with several androgens which are present in the general circulation of this species [T (12,13,29); DHT (12,13); 3α-diol (8,29,45); 3β-diol (8,45)]. Adult male rats were castrated under light ether anesthesia 5 weeks before the beginning of the experiment. Animals were treated for 6 days with 2 mg/day of the various androgens. Controls received the vehicle only (0.2 ml peanut oil). All steroids were administered in the propionate form (monoester in the case of T and DHT, or diesters in the case of 3α- and 3β-diol). With the exception of T propionate, all esters were prepared in the laboratory as previously described (5).

Figure 5 shows that the *in vivo* treatment with either T or DHT significantly increases the quantities of DHT formed in the ventral prostate following incubation with labeled T. Treatment with the dipropionates of 3α- and 3β-diol induces only a slight (but not significant) increase in the *in vitro* formation of DHT. The formation of the "diols" is significantly inhibited by all exogenous steroids tested. These results are the mirror image of the data obtained after castration,

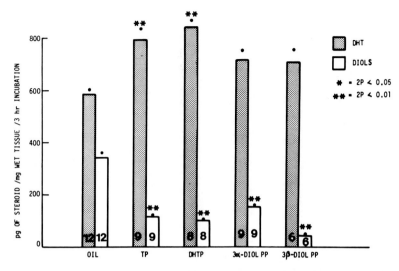

FIG. 5. Effects of different androgens on T metabolism in the ventral prostate of castrated rats.

and suggest that, in the prostate, androgens exert a major inhibitory effect on the 3-hydroxysteroid dehydrogenase. The stimulatory effect of exogenous androgens on the formation of DHT might only be indirect, resulting from the smaller utilization of DHT as the substrate for the formation of the "diols." However, the stimulatory effect of T propionate on the 5α-reductase activity of the prostate of the rat is in agreement with previous results (22,44). To the authors knowledge, no data on the effects on this enzyme of the other androgens included in this study have been reported so far. Shimazaki et al. (37) have demonstrated that, in the prostate of the rat, the 3-hydroxysteroid dehydrogenase system is not affected by the administration of exogenous T propionate. These results are in disagreement with the present data. The discrepancy may result from differences in the experimental conditions used, such as the beginning of treatment after castration (1 week versus 5 weeks) and the preparation of the tissues (homogenization versus fragmentation).

To substantiate the hypothesis that androgens in the prostate might mainly affect the 3-hydroxysteroid dehydrogenase, an experiment was performed in which labeled DHT was used as the substrate. Treatments were performed as in the preceding experiment. It is apparent from the data (Fig. 6) that pretreatment with T and DHT propionates, 3α-diol and 3β-diol dipropionates decreased the formation of the "diols." T and 3α-diol were particularly effective. These results certainly support the view that androgens directly affect the activity of this enzymatic system, and reinforces the hypothesis that their activity on the 5α-reductase of the prostate is probably only an indirect one.

Figure 7 shows that the administration of exogenous androgens brings about

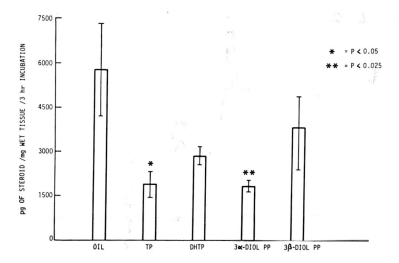

FIG. 6. Effects of different androgens on DHT metabolism in the ventral prostate of castrated male rats.

a significant increase in the formation of DHT in the seminal vesicles of orchidectomized rats. DHT propionate and 3α-diol dipropionate seem also able to increase the formation of the "diols." These data may appear surprising, since castration did not exert any significant effect on T metabolism in the seminal vesicles. It is possible that the T converting enzymes of this structure, although sensitive to androgens, need supraphysiological doses in order to be activated.

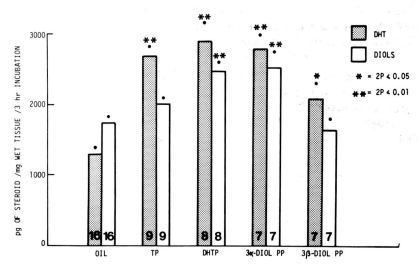

FIG. 7. Effects of different androgens on T metabolism in the seminal vesicles of castrated rats.

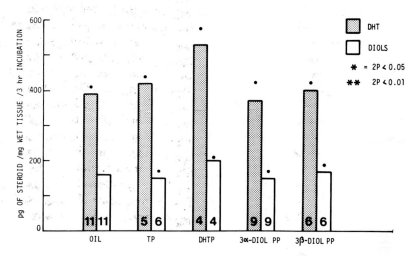

FIG. 8. Effects of different androgens on T metabolism in the hypothalamus of castrated male rats.

It is however interesting to note that the seminal vesicles respond to androgen treatment in a fashion totally different from the prostate. Androgen treatment did not influence the formation of DHT and of "diols" in the hypothalami (Fig. 8). This is analogous to what it has been observed following castration, and shows the total insensitivity to T and its derivatives of the androgen metabolizing enzymes of this structure.

Figure 9 indicates that, at the level of the anterior pituitary, the formation of DHT is inhibited by all the steroids used and significantly so by T propionate,

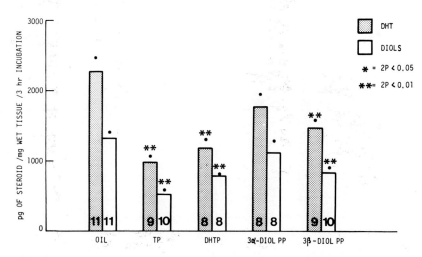

FIG. 9. Effects of different androgens on T metabolism in the anterior pituitary of castrated male rats.

DHT propionate, and 3β-diol dipropionate. Also, the formation of the "diols" was decreased by all steroids tested; the decrease, however, was not significant in the case of 3α-diol dipropionate. The inhibitory effect of androgens on the 5α-reductase-3-hydroxysteroid dehydrogenase system of the anterior pituitary is consistent with previous observations made administering T (10,11,19,20,28). At variance with the present results in which T and DHT had comparable inhibitory effects, Denef et al. (11) have reported DHT to be less effective than T in decreasing the 5α-reductase activity of the anterior pituitary. It must however be noted that the experiments of Denef et al. (11) have been performed in prepuberal rats, while those here reported have utilized mature animals. In agreement with the interpretation provided when considering the effects of castration at anterior pituitary level, it is possible that the results obtained following androgen treatment only reflect the disappearance (or the return to normal) of the gonadotrophs in which, as previously mentioned, the T-metabolizing machinery is predominantly localized (4,9,23).

Effect of Prolactin

In this study, rat prolactin (rPrl) has been administered subcutaneously for 5 days to adult male rats (castrated since 20 days) in the daily dose of 800 μg/rat. It was decided to use orchidectomized animals in order to avoid the possibility of indirect effects due to the actions of prolactin on the testis. This hormone potentiates the activity of luteinizing hormone in inducing the secretion of T and of other androgens from the testis (1,14). In these experiments, the

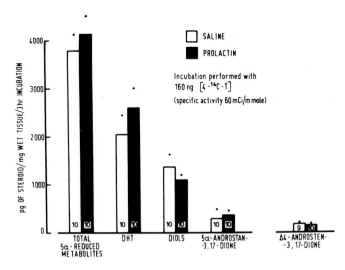

FIG. 10. Effect of *in vivo* treatment with rat prolactin (400 μg/rat twice daily s.c. for 5 days) on T metabolism *in vitro* in the ventral prostate of castrated male rats.

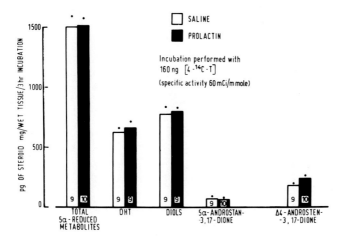

FIG. 11. Effect of *in vivo* treatment with rat prolactin (400 μg/rat twice daily s.c. for 5 days) on T metabolism *in vitro* in the seminal vesicles of castrated male rats.

amounts of 5α-androstan-3,17-dione and of Δ₄-androstene-3,17-dione formed by the various tissues have also been quantitated.

Figures 10, 11, and 12 clearly indicate that, at the dose used, rPrl did not significantly alter the conversion of T into its various metabolites in the prostate, in the seminal vesicles, and in the anterior pituitary. By contrast, the treatment was able to significantly diminish the total amounts of the 5α-reduced metabolites formed by the hypothalamus (Fig. 13). The quantities of DHT, "diols" and 5α-androstan-3,17-dione were all proportionally decreased by the treatment.

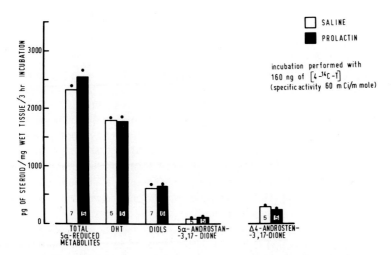

FIG. 12. Effect of *in vivo* treatment with rat prolactin (400 μg/rat twice daily s.c. for 5 days) on T metabolism *in vitro* in the anterior pituitary of castrated male rats.

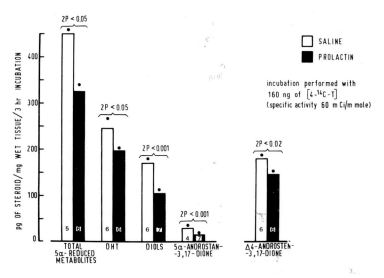

FIG. 13. Effect of *in vivo* treatment with rat prolactin (400 μg/rat twice daily s.c., for 5 days) on T metabolism *in vitro* in the hypothalamus of castrated male rats.

The production of Δ_4-androstene-3,17-dione was also diminished. These data suggest that the 5α-reductase 3-hydroxysteroid dehydrogenase system is sensitive to the inhibitory effect of Prl only at hypothalamic level, but not in the anterior pituitary, the prostate, and the seminal vesicles. Evidence supporting the possibility of an action of prolactin on the hypothalamus is already available. Prl, when implanted into the median eminence, has been shown to decrease the release of endogenous prolactin via a "short feedback" effect (see 30 and 32 for refs.). Systemically administered prolactin has also been reported to modify the firing rate of hypothalamic neurons (7,43).

CONCLUSIONS

The results of the present experiments indicate that androgens participate in the control of the metabolism of T in the prostate, in the seminal vesicles, and in the anterior pituitary but that they do not intervene in such a regulation at hypothalamic level. The effect of androgens, however, seems to be different in the various organs. In the prostate, androgens seem to exert mainly an inhibitory effect on the 3-hydroxysteroid dehydrogenase; as a consequence of this, an indirect stimulation of the 5α-reductase activity may be observed. In contrast, in the seminal vesicles (which on the basis of the results obtained following castration seem to be less sensitive to androgens) exogenous androgens, when given in supraphysiological doses, seem to exert a stimulatory effect on both the 5α-reductase and the 3-hydroxysteroid dehydrogenase. Finally, androgen decreases the formation of DHT and of the "diols" in the anterior pituitary.

Prl, on the other hand, does not affect the metabolism of T in the prostate, the seminal vesicles, or the anterior pituitary. This hormone seems to intervene in the regulation of T metabolism only at hypothalamic level, i.e., in the only structure which has been found to be refractory to the effect of androgens.

It is obvious that the present results must be considered preliminary because the kinetics of the various reactions involved have not been studied in detail. The data presented suggest that a further analysis of the effect of different androgens and of Prl on the 5α-reductase 3-hydroxysteroid dehydrogenase of various androgen dependent-structures may be fruitful.

ACKNOWLEDGMENTS

The experiments reported here have been supported by grants of the Ford Foundation, New York, and of the Consiglio Nazionale delle Ricerche through the projects "Control of Neoplastic Growth" and "Biology of Reproduction."

REFERENCES

1. Bartke, A. (1971): *J. Endocrinol.*, 49:311–316.
2. Becker, H., Kaufmann, J., Klosterhalfen, H., and Voigt, K. D. (1972): *Acta Endocrinol. (Kbh.)*, 71:589–599.
3. Bruchovsky, N., and Wilson, J. D. (1968): *J. Biol. Chem.*, 243:2012–2021.
4. Celotti, F., Farina, J., Cresti, L., and Martini, L. (1976): *Program 5th International Congress of Endocrinology*, p. 44.
5. Celotti, F., Farina, J. M. S., Santaniello, E., Martini, L., and Motta, M. (1979): *J. Steroid Biochem.*, 11:215–219.
6. Celotti, F., Massa, R., and Martini, L. (1979): In: *Endocrinology*, edited by L. J. De Groot, pp. 41–53, Grune & Stratton, New York.
7. Clemens, J. A., Gallo, R. V., Whitmoyer, D. I., and Sawyer, C. H. (1971): *Brain Res.*, 25:371–379.
8. Corpechot, C., Eychenne, B., and Robel, P. (1977): *Steroids*, 29:503–515.
9. Denef, C. (1979): *Neuroendocrinology*, 29:132–139.
10. Denef, C., Magnus, C., and McEwen, B. S. (1973): *J. Endocrinol.*, 59:605–621.
11. Denef, C., Magnus, C., and McEwen, B. S. (1974): *Endocrinology*, 94:1265–1274.
12. Ganadian, R., Lewis, J. G., and Chisholm, D. C. (1975): *Steroids*, 25:753–762.
13. Gupta, D., Zarzycki, J., and Rager, K. (1975): *Steroids*, 25:33–42.
14. Hafiez, A. A., Bartke, A., and Lloyd, C. W. (1972): *J. Endocrinol.*, 53:223–230.
15. Inano, H., Hayashi, S., and Tamaoki, B. (1977): *J. Steroid Biochem.*, 8:41–46.
16. Jacobi, G. H., and Wilson, J. D. (1976): *Endocrinology*, 99:602–610.
17. Jacobi, G. H., and Wilson, J. D. (1977): *J. Clin. Endocrinol. Metab.*, 44:107–115.
18. Kao, L., Lloret, A. P., and Weisz, J. (1977): *J. Steroid Biochem.*, 8:1109–1115.
19. Kniewald, Z., Massa, R., and Martini, L. (1971): In: *Hormonal Steroids*, edited by V. H. T. James and L. Martini, pp. 784–791. Excerpta Medica, Amsterdam.
20. Kniewald, Z., and Milkovic, S. (1973): *Endocrinology*, 92:1772–1775.
21. Leav, I., Morfin, R., Ofner, P., Cavazos, L. F., and Leeds, E. B. (1971): *Endocrinology*, 89:465–483.
22. Lee, D. K. H., Bird, C., and Clark, A. (1974): *J. Steroid Biochem.*, 5:609–617.
23. Lloyd, R. V., and Karavolas, J. H. (1975): *Endocrinology*, 97:517–526.
24. Martini, L., Celotti, F., Massa, R., and Motta, M. (1978): *J. Steroid Biochem.*, 9:411–417.
25. Massa, R., Cresti, L., and Martini, L. (1977): *J. Endocrinol.*, 75:347–354.
26. Massa, R., and Martini, L. (1971/1972): *Gynecol. Invest.*, 2:253–270.
27. Massa, R., Mas Garcia, M., and Martini, L. (1978): *J. Endocrinol.*, 79:143–144.

28. Massa, R., Stupnicka, E., Kniewald, Z., and Martini, L. (1972): *J. Steroid Biochem.,* 3:385–399.
29. Moger, W. H. (1977): *Endocrinology,* 100:1027–1032.
30. Motta, M., Fraschini, F., and Martini, L. (1969): In: *Frontiers in Neuroendocrinology,* edited by W. F. Ganong and L. Martini, pp. 211–253. Oxford University Press, New York.
31. Noma, K., Sato, B., Yano, S., and Yamamura, Y. (1975): *J. Steroid Biochem.,* 6:1261–1266.
32. Piva, F., Motta, M., and Martini, L. (1979): In: *Endocrinology,* edited by L. J. De Groot, pp. 21–33. Grune & Stratton, New York.
33. Robel, P., Lasnitzki, I., and Baulieu, E. E. (1971): *Biochimie,* 53:81–96.
34. Rommerts, F. F. G., and Van der Molen, H. J. (1971): *Biochim. Biophys. Acta,* 248:489–502.
35. Schmidt, H., Giba-Tziampiri, O., Rotteck, G. V., and Voigt, K. D. (1973): *Acta Endocrinol. (Kbh.),* 73:599–611.
36. Schmidt, H., Noack, I., and Voigt, K. D. (1972): *Acta Endocrinol. (Kbh.),* 69:165–173.
37. Shimazaki, J., Kato, N., Nagai, H., Yamanaka, H., and Shida, K. (1972): *Endocrinol. Jpn.,* 19:97–106.
38. Taurog, J. D., Moore, R. J., and Wilson, J. D. (1975): *Biochemistry,* 14:810–817.
39. Thien, N. C., Samperez, S., and Jouan, P. (1975): *J. Steroid Biochem.,* 6:1165–1169.
40. Thieulant, M. L., Samperez, S., and Jouan, P. (1973): *J. Steroid Biochem.,* 4:677–685.
41. Whalen, R. E., and Rezek, D. L. (1972): *Steroids,* 20:717–725.
42. Wilson, J. D., and Gloyna, R. (1970): *Rec. Prog. Horm. Res.,* 26:309–336.
43. Yamada, Y. (1975): *Neuroendocrinology,* 18:263–271.
44. Yamanaka, H., Kirdani, R. Y., Saroff, J., Murphy, G. P., and Sandberg, A. A. (1975): *Am. J. Physiol.,* 229:1102–1109.
45. Zamecnik, J., Barbe, G., Moger, W. H., and Armstrong, D. T. (1977): *Steroids,* 30:679–689.

Hormones and Cancer, edited by S. Iacobelli et al.
Raven Press, New York © 1980.

Hormonal Dependence of Endometrial Adenocarcinoma and Its Hormonal Sensitivity to Progestogens and Antiestrogens

J. Bonte

*Gynecologic Cancerology, Sint Rafaël Hospital, University of Louvain,
B-3000 Louvain, Belgium*

The generally accepted hypothesis of hormonal dependence of uterine adenocarcinoma on estrogens and the rational corollary of hormonal sensitivity to progestogens and antiestrogens has been studied *in vivo* on 341 patients and *in vitro* on organotypic cultures.

RESEARCH DATA

Histological Data

Histological data were obtained *in vivo* by pathological examination of tissue from successive curettages in stage I endometrial adenocarcinoma and of material collected by successive biopsies from vaginal recurrences in advanced cancers under progestational or antiestrogenic treatment. Except for extremely well differentiated and totally anaplastic tumors, most uterine adenocarcinomas exhibit histological polymorphism. Such tumors are subdivided for experimental purposes according to the dominant histological entity into differentiated and undifferentiated adenocarcinomas.

There is a striking correlation between the histological type of the adenocarcinoma and the hormonal status of the patient: in our study postmenopausal patients, presenting an estrogenic vaginal smear, bear the more differentiated adenocarcinomas, characterized by pseudostratification and a high mitotic index, whereas those with an atrophic vaginal smear have a rather undifferentiated tumor (20). These data evidence a certain hormonal dependence of the tumor on estrogens. Moreover, in practically all our postmenopausal patients bearing either primary or metastatic uterine adenocarcinoma, plasma estradiol levels are statistically elevated as compared with normal postmenopausal values.

The hormonal sensitivity of uterine adenocarcinoma to progestogens and antiestrogens was studied in short-term experiments in stage I cases by the administration per os of either 150 mg medroxyprogesterone acetate (MPA; Provera®), 10 mg 18-methylnorethisterone (*d*-norgestrel), or 60 mg tamoxifen (Nolvadex®) a day for 7 days. In long-term experiments in advanced, metastatic, or recurrent adenocarcinoma either 150 mg MPA or 40 mg tamoxifen/day was administered per os over many months or years.

The response of differentiated endometrial adenocarcinomas (19) to progestogens is characterized by the transformation of pseudostratified to monolayered glands, presenting a secretory activity; by marked epithelial metaplasia of the glandular structures, especially in adenoacanthomatous tumors; by pseudodecidualization of the stroma; and finally by atrophy of the epithelium and fibrosis of the stroma, representing the disappearance of the tumoral structures.

In undifferentiated adenocarcinomas (21) progestogens induce polarization and centralization of the cells, suggesting acinus formation in massive anaplastic tumors and producing endopapillary acinus formation in poorly differentiated ones.

Analogous, more rapidly appearing histological responses of endometrial adenocarcinoma are found under influence of antiestrogens: transformation of pseudostratified carcinomatous glands to monolayered structures constituted by high, cylindrical and even atrophic cells.

Some endometrial adenocarcinomas, unresponsive to progestogens from the beginning or becoming resistent after a long period of responsiveness, still evidence marked histological regression phenomena with antiestrogen treatment. However, they maintain a high mitotic index, perhaps explaining the transitory nature of the response.

The original polymorphism and the hormonal-induced structural changes indicate that endometrial adenocarcinoma responds to estrogens by extreme proliferation, and to progestogens and antiestrogens by transformation to reserve cells, by secretion, and finally by atrophy. Studied separately, estrogens on one side, and progestogens and antiestrogens on the other side exert an antagonistic effect on the endometrial adenocarcinoma; moreover, progestogens and antiestrogens illustrate at least partly different aspects of hormonal sensitivity of endometrial adenocarcinoma.

Clinical Data

While on histological, and certainly on cytological evaluation, all endometrial adenocarcinomas seem to be responsive to progestogens and antiestrogens to some extent, only a proportion can be considered as hormonal sensitive on a clinical basis. This clinical evaluation of the therapeutic efficiency of progestogens and antiestrogens alone or as an adjuvant in a treatment scheme is founded on anatomoclinical and radiological data.

Hormonal Therapy

In approximately 60% of the patients with endometrial adenocarcinoma *in situ* treated by means of progestogens, no residual cancer could be detected. The same oral or parenteral administration of progestogens in invasive stage I endometrial adenocarcinoma completely destroyed the tumor in not more than 20% of the cases (15,16).

Local intracavitary application of progestogens was more effective in eradication of invasive stage I endometrial adenocarcinoma. After intrauterine instillation of progestogens, the tumor completely disappeared in approximately 35% of the cases. Intrauterine insertion of a medroxyprogesterone-releasing silastic device achieved total destruction of cancer tissue in 60% of uteri having no myometrial invasion (22).

Since the first publication by Kelley and Baker (24) on the treatment of advanced or recurrent uterine adenocarcinoma by means of progestogens, 84 reports have provided data on responses to 11 different progestogens and have analyzed the remission rate in about 3,700 patients. In the five collaborative reports, more than half of the 2,018 patients were treated by 17α-hydroxy progesterone caproate (17α-OHPC) and the mean objective remission rate lies between 30 and 35%. A total of 1,670 patients was studied in 59 individual reports: 550 patients were treated with MPA and 586 with 17α-OHPC. Considering the mean objective remission rate calculated per individual report, one observes a difference between the responses to the various progestogens: 47% with MPA and 28% with 17α-OHPC (9) (Table 1).

In the most recent analysis of our series of 115 patients treated with 150 mg MPA/day p.o., the objective remission rate was 51%. The average duration of remissions obtained by MPA therapy was 11 months (Fig. 1). The mean survival of the total patient group amounts to 7 months, while the duration of survival reaches 20 months in the subgroup of more hormone-responsive cases (Fig. 2).

In one case report, in 4 of 11 patients with endometrial adenocarcinoma, objective regressions were obtained following the administration of clomiphene citrate. Taking these data into account, we have carried out a preliminary study of secondary tamoxifen therapy in advanced or recurrent endometrial adenocarcinomas. Tamoxifen at a daily dosage of 40 mg was administered orally to a series of 10 patients who either failed to respond or relapsed after significant remission under MPA treatment. Six patients showed tumor regression (two showed complete regression, two partial regression). The patients who were sensitive to tamoxifen were those who had previously responded to MPA, but under tamoxifen the duration of the remission seems markedly shorter (Table 2).

TABLE 1. *Treatment of advanced or recurrent endometrial adenocarcinoma with progestogens*

Type of progestogen	Mean significant remission rate %	No. cases
Progesterone	56	4
MPA	47	22
6,17α-Dimethyl-6-dehydroprogesterone	33	4
17α-OHPC	28	15

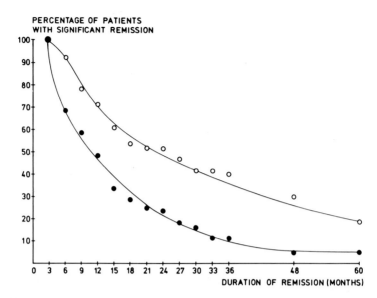

FIG. 1. Advanced or recurrent endometrical adenocarcinoma patients treated with MPA alone *(closed circles)* or with MPA followed by radiotherapy *(open circles)* presenting significant remission.

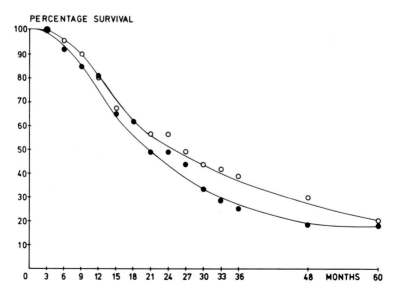

FIG. 2. Advanced or recurrent endometrial adenocarcinoma patients treated with MPA alone *(closed circles)* or with MPA followed by radiotherapy *(open circles)* presenting significant remission.

TABLE 2. *Response of advanced endometrial adenocarcinoma to successive MPA and tamoxifen treatment*

Patient	Histolog. Type	Response to MPA treatment		Response to tamoxifen treatment			
				Clinical		Cytological	
		Type	Duration	Type	Duration	PAP smear evolution	Cytohormonal evolution
75/1067	Diff	Stabil	4 mos.	Part. regres	2 mos.	PAP V → PAP V	Atrophic → Estrog
75/1117	Undiff	Progres	2 mos.	Stabil	2 mos.	PAP V → PAP V	Subatr → Estrog
73/1136	Well diff	Compl. regres	6 mos.	Part. regres	5 mos.	PAP V → PAP V	Atrophic → Subatr
76/1247	Mod. diff	Unsucc. adj.	6 mos.	Progres	2 mos.	PAP II → PAP II	Subatr → Estrog
76/1048	Well diff	Stabil	4 mos.	Progres	1½ mos.	PAP V → PAP V	Subatr → Estrog
75/1706	Well diff	Progres	5 mos.	Stabil	1 mos.	PAP V → PAP V	Atrophic → Atrophic
69/1151	Well diff	Compl. regres	9 yr	{ Part. regres / Stabil	3 mos. / 5 mos.	PAP V → PAP I	Subatr → Estrog
72/1618	Diff	Compl. regres	5 yr	Part. regres	1 mos.	PAP V → PAP V	Subatr → Subatr
77/1312	Mod. diff	Unsucc. adj.	1 yr	Stabil	3 mos.	PAP V → PAP V	Subatr → Estrog
77/1156	Well diff	I { Adj	1 yr	{ Compl. regres / Stabil	2 mos. / 2 mos.	PAP V → PAP V	Atrophic → Estrog
		II { Compl. regres / Stabil	3 mos. / 12 mos.	Compl. regres	3 mos.		Atrophic → Estrog

Because the complete cure rate in endometrial adenocarcinoma *in situ* and stage I achieved by means of progestogens alone is limited to 60%, this exclusive hormonal therapy is only indicated in selected cases such as a carcinoma *in situ* in the endometrium of a younger woman, still having pregnancy expectations. In stage I endometrial adenocarcinoma, peroral or parenteral progestational therapy can be used as an adjuvant to the radiosurgical treatment of this cancer, while intrauterine insertion of a silastic device impregnated with MPA replaces presurgical radiumpacking with a view to radioprotection.

In advanced and recurrent endometrial adenocarcinomas, administration of progestogens or antiestrogens represents the treatment of choice, because these hormonal treatments never induce significant side effects, exhibit cross-efficiency, and can be complemented by radiotherapy.

Adjuvant Hormonal Therapy

Progestogens are also used as adjuvant therapy to the radiosurgical management of stage I endometrial adenocarcinoma either prior to radium applications or hysterectomy, or during the postoperative period (5).

Radical hysterectomy has of course a very important place in primary treatment of localized endometrial carcinoma. Preparing patients 4 weeks in advance by means of intracavitary radiumtherapy results in a 5-year survival rate of 72%. In a randomized study we have tried to evaluate the contribution of three different types of progestogen prophylaxis. The first type of progestogen prophylaxis consisted of 1 g MPA/week during 4 weeks prior to radiumpacking and increased the 5-year survival rate in this group to 90%. This progestogen adjuvant therapy represents a radiosensitization of the adenocarcinoma (13): MPA makes the tumor more sensitive to the antitumoral effect of ionizing radiation and thus potentiates the radiotherapy. Pathological examination of resected material reveals a significant decrease of apparently viable adenocarcinomatous tissue in patients receiving progestogen adjuvant therapy, as compared with those treated with radiation and surgery alone. For the same hormonal prophylactic purposes, more recently we have used norgestrel (10 mg/day p.o.) and tamoxifen (60 mg/day p.o.) during the week immediately preceding radiumpacking.

In another type of progestogen prophylaxis we administered 1 g MPA/week during 2 years following radiumpacking and hysterectomy in order to prevent recurrences and metastatic dissemination; this approach resulted in an increase of the 5-year survival rate to 86%. Finally, combining postsurgical progestogen prophylaxis with progestogen prophylaxis prior to radiumpacking yielded a 5-year survival rate of nearly 100%.

In a retrospective study the influence of adjuvant progestogen therapy on recurrence rate and 5-year survival rate of patients treated with different therapeutic schemes is evaluated. After correction for death from intercurrent disease, the recurrence rate remains 0 and the 5-year survival rate 100% (7) (Fig. 3).

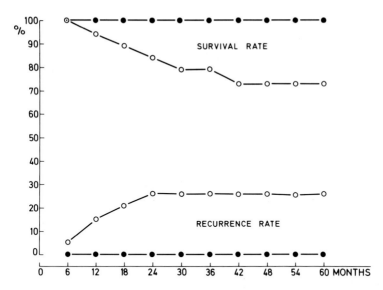

FIG. 3. Endometrial adenocarcinoma—stage I. 71 patients treated with radiumtherapy and/ or hysterectomy without adjuvant hormonotherapy *(open circles)* or with adjuvant medroxypro- gesterone therapy *(closed circles)*. Numbers have been corrected for deaths from intercurrent disease.

Adjuvant progestational treatment seems to be effective not only in stage I endometrial adenocarcinoma but even in advanced (III–IV) stages (4). Radio- therapy used in combination with the MPA treatment in a selected patient group further improved the objective remission rate achieved by radiotherapy alone (25%) and by MPA treatment alone (51%) by elevating the remission rate to 91%; in that way the average duration of remissions can be extended to 25 months, and the mean survival to 27 months for the total selected patient group and to 26 months for the hormone-sensitive cases.

FUNDAMENTAL MECHANISMS

The factors influencing the response of endometrial adenocarcinoma to proges- togen and antiestrogen therapy can be divided into two groups: (a) those relating to the administration of the hormonal compound, and (b) those relating to the responsiveness of the tumor and the host. Moreover, these factors elucidate the mechanism of action of this hormonal cancer therapy and have a prognostic value, permitting monitoring of the response during the treatment.

Pharmacological Data

Response to the progestational agent is conditioned by the type of drug and its route, dosage, and duration. These factors will determine progestational levels in the serum.

Comparison of the mean objective remission rates obtained with the progestational compounds most frequently used in the treatment of advanced or recurrent adenocarcinoma proves the influence of the type of compound on the response and permits their listing in relation to cancericidal effectiveness. Taking into account the difficulties of injecting progesterone at sufficient dosage for long periods of time, the practical superiority of MPA for cancer therapy is evident. In our experience with MPA the route of administration first appears to affect remission rate. For the same dosage of 1 g/week, oral administration achieved a 53% objective remission rate in the advanced disease compared with 31% by intramuscular injection (18,21). On the other hand, stage I endometrial adenocarcinoma seems to respond better to local intracavitary progestational therapy than to oral or parenteral administration.

Although many reports point out better results with higher dosage of the progestogen and advocate very high "loading doses" during the first weeks of treatment, our survey on the remission rates obtained by increasing doses of progesterone, MPA, and 17α-OHPC therapy did not indicate a direct dose–response relationship.

Progestational therapy should be continued for as long as the remission lasts; after discontinuing MPA treatment striking relapses are often observed. Continuous progestational administration should also be made a rule for adjuvant therapy in order to avoid the risk of sudden recurrence.

In our experience, the serum level of the administered progestogen correlates with an influence on the tumor cells. (Table 3). With MPA therapy, serum levels above 90 ng/ml radioimmunoassayable MPA are necessary to obtain a good response (6). An elevation of serum MPA levels beyond 90 ng/ml occurs within 10 days of oral MPA treatment, while it takes 5 weeks of intramuscular administration for MPA serum levels to attain the 90 ng/ml threshold (10,17). The serum MPA levels registered during intrauterine MPA insertion remain extremely low (< 10 ng/ml) and evidence the importance of the local mechanism of progestational cancericidal action.

Although this progestogen therapy was based on very high doses which have, in some instances, been administered for long periods, we have never observed

TABLE 3. *Disseminated or recurrent uterine adenocarcinoma*[a]

MPA-serum concentration (ng/ml)	Responsive group %	Nonresponsive group %
< 5	0	35
5–29	12	15
30–90	35	50
> 90	53	0

[a] 115 cases treated by means of MPA. Value of reached MPA-serum concentration as a predictive factor of good response.

any significant side effects of hepatic, thrombotic, steroid, or mammary nature. With respect to mammary changes both retrospective and prospective, mammographic studies have proven the innocuous nature of MPA (8,11).

In all endometrial adenocarcinoma patients the serum follicle stimulating hormone (FSH) and luteinizing hormone (LH) levels are elevated, corresponding to generally accepted menopausal levels or often beyond these limits. Parenteral or peroral administration of 1 g MPA/week provokes an early and abrupt fall of FSH and LH levels (14). In the progestogen-sensitive patients the LH but not FSH fall is statistically significant (Fig. 4). Our patients have low serum estrone levels within generally accepted menopausal limits; serum estradiol levels on the contrary are significantly higher than menopausal levels.

Progestogen responsiveness is not related to a significant variation of serum estrone levels under MPA treatment, while estradiol level elevation seems to be not significant.

About 60% of our endometrial adenocarcinoma patients have an estrogenic vaginal smear and, at the same time, represent the progestogen-sensitive group (20,23). Later on, progestogen responsiveness is characterized by a sudden change toward atrophy in the vaginal smear, appearing earlier under oral than under parenteral MPA administration.

Partial inhibition of the hypothalamo–hypophyseal axis by the administration

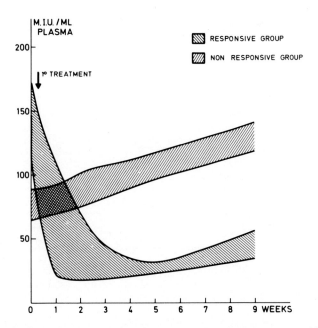

FIG. 4. Disseminated or recurrent uterine adenocarcinoma. 115 postmenopausal (hyster-) ovarectomized patients treated by mean of 1 g MPA/week. Hypophysial LH-response to progestational treatment.

of 1 g MPA/week could represent the indirect mechanism of action of progestogens on endometrial adenocarcinoma.

In endometrial adenocarcinoma treatment, we administered 20 to 60 mg/day tamoxifen p.o. Within these limits no direct dose–response relationship was seen. Slight, possible side effects were exceptionally observed, but disappeared after diminishing the dose and stopping the treatment.

Under tamoxifen therapy, serum estradiol levels mostly fluctuate around the original level; in some patients they fell; serum FSH, LH, and estrone levels remain unchanged or fluctuate. The vaginal smear of adenocarcinoma patients treated with tamoxifen remains or becomes estrogenic; this cytohormonal change is constant and without any relation (Table 4) to hormonal responsiveness. These data for tamoxifen do not evidence at all an indirect mechanism of action on endometrial adenocarcinoma.

Tumor/Host Factors

Good responsiveness of endometrial adenocarcinoma to MPA is characterized by an objective, anatomoclinically or radiologically evaluative tumor regression appearing within 4 to 6 weeks of treatment, provided serum MPA levels reach at least 90 ng/ml. This responsiveness is directly related to the hormone dependency of the adenocarcinoma and to the metabolic and hormonal status of the patient.

There is general agreement on the prognostic value of some tumoral factors (2,3,12): well-differentiated adenocarcinomas tend to show the best response; in the case of advanced or recurrent cancers, it is the slowly growing primary or disseminated lesions that provide the most dramatic remissions. In our experience, adenocarcinomas with a primary endocervical origin are very sensitive to progestogens. The localization of the tumor masses influences their responsiveness: mobile vaginal recurrences, and pulmonary and lymphatic metastases seem

TABLE 4. *Cytohormonal evolution in stage I endometrial adenocarcinoma patients under short-term (7 days) preradium tamoxifen treatment (60 mg/day)*

Patient	Age (yr)	Hormonal status	Cytohormonal evolution
77/1157			Estrogenic → Estrogenic
78/1577	53	Premenopausal	Estrogenic → Estrogenic
78/1633	64	Postmenopausal	Estrogenic → Estrogenic
78/1677	55	Menopausal	Estrogenic → Estrogenic
78/1869	60	Postmenopausal	Estrogenic → Estrogenic
78/1703	47	Premenopausal	Estrogenic → Estrogenic
78/1849	55	Postmenopausal	Estrogenic → Subatrophic
79/G004	69	Postmenopausal	Estrogenic → Subatrophic
79/G041	64	Postmenopausal	Estrogenic → Estrogenic
79/G043	70	Postmenopausal	Estrogenic → Estrogenic
79/G046	72	Postmenopausal	Atrophic → Atrophic

to be very responsive, while pelvic and abdominal tumors hardly respond at all. The type of primary treatment seems to have little influence on the results of subsequent progestational therapy.

In our MPA study we were able to discern the host factors favoring clinical response by the tumor. Older patients tend to be the best responders (2,3,12). Obesity, diabetes and estrogenic milieu (all of which affect the hormonal and metabolic environment of the tumor) seem to be related to good remission rates. Patients having an initial estrogenic vaginal smear have a higher response rate to progestational therapy.

In order to study separately the tumor and host factors influencing the responsiveness of endometrial adenocarcinoma to progestogens and antiestrogens, differentiated and undifferentiated endometrial adenocarcinomas were grown in organotypic cultures, permitting the addition to the medium of the different hormones (1). By adding estrogens, progestogens, or antiestrogens we were able to reproduce in these organotypic cultures of the different types of adenocarcinoma the same histological transformations as described *in vivo* for the treated patients. These data prove that certainly progestogens, and perhaps antiestrogens, locally attack the adenocarcinoma by a direct mechanism of action at a cellular level. The cancericidal efficiency of intrauterine progestogen applications confirms this hypothesis.

The essentially direct mechanism of action of steroid hormones and antihormones on the endometrial adenocarcinoma cells hits, by way of the steroid receptors, the mitotic and secretory activity, as demonstrated by labeled thymi-

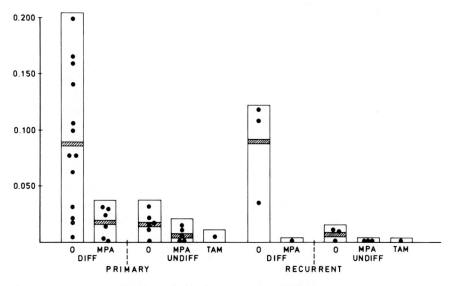

FIG. 5. Cytosolic estradiol receptor binding capacity in pmoles/mg protein of primary or recurrent endometrial adenocarcinoma under MPA of tamoxifen treatment.

dine incorporation and mucopolysaccharide and glycogen accumulation in the tumor maintained in organotypic culture.

In all differentiated adenocarcinomas, addition of estrogens to the culture medium suppresses secretory activity and mucopolysaccharide and glycogen accumulation, while it enhances thymidine incorporation. On the contrary, addition of progestogens (MPA, *d*-norgestrel) or antiestrogens enhances secretory activity and mucopolysaccharide and glycogen accumulation, but inhibits thymidine incorporation. These phenomena were seen in only 75% of undifferentiated adenocarcinoma cultures.

Cytosolic estrogen receptor levels are highest in differentiated endometrial adenocarcinomas and lowest in the undifferentiated tumors. In all these adenocarcinomas, administration of progestogens as well as antiestrogens induced a rapid and significant fall of ER levels, even to 0 in undifferentiated tumors (Fig. 5).

Cytosolic progestogen receptor levels seem to be reduced by progestogen treatment and raised by antiestrogen administration.

PERSPECTIVES

Endometrial adenocarcinomas are, to some extent, dependent on estrogens and sensitive to progestogens and antiestrogens. Clinical response to hormonal therapy may be expected in about half of the tumors. Hormonal dependence and sensitivity appears in the differentiation grading of the adenocarcinoma and in the cytohormonal evolution of the vaginal smear. Finally, this hormonal dependence and responsiveness could be determined by the presence and the binding capacity of the cytosolic estrogen and progestogen receptors.

Studied separately, progestogens and antiestrogens on one side, estrogens on the other side, exert an antagonistic effect on the endometrial adenocarcinoma. Moreover, combination of progestogen with either estrogen or antiestrogen produces a synergistic effect. In practice, originally responsive adenocarcinomas, which become insensitive after a period of progestational therapy, still retain an appreciable responsiveness to antiestrogens. Finally, steroid receptor analyses indicate a striking difference in the mechanism of action of these three classes of hormones and antihormones: Estrogens stimulate progestogen receptor synthesis; progestogens neutralize the estrogen receptor system; antiestrogens block the estrogen receptor system and induce progestogen receptor synthesis.

Taking into account these data together with a possible classification of endometrial adenocarcinomas into three types, hormonal manipulations of the cytosolic steroid receptor system could open new perspectives in the treatment of this tumor. In the first type of endometrial adenocarcinoma, the well-differentiated tumor contains both estrogen and progestogen receptors, but with a PR:ER ratio lower than in normal endometrium. These tumors are usually fully responsive to progestogen treatment. The second type is poorly differentiated and devoid of both ER and PR. The tumors are generally not responsive to endocrine therapy. In the third type, the adenocarcinoma is either anaplastic or moderately differentiated but typically shows only one of the receptors. The presence of ER alone seems to be an indication for priming the tumor with tamoxifen in order to reduce ER binding and stimulate synthesis of PR sites. On the other hand, the presence of PR alone may suggest the need for estrogen pretreatment before the administration of progestogens.

REFERENCES

1. Billiet, G., Bonte, J., and Ide, P. (1971): *Basic Actions of Sex Steroids on Target Organs,* edited by P. O. Hubinont, F. Leroy, and P. Galand, pp. 280–283. Karger, Basel.
2. Bonte, J. (1972): *Cancro,* XXV:11–15.
3. Bonte, J. (1972): *Acta Obstet. Gynecol. Scand.* [*Suppl.*], 19:21–24.
4. Bonte, J. (1973): In: *Symposium on Endometrial Cancer,* edited by M. G. Brush, R. W. Taylor, and D. C. Williams, pp. 203–211. Heinemann, London.
5. Bonte, J. (1974): *Med. Hyg.,* 1107:1106–1107.
6. Bonte, J. (1975): *Med. Hyg.,* 1173–1831.
7. Bonte, J. (1977): *Med. Hyg.,* 1266:4193–4197.
8. Bonte, J. (1977): In: *Gynecology and Obstetrics,* edited by L. Castelazo-Ayala and C. MacGregor, pp. 139–154. Excerpta Medica, Amsterdam.
9. Bonte, J. (1978): In: *Hormonal Biology of Endometrial Cancer,* edited by G. S. Richardson, and D. T. MacLaughlin, pp. 155–187. UICC Technical Report Series, Vol. 42, Geneva.
10. Bonte, J. (1978): *Gynaekol. Rundsch.,* 18:172–182.
11. Bonte, J. (1978): *Gynaekol. Rundsch.,* 18:220–245.
12. Bonte, J., Decoster, J. M., Drochmans, A., Ide, P., and Billiet, G. (1970): *C.R. Soc. Franc. Gynecol.,* 1:1–7.
13. Bonte, J., Decoster, J. M., and Ide, P. (1970): *Cancer,* 25(4):907–910.
14. Bonte, J., Decoster, J. M., and Ide, P. (1977): *Acta Cytol.,* 21(2):218–224.
15. Bonte, J., Decoster, J. M., Ide, P., and Billiet, G. (1978): *Gynecol. Oncol.,* 6:60–75.
16. Bonte, J., Decoster, J. M., Ide, P., and Billiet, G. (1978): In: *Endometrial Cancer,* edited by M. G. Brush, R. J. B. King, and R. W. Taylor, pp. 192–205. Baillière, Tindall & Cox, London.
17. Bonte, J., Decoster, J. M., Ide, P., Wynants, P., and Billiet, G. (1974): In: *Recent Progress in Obstetrics and Gynaecology,* edited by L. S. Persianinov, T. V. Chervakova, and J. Presl, pp. 285–297. Excerpta Medica, Amsterdam.
18. Bonte, J., Drochmans, A., and Ide, P. (1966): In: *Excerpta Medica International Congress Series,* No. 111:307, Excerpta Medica, Amsterdam.
19. Bonte, J., Drochmans, A., and Ide, P. (1966): *Acta Obstet. Gynecol. Scand.,* 45:121–129.
20. Bonte, J., Drochmans, A., and Ide, P. (1970): *Acta Cytol.,* 14(6):353–355.
21. Bonte, J., Drochmans, A., and Lassance, M. (1966):*Gynecol. Obstet. (Paris),* 65(2):179–185.
22. Decoster, J. M., Bonte, J., and Marcq, A. (1977): *Gynecol. Oncol.,* 5:189–195.
23. Ide, P., and Bonte, J. (1974): *Br. J. Cancer,* 30:175.
24. Kelley, R. M., and Baker, W. H. (1961): *N. Engl. J. Med.,* 264:216–222.

Hormones and Cancer, edited by S. Iacobelli et al.
Raven Press, New York © 1980.

Cellular Factors Contributing to the High Concentration of Dihydrotestosterone in Hyperplastic and Carcinomatous Human Prostates

Nicholas Bruchovsky, Paul S. Rennie, and *Theodor K. Shnitka

*Department of Cancer Endocrinology, Cancer Control Agency of British Columbia, Vancouver, British Columbia V5Z 3J3; and *Department of Pathology, University of Alberta, Edmonton, Alberta T6G 2G3, Canada*

Dihydrotestosterone is accumlated in the prostate by a complex process sustained by stroma–epithelial interactions, steroid-converting enzymes, binding reactions between androgen receptors and DNA, and possibly receptor-independent transport mechanisms within the cell. Fully integrated, this system yields a whole-tissue concentration of dihydrotestosterone of 130 to 210 ng/100 g tissue in normal prostate (10,18). The resultant concentration in benign prostatic hyperplasia (BPH), however, is considerably higher at 400 to 1,300 ng/100 g tissue (8,10,12,13,18), while in carcinoma it falls at an intermediate level (8, 11,12). Concerning the excessive capacity of BPH to retain dihydrotestosterone, Bruchovsky and Lieskovsky (1) have suggested that this is due to an approximate threefold increase in the activity of 5α-reductase.

In studying the pathogenesis of BPH, Cowan et al. (6) found that the greater part of the 5α-reductase activity in BPH tissue was localized in stroma. Their data, taken together with the results of Bruchovsky and Lieskovsky (1), imply that BPH stroma is characterized by a raised level of 5α-reductase activity. The experiments described in our present report were designed to test this premise. In addition, we examined two other aspects of the disposition of androgen in the prostate, namely the relationship between the quantity of receptor and the steady state concentration of dihydrotestosterone, and the role of DNA in fostering the nuclear retention of androgen receptor.

MATERIALS AND METHODS

Tissue Specimens

Normal prostates were obtained either at autopsy 2 to 15 hr after death or from brain-dead kidney donors. The age range of this group was 17 to 71 years. Hyerplastic prostates were obtained within 1 hr of suprapubic or retropubic extirpation. The age of the patients with BPH ranged from 53 to 90 years. Carcinomatous tissue was obtained at the time of radical prostatectomy. The age range of the cancer patients was 59 to 73 years. In each instance the diagnosis was confirmed by pathological examination. Studies on malignant tissue were confined to well-differentiated carcinoma.

Stroma and Epithelium

Separation of prostate into stromal and epithelial fractions was accomplished by forcing finely minced tissue through a stainless steel wire screen with a Teflon pestle, as described in previous reports (3,20).

Incubation Conditions

Following homogenization of the stroma and epithelium (3) incubation mixtures (final volume 2 ml) were prepared with the following components: 1.6 ml homogenate, 50 nM radioactive androgen and either a reduced nicotinamide-adenine dinucleotide phosphate (NADPH)-generating system for measuring 5α-reductase and 3α(β)-hydroxysteroid dehydrogenase (reductive) activities or 5×10^{-4} M NAD for measuring 3α(β)-hydroxysteroid dehydrogenase (oxidative) activity. A full outline of this procedure is given in ref. 1.

Estimation of 5α-reductase activity was based on the percentage formation of dihydrotestosterone and 3α(β)-androstanediol from testosterone. 3α(β)-Hydroxysteroid dehydrogenase (reductive) activity was estimated from the percentage formation of 3α(β)-androstanediol from dihydrotestosterone. The oxidative activity of the dehydrogenase reaction was examined with 3α-androstanediol as substrate, estimating the percentage formation of dihydrotestosterone.

Purification of Nuclei

Detailed description of the methods used for purifying nuclei have been reported by Bruchovsky et al. (2) and more recently by Rennie (17).

Extraction of Nuclei

Purified nuclei were disrupted by sonication and extracted directly with 0.6 M NaCl or, alternatively, first treated with micrococcal nuclease and then extracted with salt. These procedures have been described in an earlier report by Bruchovsky et al. (3).

Studies on Chromatin

Methods for the isolation and labeling of chromatin with [1,2-³H] dihydrotestosterone and for the preparation of oligomeric nucleosomes using micrococcal nuclease have been described recently by Rennie (17).

Assay of Nuclear Receptor

About 0.5 ml of nuclear extract was incubated with 20 nM [1,2-³H] dihydrotestosterone or 17β-hydroxy-17α-methylestra-4,9,11-trien-3-one ([17α-methyl-³H]methyltrienolone) at 4°C for 16 to 20 hr. Another 0.5 ml was treated similarly except that the sample also contained a 1,000-fold excess of nonradioactive dihydrotestosterone or methyltrienolone. After incubation both samples were analyzed for binding of ³H-steroid by gel exclusion chromatography using a dual-column apparatus (2,14). The amount of specific binding was calculated as the difference between total and nonspecific binding in the receptor peak.

Sucrose density-gradient centrifugation (17) was also used to detect the presence of androgen–receptor complexes.

Radioimmunoassay

Homogenates of whole tissue, stroma, and epithelium were extracted with 10% (volume/volume) ethylacetate:hexane. The organic phase of the extract was chromatographed on Al_2O_3 (9) and the fractions containing dihydrotestosterone were pooled. The amount of dihydrotestosterone recovered was measured by radioimmunoassay using a rabbit antiserum. Information concerning the sensitivity, accuracy, and precision of the assay has been published elsewhere (3).

Electron Microscopy

Pellets of samples of stromal homogenates were fixed in 3% glutaraldehyde in 0.1 M cacodylate buffer, pH 7.3, and postfixed in Caufield's osmium tetroxide (5) for 2 hr at 4°C. The tissue was dehydrated by rapid changes in graded alcohols followed by propylene oxide, and was embedded in Epon 812 modified from Luft (16). Silver sections were cut on a Reichert Om-42 ultramicrotome equipped with a diamond knife, and were placed on 400-mesh uncoated upper grids. Sections stained with uranyl acetate (19) followed by Fahmy's lead citrate (7) were viewed in a Siemens Elmiskop IA electron microscope at an accelerating voltage of 30 kV with a 30μm objective aperture.

Other Analytical Procedures

Protein was measured by the method of Lowry et al. (15) using bovine serum albumin as the reference standard, or by the Bio-Rad Protein Assay with bovine gamma globulin as standard. DNA was measured by the method of Burton (4) using calf thymus DNA as standard.

Radioactivity was counted in a Beckman LS-250 liquid scintillation system using a diphenyloxazole/toluene solution which contained 6 g diphenyloxazole, 75 ml water, and 126 g Bio-solv BBS-3 per liter toluene. The counting efficiency for ³H was 35%.

Chemicals and Reagents

Reagents used to prepare buffers and other solutions were purchased from Sigma Chemical Co., St. Louis, Missouri. Micrococcal nuclease was also obtained from Sigma. Stains-all was supplied by Eastman Kodak, Rochester, New York, and Bio-solv by Beckman Instruments, Fullerton, California. Steroids were obtained from Steraloids, Pawling, New York. Chromatographic Al_2O_3 and the Bio-Rad Protein Assay were purchased from Bio-Rad Laboratories, Mississauga, Ontario, Canada. The supplier of the dihydrotestosterone antiserum (DT 3–154) was Endocrine Sciences, Tarzana, California.

[1,2-^{3}H]Dihydrotestosterone (40 Ci/mmole) and [17α-methyl-^{3}H]methyltrienolone (87 Ci/mmole) were purchased from New England Nuclear, Boston, Massachusetts. Purity was checked by thin-layer chromatography (TLC), and the steroids were considered acceptable only if they were 95 to 100% pure.

RESULTS

Morphology of Stroma and Epithelium

The histological appearance of the stroma is shown in Fig. 1 (top) and that of the epithelium in Fig. 1 (bottom). The former consists of spindle-shaped fibromuscular cells and collagen, while the latter is made up of sheets of densely packed cuboidal cells with round, darkly staining nuclei. From a detailed microscopic analysis of such fractions from eight different prostates, it was established that the purity of the stroma was virtually 100% in all cases; in contrast, the purity of the epithelium ranged from 50 to 100% owing to contamination by stromal debris. About 40% of the whole-tissue DNA and protein was recovered in the stromal fraction (data not shown).

Examination of the stroma by electron microscopy showed that it consists of portions of smooth muscle cells containing actin filaments and dense bodies (Fig. 2, top). The interstitial spaces contain collagen fibers and fragments of basilar lamina (Fig. 2, top). An occasional nucleus with a folded irregular membrane is observed (Fig. 2, bottom). It is likely that such nuclei originate from stromal fibroblasts.

Stromal Versus Epithelial Localization of 5α-Reductase

The data in Table 1 indicate that the localization of 5α-reductase is predominantly in stroma, irrespective of the condition of the prostate (normal or abnormal). Moreover, the proportion of 5α-reductase activity associated with BPH stroma, *viz.* 84.4 ± 2.3% (mean ± SEM) relative to the normal value of 71.2 ± 1.5%, is significantly elevated (Student's *t*-test, $p < 0.005$). In contrast to the predominantly stromal distribution of 5α-reductase activity, the reductive

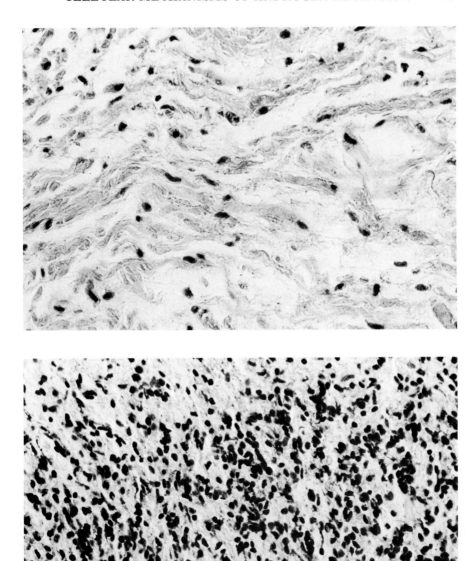

FIG. 1. Histology of prostatic stroma and epithelium. Separated stroma and epithelium were fixed 4% formaldehyde, stained with hematoxylin and eosin, and examined by light microscopy. **Top.** stroma; **bottom:** epithelium. ×300.

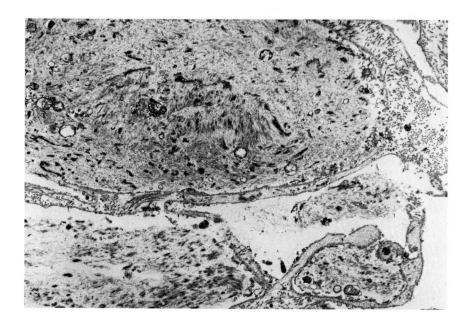

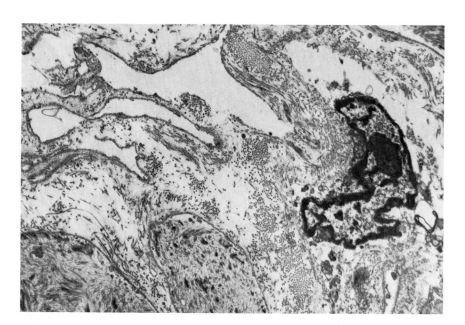

FIG. 2. Electron microscopy. Details of carcinomatous stroma as visualized by electron microscopy. **Top:** smooth muscle cell with actin filaments and dense bodies; **bottom:** abundant collagen fibrils and nucleus of unidentified origin. ×11,250.

TABLE 1. *Stromal vs epithelial localization of 5α-reductase and 3α(β)-hydroxysteroid dehydrogenase in human prostate[a]*

Tissue	% Total enzyme activity in stroma		
	5α-Reductase	Dehydrogenase (r)	Dehydrogenase (o)
Normal	71.2 ± 1.5 (3)	35.5 ± 4.3 (3)	46.4 ± 5.6 (3)
BPH	84.4 ± 2.3 (9)	59.9 ± 6.1 (8)	71.5 ± 7.8 (8)
Carcinoma	71.0 (2)	36.6 (2)	49.9 (2)

[a] Homogenates of stroma and epithelium were analyzed for activity of 5α-reductase and 3α(β)-hydroxysteroid dehydrogenase [both oxidative (o) and reductive (r) pathways] as described in the text. Total enzyme activity was determined on the basis of the combined protein content of the stromal and epithelial fractions. The percentage of the total enzyme activity in each fraction was then calculated. Values are presented as the mean ± SEM; the number of prostates examined is shown in parentheses.

and oxidative activities of 3α(β)-hydroxysteroid dehydrogenase are more evenly divided between stroma and epithelium.

Data on the specific activities of the various enzymes in stroma and epithelium are presented in Table 2. As might be expected, the specific activity of 5α-reductase is uniformly higher in the stromal than in the epithelial fractions of all prostates examined. Comparing stromal fractions alone, it is clear that the mean specific activity of 5α-reductase in BPH stroma at 84.6 ± 13.1 pmoles/mg protein/30 min is significantly greater than the corresponding value in normal stroma, 31.6 ± 7.2 pmoles/mg protein/30 min (Student's t-test, $p < 0.05$). On the other hand, stroma from the two carcinomatous prostate samples studied was relatively poor in 5α-reductase activity.

TABLE 2. *5α-Reductase and 3α(β)-hydroxysteroid dehydrogenase activities in stroma and epithelium of human prostate[a]*

Tissue	Enzyme activity (metabolites formed, pmoles/mg protein/30 min)		
	5α-Reductase	Dehydrogenase (r)	Dehydrogenase (o)
Normal			
Stroma	31.6 ± 7.2 (3)	15.0 ± 4.5 (3)	7.8 ± 1.3 (3)
Epithelium	9.2 ± 3.0 (3)	19.7 ± 5.5 (3)	7.2 ± 2.5 (3)
BPH			
Stroma	84.6 ± 13.1 (9)	20.9 ± 2.6 (8)	12.7 ± 1.7 (8)
Epithelium	11.3 ± 1.9 (9)	11.7 ± 2.5 (9)	4.9 ± 2.1 (8)
Carcinoma			
Stroma	12.4 (2)	13.2 (2)	8.4 (2)
Epithelium	3.7 (2)	17.8 (2)	6.8 (2)

[a] Homogenates of stroma and epithelium were analyzed for activities of 5α-reductase and 3α(β)-hydroxysteroid dehydrogenase [both reductive (r) and oxidative (o)] pathways as described in Materials and Methods. Mean ± SEM for each set of results is shown for the number of experiments in parentheses.

Concentration of Dihydrotestosterone in Stroma and Epithelium

To examine the effect of the high level of 5α-reductase activity in BPH stroma on the tissue distribution of dihydrotestosterone, we measured the concentration of dihydrotestosterone in stroma and epithelium by radioimmunoassay. The preliminary observations recorded in Table 3 suggest that BPH stroma and epithelium are both characterized by an above-normal level of dihydrotestosterone. The concentration appears to be highest in the epithelium, a change which is consistent with a trend towards an elevated epithelial:stromal ratio of the concentrations of dihydrotestosterone in the separated fractions of BPH tissue.

Subcellular Distribution and Nuclear Abundance of Dihydrotestosterone

Since BPH tissue manifests an unusual propensity for accumulating dihydrotestosterone, it was of interest to determine whether there is a specific location within the prostatic cell where pooling of dihydrotestosterone occurs. This was done by measuring the concentraion of dihydrotestosterone in homogenates of whole tissue and also in fractions of purified nuclei, and calculating the results on the basis of DNA content of the samples. The difference between the whole-tissue concentration and the nuclear concentration of dihydrotestosterone gives the quantity of the steroid in the cytoplasm. From the data presented in Table 4, it is clear that in normal and BPH tissues about 45% of the dihydrotestosterone is held in the nucleus compared with only about 20% in carcinoma, per unit DNA. The proportion differs considerably in rat ventral prostate where all of the dihydrotestosterone is stored in the nucleus. Castration, while causing a

TABLE 3. *Concentration of dihydrotestosterone in stroma and epithelium[a]*

Tissue	Concentration of dihydrotestosterone (pmoles/mg DNA)		Ratio (e/s)
	Stroma	Epithelium	
Normal			
1	4.3	4.9	1.1
2	3.0	3.5	1.2
BPH			
1	5.4	7.1	1.3
2	11.8	20.0	1.7
3	6.4	9.1	1.4
4	6.0	9.0	1.5
Carcinoma			
1	5.6	5.1	0.9
2	5.9	15.0	2.5

[a] The concentration of dihydrotestosterone was measured in separated stroma and epithelium by radioimmunoassay as described in Materials and Methods. Dividing the concentration in epithelium by that in stroma gives the e/s ratio.

TABLE 4. *Subcellular distribution and nuclear abundance of dihydrotestosterone[a]*

| | Concentration (pmoles/mg DNA) | | |
| | Dihydrotestosterone | | Nuclear receptor |
Tissue	Whole tissue	Nucleus	
Human			
Normal	3.7 ± 0.5 (4)	1.5 ± 0.4 (5)	0.11 ± 0.02 (7)
BPH	9.3 ± 1.2 (8)	4.3 ± 0.7 (14)	0.14 ± 0.02 (17)
Carcinoma	8.5 ± 1.5 (6)	1.7 ± 0.4 (7)	0.11 ± 0.01 (7)
Rat			
Normal	13.7 ± 0.6 (20)	18.2 ± 0.8 (5)	3.6 ± 0.7 (4)
Castrated	2.3 ± 0.3 (6)	2.0 ± 0.7 (4)	0.27 ± 0.05 (4)

[a] The concentration of dihydrotestosterone in homogenates of whole tissue and in preparations of purified nuclei was measured by radioimmunoassay. Nuclear extracts were also analyzed for the presence of androgen receptor by exchange labeling with [1,2-³H]dihydrotestosterone and [17α-methyl-³H]methyltrienolone, and Sephadex G25:G100 dual column chromatography, as described in Materials and Methods. The time after castration of the rats was 24 hr. Results were normalized on the basis of the DNA content of the various fractions. In the case of carcinoma the method of calculating results did not take into account the fact that the carcinomatous nucleus contains twice the normal amount of DNA. Values are presented as the mean ± SEM; the number of prostates examined is shown in parentheses.

marked reduction in the concentration, does not change the relative distribution of this steroid.

Despite the differences in the nuclear concentrations of dihydrotestosterone in human prostates, no significant variation is obvious in the amounts of nuclear receptor. The finding that the concentration of receptor is 13 to 30 times lower than the concentration of dihydrotestosterone suggests that the nucleus of the prostatic cell is characterized by an abundance of free (nonreceptor-bound) steroid. The concentration of nuclear receptor in rat ventral prostate, while almost 30 times greater than the concentration in human prostate, is nevertheless exceeded fivefold by the concentration of dihydrotestosterone.

Effect of DNA Content on the Nuclear Concentration of Dihydrotestosterone and Androgen Receptor

The data in Table 4 suggest that there is no difference between the concentrations of dihydrotestosterone in normal and carcinomatous nuclei and that nuclei from the three types of human prostate contain the same amount of receptor. However, when the data are adjusted to compensate for the varying amounts of DNA/nucleus,[1] as is done by normalizing on the basis of nuclear counts, a different perspective is obtained. Owing to the twofold increase in the DNA

---

[1] Normal 13.7 ± 1.7 pg (mean ± SEM, $N = 5$); BPH 19.1 ± 1.5 pg ($N = 15$); carcinoma, 27.6 ± 2.7 pg ($N = 7$).

TABLE 5. *Relationship of DNA content to the nuclear concentration of dihydrotestosterone and androgen receptor in human prostate[a]*

Tissue	Concentration (molecules/nucleus)	
	Dihydrotestosterone	Nuclear receptor
Normal	12,000 ± 3000 (5)	900 ± 200 (7)
BPH	49,000 ± 8000 (14)	1600 ± 300 (17)
Carcinoma	29,000 ± 7000 (7)	1800 ± 200 (7)

[a] The concentrations of dihydrotestosterone and nuclear receptor were normalized on a per nucleus basis to compensate for the greater amount of DNA/nucleus in carcinomatous cells (see text). The number of molecules of receptor was estimated by assuming that one steroid molecule is equivalent to one receptor molecule. Values are presented as the mean ± SEM; the number of prostates examined is shown in parentheses.

content of carcinomatous nuclei, the actual per nucleus concentrations of dihydrotestosterone and its receptor are at least double the normal level (Table 5). These observations strongly suggest that DNA exerts a positive influence on the nuclear retention of bound and unbound steroid.

Digestion of Linker DNA and Analysis of Fragments

In view of the apparent direct relationship between the amounts of nuclear receptor and DNA, we investigated the binding reaction between the two molecules in more detail as described by Rennie (17). Extracts of nuclei from rat ventral prostate were digested with micrococcal nuclease to yield receptor–chromatin complexes of varying sizes; the complexes were separated on linear 7.6 to 76% (volume/volume) glycerol density gradients. After digestion of 5% of the DNA to acid soluble products most of the material absorbing light at 260 nm (A_{260}) and chromatin-bound radioactivity is recovered in fractions 1–28 of the gradient (Fig. 3). Approximately 18 and 16% of the A_{260} and radioactivity, respectively, are associated with the pellet fraction (data not shown).

Within the gradient five A_{260} peaks are observed, the largest having a sedimentation value of about 11 S. Almost all of the specific binding is associated with the rapidly sedimenting components. Peak 1 is characterized by the highest mean value of dpm/A_{260} unit (5,826 ± 1,173; mean ± SEM, $N = 4$) which is 15, 38, 90, and 300% greater than the mean values for peaks 2, 3, 4, and 5, respectively. Since peaks 1 and 2 contain large oligomeric forms of nucleosomes and peaks 3, 4, and 5 small forms and monomers (17), it appears that smaller fragments of DNA are less capable of binding labeled receptor.

Release of Receptor from Chromatin by the Action of Micrococcal Nuclease

Chromatin from Rat Ventral Prostate

Micrococcal nuclease was used to digest preparations of labeled chromatin from rat ventral prostate. After varying amounts of hydrolysis, the nuclease-

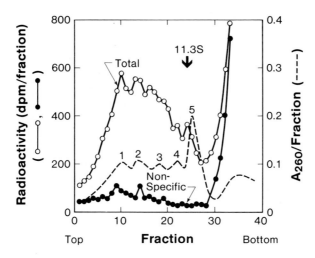

FIG. 3. Glycerol gradient separation of chromatin digests. Following digestion to 5% acid soluble with micrococcal nuclease, 200 μl of chromatin, labeled *in vitro* with 20 nM [1,2-³H]dihydrotestosterone and containing approximately five A_{260} units, were applied to 7.6–76% (vol/vol) glycerol density gradients and centrifuged at 130,000 × *g* for 16 hr. Fractions were collected from the bottom and analyzed for absorbance at 260 nm *(broken line)* and for radioactivity. The *arrow* indicates the position of the catalase sedimentation standard. Radioactivity recovered: *(open circles)* after incubation with isotope alone; *(closed circles)* after incubation with isotope and a 1,000-fold excess of nonradioactive dihydrotestosterone. Modified from Rennie (17).

treated chromatin was analyzed on 5 to 20% (weight/volume) sucrose density gradients to check for the presence of unbound nuclear receptors. As indicated by the results in Fig. 4, no peak corresponding to free receptors is observed in the undigested sample; after 5% digestion of DNA a small receptor peak appears in the gradient. The peak is considerably augmented after 15% of the DNA is digested to acid soluble products. Thus, the binding of androgen receptors to chromatin seems to depend on the region of DNA sensitive to nuclease attack.

Chromatin from Human Prostate

Nuclear receptors are usually recovered from human prostatic nuclei in a free form if the nuclei are extracted with 0.6 M NaCl (14). However, we have noted that this treatment is occasionally ineffective and that the receptor remains associated with chromatin. The failure to achieve the release of receptor with the use of salt is illustrated by the results in Fig. 5A. However, if the purified nuclei are disrupted and treated with micrococcal nuclease until 20% of the DNA is hydrolyzed to acid-soluble products, the presence of free receptor is demonstrated as a peak of radioactivity in fractions 20–30 (Fig. 5B). These findings reinforce the idea that there is a direct relationship between the amount of intact linker DNA and the amount of binding of receptor to chromatin. The relationship appears to hold for both rat and human prostates.

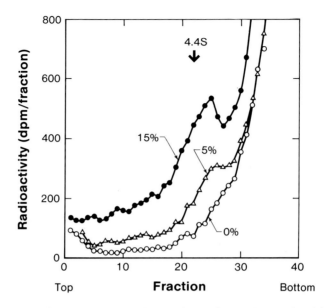

FIG. 4. Sucrose gradient analysis of nuclease digests. Chromatin samples, labeled *in vitro* with 20 nM [1,2-³H]dihydrotestosterone and containing approximately four A_{260} units, were digested to a predetermined extent (0, 5, or 15% acid soluble) with micrococcal nuclease and centrifuged at 12,000 × *g* for 10 min. The supernatant fractions (200 μl) were applied to 5–20% (wt/vol) sucrose density gradients and centrifuged at 246,000 × *g* for 18 hr. Fractions were collected from the bottom and assayed for radioactivity. The *arrow* indicates the hemoglobin sedimentation standard. Modified from Rennie (17).

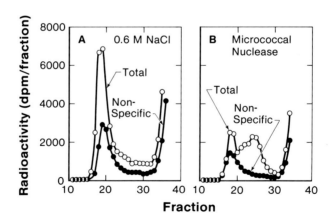

FIG. 5. Release of receptor from chromatin of normal human prostate by the action of micrococcal nuclease. Purified nuclei were either extracted with 0.6 M NaCl or disrupted and digested with micrococcal nuclease until 20% of the DNA was hydrolyzed. Concerning the latter procedure, the receptor-containing extract was prepared by solubilizing the precipitate formed during hydrolysis. The final extracts were incubated at 4°C for 16–20 hr in the presence of 20 nM [17α-methyl-³H]methyltrienolone. Nonspecific binding was measured in duplicate samples. After incubation the extracts were analyzed by Sephadex G25:G100 dual-column chromatography. Total *(open circles)* and nonspecific *(closed circles)* binding of radioactivity in nuclei treated with 0.6 M NaCl **(A)** or micrococcal nuclease **(B)**.

DISCUSSION

Several processes contributing to the formation and retention of dihydrotestosterone by prostatic tissue have been studied. Concerning the function of different regions of the prostate, our results indicate that stroma is the primary site of conversion of testosterone to dihydrotestosterone in the human prostate owing to the prevalence in stroma of 5α-reductase. This finding is harmonious with the original conclusion of Cowan et al. (6) as based on their experiments with BPH tissue. In the present report we show that 5α-reductase activity is largely confined to stroma in normal and carcinomatous prostates as well. We also demonstrate that the threefold elevation of 5α-reductase activity previously observed in homogenates of whole BPH tissue (1) is mirrored by an increase of almost similar magnitude in the specific activity of the enzyme in BPH stroma. In analyzing the degree of linear association between the variables of 5α-reductase activity and age, Bruchovsky and Lieskovsky (1) obtained a correlation coefficient that was consistent with a weakly positive relationship only; as a result they inferred that the rise in 5α-reductase activity is symptomatic of BPH and not exclusively of age. Allowing that age is indeed a negligible factor, our present findings support the conclusion that BPH is characterized by an abnormally high level of stromal 5α-reductase activity.

In studying the postformation disposal of dihydrotestosterone, we observed that BPH stroma and epithelium are both characterized by an above-normal level of dihydrotestosterone. Also, the tendency for BPH to accumulate dihydrotestosterone appears to be equally pronounced in both the cytoplasm and the nucleus. A striking property of the nucleus is its ability to accumulate dihydrotestosterone well in excess of the quantity of receptor (Tables 4 and 5); no exceptions to this were noticed in any of the tissues examined. The simplest interpretation of this finding is that a large amount of dihydrotestosterone is transported into the nucleus by a nonreceptor-mediated process.

Despite the high nuclear concentration of dihydrotestosterone in BPH, the mean level of receptor, although somewhat elevated, is not significantly different from normal (Tables 4 and 5). However, owing to a twofold greater concentration of DNA, whole nuclei recovered from prostatic carcinoma are characterized by a proportional increase in the concentrations of both dihydrotestosterone and nuclear receptor (Table 5). It is possible, therefore, that the DNA content of the cell influences the nuclear concentration of these molecules.

The inferred relationship between the amount of nuclear receptor and DNA is supported by experimental evidence that nuclear receptor is bound to linker DNA both in rat and in human prostates. Three lines of evidence are presented: first, more receptor is bound to large oligomeric nucleosomes than to small ones (Fig. 3); second, more receptor is released from chromatin as hydrolysis of DNA with micrococcal nuclease is allowed to proceed (Fig. 4); third, in cases where salt is ineffective, free receptor is generated in preparations of nuclei by the action of micrococcal nuclease (Fig. 5).

The kinetics of androgen production and turnover are apparently quite different in BPH and carcinoma. While both tissues are characterized by a high concentration of dihydrotestosterone, stromal 5α-reductase activity is grossly elevated in BPH but was abnormally low in the carcinoma cases studied (Table 2). Hence, either 5α-reductase activity does not influence the accumulation of dihydrotestosterone, or this process is controlled by disparate mechanisms in the two tissues.

ACKNOWLEDGMENTS

Gillian Birt provided valuable assistance in preparing this manuscript. Dr. T. K. Shnitka performed the histological and pathological examinations of the experimental tissues and gave generously of his time for this critical aspect of the study. Trudy Comeau was instrumental in supervising the performance of the various assays. The project was supported by grants from the Medical Research Council of Canada and the National Cancer Institute of Canada; P.S.R. is a Scholar of the latter agency.

REFERENCES

1. Bruchovsky, N., and Lieskovsky, G. (1979): *J. Endocrinol.,* 80:289–301.
2. Bruchovsky, N., Rennie, P. S., and Vanson, A. (1975): *Biochim. Biophys. Acta,* 394:248–266.
3. Bruchovsky, N., Rennie, P. S., and Wilkin, R. P. (1980): In: *Steroid Receptors, Metabolism and Prostatic Cancer,* edited by H. J. de Voogt, F. A. G. Teulings, and Schroder, F. H. Excerpta Medica, Amsterdam *(in press).*
4. Burton, K. (1956): *Biochem. J.,* 62:315–323.
5. Caulfield, J. B. (1957): *J. Biophys. Biochem. Cytol.,* 3:827–830.
6. Cowan, R. A., Cowan, S. K., Grant, J. K., and Elder, H. Y. (1977): *J. Endocrinol.,* 74:111–120.
7. Fahmy, A. (1967): In: *Proceedings 25th Anniversary Meeting, Electron Microscopy Society of America,* edited by C. J. Arceneaux, pp. 148–149. Claitor's Book Store, Baton Rouge, Louisiana.
8. Farnsworth, W. E., and Brown, J. R. (1976): *Endocr. Res. Commun.,* 3:105–117.
9. Furuyama, S., Mayes, P., and Nugent, C. A. (1970): *Steroids,* 16:415–428.
10. Geller, J., Albert, J., Lopez, D., Geller, S., and Niwayama, G. (1976): *J. Clin. Endocrinol. Metabol.,* 43:686–688.
11. Geller, J., Albert, J., Loza, D., Geller, S., and Stoltzing, W. (1978): *J. Clin. Endocrinol. Metab.,* 46:440–444.
12. Habib, F. K., Lee, S. R., Stitch, S. R., and Smith, P. H. (1976): *J. Endocrinol.,* 71:99–107.
13. Krieg, M., Bartsch, W., Herzer, S., Becker, H., and Voigt, K. D. (1977): *Acta Endocrinol. (Copenh.),* 86:200–215.
14. Lieskovsky, G., and Bruchovsky, N. (1979): *J. Urol.,* 121:54–58.
15. Lowry, O. H., Rosebrough, N. J., Farr, A. L., and Randall, R. H. (1951): *J. Biol. Chem.,* 193:265–275.
16. Luft, J. H. (1961): *J. Biophys. Biochem. Cytol.,* 9:409–414.
17. Rennie, P. (1979): *J. Biol. Chem.,* 254:3947–3957.
18. Siiteri, P. K., and Wilson, J. E. (1970): *J. Clin. Invest.,* 49:1737–1745.
19. Stempak, J. G., and Ward, R. T. (1964): *J. Cell Biol.,* 22:697–701.
20. Wilkin, R. P., Bruchovsky, N., Shnitka, T. K., Rennie, P. S., and Comeau, T. L.: *Acta Endocrinol. (in press).*

Hormones and Cancer, edited by S. Iacobelli et al.
Raven Press, New York © 1980.

Steroid Hormones and Human Cancer

V. H. T. James and M. J. Reed

*Department of Chemical Pathology, St. Mary's Hospital Medical School,
London W2 1PG, England*

During the last three decades, a substantial proportion of endocrine research has been devoted to the possible role of steroid hormones in human cancer. More recently, the field has been dominated by the important advances in the area of steroid receptors and their significance in hormone-dependent cancer, and these advances have been particularly significant in relation to prognosis and treatment. However, the extent of steroid hormone involvement in this major disease is potentially much wider than that delineated by receptor studies, and so this chapter will attempt to consider metabolism in a broader sense and will try to review particularly the advances in the last few years. Limitations of space enforce some selectivity and so we shall consider specifically steroid metabolism in breast cancer and endometrial cancer, and will limit discussion entirely to the problem of human cancer.

Cancer of the breast and uterus account for a substantial number of cancer deaths each year. Since these are hormone-dependent tissues, and in some cases the growth of the tumor can be markedly influenced by manipulation of the hormone environment, there is strong circumstantial evidence to suggest that steroids directly or indirectly may be involved in some way in the genesis of these tumors. As far as human cancer is concerned though, the direct evidence that steroids themselves may be carcinogenic is very limited. The view of many investigators is that steroids exert in this regard only a permissive role. Thus, steroids may operate by allowing or facilitating the primary action of other agents, such as viruses, or other hormones; or by promoting cell proliferation, providing greater opportunity for carcinogens to initiate neoplastic change, or their main role may be to maintain tumor growth, once initiated (35).

What are the reasons for studying steroid metabolism in cancer? What positive results could we hope to achieve from further research in this field?

First, to seek a better understanding of the role that steroids might play in carcinogenesis, and perhaps particularly in relation to the control of tumor growth. Second, to look for specific abnormalities in steroid metabolism which might serve as cancer "markers," and may thus be of value for population screening. Third, to detect, and then possibly repair or modify an unfavorable hormonal environment.

A considerable amount of work has been carried out to try to reach these objectives, but before discussing some of these studies, it is relevant to consider some of the difficulties in this field. Failure to do so may make it impossible to assess the real significance of a particular study.

Unfortunately, a variety of factors influence steroid metabolism and many of these are difficult to evaluate quantitatively, or to control. These include diet, nutritional status, age, sex, race, posture, hormonal status, drug therapy, nonspecific disease, and "stress" (e.g., due to trauma or surgery).

It is not possible here to consider all these points in detail, but, for example, nutritional state markedly affects adrenocortical function, and does so not only quantitatively but can also alter the qualitative pattern of steroid secretion, particularly corticosteroids in relation to androgens (16,74). Patients studied just prior to surgery cannot fairly be compared with unstressed volunteers (66), and drugs can both affect steroid metabolism and may cause analytical interference (20). These factors can hardly be overemphasized, and make it essential to choose both patient and control populations very carefully.

Another very real difficulty is the long-term nature of any possible effect which steroid hormones may exert. Many of the epidemiological data suggest that the delay between a significant endocrine event and the onset of recognizable neoplastic change may be 10 to 20 years or more (27), and thus it may be inappropriate to study patients with established disease, and more relevant to investigate women who are at cancer risk.

Lastly, the technique of studying steroid metabolism has to be considered critically. For example, single blood samples are often a poor indicator of hormone production (30) and thus tissue exposure, and if, as one might expect, we are seeking only subtle changes in steroid metabolism, our techniques must be suitably designed.

There have been many investigations of urinary steroid excretion by cancer patients, well reviewed elsewhere (19). Most of the published data have dealt with the excretion of steroids containing 19 carbon atoms (the so-called urinary androgens, C_{19} steroids) by patients with breast cancer, and these studies followed the initial report in 1960 that a statistical relationship existed between urinary steroid metabolite levels and the response of breast cancer patients to ablative endocrine therapy. The original findings suggested that a high ratio of 11-deoxy carbon-19 steroids to 17-hydroxycorticosteroids was associated with a better response to treatment (10). Figure 1 illustrates the origin and significance of these steroid fractions.

Further work, particularly by Bulbrook and colleagues (13,25) focused attention on the individual urinary steroids (dehydroepiandrosterone, etiocholanolone, and androsterone) and suggested that a low excretion of these individual metabolites was prognostically unfavorable. In the 20 years or so since these studies commenced, there is still no clear agreement between all investigators, and whilst some have confirmed the original findings in patients with advanced disease (14,36), others have not been able to do so (71).

A major criticism of these studies has always been that a large number of

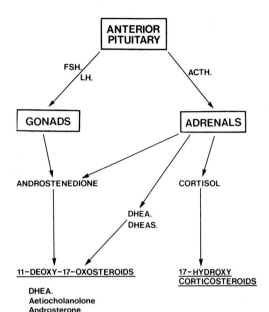

FIG. 1. Origin of urinary steroid metabolites.

factors influence the production and excretion of urinary steroids, and in particular, for poorly understood reasons, illness is generally associated with diminished excretion of 17-oxosteroids (74). It may reasonably be argued that since some patients with breast cancer, especially those with advanced disease, may be seriously ill, the observed diminution in C_{19} steroid excretion is only a nonspecific effect of illness. However, against this view has to be weighed the apparent predictive value of measuring urinary steroid excretion. In the only study of its kind so far carried out, Bulbrook and his colleagues obtained urine samples from a population of women in Guernsey (11), and retrospectively analyzed those from the women who subsequently developed breast cancer, measuring urinary etiocholanolone. The results, when compared against matched controls, show that the mean steroid excretion of these women was significantly lower than the noncancer controls, although the amounts excreted were still within the control range.

In contrast, Poortman and colleagues (50) investigated the excretion of urinary androgens by nearly 4,000 women over 50 years of age who were being screened for breast cancer and were unable to detect any difference in steroid excretion by the women found to have cancer and the matched controls. At the present time, the prospects for screening for breast cancer using urinary androgen excretion still seem unpromising.

Although most of the work reported to date has involved urinary "androgens," estrogen excretion has also been investigated essentially as a crude index of estrogen exposure.

Investigation of the excretion of the three so-called classic estrogens—estradiol, estrone, and estriol—led to the observation that the ratio of estriol to estradiol plus estrone was lower in patients with breast cancer. These data formed the basis of the postulate by Lemon and his colleagues (37) that estriol is protective against breast cancer if production is elevated during early reproductive life. This would explain the diminished risk for women who had an early pregnancy. The original experimental data from animal studies were also exciting, since they suggested that estriol did not promote a typically estrogenic response in target tissues, and they appeared to confirm the idea that estriol is able to attenuate the biological effect of other estrogens (28).

Attractive though the theory is, it has major deficiencies. Thus, urinary estriol excretion does not necessarily reflect the plasma level of free steroid, neither does the estriol ratio reflect the plasma level or production rate (39). Not all investigators have found low ratios in breast cancer; indeed, some find elevated ratios in their patients (7,26). Most important though, are the recent data from animal studies, and from *in vitro* work, which demonstrate that estriol *is* biologically active and can and does initiate the intracellular events associated with estrogen action (3). Thus, although many of the data suggest that in some way estriol metabolism may be altered in some cancer patients, the conclusion drawn from a recent study (15) that "The hypothesis that a low oestriol ratio is a cause of breast cancer is given only minimal support," seems appropriate at the present time.

It has been pointed out by Zumoff and his colleagues (75) that a low estriol ratio can also be due to a high excretion rate of estrone and estradiol relative to estriol. However, such data as are available do not offer much support for this view, and indeed, in one study, compared with controls, breast cancer patients excreted less estrone and estradiol (5). The choice of appropriate controls, the timing of the collection in the menstrual cycle and the low urinary levels in postmenopausal patients pose problems which are not easily overcome, and still require solutions.

It is interesting and possibly significant that abnormalities similar to those seen in breast cancer patients have also been reported in other types of cancer. Poortman and Thijssen (48) reported that patients with endometrial cancer excreted less etiocholanolone and androsterone than did controls. There is also a report by Rao (52), who found that there was a significant relationship between the excretion ratio of C_{19} steroids by lung cancer patients and their subsequent clinical progress, but this observation does not appear to have been pursued.

Because of the inference from the urinary data that in some way diminished androgen production or metabolism is an unfavorable factor, a number of attempts to investigate plasma androgen levels have been made. Such studies in breast cancer patients have revealed no consistent abnormality. Some, but not all investigators, have found that plasma dehydroepiandrosterone sulfate levels are lower than normal (9), particularly in advanced breast cancer, but there does not appear to be any significant depression of the levels of plasma androstenedione (49,72).

It is difficult to try to tie together in a working hypothesis these data which suggest some involvement of androgen metabolism in endocrine cancer. Some clue may come from the observations of Poortman and his colleagues (49) who found diminished production of dehydroepiandrosterone and its sulfate in patients with breast cancer. These authors suggested a major role for androstenediol, which is produced from dehydroepiandrosterone, and showed that it competes with estradiol for estrogen receptor, thus acting as an antiestrogen. Diminished production of androstenediol would be unfavorable because of the antiestrogenic role of this steroid (48).

Other workers have focused attention on androstenediol. Maynard et al. (45) showed significant amounts of this steroid accumulated in breast tumors. Adams et al. (1), using a rat mammary tumor, showed that androstenediol can translocate estrogen receptor to the nucleus, and also inhibit estrogen sulfotransferase activity.

It is clear then, that androstenediol may well be able to modulate intracellular estrogen activity, within the tumor cell, but whether it acts as an antiestrogen in the human or potentiates estrogenic activity (69) is still unclear and is an important area for further study.

Studies of total plasma estrogens in breast cancer have not revealed obvious differences from normal (32), although very recently Siiteri *(this volume)* has reported that there are clear differences in the free or unbound estradiol plasma levels between postmenopausal women with and without breast cancer.

Progesterone levels measured on single blood samples in the luteal phase of the cycle were found to be depressed in the highest breast cancer risk group (12), and it has been shown by Sitruk-Ware and colleagues (63) that women with benign breast disease, another risk factor, have luteal phase plasma progesterone levels which are considerably lower than normal.

These data fit well with the attractive postulate by Sherman and Korenman (58) that luteal insufficiency is an important factor in the pathogenesis of breast cancer, possibly because of the continuing exposure of breast tissue to the stimulus of unopposed estrogen.

Recently too, there is an interesting report that 17β-hydroxysteroid dehydrogenase activity is present in normal human breast tissue and furthermore, that the activity is dependent on the phase of the menstrual cycle, being highest in the secretory phase (47). This is, therefore, possibly a progesterone-dependent phenomenon, and it may be similar to the biochemical events described by Gurpide et al. (23) in the endometrium. Progesterone may in this way diminish the exposure of breast tissue to estradiol by increasing the conversion of estradiol to estrone and to estrone conjugates. It is interesting too, to note that enzyme activity is less in breast tumor tissue (47). In a study of 10 patients with breast cancer, infused with [³H]estradiol for 12 hr prior to surgery, we found that in most cases the tumor accumulates estradiol, and in only 2 patients is there substantial conversion to estrone (29). It is interesting to speculate that the favorable response to progesterone therapy by some tumors may be due, by analogy with uterine tissue, to activation of this mechanism. This is an exciting area for further work, but attractive though the concept of progesterone deficiency is, one has to note that another group has found almost completely opposing results: plasma progesterone levels in benign disease were found to be normal, or even elevated in the luteal phase, and slightly, but significantly raised in premenopausal women with breast cancer (17). These data typify the problem in this field; while one group find apparently convincing differences in their patients, others fail to do so. Whether this is methodological or due to inadvertent patient selection in some way is quite unclear, but it is a problem urgently requiring solution.

Let us consider now in more detail some aspects of estrogen production in women, and its possible relationship to cancer, particularly in postmenopausal women. This is a population which has attracted detailed study for various reasons. In this age group, there is the highest incidence of supposedly endocrine associated cancer, especially breast and endometrial cancer and yet the situation carries the apparent anomaly that it is at this time of her life that the human female is exposed to relatively low levels of estrogen. Equally though, this exposure is no longer opposed by progesterone, and the endocrine environment is radically different from that which occurs through the normal menstrual cycle. It is also at this stage of life, that increasing numbers of women are being offered estrogen replacement therapy. Given incautiously, this can lead to endometrial hyperplasia (41) and there is at least suggestive evidence for an association of estrogen therapy with the development of endometrial carcinoma (4,18,44). The incidence of this condition is also higher in older women bearing estrogen secreting tumors (43). These data support the view that continuing exposure to unopposed estrogen in, perhaps, predisposed women, may be an important factor in the development of endometrial cancer. Finally, the estrogen dependence of many uterine and breast cancers is a strong additional reason for seeking to enlarge our knowledge of this area of cancer endocrinology.

Through the menopause, estrogen secretion by the ovary declines and eventually ceases, and indirect production of estrogen starts to assume major importance. It is for this reason that extragonadal production of estrogens has attracted attention (62).

Figure 2 illustrates some of the factors which will control estrogen production in the postmenopausal female. The major estrogen produced is estrone derived from androstenedione. This latter steroid is produced by both adrenals and ovaries, and in the premenopausal woman the ovarian contribution is quite substantial. The postmenopausal ovary is much less active and although both androstenedione and testosterone are secreted, the blood flow through the ovary is small. Compared with the adrenal gland, ovarian contribution is minimal and after the menopause it is the pituitary–adrenal axis which assumes prominence. The amount of estradiol produced by postmenopausal women is relatively small and in part arises from estrone (22). The production of estrogen in the postmenopausal woman, both overall, and perhaps what is even more important,

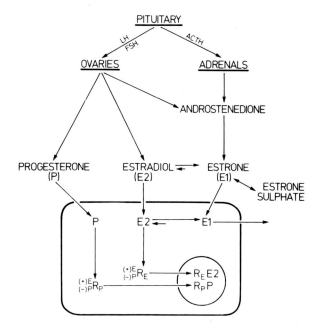

FIG. 2. Estrogen production and action in the female. (Adapted from Siiteri, ref. 59.)

locally in individual tissues, will therefore be affected by a variety of factors, all of which merit consideration.

Production of androstenedione is obviously an important factor, and since this is predominantly adrenocortical in origin, it is indirectly the level of adrenal activity which will be significant. It is true that subsequent conversion stages are relatively inefficient, but there is no question of the relevance of this phenomenon, since even physiological stimulation of the adrenal will rapidly and significantly increase peripheral estrogen levels (31) (see Fig. 3).

It is relevant to consider therefore, whether androstenedione production may be abnormal in endometrial cancer, both because of its direct relationship to estrogen production and also because of the reports referred to earlier of apparent alterations in urinary androgen excretion in this condition (48).

The best estimate we can make of androstenedione production is from the plasma level and the clearance rate, both of which can be determined experimentally. Androstenedione secretion though is episodic (30,31) and is mediated very closely by adrenocorticotropic hormone, exactly like cortisol. A single blood level reflects very poorly the 24-hr production, and is no more meaningful in this respect than a single plasma cortisol reading is as an indication of cortisol production. If one takes, as some investigators do, one or two readings, the error in estimating 24-hr secretion may be very large. Ideally, a mean level should be taken from a 24-hr study. Thus, the best estimate we can make of

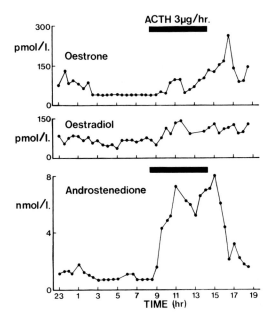

FIG. 3. Effect of corticotropin on plasma steroid levels. Subject is postmenopausal.

the androstenedione production rate is to determine the metabolic clearance rate using an isotope procedure, and the mean plasma level from a 24-hr sampling study.

With these techniques, can we detect any abnormality in patients with endometrial cancer? Figure 4 shows the results of such a study in a small group of patients carefully selected with regard to their weight. Five were postmenopausal and one was premenopausal. There is no obvious abnormality in plasma level, metabolic clearance rate, or plasma production rate of androstenedione. All the patients were studied again 3 months after ovariectomy and hysterectomy.

Removal of the ovaries produced a significant change in the production of androstenedione only in the premenopausal female, confirming the negligible contribution made by the postmenopausal ovary to androstenedione production (53).

In the basal state, then, we have not found any obvious difference from normality in the secretion of androstenedione in the patients with endometrial cancer, but this type of investigation obviously permits no comment on nonbasal conditions which in fact may be much more relevant.

The conversion of androstenedione to estrone is a key step in the production of estrogens, and this process takes place in the peripheral, that is, the extragonadal tissues. Although only about 2 to 4% of the androstenedione is converted to estrone, this is a very substantial proportion of the total estrone produced in the postmenopausal woman. This aspect of steroid metabolism has attracted a good deal of attention, mostly because of the interesting work of Siiteri and McDonald (60), whose provocative hypotheses have been a major stimulus in

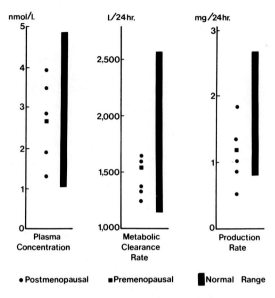

FIG. 4. Production rates of androstenedione calculated from the plasma concentration of androstenedione and metabolic clearance rate in women with endometrial cancer. Ranges for women without endometrial cancer are indicated by the *solid bars* (data from Grodin et al., ref. 21).

this field. These investigators drew attention to the fact that certain conditions which are risk factors for endometrial cancer, e.g., obesity and perhaps liver disease, are also those in which increased peripheral aromatization occurs. They suggested that this may result in a chronically elevated production of estrone. If estrone has directly (61), or even indirectly, specifically undesirable effects on the endometrium, this mechanism may be fundamentally involved in the pathogenesis of the disease. It is relevant, therefore, to consider whether the peripheral aromatization of androstenedione to estrone is altered in patients with endometrial cancer, and what role estrone plays at the tissue level. There are three ways to approach this problem—by attempting to examine tissue inter-conversion directly, and by looking at the overall conversion *in vivo* using isotopic or nonisotopic methods.

If physiological amounts of androstenedione are infused (Fig. 5) into a post-menopausal woman, we can demonstrate rapid and efficient conversion to es-trone. In this subject, there is also a small increase in estradiol levels, although this may not be detected in all subjects (31). However, the site or sites at which these conversions occur are not known with certainty; even less do we know what factors are involved in controlling this conversion.

A number of studies have demonstrated that adipose tissue, muscle, and possibly liver are all potentially important sites of aromatization, but there are relatively few reports on human tissue (40,46,57,64). We have therefore started

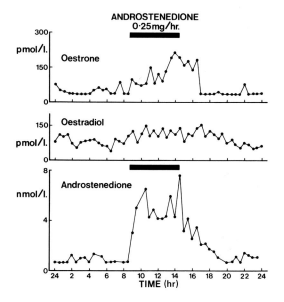

FIG. 5. Effect of infusion of androstenedione on plasma steroid levels in a postmenopausal female.

to re-examine this problem and Table 1 shows some preliminary data (Frost et al., *unpublished data*). It represents the percentage conversion of androstenedione to estrone by various human tissues *in vitro*. In many cases, aromatization is barely detectable, but the type of adipose tissue may be important. There is (64) only one other report in the literature of aromatization of androstenedione by human liver and Table 1 shows how efficient liver is in this respect compared with adipose tissue. In two patients the adipose tissue appeared to be highly efficient in aromatizing the substrate. One patient had hyperprolactinemia and the other was the only patient so far studied with endometrial cancer. It would be very unwise to speculate further, but it is noteworthy that in an earlier study, Schindler and his colleagues (57) reported increased conversion in adipose tissue from patients with endometrial cancer.

Can we demonstrate then, that in patients with endometrial cancer there is altered aromatization, or increased production of estrone? The initial results from various groups of investigators looked exciting in this respect, since some workers found undoubtedly higher than normal conversion rates of androstenedione to estrone in their patients with endometrial cancer (24). Recently, though, particularly from the work of Judd et al. (34) and McDonald et al. (42), it has become clear that it is extremely important to exclude the influence of excess weight in studies of this type, and when this is done, the results in patients with endometrial cancer do not appear to be significantly different from normal.

Figure 6 shows our own data. When careful allowance is made for the effect of excess weight, there is no obvious increase in the cancer patients in estrone

TABLE 1. In vitro conversion of androstenedione to estrone[a]

Subject	Age	LMP or yr postmenopausal	Condition	Tissue	Conversion of A → E1 (%)
A.S.	4	—	Herpes encephalitis (sample obtained at necroscopy)	AT from abdominal wall	nd
A.S.	4	—	Herpes encephalitis (sample obtained at necroscopy)	Liver	0.18
J.S.	26	Intermittent bleeding	Infertility—treatment with stilbestrol pessary	AT from abdominal wall	nd
S.W.	28		Stein Levanthal syndrome	AT from abdominal wall	nd
S.W.	28		Stein Levanthal syndrome	AT from intraperitoneal cavity	0.05
H.P.	34	5 days before sample obtained	Secondary infertility. Previously hyperprolactinemic. Bromocriptine therapy until 2 weeks before sample obtained.	AT from abdominal wall	0.6
N.MG	34	10 days before sample obtained	Primary infertility	AT from abdominal wall	0.07
E.G.	38	10 days before sample obtained	Ovarian cyst	AT from abdominal wall	nd
E.L.	59	12 yr	Cystic adenocarcinoma	AT from abdominal wall	nd
H.M.	59	Frequent irregular periods	Polymenorrhea—3 years earlier had cystic hyperplasia	AT from abdominal wall	0.02
S.W.	62	15 yr	Leiomyosarcoma	AT from abdominal wall	0.05
E.C.	66	18 yr	Endometrial cancer	AT from abdominal wall	0.55
E.C.	66	18 yr	Endometrial cancer	AT from intraperitoneal cavity	0.02

[a] nd, not detectable; AT, adipose tissue; LMP, last menstrual period; A, androstenedione; E1, estrone.

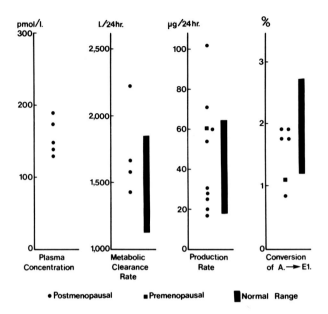

FIG. 6. Estrone metabolism in patients with endometrial cancer. All patients were of normal weight except one, who had the highest metabolic clearance rate and highest production rate, shown in the figure. Ranges for normal women are indicated by the *solid bars* (data from Reed and Murray, ref. 54). A, androstenedione; E1, estrone.

plasma level, metabolic clearance rate, blood production rate, or conversion of androstenedione to estrone.

Although Siiteri et al. (61) originally suggested a specific culpable role for estrone, its importance may be more as a precursor of estradiol than as a hormone per se. Such human biological evidence as exists tends to support this view. When Thijssen and his colleagues (67) infused radiolabeled estrone into their patients, and then subsequently examined the uterine tissues removed at surgery, they found that labeled estradiol, not estrone, accumulated in the endometrium.

Our own data show that there is a significant correlation between vaginal cytology and plasma estradiol levels, but no such relationship exists for estrone (45a).

There is relatively little information on plasma estrogen levels in endometrial cancer, and so far as we are aware, there are no published data on production rates of estradiol in this condition. Two groups have found evidence for increased plasma estrone and estradiol levels (2,6); other workers, though, could find no difference from normal (33). Again, it is important to take note of the problem of obesity (34).

Defining the sources of estradiol in normal postmenopausal women still presents a problem which is not entirely solved.

As shown in Fig. 7, the production rate of estradiol is considerably reduced

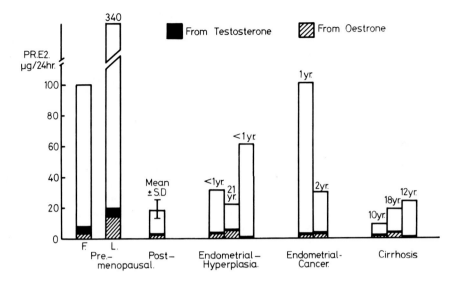

FIG. 7. Production rates of estradiol (PR.E2) and contribution to estradiol production from estrone and testosterone in female subjects. (Values for normal women are taken from Reed and Murray, ref. 54.) For subjects with endometrial hyperplasia, endometrial cancer, or cirrhosis, the number of years elapsed since the menopause are indicated. F, follicular phase; L, luteal phase.

after the menopause and, in 4 normal postmenopausal women studied by Pratt and Longcope (51), was found to range from 11 to 25 μg/24 hr. Transfer constants for the conversion of estrone and testosterone to estradiol by normal postmenopausal women have also been measured (38). Using the transfer constants obtained by Longcope, it appears that less than 20% of the estradiol produced by normal postmenopausal women is apparently derived from estrone and testosterone (Fig. 7).

In a study we have carried out, the production rates of estradiol have been measured in two menopausal women with endometrial cancer and three with endometrial hyperplasia, a possible predisposing condition to endometrial cancer, and our results are also shown in Fig. 7. In addition, production of estradiol was also measured in 3 postmenopausal women with cirrhosis, as it has been suggested that this condition is associated with a higher incidence of endometrial cancer than normal (65). However, this is a controversial topic and in one study no cases of endometrial cancer were found in a very large series of patients with cirrhosis (8).

Also shown in Fig. 7 for the subjects in our study are the number of years that have elapsed since the menopause. When several years had elapsed, estradiol production was similar to that of normal postmenopausal women. However, closer to the menopause, production of estradiol was elevated, presumably reflecting continued ovarian secretion. In one subject with endometrial cancer the production of estradiol was greatly increased, despite this subject having plasma concentrations of gonadotropins and progesterone in the postmenopausal ranges.

The conversion of estrone to estradiol was measured in 6 women (range 3.3–5.3%) and of testosterone to estradiol in 2 other women (0.25 and 0.5%), and used to calculate the contributions of estrone and testosterone to the production of estradiol, as shown in Fig. 7. As calculated for normal postmenopausal women, less than 20% of the production of estradiol by the subjects of this study can be accounted for by peripheral conversion of estrone and testosterone.

Although a significant gradient has been found between the concentrations of estradiol in ovarian and peripheral plasma (33), the difference was very small and probably contributes less than 0.5 μg/day to the total production rate of estradiol. Wasda et al. (73) recently reported evidence for direct secretion of estradiol from the adrenal cortex of postmenopausal women, although it was calculated that this would only account for 1 to 2 μg/day. Since transfer constants of 30 to 50% for the conversion of estrone to estradiol calculated from urinary metabolites (70) are much higher than those estimated from blood, it is possible that the model used for dynamic studies will have to be re-examined in order to explain the discrepancy between total estradiol production and peripheral production from precursors.

In summary, then, it appears that as judged from kinetic isotope studies, the overall production rates of androstenedione and of estrone in nonobese patients with endometrial cancer are not abnormal, although the conversion of androstenedione to estrone in fat in these patients may be altered. It is not clear yet from where all the estradiol derives in postmenopausal women, and there is an almost complete lack of information on estradiol kinetics. It may be that small increases in estradiol production, unopposed by progesterone, and possibly combined with altered plasma binding activity may be important. We obviously still need to extend our knowledge of estradiol metabolism both in normal women and in patients with cancer.

It seems appropriate to try to summarize where we stand in relation to the research objectives which we discussed at the beginning of this chapter. We still lack unequivocal and noncontroversial evidence for the hypothesis that altered endogenous steroid metabolism plays a significant role in the pathogenesis of human breast and endometrial cancer. There is evidence to suggest that in some women, diminished androgen secretion may be a cancer-associated phenomenon. Perhaps the most exciting concept for exploration is still the possibility of altered estrogen–progesterone interaction, and the best hope for further advance may be in studies at tissue or cellular level.

Screening for steroid abnormalities still seems premature; on the other hand, methods of manipulating the hormone environment based on our knowledge of steroid metabolism are already playing important therapeutic roles—for example, the use of aminoglutethimide (55,56) to inhibit the aromatization of androstenedione in breast cancer patients, and the addition of progestins to estrogen therapy (68).

Clearly though, much more still needs to be done to achieve all these objectives, but whatever contribution steroid research can make, the nature of the prize makes that contribution infinitely worthwhile.

ACKNOWLEDGMENT

This work was supported by a grant from the Cancer Research Campaign.

REFERENCES

1. Adams, J. B., Archibald, L., and Clarke, C. (1978): *Cancer Res.,* 38:4036–4040.
2. Aleem, F. A., Moukhtar, M. A., Hung, H. C., and Romney, S. L. (1976): *Cancer,* 38:2101–2104.
3. Anderson, J. N., Peck, E. J., and Clark, J. H. (1975): *Endocrinology,* 96:160–165.
4. Anon. (1977): *Br. Med. J.,* 2:209–210.
5. Arguelles, A. E., Poggi, U. L., Saborida, C., Hoffman, C., Chekherdemian, M., and Blanchard, O. (1973): *Lancet,* 1:165–168.
6. Benjamin, F., and Deutsch, S. (1976): *Am. J. Obstet. Gynecol.,* 126:638–647.
7. Brown, J. B. (1958): In: *Endocrine Aspects of Breast Cancer,* edited by A. R. Currie, p. 197. Livingstone, Edinburgh.
8. Brewer, J. I., and Foley, T. J. (1953): *Obstet. Gynecol.,* 1:67–73.
9. Brownsey, B., Cameron, E. H. D., Griffiths, K., Gleave, E. N., Forrest, A. P. M., and Campbell, H. (1972): *Eur. J. Cancer,* 8:131–137.
10. Bulbrook, R. D., Greenwood, F. C., and Hayward, J. L. (1960): *Lancet,* 1:1154–1157.
11. Bulbrook, R. D., Hayward, J. L., and Spicer, C. C. (1971): *Lancet,* 2:395–398.
12. Bulbrook, R. D., Moore, J. W., Clark, G. M. G., Wang, D. Y., Tong, D., and Hayward, J. L. (1978): *Eur. J. Cancer,* 14:1369–1375.
13. Bulbrook, R. D., Thomas, B. S., Utsonomiya, J., and Hamaguchi, E. (1967): *J. Endocrinol.,* 38:401–406.
14. Cameron, E. H. D., Griffiths, K., Gleave, E. N., Stewart, H. J., Forrest, A. P. M., and Campbell, H. (1970): *Br. Med. J.,* 4:768–771.
15. Cole, P., Cramer, D., Yen, S., Paffenbarger, R., McMahon, B., and Brown, J. (1978): *Cancer Res.,* 38:745–748.
16. Cooke, J. N. C., James, V. H. T., Landon, J., and Wynn, V. (1964): *Br. Med. J.,* 1:662–666.
17. England, P. C., Skinner, L. G., Cottrell, K. M., and Sellwood, R. A. (1975): *Br. J. Surg.,* 62:806–809.
18. Feinstein, A. R., and Horwitz, R. I. (1978): *Cancer Res.,* 38:4001–4005.
19. Fotherby, K., and James, F. (1972): In: *Endocrine Therapy in Malignant Disease,* edited by B. A. Stoll, pp. 25–51. Saunders, London.
20. Gray, C. H., Baron, D. N., Brooks, R. V., and James, V. H. T. (1969): *Lancet,* 1:124–127.
21. Grodin, J. M., Siiteri, P. K., and MacDonald, P. C. (1973): *J. Clin. Endocrinol. Metab.,* 36:207–214.
22. Gurpide, E. (1978): In: *Endocrinology of the Ovary,* edited by R. Scholler, pp. 3–21. Editions Sepe, Paris.
23. Gurpide, E., Tseng, L., and Gusberg, S. B. (1977): *Am. J. Obstet. Gynecol.,* 129:809–813.
24. Hausknecht, R. U., and Gusberg, S. B. (1973): *Am. J. Obstet. Gynecol.,* 116:981–984.
25. Hayward, J. L., and Bulbrook, R. D. (1968): In: *Prognostic Factors in Breast Cancer,* edited by A. P. M. Forrest and P. B. Kunkler, p. 383. Livingstone, Edinburgh.
26. Hellman, L., Zumoff, B., Fishman, J., and Gallagher, T. F. (1971): *J. Clin. Endocrinol. Metab.,* 33:138–144.
27. Hertz, R. (1979): *J. Steroid Biochem.,* 11:435–442.
28. Hisaw, F. L., Velardo, J. T., and Goolsby, S. M. (1954): *J. Clin. Endocrinol. Metab.,* 14:1134–1143.
29. James, F., Braunsberg, H., Irvine, W. T., and James, V. H. T. (1970): *Steroids,* 15:669–678.

30. James, V. H. T., Tunbridge, D., Wilson, G. A., Hutton, J. D., Jacobs, H. S., Goodall, A. B., Murray, M. A. F., and Rippon, A. E. (1978): *J. Steroid Biochem.,* 9:429–436.
31. James, V. H. T., Tunbridge, R. D. G., Wilson, G. A., Hutton, J. D., Jacobs, H. S., and Rippon, A. E. (1978): In: *The Endocrine Function of the Human Adrenal Cortex,* edited by V. H. T. James, M. Serio, and G. Giusti, pp. 179–192. Academic, London.
32. Jones, M. K., Ramsay, I. D., Collins, W. P., and Dyer, G. I. (1977): *Eur. J. Cancer,* 13:1109–1112.
33. Judd, H. L., Judd, G. E., Lucas, W. E., and Yen, S. S. C. (1974): *J. Clin. Endocrinol. Metab.,* 39:1020–1024.
34. Judd, H. L., Lucas, W. E., and Yen, S. S. C. (1976): *J. Clin. Endocrinol. Metab.,* 43:272–278.
35. Jull, J. W. (1977): In: *Chemical Carcinogens,* edited by C. E. Searle. ACS Monograph No. 173, American Chemical Society, Washington, D.C.
36. Juret, P., Hayem, M., and Flaisler, A. (1964): *J. Chir.,* 87:409–433.
37. Lemon, H. M., Wotiz, H. H., Parsons, L., and Mozden, P. J. (1966): *JAMA,* 196:112–120.
38. Longcope, C. (1978): In: *Endocrinology of the Ovary,* edited by R. Scholler, pp. 23–33. Editions Sepe, Paris.
39. Longcope, C., and Pratt, J. H. (1977): *Steroids,* 29:483–492.
40. Longcope, C., Pratt, J. H., Schneider, S. H., and Fineberg, S. E. (1976): *J. Clin. Endocrinol. Metab.,* 43:1134–1145.
41. Lucas, W. E. (1974): *Obstet. Gynecol. Surv.,* 29:507–528.
42. MacDonald, P. C., Edman, C. D., Hemsell, D. L., Porter, J. C., and Siiteri, P. K. (1978): *Am. J. Obstet. Gynecol.,* 130:448–455.
43. McDonald, T. W., Malkasian, G. D., and Gaffey, T. A. (1977): *Obstet. Gynecol.,* 49:654–658.
44. Mack, T. M. (1978): In: *Endometrial Cancer,* edited by M. G. Brush, R. J. B. King, and R. W. Taylor, pp. 17–28. Baillière Tindall, London.,
45. Maynard, P. V., Bird, M., Basu, P. K., Shields, R., and Griffiths, K. (1978): *Eur. J. Cancer,* 14:549–553.
45a. Morse, A. R., Hutton, J. D., Jacobs, H. S., Murray, M. A. F., and James, V. H. T. (1979): *Br. J. Obstet. Gynaecol.,* 86:981.
46. Nimrod, A., and Ryan, K. J. (1975): *J. Clin. Endocrinol. Metab.,* 40:367–372.
47. Pollow, K., Boquoi, E., Baumann, J., Schmidt-Gollwitzer, M., and Pollow, B. (1977): *Mol. Cell. Endocrinol.,* 6:333–348.
48. Poortman, J., and Thijssen, J. H. H. (1978): In: *Endometrial Cancer,* edited by M. G. Brush, R. J. B. King, and R. W. Taylor, pp. 375–382. Baillière Tindall, London.
49. Poortman, J., Thijssen, J. H. H., and Schwarz, F. (1973): *J. Clin. Endocrinol. Metab.,* 37:101–109.
50. Poortman, J., van der Smissen, J., Collette, H. J. A., and de Waard, F. (1979): *Br. J. Cancer,* 39:688–695.
51. Pratt, J. H., and Longcope, C. (1978): *J. Clin. Endocrinol. Metab.,* 46:44–47.
52. Rao, L. G. S. (1970): *Lancet,* 2:441–445.
53. Reed, M. J., Hutton, J. D., Baxendale, P. M., James, V. H. T., Jacobs, H. S., and Fisher, R. P. (1979): *J. Steroid Biochem.,* 11:905–911.
54. Reed, M. J., and Murray, M. A. F. (1979): In: *Hormones in Blood, Vol. 3,* edited by C. H. Gray and V. H. T. James, pp. 263–354. Academic, London.
55. Samojlik, E., and Santen, R. J. (1978): *J. Clin. Endocrinol. Metab.,* 47:717–724.
56. Santen, R. J., Samojlik, E., Lipton, A., Harvey, H., Ruby, E. B., Wells, S. A., and Kendall, J. (1977): *Cancer,* 39:2948–2958.
57. Schindler, A. E., Ebert, A., and Friederick, E. (1972): *J. Clin. Endocrinol. Metab.,* 35:627–630.
58. Sherman, B. M., and Korenman, S. G. (1973): *Cancer,* 33:1306–1312.
59. Siiteri, P. K. (1978): *Cancer Res.,* 38:4360–4366.
60. Siiteri, P. K., and MacDonald, P. C. (1973): In: *Handbook of Physiology, Sec. 7: Endocrinology,* edited by G. B. Astwood and R. O. Greep, pp. 615–629. American Physiological Society, Washington, D.C.
61. Siiteri, P. K., Schwarz, B. E., and MacDonald, P. C. (1974): *Gynecol. Oncol.,* 2:228–238.
62. Siiteri, P. K., Williams, J. E., and Takaki, N. K. (1976): *J. Steroid Biochem.,* 7:897–903.
63. Sitruk-Ware, R., Sterkers, N., and Mauvais-Jarvis, P. (1979): *Obstet. Gynecol.,* 53:457–460.

64. Smuk, M., and Schwers, J. (1977): *J. Clin. Endocrinol. Metab.*, 45:1009–1012.
65. Speert, H. (1949): *Cancer*, 2:597–603.
66. Strong, J. A., Brown, J. B., Bruce, J., Douglas, M., Klopper, A. I., and Loraine, J. A. (1956): *Lancet*, 2:955–959.
67. Thijssen, J. H. H., Wiegerink, M. A. H. M., and Poortman, J. (1978): *J. Steroid Biochem.*, 9:893 (abstr. 312).
68. Thom, M. H., White, P. J., Williams, R. M., Sturdee, D. W., Paterson, M. E. L., Wade-Evans, T., and Studd, J. W. W. (1979): *Lancet*, 2:455–457.
69. van Doorn, L. G., Poortman, J., and Thijssen, J. H. H. (1979): *Acta Endocrinol. [Suppl.] (Copenh.)*, 225(abstr. 265).
70. Vande Wiele, R. L. (1965): In: *Estrogen Assays in Clinical Medicine, Basis and Methodology: A Workshop Conference,* edited by C. A. Paulsen, pp. 142–155. University of Washington Press, Seattle.
71 Wade, A. P., Davis, J. C., Tweedie, M. C. K., Clarke, C. A., and Haggart, B. (1969): *Lancet*, 1:853–856.
72. Wang, D. Y., Bulbrook, R. D., and Hayward, J. L. (1977): *Eur. J. Cancer*, 13:187–192.
73. Wasda, T., Akamine, Y., Kato, K.-I., Ibayashi, H., and Nomura, Y. (1978): *Endocrinol., Jpn.*, 25:123–128.
74. Zumoff, B., Bradlow, H. L., Gallagher, T. F., and Hellman, L. (1971): *J. Clin. Endocrinol. Metab.*, 32:824–832.
75. Zumoff, B., Fishman, J., Bradlow, H. L., and Hellman, L. (1975): *Cancer Res.*, 35:3365–3373.

Hormones and Cancer, edited by S. Iacobelli et al.
Raven Press, New York © 1980.

Endometrial Morphologic Response to Endogenous and Exogenous Hormonal Stimuli in Health and Disease: Normal Endometrium During the Menstrual Cycle; Endometrial Hyperplasia and Carcinoma

Alex Ferenczy

*Department of Pathology, Sir Mortimer B. Davis Jewish General Hospital,
Montreal, Quebec H3T 1E2, Canada*

Knowledge of endometrial morphologic responses to hormonal environment in normal conditions is important not only to assess the status of the hypo-thalamo–pituitary–ovarian axis in cases of infertility but also to compare normal with pathological states. Indeed, one of the major dilemmas in endometrial pathology is related to the pathogenetic development of endometrial hyperplasia and carcinoma and to their relationship to hormonal influence. This chapter reviews the present state of knowledge of the morphological and kinetic charac-teristics of normal, hyperplastic, and neoplastic endometria and relates these to pathogenesis and to endogenous and exogenous hormonal influence. When pertinent, data derived from clinical studies and steroid biochemistry are corre-lated with morphologic alterations.

NORMAL ENDOMETRUIM

Preovulatory phase endometrium is characterized by active growth as evi-denced by an elevated labeling index (the percentage of nuclei incorporating nucleoprotein precursor-[^{3}H]thymidine) (Fig. 1) and numerous mitoses in the nuclei of gland cells, fibroblasts, and vascular endothelium (6). Ultrastructurally, the cytoplasm is rich in free and bound ribosomes, Golgi apparatus, mitochon-dria, and acid phosphatase-rich primary lysosomes. Both cilio- and surface micro-villogenesis are well developed in the proliferative endometrium (Table 1) and receptors for estradiol (E_2R) and progesterone (PR) are elevated (11,13,14). All these features depend on (estradiol) E_2-stimulated DNA-dependent RNA synthesis (2,6). During the preovulatory period, plasma (E_2) and estrone (E_1) are elevated.

In the early postovulatory endometrium, the effects of progesterone (P) are manifested by an accumulation of intracytoplasmic glycogen and the appearance

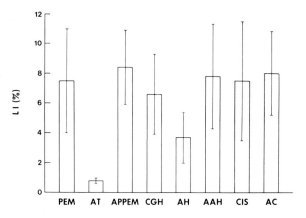

FIG. 1. Mean labeling index of normal and abnormal endometria. PEM: cyclic proliferative endometrium, 11 cases; AT: atrophic endometrium, 4 cases; APPEM: anovulatory, persistent proliferative endometrium, 6 cases; CGH: cystic glandular hyperplasia, 4 cases; AH: adenomatous hyperplasia without atypia, 5 cases; AAH: AH with severe cytologic atypia, 4 cases; CIS: carcinoma *in situ,* 6 cases; AC: invasive adenocarcinoma, 14 cases; LI: labeling index is high in APPEM, low in AH, and is similar in AAH, CIS, and AC.

of giant mitochondria and basket-like nucleolar channel systems (7). The latter are unique to the postovulatory human endometrium but their significance is presently not understood.

Later in the cycle, glycoprotein synthesis becomes prominent, involving the ergastoplasm–glycogen–mitochondria–Golgi complex. Coinciding with intraluminal gland secretion, DNA synthesis and mitoses in gland cells become negligible and absent, respectively (6). Surface microvilli become shorter and fewer in number and ciliated cells are limited almost exclusively to the endometrial surface epithelium (2,7).

From cycle day 25, the conceptus-free endometrium undergoes lysosomal enzyme-mediated involution and degeneration. P is a potent stabilizer of E_2-produced primary lysosomes. Coinciding with the fall of plasma P, lysosomal membrane integrity is no longer maintained, the acid hydrolases are thus released into cellular cavities (autophagosomes), cytoplasmic matrix, and presumably intercellular spaces resulting in enzymatic digestion and destruction of the glandular epithelium, stromal cells, and vascular system (2). Endothelial membrane injury promotes prostaglandin-mediated vascular thrombosis, anoxia, and further tissue necrosis.

HYPERPLASTIC ENDOMETRIUM

Clinical and morphologic observations suggest that about 10% of women with untreated adenomatous hyperplasia may progress to carcinoma (3). Thus, adenomatous hyperplasia is considered to be a risk factor for developing carci-

TABLE 1. *Ultrastructural characteristics of normal and abnormal endometrium*[a]

Glandular epithelium	Cyclic proliferative	APPEM	CGH	AH	AAH	CIS	Invasive carcinoma
Organelles	2+	4+	3+	3+	Increasingly pleomorphic		
Microfilaments	1+	2+	2+	3+	Increasingly disorganized		
Autophagocytosis	0/1+	1+	1+	1+	1–2+	2+	3+
Primary lysosomes	2+	4+	2–3+	3+	2+	1+	1+
Ciliogenesis	2+	4+	3+	3+	2–3+	2+	1+
Microvillogenesis	1+	4+	3+	3+	2–3+	1+	1+
Nuclear membrane	Regular			Slightly irregular	Increasingly irregular		
Plasma membrane	Regular to slightly Convoluted			Slightly convoluted	Increasingly convoluted		

[a] CGH, cystic glandular hyperplasia; AH, adenomatous hyperplasia; AAH, atypical adenomatous hyperplasia; CIS, carcinoma *in situ*.

noma (3). Also, many women with adenomatous hyperplasia have clinical and hormonal-metabolic stigmata including obesity and increased peripheral conversion of androgens into E_1 similar to those with endometrial carcinoma (10). Cystic glandular hyperplasia, adenomatous hyperplasia, atypical adenomatous hyperplasia, or carcinoma *in situ* may be found adjacent to 17 to 43% of endometrial carcinomas (2). The remainder of uterine malignancies are associated with an atrophic endometrium. In many of these cases, however, when the adjacent endometrium is thoroughly examined, it shows features of remote hyperplasia such as polyps or foci of thickened, polypoid mucosa with retrogressive atrophic features. In other instances, the carcinomatous process might have replaced the hyperplastic endometrium.

In addition to light microscopy, hyperplastic endometria have been examined by means of Feulgen-DNA microspectrophotometry (14), transmission and scanning electron microscopy (2,7), *in vitro* DNA-historadioautography (4), and specific receptor binding of E_2 and P (9,11,13,14). The results of most of these studies indicate that endometrial hyperplasia represents a spectrum of morpho-biochemical changes that are intermediate between normal, proliferative endometrium, and endometrial carcinoma. Endometrial hyperplasia may morphologically and biologically be subdivided into two pathogenetic phases: (a) proliferative phase, and (b) remodeling phase. The proliferative phase consists of an increase in the cell number and/or volume (hyperplasia-hypertrophy) of endometrial mucosa, but otherwise the general architecture of the endometrium demonstrates only minimal deviation from the normal, preovulatory endometrium. These changes are best referred to as anovulatory, persistent proliferative endometrium (APPEM) (Fig. 2a). Others may use the term "simple hyperplasia" for APPEM (9). APPEM is often associated with focal dilatation of endometrial glands. When APPEM undergoes diffuse glandular dilatation, the so-called cystic glandular hyperplasia pattern is produced. Cystic glandular hyperplasia contains essentially the same biochemical and fine structural alterations as APPEM (2,7). The proliferative phase of endometrial hyperplasia is clinically unstable. Most often it regresses following D & C but may persist or progress to the second or remodeling phase of endometrial hyperplasia.

It is conceivable, although not proven, that the genesis of APPEM in the human is related to loss of control mechanisms of E_2-dependent uterine growth, the so-called "uterine chalone" (8). In the rat, a "uterine chalone" may be present and be responsible for controlling E_2-induced uterine growth (8). Loss of uterine chalone in the human may theoretically lead to the loss of endometrial refractoriness to long-standing E_2 stimulation in the absence of P. This results in E_2-sensitive endometrial cell overgrowth producing a picture of APPEM. It is also conceivable that further E_2 stimulation may lead to the development of a gradually increasing number of E_2-independent cells as a reflection of escape from E_2-promoted growth. In these cells, architectural and cytonuclear alterations prevail and the volume of endometrial stroma decreases in favor of the glands from adenomatous hyperplasia with atypia to atypical adenomatous hy-

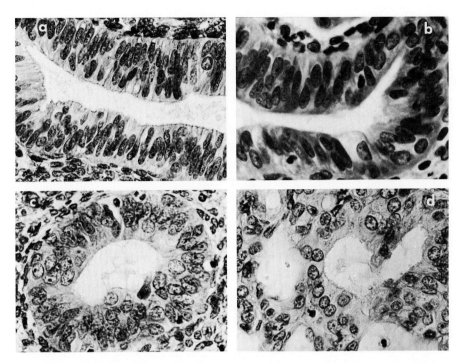

FIG. 2. a: APPEM. The volume of glands, height of lining cells, and pseudostratification of pencil-shaped nuclei are exaggerated from cyclic, proliferative endometrium. **b:** Adenomatous hyperplasia without cytologic atypia. Note slight rounding of nuclei. Nucleoli are visible. **c:** AH with severe cytologic atypia. The nuclei are round, overlapping, devoid of cohesion, and have enlarged nucleoli and aggregated nuclear chromatin. **d:** Carcinoma *in situ*. Cribriform glandular pattern associated with round, pleomorphic nuclei, macronucleoli, and clumping of nuclear chromatin. **a–d:** × 315.

perplasia. This is the remodeling stage of endometrial hyperplasia which tends to persist rather than regress and occasionally progress to carcinoma. Although a uniform terminology for this stage of endometrial hyperplasia has not yet been adapted, the changes range from adenomatous hyperplasia without atypia (Fig. 2b) to adenomatous hyperplasia with severe, atypical cytological and architectural patterns (Fig. 2c) (3). Cytological rather than architectural alterations are significant in relation to the risk of progression to carcinoma (3).

Feulgen-DNA cytophotometry of both cystic glandular hyperplasia and adenomatous hyperplasia without atypia demonstrates a diploid to tetraploid nuclear DNA content similar to normal, proliferative endometrial gland cells engaged in active DNA synthesis (14). However, when DNA synthesis is studied by DNA historadioautography, it is greater (although not statistically significant) in APPEM than in proliferative endometrium, cystic glandular hyperplasia, or adenomatous hyperplasia (Fig. 1). Furthermore, the DNA S phase is significantly shorter in APPEM than in proliferative endometrium or adenomatous hyperplasia without atypia (Fig. 3). Since DNA synthesis in the endometrium is E_2-stimulated, the kinetics of APPEM reflect its increased estrogenic responsiveness in comparison to cyclic proliferative endometrium as well as cystic glandular hyperplasia and adenomatous hyperplasia. Also, E_2-induced PR content was higher in three cases of APPEM than in proliferative endometrium or adenomatous hyperplasia (13). Others, however, found higher values in adenomatous hyperplasia than in proliferative endometrium or cystic glandular hyperplasia (9). Electron microscopy of gland cells of APPEM, cystic glandular hyperplasia, and adenomatous hyperplasia without atypia shows an increase in estrogen-related morphologic alterations compared to their normal, proliferative counterparts (2,3) (Table 1). Additional evidence of end-organ sensitivity to E_2 stimulation is offered by the suppression of E_2-related morphologic changes by pharmacologic doses of exogenous progestagens. The latter are capable of inhibiting DNA synthesis and mitotic activity as well as cilio- and microvillogenesis, and of transforming hyperplastic gland cells into normal secretory units (2,4). Such endometria have a considerably prolonged potential doubling time (5). Akin to postovulatory progestational endometrium, in gestagen-treated endometrial hyperplasia, secretory gland cell exhaustion and stromal decidualization are followed by lysosomal autodestruction (2,4). Gestagen-induced effects are produced more often in the early than in the later stages of endometrial hyperplasia (5,13) and are correlated with generally high concentrations of E_2R and PR (13,14). Also, gestagens when given to postmenopausal women in combi-

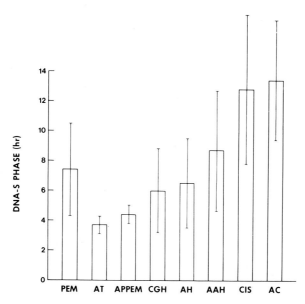

FIG. 3. Mean DNA S phase of normal and abnormal endometria. DNA S phase gradually lengthens from APPEM to CIS and AC. (See Fig. 1 legend for abbreviations.)

nation with exogenous estrogens considerably reduce the risk of developing endometrial hyperplasia compared with estrogenic replacement therapy alone (9).

Electron microscopy (2,3), DNA tracing (4), and steroid receptor analysis (13) of adenomatous hyperplasia without atypia and with varying degrees of cytonuclear and histologic abnormalities show a spectrum of alterations which are minimal in adenomatous hyperplasia without atypia and greatest in atypical adenomatous hyperplasia. There is a gradual increase in ultrastructural abnormalities (Table 1) and prolongation of the DNA S phase (Fig. 2), and the PR content gradually decreases from adenomatous hyperplasia without atypia to atypical adenomatous hyperplasia and carcinoma *in situ* and carcinoma (12). These observations support the thesis that atypical adenomatous hyperplasia is a precursor of carcinoma *in situ*. Intermediate lengths of DNA S phase are also seen in other carcinoma precursor tissue systems such as GI tract and skin (4).

NEOPLASTIC ENDOMETRIUM

Ultrastructurally, carcinoma cells *in situ* have comparatively fewer estrogen-related cellular alterations and greater pleomorphism and abnormal distribution of their intracytoplasmic organelles and microfilaments, respectively, than those of adenomatous hyperplasia and atypical adenomatous hyperplasia (2–4) (Table 1). When the findings are compared with well-differentiated adenocarcinoma cells with myometrial invasion (2,3), they are essentially identical and provide supportive submicroscopic evidence that the cells in carcinoma lesions *in situ* are indeed neoplastic and are the immediate precursors of invasive carcinoma. Such lesions characteristically demonstrate intraglandular bridges (cribriform glandular pattern) and pleomorphic nuclei with clumping of the chromatin (Fig. 2d). Such a nuclear pattern corresponds to aneuploid DNA content (15). Nuclear aneuploidy is a characteristic feature of invasive and noninvasive carcinomas in general and is a reflection of abnormal number and/or organization of chromosomes. DNA historadioautography of carcinoma *in situ* and invasive adenocarcinoma shows a significant prolongation of the DNA S phase (Fig. 3) and a considerably shorter potential doubling time compared with the adjacent hyperplastic or atrophic endometrium. Prolonged DNA S phase, like nuclear aneuploidy, is a characteristic feature of invasive and preinvasive malignant cells in general. The results provide an additional piece of evidence for the existence of endometrial carcinoma *in situ*.

The gradual decrease in estrogen-related alterations in neoplastic endometrial cells is considered to be a reflection of dedifferentiation, which presumably produces a gradually increasing number of E_2-insensitive cells rather than of reduced estrogenic influence. Indeed, despite relatively elevated endogenous or exogenous estrogens in many women with uterine carcinoma (10), steroid receptor content is comparatively lower in carcinomatous than in hyperplastic endometrium

(9,11,13,14) (Fig. 4). Furthermore, PR concentrations are correlated with cyto-histological differentiation of uterine carcinomas. In general, grade 1 well-differ-entiated carcinoma has PR more often present and at higher concentrations than the grade 3 poorly differentiated variety (9,11,13,14). Also, clinical and morphological responses to gestagen therapy are observed in only those carcino-mas in which PRs are present above 50-fmole levels (11). Although gestagens may produce redifferentiation of PR-containing tumor cells, the changes tend to be focal rather than diffuse, and following cessation of therapy, growth and/or recurrences of malignancy are observed in most cases (5). These alterations are partly due to exhaustion of PR presumably by their nuclear translocation and inhibition of their replenishment (11) and partly to the heterogeneous (E_2-sensitive–E_2-insensitive) cell population of neoplastic and hyperplastic as well as normal endometrial tissues (5). Histology and DNA tracer studies of cyclic endometrium (6) as well as gestagen-treated hyperplastic and neoplastic endome-tria (5) show geographical differences in secretory differentiation and nucleic acid synthesis in gland cells, respectively. There is a tendency toward higher [^{3}H]thymidine uptake and greater secretory differentiation in the upper than in the lower layers of the endometrium. The fact that PRs are higher in prolifera-tive endometrium than in carcinoma with intermediate values in endometrial hyperplasia (Fig. 4) supports the concept of a gradual decrease in E_2-sensitive cells and an increase in E_2-insensitive or independent cells from normal to carci-noma. The finding of labeling index in atypical adenomatous carcinoma, carci-noma *in situ* and carcinoma (Fig. 2) similar to that of normal endometrium in the face of a gradual lengthening of the DNA S phase (Fig. 1) suggests a dissociation between E_2-promoted and E_2-independent endometrial proliferations and thus reinforces this concept.

A final consideration is related to the presumed relationship between endome-trial carcinogenesis and hormone replacement therapy (HRT). Recent epidemio-logic studies found that women with endometrial carcinomas had a mean sixfold

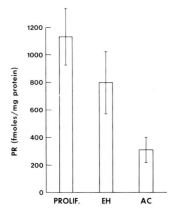

FIG. 4. PR concentrations. Cyclic proliferative endome-trium (PROLIF.), EH: endometrial hyperplasia with and without atypia; AC: well to poorly differentiated invasive adenocarcinoma.

greater probability of having received HRT than those without carcinoma (1). In the former group, however, most carcinomas are FIGO stage 1 and grade 1 well-differentiated lesions, and are associated with near 100% 5-year survival rates (1). The data may suggest that HRT-associated carcinomas are biologically different from those without HRT.

Our preliminary results derived from ultrastructure, *in vitro* DNA historadioautography, and receptor analysis of carcinomas in women on HRT for a minimum of 2 years are not significantly different from those without such therapy when matched for stage and grade as well as weight and age. Further studies of a larger number of cases are underway in our laboratory to determine whether the findings can be generalized. It is interesting to note that a recent and careful pathological analysis of endometrial carcinoma patients with and without HRT found no difference in biological behavior when survival rates were corrected for histological differentiation (12).

CONCLUSIONS

1. The normal cyclic endometrium is composed of a heterogeneous cell population characterized by E_2-sensitive and -insensitive cells, the ratio of which is largely in favor of the former. These cells respond to proliferation and secretory differentiation to E_2 and P, respectively. Withdrawal of both hormones is followed by lysosomal and prostaglandin-mediated involution and autodestruction.

2. Endometrial hyperplasia represents a disease continuum; its early development is a reflection of an increased sensitivity of the endometrium to E_2 stimulation unmodified by P. Increasing cytological and architectural atypia of endometrial hyperplasia seems to be associated with a gradual decrease in E_2-sensitive cell populations.

3. There is convincing evidence indicating the existence of carcinoma *in situ* of the endometrium as a distinct morphologic entity representing the immediate precursor of invasive carcinoma.

4. Carcinoma *in situ* of the endometrium derives from adenomatous hyperplasia with severe cytonuclear atypia.

5. In endometrial adenocarcinomas, including the carcinoma *in situ* variety, E_2-sensitive cells are further decreased or absent probably as a result of neoplastic dedifferentiation. The available data suggest that endometrial carcinogenesis per se is independent of E_2 influence. However, estrogens are likely to promote the development of an endometrial environment which, in the genetically predisposed, is susceptible to malignant transformation.

ACKNOWLEDGMENTS

Supported by Grant MA 5137 from the Medical Research Council of Canada. The author is indebted to Miss Rosemary De Marco for typing the manuscript.

REFERENCES

1. Antunes, C. M. F., Stolley, P. D., Rosenshein, N. B., Davies, J. L., Tonascia, J. A., Brown, C., Burnett, L., Rutledge, A., Pokempner, M., and Garcia, R. (1979): *N. Engl. J. Med.,* 300:9–13.
2. Ferenczy, A. (1977): In: *Biology of the Uterus,* edited by R. M. Wynn, pp. 545–585. Plenum Press, New York.
3. Ferenczy, A. (1979): In: *Hormonal Biology of Endometrial Cancer,* edited by G. S. Richardson and D. T. MacLaughlin, pp. 49–58. UICC Technical Report Series, Geneva.
4. Ferenczy, A. (1979): *Exp. Mol. Pathol.,* 31:226–235.
5. Ferenczy, A. (1980): In: *Functional Morphological Changes in Female Sex Organs Induced by Exogenous Hormones,* edited by G. Dallenbach-Hellweg, pp. 101–110. Springer-Verlag, Berlin.
6. Ferenczy, A., Bertrand, G., and Gelfand, M. M. (1979): *Am. J. Obstet. Gynecol.,* 133:859–867.
7. Ferenczy, A., and Richart, R. M. (1974): *Female Reproductive System. Dynamics of Sand and Transmission Electron Microscopy.* Wiley, New York.
8. Gorski, J., Stormshak, F., Harris, J., and Wertz, N. (1977): *J. Toxicol. Environ. Health,* 3:271–279.
9. King, R. J. B. (1978): In: *Hormonal Biology of Endometrial Cancer,* edited by G. S. Richardson and D. T. MacLaughlin, pp. 139–153, UICC Technical Report Series, Geneva.
10. MacDonald, P. C., Edman, C. D., Hemsell, D. L., Porter, J. C., and Siiteri, P. K. (1978): *Am. J. Obstet. Gynecol.,* 130:448–455.
11. Martin, P. M., Rolland, P. H., Gamerre, M., Serment, H., and Toga, M. (1979): *Int. J. Cancer,* 23:321–329.
12. Robboy, S. J., and Bradley, R. (1979): *Obstet. Gynecol.,* 54:269–277.
13. Shymala, G., and Ferenczy, A. (1980): *In preparation.*
14. Vihko, R., Robel, P., and Pollow, K. (1978): In: *Hormonal Biology of Endometrial Cancer,* edited by G. S. Richardson and D. T. MacLaughlin, pp. 63–112. UICC Technical Report Series, Geneva.
15. Wagner, D., Richart, R. M., and Turner, J. Y. (1967): *Cancer,* 20:2067–2077.

Hormones and Cancer, edited by S. Iacobelli et al.
Raven Press, New York © 1980.

Hormonal Basis of Risk Factors for Breast and Endometrial Cancer

P. K. Siiteri, J. A. Nisker, and G. L. Hammond

*Reproductive Endocrinology Center, University of California,
San Francisco, California 94143, U.S.A.*

Cancer of estrogen target tissues, including the breast, endometrium, cervix, and ovary, constitute approximately 50% of all cancer that occurs in women (12). Since the original studies which demonstrated that estrogen was capable of promoting breast cancer in animals (32), the possibility that endogenous hormone production may play a role in carcinogenesis in the human has received considerable attention. It is generally held that cancer induction in the human is a long-term process requiring 20 to 30 years for tumor expression. Thus, the hormonal influence is believed to exert itself late in tumorigenesis by stimulating an already transformed cell population to proliferate. This view, which is based on the correlation of exposure to carcinogens, such as cigarette smoke, and subsequent changes in the incidence of lung cancer, may not be accurate in hormonally related cancer. For example, breast cancer is very rare in males, but men on estrogen therapy develop this malignancy with increased frequency within the first year of estrogen intake. Similar considerations apply to the onset of endometrial cancer in postmenopausal women receiving exogenous estrogens. Indeed, other forms of cancer, such as Wilms' tumor and adrenoblastoma, which are among the most common malignancies in young children, obviously do not require long induction periods. The increase in breast and endometrial cancer that occurs following the menopause, a time of ovarian senescence, led to the traditional epidemiological view that estrogens play a minimal role in the development of these cancers. However, it is clear that postmenopausal women produce estrogens and that under certain circumstances the amounts are sufficient to fully activate target tissues. Indeed, the constitutional characteristics associated with an increased risk for development of endometrial and possibly breast cancer are those which now are known to be associated with increased estrogen production. Thus it seems reasonable to propose that cancer of these target tissues is related to inappropriate estrogen stimulation. In this view, estrogens can be considered to be promoters, whereby the action of carcinogens, viruses, or ionizing irradiation, impinge upon a population of dividing cells with a higher frequency than in unstimulated cells. This mechanism, coupled with a declining reactivity of the host immunological surveillance system, could easily account for the high frequency of cancer of estrogen and perhaps androgen target tissues observed in the aging human population.

EPIDEMIOLOGIC CONSIDERATIONS

Breast Cancer

The incidence of breast cancer rises with age throughout the postmenopausal period in most parts of the world. In Japanese women, however, it has been shown to decline (16). This difference cannot be easily ascribed to differences in genetic susceptibility, since it is well established that Japanese women who move to the United States assume the same frequency of breast cancer as observed for American women within two generations (6). Thus, environmental factors appear to be more important. Many studies have suggested that dietary fat content, in particular the proportion of saturated versus unsaturated fat, can be correlated with breast cancer incidence (10). Experimental evidence from animal studies is in agreement with this finding (8). The mechanism by which dietary fat influences the risk of breast cancer, however, is not known. Obesity has been the subject of much controversy as a risk factor in human breast cancer. DeWaard (15) has felt that this is a major consideration and indeed proposed weight reduction as a preventive measure some years ago. Wynder et al. (59) have reached the same conclusion in studies of American women. Other risk factors which have been often cited in the literature include hypothyroidism (18), nulliparity (21), late age of first pregnancy (41), and late menopause (42). Sherman and Korenman (51) have studied the menstrual histories of breast cancer patients and have found that many patients have a history of irregular menstrual cycles. Indeed, Grattarola (22) had proposed earlier that anovulation associated with polycystic ovarian disease was a risk factor for development of breast cancer because of increased androgen production.

Clearly the most important risk factor presently recognized for a young woman is a history of premenopausal maternal breast cancer (43). It is generally assumed, but not proven, that this increased risk is related to enhanced susceptibility to genetic transformation which leads to neoplastic cell development. It is equally possible that this inherited trait may be related to an endocrine abnormality, particularly one which increases the activity of the breast epithelium. The fact that hyperactivity, as reflected in benign breast disease, appears to increase the risk for cancer development is in accord with this view.

Endometrial Cancer

Obesity is the most common metabolic abnormality associated with endometrial cancer. The average weight of women with endometrial cancer is more than 50 lbs in excess of ideal weight (17). Indeed, 20% of endometrial cancer patients weigh more than 200 lbs (49). Low parity and irregular menses have been associated with endometrial carcinoma (39). This is especially striking in women who develop this malignancy while young. A recent report demonstrated nulliparity in 46% and abnormal menstrual pattern in 62% of women who develop endometrial carcinoma under 40 years of age (46). Polycystic ovarian disease, an anovulatory state, is strongly linked with endometrial carcinoma (3,29), as are estrogen-producing neoplasms (25). Diabetes mellitus and hypertension are other metabolic abnormalities associated with endometrial carcinoma (39), although these abnormalities may be purely a reflection of their association with obesity (35). Delayed menopause has also been associated with endometrial carcinoma (39). The increased relative risk of endometrial carcinoma in postmenopausal estrogen users has received much attention (4,23,38,56,61). Hypothyroidism was clinically evident in 10% of Wynder's 900 endometrial cancer patients (60), but later studies have not corroborated this association (39).

ENDOCRINE STUDIES

Breast

Early investigations which attempted to identify endocrine abnormalities in breast cancer patients dealt with the urinary excretion of steroid metabolites. Bulbrook and his associates studied the excretion of many steroids and observed abnormalities in the excretion of androgen metabolites in breast cancer patients (7). Other investigators studied androgen production by the adrenal gland and observed diminished production of dehydroepiandrosterone sulfate (48,57). However, these findings are difficult to relate to the etiology of breast cancer. More recently Poortman and his co-workers have proposed that the androgen androstenediol may be important by virtue of the fact that it can interact with the estrogen receptor and therefore at least potentially stimulate breast epithelial cells (47).

MacMahon and co-workers studied urinary excretion of various estrogens and found that the excretion of estriol, relative to estrone and estradiol, was lower in American women than in Japanese women (40). Together with earlier observations on the biological activity of estriol (27), they proposed that estriol was a protective estrogen, and therefore the difference in frequency of breast cancer in the two populations might be explained by an abnormality in estriol production (11). However, studies by Hellman et al. (26) have refuted these findings, and more recent experiments by Clark et al. (9) and others (24) have shown that estriol when administered continuously is a potent estrogen inducing breast tumors in experimental animals.

Fishman et al. (19) have proposed that differences in metabolism of the active estrogens estradiol and estrone may be important in breast cancer patients. They found that 16-hydroxylation was increased relative to 2-hydroxylation and suggested that estriol is an active estrogen as compared with 2-hydroxyestradiol or estrone, and that it could account for enhanced estrogenic activity in breast cancer patients. However, since the concentration of estriol in the circulation of normal or breast cancer patients is extremely low, it is difficult to see how this mechanism could be important, unless of course estriol is produced within the breast itself. It is of interest to point out, however, that the balance of 16-hydroxylation versus 2-hydroxylation appears to be under the control of thyroid hormone and that the hypothyroid state is associated with enhanced 16-hydroxylation (20). The mechanism underlying increased risk associated with anovulation is not clear; however, it appears likely that the anovulatory state represents a situation in which target cells are exposed continuously to estrogen without the modifying influence of progesterone from the corpus luteum.

Women with polycystic ovarian disease clearly have high levels of estrogen formed peripherally from the excessive androstenedione produced by the abnormal ovaries (2). However, it is not clear what percentage of anovulatory subjects who develop breast cancer have had polycystic ovaries. Dao et al. (13) some years ago proposed that estrogen could be formed locally within the breast from circulating androgens. Many investigators have studied the capacity of normal breast and breast tumors to produce estrogens via the aromatase enzyme and conflicting results have appeared (1,44). Studies in this laboratory have shown that only a very few breast tumors have aromatizing capacity using an extraordinarily sensitive assay for the aromatase enzyme (55). Conflicting results have also been obtained recently in studies of a human breast cancer cell line (MCF-7). Lippman and co-workers (33) failed to demonstrate aromatization of androstenedione in these cells, whereas MacIndoe (37) was able to show that testosterone was converted to estradiol by these cells. Thus, the importance of local production of estrogens by normal or breast tumor cells remains to be established. Clearly, if this process is generally active, then abnormalities of hormone production or action may not be found by analysis of serum hormones.

Many laboratory investigations have demonstrated the importance of prolactin in the initiation and maintenance of breast tumors in rodents. However, most studies to date in humans have revealed no significant differences in circulating prolactin levels between normal subjects, women at high risk, or breast cancer patients (5,28,31). However, it should be emphasized that circulating levels of prolactin fluctuate widely so that serum estimations are difficult to interpret.

POSTMENOPAUSAL ESTROGEN PRODUCTION AND METABOLISM

As the menstrual cycle becomes less regular during the menopausal transition, ovarian secretion of estradiol becomes sporadic and ultimately falls to essentially zero when ovulation no longer occurs (52). However, most postmenopausal women continue to produce low levels of estrone from androstenedione derived from the adrenals by aromatization in tissues such as the liver and fat. The production rate of androstenedione is 1 to 2 mg/day in normal postmenopausal women, and about 1.5 to 2.0% of this is converted to estrone (54). Therefore, the production rate of estrone is 30 to 40 μg/day and the serum levels of estrone and estradiol are 30 to 40 and 5 to 10 pg/ml, respectively (30). It has recently been reported that the mean serum level of estrone sulfate in postmenopausal women is considerably higher (178 pg/ml) than that of free estrone and estradiol (50). Thus estrone sulfate appears to be the principal estrogen in the blood of postmenopausal women as is the case in younger women (34,58). Studies of the origin of estrone sulfate following the menopause appear not to have been carried out, although estrone sulfate appears to arise from estrone following conversion of androstenedione in tissues.

It is now well established that several common conditions increase the efficiency of peripheral estrone production. These include obesity, hepatic disease, and hyperthyroidism. Less frequently, the production rate of androstenedione is increased due to ovarian tumors or stromal hyperplasia, which results in an increase in estrone production without an increase in the conversion from androstenedione. The conversion of androstenedione to estrone may be elevated two- to fivefold in obese postmenopausal women (36), and the production rates of estrone and serum estrogen levels are also elevated (30). This mechanism readily explains the findings of less severe atrophy of the vagina and a higher incidence of uterine bleeding in obese as compared with thin postmenopausal women.

We have recently addressed another aspect of estrogen activity in obese postmenopausal women. An early report suggested that the levels of serum sex hormone binding globulin (SHBG) are depressed in obese men and women (14). However, little information is available concerning the influences of SHBG capacity in modulating estrogen, as compared with androgen action. For these reasons we have measured the serum levels of SHBG and the percentage of free estradiol in normal and obese postmenopausal women (45). The (mean $\pm$ SEM) SHBG for women less than 5 lbs above ideal weight, between 15 and 64 lbs overweight, and more than 65 lbs above ideal weight were 53 $\pm$ 3, 27 $\pm$ 2, and 17 $\pm$ 2 pmoles/ml, respectively. These means were significantly different ($p < 0.002$). In addition, women with hyperthyroidism were shown to have an elevated SHBG capacity. SHBG is the high affinity binder of estradiol in the plasma. A decrease in its binding capacity should allow more estradiol to circulate unbound (i.e., free). This was confirmed in our laboratory (45), and obese women were shown to have significantly elevated percent of free estradiol in their blood (45). Hypothyroid women would probably also have increased free estradiol levels.

We have recently demonstrated an increase in the percentage of free estradiol in the blood of women with breast (53) and endometrial (45) cancer when compared with normal women. We have associated the increased percentage-free estradiol in endometrial cancer patients with low serum SHBG capacity, resulting essentially from their propensity to obesity. The weight and SHBG capacity of breast cancer patients did not differ from reference subjects. Therefore, a different mechanism for the increase in the serum percent-free estradiol must exist in these women. It is generally accepted that only the unbound fraction of estradiol is biologically active. An increase in this fraction demonstrated in both breast and endometrial cancer patients is highly suggestive of a common mechanism, in which free estradiol promotes target cell proliferation and susceptibility to carcinogenesis.

ACKNOWLEDGMENTS

This work was supported by NIH Grants HD 08692 and HD 12949. Dr. Nisker is a fellow of the Medical Research Council of Canada.

REFERENCES

1. Adams, J. B., and Li, K. (1975): *Br. J. Cancer,* 31:429.
2. Aiman, E. J., Edman, C. D., Siiteri, P. K., and MacDonald, P. C. (1975): *Gynecol. Invest.,* 6:21.
3. Andrews, W. C., and Andrews, M. C. (1960): *Am. J. Obstet. Gynecol.,* 80:632.
4. Artunes, C. M. F., Stolley, P. D., Rosenshein, N. B., Davies, J. L., Tunascia, J. A., Brown, C., Burnett, L., Rutledge, A., Pokempner, M., and Garcia, R. (1979): *N. Engl. J. Med.,* 300:9.
5. Boyns, A. R., Cole, E. N., and Griffiths, K. (1973): *Eur. J. Cancer,* 9:99.
6. Buell, P. (1973): *J. Natl. Cancer Inst.,* 51:1457.
7. Bulbrook, R. D., Hayward, J. L., Spicer, C. C., and Thomas, B. S. (1962): *Lancet,* 2:1235.
8. Carroll, K. (1975): *Cancer Res.,* 35:3374.
9. Clark, J. H., Pasko, Z., and Peck, E. J., Jr. (1977): *Endocrinology,* 100:91.
10. Cole, P., and Cramer, D. (1977): *Cancer,* 40:434.
11. Cole, P., and MacMahon, B. (1969): *Lancet,* 1:604.
12. Culter, S. J., and Young, J. L., editors (1975): *Natl. Cancer Inst. Monogr.,* 41:75–787.
13. Dao, T. L., Varela, R., and Morreal, C. (1972): In: *Estrogen Target Tissues and Neoplasia,* edited by T. L. Dao, p. 163. University of Chicago Press, Chicago.
14. DeMoor, P., and Joossens, J. V. (1970): *Steroidologia,* 1:129.
15. DeWaard, F. W. (1975): *Cancer Res.,* 35:3351.
16. Doll, R., Mari, C., and Waterhouse, J. (1970): *Cancer Incidence in Three Continents, Vol. 2.* Springer-Verlag, New York.
17. Dunn, L. J., and Bradbury, J. T. (1967): *Am. J. Obstet. Gynecol.,* 97:465.
18. Edelstyn, G. A., Lyons, A. R., and Welbourn, R. B. (1958): *Lancet,* 1:670.
19. Fishman, J., and Martucci, C. (1978): *Pediatrics,* 62:1128.
20. Fishman, J., Hellman, L., Zumoff, B., and Gallagher, T. F. (1965): *J. Clin. Endocrinol. Metab.,* 25:365.
21. Gagnon, F. (1950): *Am. J. Obstet. Gynecol.,* 60:516.
22. Grattarola, R. (1964): *Cancer,* 17:1119.
23. Gray, L. A., Christopherson, W. M., and Hoover, R. N. (1977): *Obstet. Gynecol.,* 49:385.
24. Gross, J., Modan, B., Bertini, B., Spira, O., de Waard, F., Thijssen, J. H. H., and Vestergaard, P. (1977): *J. Natl. Cancer Inst.,* 59:7.
25. Gusberg, S. B., and Kardon, P. (1971): *Am. J. Obstet. Gynecol.,* 111:633.
26. Hellman, L., Zumoff, B., Fishman, J., and Gallagher, T. F. (1971): *J. Clin. Endocrinol. Metab.,* 33:138.
27. Huggins, C., Grand, L. C., and Brillantes, F. P. (1961): *Nature,* 189:204.
28. Wilson, R. G., Buchan, R., Roberts, M. M., Forrest, A. P. M., Boynes, A. R., Cole, E. N., and Griffiths, K. (1974): *Cancer,* 33:1325.
29. Jackson, R. L., and Dockerty, M. B. (1957): *Am. J. Obstet. Gynecol.,* 73:161.
30. Judd, H. L. (1976): *Clin. Obstet. Gynecol.,* 19:775.
31. Kwa, H. G., Engelsman, De Jong-Bakken, M., and Cuton, F. J. (1974): *Lancet,* 1:433.
32. Lacassagne, A. (1933): *C. R. Acad. Sci. Paris,* 195:630.
33. Lippman, M., Monaco, M. E., and Bolan, G. (1977): *Cancer Res.,* 37:1901.

34. Loriaux, D. L., Ruder, H. J., and Lipsett, M. B. (1971): *Steroids,* 18:463.
35. Lucus, W. E. (1974): *Obstet. Gynecol. Surv.,* 29:507.
36. MacDonald, P. C., Edman, C. D., Hemsell, D. C., Porter, J. C., and Siiteri, P. K. (1978): *Am. J. Obstet. Gynecol.,* 130:448.
37. MacIndoe, J. H. (1979): *J. Clin. Endocrinol. Metab.,* 49:272.
38. Mack, T. M., Pike, M. C., Henderson, B. E., Pfeffer, R. I., Gerkins, V. R., Arthur, M., and Brown, S. E. (1976): *N. Engl. J. Med.,* 294:1262.
39. MacMahon, B. (1974): *Gynecol. Oncol.,* 2:122.
40. MacMahon, B., Cole, P., and Brown, J. B. (1974): *Int. J. Cancer,* 14:161.
41. MacMahon, B., Cole, P., and Lin, T. M. (1970): *Bull. WHO,* 43:209.
42. MacMahon, B., and Feinleib, M. (1960): *J. Natl. Cancer Inst.,* 24:733.
43. Miller, A. B. (1978): *Cancer Res.,* 38:3985.
44. Miller, W. R., Forrest, A. P. M., and Hamilton, T. (1974): *Steroids,* 23:379.
45. Nisker, J. A., Hammond, G. L., Davidson, B. J., Frumar, A. M., Takaki, N. K., Judd, H. L., and Siiteri, P. K. (1980): *Am. J. Obstet. Gynecol. (in press).*
46. Nisker, J. A., Ramzy, I., and Collins, J. A. (1978): *Am. J. Obstet. Gynecol.,* 130:546.
47. Poortman, J., Prenen, J. A. C., Schwarz, F., and Thijssen, J. H. H. (1975): *J. Clin. Endocrinol. Metabl.,* 40:373.
48. Poortman, J., Thijssen, J. H. H., and Schwarz, F. (1973): *J. Clin. Endocrinol. Metab.,* 37:101.
49. Prem, K. A., Mensheha, N. M., and McKelvey, J. L. (1965): *Am. J. Obstet. Gynecol.,* 71:718.
50. Roberts, K. D., Rochefort, G., Bleau, G., and Chapdelaine, A. (1980): *Steroids,* 35:179.
51. Sherman, B. M., and Korenman, S. G. (1974): *Cancer,* 33:1306.
52. Sherman, B. M., and Korenman, S. G. (1975): *J. Clin. Invest.,* 55:699.
53. Siiteri, P. K., Hammond, G. L., and Nisker, J. A. (1980): *Submitted for publication.*
54. Siiteri, P. K., and MacDonald, P. C. (1973): In: *Handbook of Physiology, Sect. 7,* edited by S. R. Geiger, E. B. Astwood, and R. O. Greep, pp. 615–629. American Physiological Society, New York.
55. Siiteri, P. K., Williams, J. E., and Takaki, N. K. (1976): *J. Steroid Biochem.,* 7:897.
56. Smith, D. C. (1975): *N. Engl. J. Med.,* 293:1164.
57. Wang, D. Y., Hayward, J. L., and Bulbrook, R. D. (1966): *Eur. J. Cancer,* 2:373.
58. Wright, K., Collins, D. C., Musey, P. I., and Preedy, J. R. K. (1978): *J. Clin. Endocrinol. Metab.,* 47:1092.
59. Wynder, E. L., Bross, I. J., and Hirajama, T. (1960): *Cancer,* 13:559.
60. Wynder, E. L., Escher, G. C., and Mantel, N. (1966): *Cancer,* 19:489.
61. Ziel, H. K., and Finkle, W. D. (1975): *N. Engl. J. Med.,* 293:1167.

New Therapeutic Approaches

Hormones and Cancer, edited by S. Iacobelli et al.
Raven Press, New York © 1980.

Inhibition of Estrogen Biosynthesis: An Approach to Treatment of Estrogen-Dependent Cancer

Angela M. H. Brodie

Department of Pharmacology and Experimental Therapeutics, University of Maryland School of Medicine, Baltimore, Maryland 21201, U.S.A.

Over the past few years, with the advent of steroid receptor biochemistry, there has been considerable interest in diagnosing breast cancer patients with tumors that are likely to respond to hormone manipulations so that these patients can then be selected for appropriate treatment (21).

Our laboratory has been interested in developing compounds which may be able to provide effective therapy for this type of cancer as well as other estrogen-dependent cancers and diseases, for example, endometrial cancer and endometriosis.

The aromatase inhibitors we have developed to date compete with the androgen substrate for the enzyme in the aromatization reaction and thereby prevent estrogen biosynthesis (25). Aromatization is the terminal sequence in the biosynthesis of estrogen and is a unique reaction in steroid metabolism. Thus, inhibition of aromatase may be a more specific means of regulating estrogen synthesis than others presently available.

Although the major source of estrogen production is removed by ovariectomy, long used in the treatment of advanced breast cancer, there is now substantial evidence to show that estrogen is produced by extragonadal tissue, such as fat and muscle (19,20) and contributes to tumor recurrence. The substrate for peripheral aromatization is adrenal androstenedione and although adrenalectomy is often performed, both this type of surgery and ovariectomy have associated morbidity and mortality rates.

There are now numerous reports that aromatization also takes place in many breast tumors (1,13,18,23,28).

Endometrial cancer is highly correlated with obesity (29). Not only does this increase the risk of surgery for these patients, but also the production of peripherally formed estrogen is enhanced (26).

Endometriosis, a common gynecological disorder, in which ectopic endometrial tissue under ovarian steroidal control can be debilitating, might also be effectively treated by a systemic and reversible means of preventing estrogen production.

Peripherally produced estrogen is mainly estrone, a weaker estrogen than estradiol-17β. Since the binding affinity of estrone to steroid-binding protein is less than that of estradiol, the availability to the target cell may be quite great under conditions of increased estrone production (26). Clark et al. (12) report evidence which suggests that there may be little difference between the biological activity of the estrogens when "weaker" estrogens, such as estriol, are continuously present, in contrast to being given as a single injection. Recently, Brooks et al. (3) observed that estrone is bound with high affinity to a cytosolic macromolecule and enters the nucleus of breast tumor cells. These findings suggest that estrone may play a significant role in estrogen–receptor interactions.

Thus, compounds that would inhibit aromatization at all tissue sites could be more effective than surgical means for preventing biologically active estrogens from reaching the tumor.

STUDIES WITH AROMATASE INHIBITORS *IN VITRO*

Over the past few years, we have evaluated a number of compounds for aromatase inhibition *in vitro*, first using human placental microsomes as a source of aromatase (25) and later a highly active microsomal preparation from ovaries of rats stimulated with pregnant mare serum gonadotropin (PMSG) (9). Our studies of the two microsomal preparations suggest that subtle differences may exist between aromatases from the two sources. For evaluating inhibitors of estrogen synthesis, the ovarian microsomal preparation has been preferred, as it appears to be more appropriate for predicting *in vivo* activity in the rat.

Compounds were evaluated by comparing the extent of aromatization with and without the test compound incubated *in vitro*. The conversion of androstenedione to estrogen by the microsomal preparation can easily be estimated by measuring the loss of tritium from the C-1β and C-2β positions (2) during aromatization of [1,2-^{3}H(70%β)]androstenedione. The tritium released as ^3H_2O is measured in the incubation medium after extraction of steroids by organic solvent (27).

The most active aromatase inhibitors we have studied in detail are 4-hydroxyandrostene-3,17-dione (4-OH-A) (10), 4-acetoxyandrostene-3,17-dione (4-acetoxy-A) (4,6), and 1,4,6-androstatriene-3,17-dione (ATD) (8). All show Lineweaver-Burke plots typical of competitive inhibition (25).

We recently prepared [6,7-^{3}H]4-OH-A and determined that this compound is not aromatized to estradiol or estrone. Conversion to 4-hydroxyestrone occurs only in trace amounts. We have also determined that 4-OH-A does not appear to interfere with metabolism of progesterone or dehydroepiandrosterone *in vitro* (22).

IN VIVO STUDIES WITH AROMATASE INHIBITORS

In order for the compounds to be useful clinically, it is important that they have little or no significant intrinsic hormonal or antihormonal activity which could lead to undesirable side effects. Evaluated in bioassay, 4-OH-A (10) and ATD (8) had no estrogenic or progestational activity, nor did they have any antihormonal activity in relation to estrogen, progesterone, or testosterone. 4-Acetoxy-A has not yet been evaluated for these activities.

ATD had no detectable androgenic activity at the dose levels tested. 4-OH-A and 4-acetoxy-A (5) had approximately 1% or less the androgenic activity of testosterone.

To determine whether these *in vitro* inhibitors are active *in vivo*, we have evaluated them in PMSG-stimulated rats (6). PSMG increases the secretion of estradiol, estrone, and other steroids (progesterone, androstenedione, and testosterone). The steroid levels reach a maximum on about the 10th day during PMSG treatment and remain constant for the next few days, at least to day 13. As the ovary is presumably maximally stimulated by the exogenous gonadotropin (PMSG), it will be unresponsive to changes in endogenous gonadotropins that might be caused by aromatase inhibitor treatment.

Groups of rats pretreated for 12 days with PMSG were injected with either vehicle or 4-OH-A (5 mg/rat at 8 A.M. and 5 P.M.). Peripheral blood samples were collected prior to inhibitor treatment and at 9 A.M. the following day.

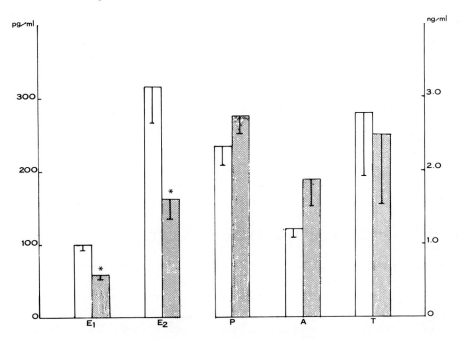

FIG. 1. Effect of 4-OH-A on peripheral steroid levels in PMSG-stimulated rats. On day 12 of PMSG treatment, rats were injected with a suspension of 4-OH-A (2.5 mg/100 g), or vehicle for controls, at 8 A.M. and 5 P.M. Peripheral blood was collected at 9 A.M. the following day (day 13). There was significant reduction in estrone (E_1) ($p < 0.01$) and estradiol (E_2) ($p < 0.05$) levels compared with controls. Levels of progesterone (P), androstenedione (A), and testosterone (T) were not significantly affected by 4-OH-A treatment. Vertical brackets indicate SEM.

Both estradiol and estrone levels were significantly reduced following inhibitor treatment as shown in Fig. 1. There was no significant difference in progesterone, androstenedione, or testosterone levels before or after 4-OH-A treatment. Lack of effect on other steroids suggests that the compound probably does not act on enzymes controlling their biosynthesis. Also, as changes in estrogen levels can not be due to gonadotropin action in this experiment, and as the compounds do not compete with estradiol for its receptor (6; *unpublished in vitro studies*), the results indicate that reduced estrogen levels are probably due to inhibition of estrogen biosynthesis.

In related studies with normal rats, the preovulatory estrogen surge can be prevented by injection of aromatase inhibitors [4-OH-A (16), 4-acetoxy-A (7), and ATD (8)] on the morning of proestrus, also indicating inhibition of estrogen production, presumably through inhibition of estrogen synthesis.

MAMMARY TUMOR STUDIES WITH AROMATASE INHIBITORS

We have studied the effects of aromatase inhibitors on mammary tumors induced in the rat with the carcinogen 7,12-dimethylbenz[a]anthracene (DMBA). Approximately 80% of the tumors produced are dependent on hormones for their induction and growth and are considered to have many similarities to those of the human (15,16). Treatment with all three compounds (4-OH-A, 4-acetoxy-A, or ATD) daily for 4 weeks caused marked regression and 90 to 95% of tumors decreased to less than half their original size. When estradiol was given in addition to aromatase inhibitor treatment, tumor regression did not occur. This finding is consistent with tumor regression resulting from reduced estrogen production. ATD and 4-acetoxy-A were more effective when administered from subcutaneous silastic wafers and up to 65% of tumors completely regressed during 4-acetoxy-A treatment (5).

At the end of 4 weeks' treatment with 4-acetoxy-A, blood samples were collected by ovarian vein cannulation for steroid estrogen measurements and by heart puncture for gonadotropin measurements. Ovarian estradiol secretion of treated animals was significantly reduced to 28% of values for control rats sampled during diestrus, when estrogen levels are normally low (5). Thus, tumor regression probably resulted from reduced estrogen production. However, there was no significant difference between luteinizing hormone (LH), follicle-stimulating hormone (FSH), and prolactin values for controls and 4-acetoxy-A treated rats. Since estrogen levels were reduced, increases in LH and FSH would be expected to occur as after ovariectomy. Similar results were also obtained with 4-OH-A (*unpublished observations*). We, therefore, studied the effect of 4-OH-A treatment on gonadotropin levels in ovariectomized rats.

Normal cycling rats were ovariectomized and six animals per group were injected with 4-OH-A (2.5 mg/100 g/day) or vehicle for controls, beginning on the day of surgery and continuing for 4 weeks. Blood samples were taken from the carotid artery of each animal 4 days after surgery and once each week thereafter. As expected, LH levels increased dramatically in the controls throughout the 4 weeks, but no increase occurred with 4-OH-A treatment (Fig. 2). FSH levels in controls also increased following ovariectomy. During the first week, FSH values rose to the same extent in treated rats as in controls. Thereafter, they declined and returned to levels similar to those measured before ovariectomy. There was no effect on prolactin levels by either ovariectomy or 4-OH-A treatment. These results suggest that the compounds not only act as aromatase inhibitors *in vivo,* but they also affect gonadotropin secretion. Celotti et al. (11) have reported evidence that a C3-ketone group is required for negative feedback action of gonadotropins. 4-OH-A, 4-acetoxy-A, and ATD are all 3-keto steroids. Maintaining gonadotropins at basal levels with aromatase inhibitors would be advantageous: since LH and FSH promote estrogen biosynthesis, increased secretion of these gonadotropins would oppose the goal of reducing estrogen production in estrogen-dependent cancer.

In further studies with DMBA-induced hormone-dependent tumors, we have

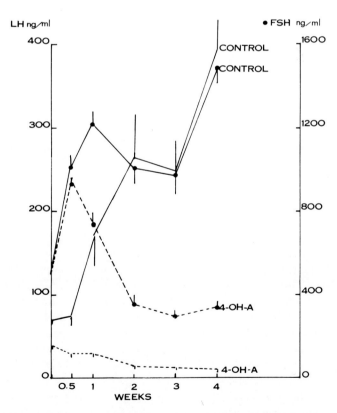

FIG. 2. Effect of 4-OH-A on LH and FSH levels in ovariectomized rats. Rats were injected with a suspension of 4-OH-A (2.5 mg/100 g/day), or vehicle for controls, s.c. twice daily for 4 weeks. Peripheral blood samples were collected from the carotid artery.

compared other agents used for breast cancer treatment with 4-OH-A. Testolo-lactone (Teslac®) is a compound used in the treatment of breast cancer for 20 years and reported by Siiteri and Thompson (27) to be an aromatase inhibitor. Incubated *in vitro* with human placental microsomes or rat ovarian microsomes at 12 times the substrate concentration, Testololactone has rather weak activity, 2 and 24% respectively. Administered daily (2.5 mg/100 g/day) for 4 weeks to rats with DMBA-induced tumors, this compound proved to have no significant effect in bringing about regression of mammary tumors.

The antiestrogen tamoxifen (ICI-46,474) caused regression of mammary tu-mors in the rat (17) at a dose of 200 µg/rat/day, but was less effective than 4-OH-A (2.5 mg/100 g/day). The combined effect of the above doses of aroma-tase inhibitor (4-OH-A) and antiestrogen (tamoxifen) was not as great as that of 4-OH-A alone and was only slightly better than that of tamoxifen alone (6).

INHIBITION OF PERIPHERAL AROMATIZATION

As indicated in the introduction, aromatase inhibitors could be effective treat-ment for estrogen-dependent cancer by acting on aromatization in peripheral tissue as well as in the ovary. Recently, in collaboration with C. Longcope, we studied the effect of 4-OH-A and 4-acetoxy-A on peripheral aromatization in the male rhesus monkey (4). This species was selected as it had previously been found to be a useful model for studying androgen and estrogen metabolism and dynamics (14).

To measure peripheral aromatization, each monkey was infused with [7-^{3}H]androstenedione and [4-^{14}C]estrone at a constant rate via the brachial vein. Blood samples were drawn from the femoral vein during infusion at 0, 2.5, 3, and 3.5 hr, and steady state conditions were verified. The conversion of andro-stenedione to estrone was measured in the samples.

Four of the monkeys were treated with injections of 4-OH-A (50 mg/kg) at 5 P.M. the day before infusion of radiolabeled androstenedione and at 1.5 hr before beginning the infusion. Each animal served as its own control, being injected with vehicle at the above times before infusion: two monkeys had control infusions 1 week before and two monkeys 1 week after 4-OH-A treatment.

Two other monkeys were implanted with silastic wafers containing 4-acetoxy-A 24 hr before the infusion. Each was also injected with 4-acetoxy-A at 9 A.M. and 5 P.M. on the day before infusion and 15 to 30 min before infusion began. Control infusions were performed 1 month after 4-acetoxy-A treatment.

Analysis of the samples revealed no specific effects on the metabolic clearance rates of androstenedione and estrone, the interconversion of the androgens or of the estrogens or on androstenedione conversion to dihydrotestosterone (DHT). Perel et al. (24), however, using very high doses (90 µM) of 4-OH-A, recently reported *in vitro* inhibition of the conversion of androstenedione to DHT and of androstenedione to testosterone in breast fat and tumor tissue.

In five of the six monkeys treated with aromatase inhibitors, aromatization rates were reduced by up to 97% of control values. In the sixth monkey there was little effect on aromatization. However, the implants containing 4-acetoxy-A had become surrounded with purulent fluid, suggesting that transport of the inhibitor from the wafer had been impaired in this animal.

In summary, our studies demonstrate that 4-OH-A, 4-acetoxy-A, and ATD, inhibitors of aromatase *in vitro,* cause marked regression of DMBA-induced hormone-dependent mammary tumors in the rat. The evidence indicates that tumor regression results from reduced estrogen production. The compounds probably act mainly by inhibiting estrogen biosythesis *in vivo.* They also prevent the increased secretion of gonadotropins which usually accompanies reduced estrogen levels. Peripheral aromatization was also inhibited by 4-OH-A and 4-acetoxy-A. Taken together, these results suggest that aromatase inhibitors may offer novel and effective treatment for estrogen-dependent cancer.

ACKNOWLEDGMENTS

This work was supported by Contract NICHD 1-HD-0-2059 and Grants CA-18595 and HD-10269, all from the National Institutes of Health.

REFERENCES

1. Abdul-Hajj, Y. J., Iverson, R., and Kiang, D. T. (1979): *Steroids,* 33:205–222.
2. Brodie, H. J., Kripalani, K. J., and Possanza, G. (1969): *J. Am. Chem. Soc.,* 91:1241–1242.
3. Brooks, S. C., Locke, E. R., and Horn, L. (1978): *Cancer Res.,* 38:4238–4242.
4. Brodie, A. M. H., and Longcope, C. (1980): *Endocrinology,* 106:19–21.
5. Brodie, A. M. H., Marsh, D. A., and Brodie, H. J. (1979): *J. Steroid Biochem.,* 10:423–429.
6. Brodie, A. M. H., Marsh, D. A., Wu, J. T., and Brodie, H. J. (1979): *J. Steroid Biochem.,* 11:107–112.
7. Brodie, A. M. H., Marsh, D. A., Wu, J. T., and Brodie, H. J. (1978): *Biol. Reprod.,* 18:365–370.
8. Brodie, A. M. H., Wu, J. T., Marsh, D. A., and Brodie, H. J. (1978): *Endocrinology,* 104:118–121.
9. Brodie, A. M. H., Schwarzel, W. C., and Brodie, H. J. (1976): *J. Steroid Biochem.,* 7:787–793.
10. Brodie, A. M. H., Schwarzel, W. C., Shaikh, A. A., and Brodie, H. J. (1977): *Endocrinology,* 100:1684–1695.
11. Celotti, F., Massa, R., Martini, L., and Motta, M. (1977): *59th US Endocrine Society Annual Meeting,* Chicago, Illinois, June 8–10, 1977, p. 188. Abstr. 266.
12. Clark, J. H., Paszko, Z., and Peck, E. J., Jr. (1977): *Endocrinology,* 100:91–96.
13. de Thibault de Boesinghe, L., Lacroix, E., Eechaute, W., and Leusen, I. (1974): *Lancet,* 2:1268.
14. Franz, C., and Longcope, C. (1979): *Endocrinology,* 105:869–874.
15. Huggins, C., Briziarelli, G., and Sutton, H. (1959): *J. Exp. Med.,* 109:25–42.
16. Huggins, C., Grand, L. C., and Brillantes, F. P. (1961): *Nature,* 189:204–207.
17. Jordan, V. C. (1976): *Cancer Treat. Rep.,* 60:1409–1419.
18. Li, K., Chandra, D. P., Foo, T., Adams, J. B., and McDonald, D. (1976): *Steroids,* 28:561–574.
19. Longcope, C., Pratt, J. H., Schneider, S. H., and Fineberg, S. E. (1978): *J. Clin. Endocrinol. Metab.,* 46:146–152.
20. MacDonald, P. C., Rombaut, R. P., and Siiteri, P. K. (1967): *J. Clin. Endocrinol. Metab.,* 27:1103–1111.

21. McGuire, W. I.. (1978): *Semin. Oncol.,* 5:428–433.
22. Marsh, D. H., Brodie, A. M. H., Romanoff, L., Williams, K. I. H., and Brodie, H. J. (1980): *In preparation.*
23. Miller, W. R., and Forrest, A. P. M. (1974): *Lancet,* 2:866–868.
24. Perel, E., Wilkins, D., and Killinger, D. W. (1979): *61st US Endocrine Society Annual Meeting,* Anaheim, California, June 13–15, 1979, p. 148. Abstr. 303.
25. Schwarzel, W. C., Kruggel, W., and Brodie, H. J. (1973): *Endocrinology,* 92:866–880.
26. Siiteri, P. (1978): *Cancer Res.,* 38:4360–4366.
27. Siiteri, P., and Thompson, E. A. (1975): *J. Steroid Biochem.,* 6:317–322.
28. Valera, R. M., and Dao, T. L. (1978): *Cancer Res.,* 38:2429–2433.
29. Wynder, E. C., Escher, G. C., and Mantel, N. (1966): *Cancer,* 19:489–520.

Hormones and Cancer, edited by S. Iacobelli et al.
Raven Press, New York © 1980.

Prostaglandins and Their Synthesis Inhibitors in Cancer

Alan Bennett

*Department of Surgery, King's College Hospital Medical School,
London SE5 8RX, England*

To those not familiar with prostaglandins the subject must seem bewildering. Although the full details are undoubtedly complex, the basic schemes of prostaglandin metabolism and the effects of therapeutic agents are relatively simple. In brief, prostaglandins (PG) are 20-carbon acidic lipids formed from precursor essential fatty acids incorporated mainly into phospholipids of cell membranes. When the precursor (predominantly arachidonic acid) is released, it can be metabolized by two main pathways into (a) prostaglandins and related substances (collectively called prostanoids), and (b) straight-chain hydroperoxy and hydroxy acids, as shown in Fig. 1.

There are numerous prostanoids, but some tissues may preferentially form one type from the endoperoxide intermediates. The prostanoids have physiological roles, but amounts formed in excess contribute to diseases. Two important therapeutic considerations are that antiinflammatory adrenocorticosteroids inhibit the release of prostaglandin precursors, and that nonsteroidal anti-inflammatory drugs, such as aspirin, indomethacin, and flurbiprofen, inhibit the conversion of released precursors into prostanoids. These actions of the inhibitors contribute to their beneficial effects in inflammation, pain, fever, and various other pathological conditions. More detailed accounts of the biochemistry, pharmacology, and pathology can be found in various texts (e.g., refs. 17,18).

The following brief discussions include various aspects of prostaglandins and inhibitors of their synthesis on tumor growth and spread in man and laboratory animals. For further details, readers are referred to ref. 2.

PROSTAGLANDINS AND TUMOR GROWTH

The relationship of prostaglandins to tumor growth is controversial, with effects on cells in culture often seeming to be different from tumor growth *in vivo*. Some possible explanations of the discrepancies are discussed below.

Only a few prostanoids have so far been studied on cell growth and, as in many systems, their effects can vary with the different types. Most studies with malignant or transformed cells in tissue culture show an inhibition of prolifera-

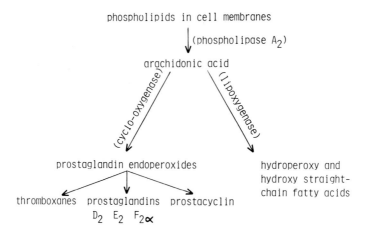

FIG. 1. Metabolism of precursor essential fatty acids into prostanoids and straight-chain hydroperoxy and hydroxy acids.

tion by PGE_1 or PGE_2, whereas $PGF_{2\alpha}$ can initiate cell proliferation in cultured mouse fibroblasts (see ref. 2). Consistent with the PGE results is the finding that low concentrations of the prostaglandin synthesis inhibitor indomethacin (0.1–100 nM) stimulated the growth of cultured cells (33). In contrast, a high concentration of indomethacin (0.1 mM) inhibited cell growth (16). Perhaps low concentrations of indomethacin do not inhibit prostaglandin synthesis sufficiently to inhibit cell growth, or at higher concentrations another action of the drug may be involved (see below).

Cyclic adenosine monophosphate (AMP) is thought to be important in cell growth, and certain prostanoids can stimulate adenylate cyclase in many types of cell. However, studies on cyclic AMP in cell growth have confused our understanding of its importance by using high concentrations of the nucleotide and its dibutyryl derivative, because the adenylate cyclase activity and/or the cyclic AMP content of tumors vary, and the importance of cell calcium (22,35) has often been ignored.

In vivo, the growth of mouse adenocarcinomas correlated with their content of arachidonic acid (1), and the inhibitors of prostaglandin synthesis indomethacin or flurbiprofen usually reduced tumor size (see ref. 2). However, the reverse occurred with melanoma (see ref. 2). A reduction of tumor size could be due to many factors apart from inhibition of tumor cell growth, such as a reduction of inflammation (30), and stimulation of the immune system (24). Furthermore, the drugs inhibit the whole cascade of prostanoid synthesis, and so increase the availability of precursors for metabolism by lipoxygenase. An effect therefore cannot be attributed to the reduced formation of any one prostanoid, and we cannot exclude the possible importance of increased metabolism of precursors by lipoxygenase, or drug actions unrelated to inhibition of prostanoid synthesis.

HUMAN BREAST CANCER

Our interest in human breast cancer was stimulated by the finding that bone destruction by benign dental cysts may involve prostaglandins (14). Previous work had also shown that some prostaglandins are potent bone-resorbing agents. Thus there might be a similar link with cancers that spread to the skeleton and cause destruction of bone.

Samples of malignant and benign breast tumors removed at surgery were assessed for their content and ability to synthesize prostaglandin-like material (6). The term "prostaglandin-like" is used to indicate that there exists a resemblance to prostaglandins in extraction characteristics and chromatographic behavior, but that formal identification which requires highly sophisticated techniques has not been made.

The first striking finding was that extracts of homogenized human mammary carcinomas usually contained substantially more prostaglandin-like material than was obtained from benign tumors or from normal breast tissue obtained at mastectomy (4,6). Similarly, incubated slices of breast carcinomas can release substantial amounts of PGE- and PGF-like material (9).

The second striking finding was that more patients whose tumors produced large amounts of prostaglandin-like material had bone metastases, as assessed by skeletal scanning with ^{99}Tc-ethanehydroxydiphosphonate in the immediate pre- or postoperative period, than did patients whose tumors produced low amounts (4,6). Since PGE and PGF compounds in blood are substantially inactivated on passage through the lungs and other tissues, we thought that the minute amounts of prostaglandins remaining unmetabolized after release from primary tumors would have little effect on the bone. A more likely explanation is that malignant cells which lodge in the bone after release from the primary breast tumor might cause osteolysis by releasing prostaglandins locally, and those cells which produce most prostaglandins are most likely to form metastases. This possibility is supported by the animal studies discussed below, but another is suggested by histological studies of tumors and resected lymph nodes. Tumor "invasiveness" tended to correlate with the prostaglandin measurements, since malignant cells escaping from the tumor into blood vessels, lymphatics, or lymph nodes tended to occur more frequently in tumors which yielded most prostaglandin-like material on homogenization (4). Perhaps prostaglandin-induced vasodilatation allows a greater escape of malignant cells from the tumor, so that more cells are available to form metastases.

Although there is good evidence for the involvement of prostaglandins in bone destruction by some tumors, the initiation or continuance of bone destruction may involve other factors. Human breast tumors can also produce nonprostaglandin bone-resorbing material which acts by stimulating osteoclasts; this has not been identified but may be osteoclast-activating factor (9). When gross bone destruction has occurred prostaglandins do not seem to contribute to the continued bone destruction, since osteoclasts are no longer present (12).

Another factor aiding the growth of tumor in bone may be the calcium made available to the malignant cells by prostaglandin-induced osteoclast stimulation (35). Furthermore, certain prostaglandins may act as calcium ionophores (19,27).

The increased spread of malignant cells would be expected to reflect a worse prognosis. This is indeed the case, since death from cancer following breast surgery occurred most quickly in those patients whose tumors produced most prostaglandin-like material (3).

HYPERCALCEMIA AND DESTRUCTION OF BONE BY TUMORS

PGE_2, which is a potent bone-resorbing agent, has been identified in extracts of various tumors. Indomethacin inhibited tumor-induced hypercalcemia in mice (32) and rabbits (34), and the *in vivo* destruction of bone in rats (26) and rabbits (11,12). The timing of indomethacin administration in relation to tumor transplantation is important. The inhibition of bone destruction induced by VX2 tumor in rabbits was statistically significant only when treatment was started within a week of tumor transplantation (12). In male patients with various solid tumors, indomethacin or aspirin can correct hypercalcemia (31), and we have preliminary unpublished evidence that flurbiprofen may reduce the size or halt the further growth of bone metastases in breast cancer patients. In contrast, however, the relatively weak prostaglandin synthesis inhibitor benorylate did not reduce the incidence of bone metastases in breast cancer patients (25), and indomethacin did not significantly alter the hypercalcemia in four other women (8). Perhaps this hypercalcemia was at the advanced stage which does not involve osteoclasts (10) or was due to nonprostaglandin-stimulated osteoclast activation (9).

BENEFICIAL EFFECTS OF PROSTAGLANDIN SYNTHESIS INHIBITORS IN TREATING ANIMALS WITH TUMORS

Indomethacin can reduce the size of tumors in mice (see ref. 2), but at least part of this effect in some cases could merely reflect a smaller local inflammatory response (30). In other cases this cannot be the whole explanation, such as the complete suppression of tumor growth (30), the complete regression of established tumors (21), or the failure of hydrocortisone to reduce tumor size significantly (21). However, prostaglandins can inhibit the immune response (24) and indomethacin may merely restore the host's immune protection. Lynch et al. (21) thought this explanation unlikely because they did not detect immunogenicity in their mouse tumors. Furthermore, flurbiprofen reduced the growth of a mouse tumor (5) which the discoverers thought was nonimmunogenic (15). This may no longer be entirely true, since there was some tendency for lymphocytic infiltration of tumors to increase in mice treated with flurbiprofen (20).

In mice with established tumors treated by radiotherapy with or without chemotherapy, the tumor size was much less when flurbiprofen was also given

(5). The drug may have reduced the inflammation caused by other treatments, or stimulated an immune response, but an action on tumor cells cannot be excluded. A concentration of aspirin or sodium salicylate, within the range obtained in blood with therapeutic doses, inhibited the proliferation of rat hepatoma and human fibroblasts in culture, and reduced protein and nucleic acid synthesis (16). Since the dose of aspirin is higher than that needed to inhibit prostanoid synthesis substantially in at least some tissues *in vivo,* and salicylate has little effect on prostaglandin synthesis *in vitro,* at least part of the reduction of growth might not involve prostanoids. Nonsteroidal anti-inflammatory drugs also affect calcium transport (23), which may be important for tumor growth (22). Even though added PGE_2 can overcome the effect of indomethacin (21,33), this does not prove that indomethacin acts by inhibiting prostaglandin synthesis: indomethacin might cause an inhibition of calcium transport which PGE_2 reverses by acting as a calcium ionophore.

Nonsteroidal anti-inflammatory drugs can also inhibit distant (13) and local (7) spread of tumors in mice, but indomethacin did not reduce distant spread in rats (26) or rabbits (11). The effect of such drugs in man must await the clinical trials that are now in progress. However, one piece of evidence consistent with their safety is the use of corticosteroids in cancer therapy, and the beneficial effect of tamoxifen which also inhibits prostaglandin synthesis (28).

Perhaps our mouse experiments of greatest interest are those designed to mimic the clinical situation by starting treatment with chemotherapy (methotrexate + melphalan) and flurbiprofen just prior to tumor excision. The combined treatment increased the survival time (7). Bioavailability of the chemotherapeutic drugs did not seem to increase since flurbiprofen neither displaced methotrexate from plasma binding sites nor increased the toxicity of large doses of chemotherapeutic drugs given to mice without tumors *(unpublished).* The mechanism is therefore not understood but might involve the various suggestions about tumor growth discussed previously. Another intriguing possibility is that prostaglandins protect cells from damage. This seems to occur in rat gastric mucosa (29) and perhaps flurbiprofen removes a similar protective effect of prostaglandins on tumor cells, thereby increasing their susceptibility.

Double-blind trials are now in progress with flurbiprofen and chemotherapeutic drugs in cancer patients. If the results are similar to those obtained in mice, cancer therapy may be substantially improved.

REFERENCES

1. Abraham, S., and Rao, G. A. (1976): In: *Control Mechanisms in Cancer,* edited by W. E. Criss, pp. 363–378. Raven Press, New York.
2. Bennett, A. (1979): In: *Practical Applications of Prostaglandins and Their Synthesis Inhibitors,* edited by S. M. M. Karim, pp. 149–188. MTP Press, Lancaster.
3. Bennett, A., Berstock, D. A., Raja, B., and Stamford, I. F. (1979): *Br. J. Pharmacol.,* 66:451P.
4. Bennett, A., Charlier, E. M., McDonald, A. M., Simpson, J. S., Stamford, I. F., and Zebro, T. (1977): *Lancet,* 2:624–626.

5. Bennett, A., Houghton, J., Leaper, D. J., and Stamford, I. F. (1979): *Prostaglandins,* 17:179–191.
6. Bennett, A., McDonald, A. M., Simpson, J. S., and Stamford, I. F. (1975): *Lancet,* 1:1218–1220.
7. Berstock, D. A., Houghton, J., and Bennett, A. (1979): *Cancer Treat. Rev. (Suppl.),* 6:69–71.
8. Coombes, R. C., Neville, A. M., Bondy, P. K., and Powles, T. J. (1976): *Prostaglandins,* 12:1027–1035.
9. Dowsett, M., Easty, G. C., Powles, T. J., Easty, D. M., and Neville, A. M. (1976): *Prostaglandins,* 11:447–455.
10. Galasko, C. S. B. (1976): *Nature,* 263:507–508.
11. Galasko, C. S. B., and Bennett, A. (1976): *Nature,* 263:508–510.
12. Galasko, C. S. B., Rawlins, R., and Bennett, A. (1979): *Br. J. Cancer,* 40:360–364.
13. Gasic, G. J., Gasic, T. B., Galanti, N., Johnson, T., and Murphy, S. (1973): *Int. J. Cancer,* 11:704–718.
14. Harris, M., Jenkins, M. V., Bennett, A., and Wills, M. R. (1973): *Nature,* 245:213–215.
15. Hewitt, H. B., Blake, E. R., and Walder, A. S. (1976): *Br. J. Cancer,* 33:241–259.
16. Hial, V., de Mello, M. C. F., Horakova, Z., and Beavan, M. A. (1977): *J. Pharmacol. Exp. Ther.,* 202:446–454.
17. Karim, S. M. M., editor (1976): *Advances in Prostaglandin Research. Prostaglandins: Physiological, Pharmacological and Pathological Aspects.* MTP Press, Lancaster.
18. Karim, S. M. M., editor (1976): *Advances in Prostaglandin Research. Prostaglandins: Chemical and Biochemical Aspects.* MTP Press, Lancaster.
19. Kirtland, S. J., and Baum, H. (1972): *Nature (New Biol.),* 236:47–49.
20. Leaper, D. J., French, B., and Bennett, A. (1979): *Br. J. Surg.,* 66:683–686.
21. Lynch, N. R., Castes, M., Astoin, M., and Salomon, J. C. (1978): *Br. J. Cancer,* 38:503–512.
22. MacManus, J. P., and Whitfield, J. F. (1974): *Prostaglandins,* 6:475–487.
23. Northover, B. J. (1973): *Br. J. Pharmacol.,* 48:496–504.
24. Plescia, O. J., Smith, A. H., and Grinwich, K. (1975): *Proc. Natl. Acad. Sci. USA,* 72:1848–1851.
25. Powles, T. J., Dady, P. J., Williams, J., Easty, G. C., and Coombes, R. C. (1980): In: *Advances in Prostaglandin and Thromboxane Research, Vol. 6,* edited by B. Samuelsson, P. W. Ramwell, and R. Paoletti, pp. 511–516. Raven Press, New York.
26. Powles, T. J., Clark, S. A., Easty, D. M., Easty, G. C., and Neville, A. M. (1973): *Br. J. Cancer,* 28:316–321.
27. Reed, P. W. (1977): *Fed. Proc.,* 36:673.
28. Ritchie, G. (1978): *Rev. Endocrine-Related Cancer,* Suppl. (Oct. 1978):35–39.
29. Robert, A. (1977): In: *Prostaglandins and Thromboxanes,* edited by F. Berti, B. Samuelsson, and G. P. Velo, pp. 287–313. Plenum Press, New York.
30. Strausser, H., and Humes, J. (1975): *Int. J. Cancer,* 15:724–730.
31. Seyberth, H. W., Segre, G. V., Morgan, J. L., Sweetman, B. J., Potts, J. T., and Oates, J. A. (1975): *N. Engl. J. Med.,* 293:1278–1283.
32. Tashjian, A. H., Voelkel, E. F., Goldhaber, P., and Levine, L. (1973): *Prostaglandins,* 3:515–524.
33. Thomas, D. R., Philpott, G. W., and Jaffe, B. M. (1974): *J. Surg. Res.,* 16:463–465.
34. Voelkel, E. F., Tashjian, A. H., Franklin, R., Wasserman, E., and Levine, L. (1975): *Metabolism,* 24:973–986.
35. Whitfield, J. F., Rixon, R. H., MacManus, J. P., and Balk, S. D. (1973): *In Vitro,* 8:257–278.

Hormones and Cancer, edited by S. Iacobelli et al.
Raven Press, New York © 1980.

Estrogen-Linked Cytotoxic Agents of Potential Value for the Treatment of Breast Cancer

G. Leclercq, N. Devleeschouwer, N. Legros, and J. C. Heuson

Medical Service and H. J. Tagnon Laboratory of Clinical Investigation (Breast Cancer Laboratory), Jules Bordet Institute, 1000 Brussels, Belgium

Since most breast cancers contain estrogen receptors (ER), it may be of interest to use estrogen-linked cytotoxic agents for the treatment of this tumor. Under appropriate conditions, such compounds might bind to the ER in the tumor cells and alter their physiologic mechanisms.

Along this line, we have initiated a screening program for assessing the potential therapeutic value of new estrogen-cytotoxic molecules (6). This program involves three successive steps: (a) *in vitro* assessment of drug binding affinity for cytoplasmic ER; (b) drug effect on the growth of two human breast cancer cell lines, one containing ER (MCF-7), the other lacking them (Evsa-T) (7); (c) toxicology studies and investigation of drug antitumor effectiveness, using dimethylbenz[a]anthracene (DMBA)-induced rat mammary tumors (2) and the hormone-dependent MXT-mouse mammary tumor (8).

In a first phase of our study, we reported that significant binding to ER occurred only when the cytotoxic-substituted estrogens had kept their original free oxygen functions (5,6). Assuming that this was a general rule, organic chemists kindly prepared for us five molecules meeting this criterion. One was an aziridine derivative of estrone (E_1; E_1-Azi) and four were nitrogen mustard derivatives of hexestrol (HEX; Ha IV), diethylstilbestrol (DES; Ha V), and E_1 (Ha VI and Ha VII), respectively (formulas and origins in Table 1). We wish to present here preliminary results on these molecules pertaining to the first two steps of our screening program.

INTERACTION OF THE DRUGS WITH ESTROGEN RECEPTORS

Apparent Binding Affinity

Cytosol preparations from immature rat uterus were used for evaluating the apparent binding affinity (4) of the drugs. Similar results were obtained with cytosols from DMBA rat mammary tumors, human breast cancer, or MCF-7 cells. Cytosol was incubated at 18°C for 30 min with 5×10^{-9} M [³H]estradiol ([³H]E_2) together with increasing amounts of unlabeled E_2 (control) or drug.

521

TABLE 1. *Origins and formulas of the drugs*

Obtained from	Drug	Structure
F. J. Zeelen (Organon, Oss, The Netherlands)	E_1-Azi	
H. Hamacher (B.G.A., Berlin)	Ha IV	
	Ha V	
	Ha VI	
	Ha VII	

At the end of incubation and after removal of unbound compounds by dextran-coated charcoal (DCC), bound $[^3H]E_2$ was measured. The relative concentration of drug and unlabeled E_2 achieving a 50% decrease of $[^3H]E_2$ binding was used as the estimate of the apparent binding affinity of the test compound. For cytotoxic derivatives of E_1, HEX, or DES, the parent estrogen was used as an additional control.

Aziridine Derivative

The aziridine derivative of E_1 was shown to produce a 50% reduction of [^{3}H]E_2 binding at a concentration close to 7×10^{-7} M (Fig. 1A). Its apparent binding affinity was estimated as 7% that of E_1.

Nitrogen Mustard Derivatives

The binitrogen mustard compounds Ha IV and Ha V were found to produce a reduction of [^{3}H]E_2 binding only at very high concentrations ($>10^{-5}$ M) (Fig. 1B). Estimated apparent binding affinities were about 0.01% relative to E_2 and parent estrogens. These affinities, although very low, were shown to be due to the compounds themselves and not to contaminating parent estrogens. Thus, unlike the latter, Ha compounds were found to form very stable complexes which were not displaced by [^{3}H]E_2 in exchange experiments (see below).

In contrast, the mononitrogen mustard compounds Ha VI and Ha VII produced a 50% reduction of [^{3}H]E_2 binding at relatively low concentrations (10^{-6}– 10^{-5} M) (Fig. 1C). Their apparent binding affinities were 3% relative to their parent estrogen (E_1).

Reversibility of Binding

The reversibility of binding (3,4) was studied after overnight incubation of the cytosol with 5×10^{-9} M [^{3}H]E_2 in the absence or presence of excess unlabeled E_2, E_1, DES, HEX, or drug. At the end of incubation and after removal of unbound compounds with DCC, bound [^{3}H]E_2 was measured. Aliquots were further incubated with [^{3}H]E_2 to permit its exchange with reversibly bound ligands. At the end of incubation (7 hr) and removal of excess [^{3}H]E_2 with DCC, bound [^{3}H]E_2 was again measured. An increase in bound [^{3}H]E_2 over the initial measurement indicates reversible binding of the drug (3).

Aziridine Derivative

Fig. 2A shows that E_2, E_1, and E_1-Azi inhibited [^{3}H]E_2 binding in the first step of the experiment (closed columns). During the second phase of the experiment (open columns) bound E_1-Azi was exchanged by [^{3}H]E_2 to the same extent as E_2 and E_1. A totally reversible interaction must therefore be ascribed to this drug.

Nitrogen Mustard Derivatives

In the first step of the experiment, all nitrogen mustard derivatives inhibited [^{3}H]E_2 binding (Fig. 2, B = Ha IV and Ha V; C = Ha VI and Ha VII). As

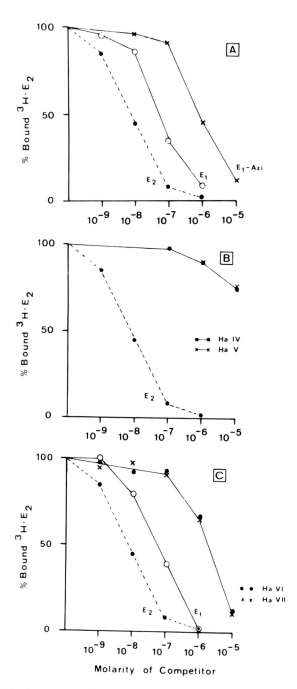

FIG. 1. Competition between ^3H-E_2 and unlabeled E_2, E_1, or drug for binding to cytoplasmic ER. Drugs: **A:** E_1-Azi; **B:** Ha IV and Ha V; **C:** Ha VI and Ha VII. Bound ^3H-E_2 in the absence of any competitor is taken as 100%.

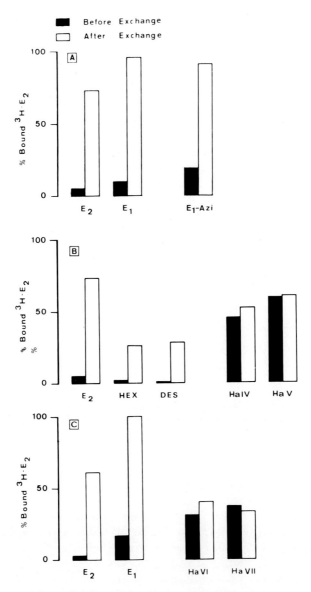

FIG. 2. Reversibility of binding of E_1-Azi **(A)** and irreversibility of binding of Ha compounds **(B,C)** with cytoplasmic ER (exchange experiment). Unlabeled E_2, E_1, DES, and HEX (control of reversibility of binding) were at a concentration of 10^{-6} M; E_1-Azi, Ha VI, and Ha VII at 10^{-5} M; and Ha IV and Ha V at 10^{-4} M. Activity is expressed as percent bound ^3H-E_2 in the absence of any competitor.

expected, this inhibition was less with Ha compounds than with parent estrogens in view of their lower apparent binding affinity. During the second phase of the experiment there was a significant exchange of bound unlabeled estrogens by $[^3H]E_2$. This phenomenon did not occur with the nitrogen mustard derivatives, suggesting that they formed very stable complexes (apparently irreversible) with the receptors. Another explanation would be that these compounds denaturate the receptors and make them unable to bind $[^3H]E_2$.

EFFECT OF THE DRUGS ON THE GROWTH OF MCF-7 AND Evsa-T CELL LINES

The effects of the drugs were tested on the growth of MCF-7 (ER+) and Evsa-T (ER−) cell lines. Growth was estimated by measuring the increase in DNA after 120 hr of culture in the presence of the drugs at concentrations of 10^{-8}, 10^{-7}, and 10^{-6} M (5). These concentrations were chosen because they cover the range reported to produce effects on MCF-7 cells with estrogens and antiestrogens (7,9). In our laboratory, 10^{-8} M E_2 was found to stimulate growth slightly (0–20%); nafoxidine at 10^{-6} M and 5×10^{-7} M was always inhibitory (60−80% and 40−60%, respectively).

Aziridine Derivative

The aziridine derivative E_1-Azi induced distinct modifications of growth of the MCF-7 cells. Concentrations of 10^{-8} and 10^{-7} M appeared stimulatory ($\sim$ 40 and 30%, respectively) whereas 10^{-6} M was slightly inhibitory (23%). On the Evsa-T cells, no effect was observed at any concentration (Table 2).

Nafoxidine at 10^{-7} M was found to reverse the stimulating effect of the drug at 10^{-8} M; 10^{-8} M E_2 reversed its inhibitory effect at 10^{-6} M (Table 3).

Nitrogen Mustard Derivatives

At the concentration of 10^{-6} M, all nitrogen mustard derivatives inhibited the growth of the MCF-7 cells (Table 4). The two disubstituted alkylating drugs

TABLE 2. Action of E_1-Azi on growth of MCF-7 and Evsa-T cells[a]

Molarity of E_1-Azi	DNA ($\mu g \pm$ SD)	
	MCF-7	Evsa-T
None	6.9 ± 1.0 (100)	12.8 ± 0.8 (100)
10^{-8} M	9.5 ± 0.5 (138)	12.8 ± 1.4 (100)
10^{-7} M	8.8 ± 1.3 (128)	13.6 ± 0.8 (106)
10^{-6} M	5.3 ± 1.0 (77)[b]	12.0 ± 1.8 (94)

[a] Experiments were performed in quadruplicate. Percent of control value shown in parentheses.
[b] Not significantly different from control.

TABLE 3. *Reversibility of effects of E_1-Azi on growth of MCF-7 cells*[a]

Effect	DNA ($\mu g \pm$ SD)
Control	7.0 ± 0.6 (100)
Stimulatory[b]	
E_1-Azi	9.8 ± 0.6 (140)
E_1-Azi + nafoxidine	7.3 ± 0.7 (104)
Inhibitory[c]	
E_1-Azi	5.2 ± 0.8 (74)
E_1-Azi + E_2	6.8 ± 0.9 (97)

[a] Experiments were performed in quadruplicate. Percent of control values is given in parentheses.
[b] E_1-Azi, 10^{-8} M; nafoxidine, 10^{-7} M.
[c] E_1-Azi, 10^{-6} M; E_2, 10^{-8} M.

Ha IV and Ha V produced an inhibition effect of about 35 to 40%; the monoalkylating drugs Ha VI and Ha VII produced stronger inhibition (about 80–90%). At lower concentrations, all drugs were devoid of significant effect except Ha VII which markedly inhibited growth at 10^{-7} M (45%). With regard to the Evsa-T cells, only Ha VII was found to inhibit growth ($\sim$ 80%) at 10^{-6} M, indicating that these drugs had a weaker effect on this line than on the MCF-7 line.

With regard to the MCF-7 cells, a series of E_1 and HEX derivatives linked with noncytotoxic agents ($-N_3$, $-NH_2$) in the same position as the nitrogen mustard group (compounds produced by Dr. G. Van Binst, Vrije Universiteit, Brussels, Belgium) were tested. All had a significant apparent binding affinity ($\sim$ 1–15% of their parent estrogen). None produced an inhibition of cell growth at the concentration of 10^{-6} M (Table 5), suggesting that the nitrogen mustard residue of Ha compound was involved in their cytotoxic action.

Finally, we tested in the MCF-7 cells the possibility that estrogens might reverse the inhibitory effect of these nitrogen mustard derivatives. E_2 and 11-chloromethyl estradiol (ORG 4333) were used for that purpose. The latter estrogen was selected in view of its very high and stable interaction with ER as well as its efficiency in antagonizing the inhibitory action of nafoxidine on the MCF-7 cell growth. Table 6 shows that E_2 as well as ORG 4333 at 10^{-8} M failed to reverse the inhibitory effect of all nitrogen mustard derivatives at 10^{-6} M.

DISCUSSION

The results reported here show that the five drugs tested bind to ER. This is consistent with our assumption that binding is likely to occur with substituted estrogens having free oxygen functions. Estimation of the apparent binding affinity of these drugs revealed a very large spectrum of values ($\sim$ 0.01–7% relative to their parent estrogen). In this regard the high difference in binding affinity

TABLE 4. Action of nitrogen mustard derivatives on growth of MCF-7 Evsa-T cells[a]

Molarity of drug	DNA (μg ± SD)							
	MCF-7				Evsa-T			
	Ha IV	Ha V	Ha VI	Ha VII	Ha IV	Ha V	Ha VI	Ha VII
None	10.4 ± 1.4 (100)	14.8 ± 0.5 (100)	10.4 ± 1.5 (100)	12.1 ± 1.8 (100)	22.6 ± 2.5 (100)	8.8 ± 1.0 (100)	11.4 ± 0.8 (100)	25.7 ± 2.5 (100)
10^{-8} M	10.0 ± 0.8 (96)	13.6 ± 0.1 (92)	10.5 ± 0.4 (101)	12.7 ± 1.4 (105)	20.0 ± 2.1 (88)	10.0 ± 1.0 (114)	13.2 ± 0.6 (116)	26.1 ± 0.5 (102)
10^{-7} M	9.4 ± 0.9 (90)	13.6 ± 1.8 (92)	9.2 ± 0.7 (88)	6.7 ± 1.2 (55)	19.6 ± 2.6 (87)	9.1 ± 0.8 (103)	9.8 ± 0.8 (86)	23.7 ± 2.9 (92)
10^{-6} M	6.6 ± 1.3 (64)	9.1 ± 1.6 (62)	2.4 ± 0.5 (23)	1.2 ± 0.2 (10)	19.2 ± 2.3 (85)	9.5 ± 1.2 (108)	12.6 ± 0.6 (110)	4.5 ± 1.1 (18)

[a] Experiments were performed in quadruplicate. Percent of control value shown in parentheses.

TABLE 5. *Comparison of noncytotoxic analogs of nitrogen mustard derivatives on growth of MCF-7 cells[a]*

		DNA (µg ± SD)			
Ha compound	Analog	Control	Ha compound[b]	Control	Analog
Ha IV	(structure)	10.4 ± 1.4	6.6 ± 1.3 (64)	10.9 ± 1.0	11.4 ± 0.5 (104)
Ha VI	(structure)	10.4 ± 1.5	2.4 ± 0.5 (23)	12.4 ± 0.8	14.1 ± 1.5 (114)
Ha VI	(structure)	10.4 ± 1.5	2.4 ± 0.5 (23)	12.4 ± 0.8	12.0 ± 1.0 (97)
Ha VII	(structure)	12.1 ± 1.8	1.2 ± 0.2 (10)	12.4 ± 0.8	11.7 ± 0.7 (94)
Ha VII	(structure)	12.1 ± 1.8	1.2 ± 0.2 (10)	12.4 ± 0.8	12.0 ± 0.8 (97)

[a]Experiments were performed in quadruplicate. Percent of control values is given in parentheses.
[b]Compounds 10^{-6} M.

TABLE 6. *Irreversibility of inhibitory effect of nitrogen mustard derivatives on growth of MCF-7 cells*[a]

	DNA (µg ± SD)			
		Ha compound[b]		
	Control	Alone	+ E₂	+ ORG 4333
Ha IV	12.3 ± 0.6	10.0 ± 0.2 (81)	9.4 ± 0.6 (76)	8.7 ± 1.6 (71)
Ha V	12.3 ± 0.6	9.5 ± 1.0 (77)	8.8 ± 1.1 (72)	9.1 ± 0.8 (74)
Ha VI	12.9 ± 1.2	9.0 ± 0.3 (70)	6.8 ± 1.2 (53)	6.8 ± 0.9 (53)
Ha VII	17.2 ± 1.2	1.6 ± 0.3 (9)	1.6 ± 0.4 (9)	0.9 ± 0.5 (5)

[a] Experiments were performed in quadruplicate. Percent of control values is given in parentheses.
[b] Ha, 10^{-6} M; E₂ and ORG 4333, 10^{-8} M.

between the mono- and the binitrogen mustard derivatives suggests that substitution near each oxygen function has additive effects on the decrease in binding affinity. Therefore, one should consider for future syntheses the possibility of linking the cytotoxic agent to an estrogen moiety through a long spacer chain (1).

As most estrogens and antiestrogens, the aziridine derivative of estrone interacted reversibly with ER. In contrast, all the nitrogen mustard interacted very strongly, in an apparent irreversible manner. This high stability of interaction suggests an alkylation of the receptors by the cytotoxic groups.

Assessment of the action of these drugs on the growth of the two breast cancer cell lines MCF-7 (ER+) and Evsa-T (ER−) revealed a marked inhibitory effect on the former. The aziridine derivative (E_1-Azi) had a biphasic effect on the growth of MCF-7, either stimulating at low dose or inhibiting at higher concentration. It seems likely that ER was the mediator of this biphasic effect, since it was suppressed by either nafoxidine or estradiol. The four nitrogen mustard derivatives produced a stronger inhibition of the growth of MCF-7 cells. The compounds having the highest apparent binding affinities (Ha VI and Ha VII) produced the strongest inhibition, suggesting a participation of ER in the cytotoxic action of these nitrogen mustard derivatives. Estradiol and 11-chloromethyl estradiol, however, were unable to reverse this inhibition. This is in contrast with the behavior of conventional antiestrogens, but may be explained by the fact that the interaction with ER is much stronger with these nitrogen mustard derivatives than with antiestrogens. An alternative explanation would be that these nitrogen mustard derivatives exert a high nonspecific cytotoxicity on the MCF-7 cell line. Indeed, additional studies are required to elucidate the specificity of these inhibitory effects and their possible mediation through ER.

Finally, the present results highlight the potential interest of the *in vitro* tests described here for the purpose of defining guidelines for the production of other cytotoxic-linked estrogens. A definite advantage of these procedures is that they require only small amounts of drug (1–10 mg), which makes them especially suitable for the screening of a large number of compounds.

ACKNOWLEDGMENTS

We wish to thank Drs. H. Hamacher (B. G. A., Berlin, Germany), G. Van Binst (Vrije Universiteit Brussel, Brussels, Belgium), and F. J. Zeelen (Organon, Oss, The Netherlands). This work was supported by a grant from the "Fonds Cancérologique de la Caisse générale d'Epargne et de Retraite," Belgium, and by Contract 1-CM-53840 from the National Cancer Institute, Bethesda, Maryland.

REFERENCES

1. Bucourt, R., Vignau, M., Torelli, V., Richard-Foy, H., Geynet, C., Secco-Millet, C., Redeuilh, G., and Baulieu, E. E. (1978): *J. Biol. Chem.*, 253:8221–8228.

2. Heuson, J. C., Legros, N., Heuson-Stiennon, J. A., Leclercq, G., and Pasteels, J. L. (1976): In: *Breast Cancer: Trends in Research and Treatment (EORTC, Vol. 2),* edited by J. C. Heuson, W. H. Mattheiem, and M. Rozencweig, pp. 81–93. Raven Press, New York.
3. Katzenellenbogen, J. A., Johnson, H. J., Jr., and Carlson, K. E. (1973): *Biochemistry,* 12:4092–4099.
4. Leclercq, G., Deboel, M. C., and Heuson, J. C. (1976): *Int. J. Cancer,* 18:750–756.
5. Leclercq, G., Devleeschouwer, N., Legros, N., and Heuson, J. C. (1980): *Eur. J. Cancer (in press).*
6. Leclercq, G., and Heuson, J. C. (1980): In: *Pharmacological Modulation of Steroid Action,* edited by E. Ganazzani, F. di Carlo, and W. I. P. Mainwaring, pp. 217–226. Raven Press, New York.
7. Lippman, M. E., Bolan, G., and Huff, K. (1976): *Cancer Res.,* 36:4595–4601.
8. Watson, S., Medina, D., and Clark, J. H. (1977): *Cancer Res.,* 37:3344–3348.
9. Zava, D. T., Chamness, G. C., Horwitz, K. B., and McGuire, W. L. (1977): *Science,* 196:663–664.

Hormones and Cancer, edited by S. Iacobelli et al.
Raven Press, New York © 1980.

LHRH and LHRH-Like Synthetic Agonists: Paradoxical Antifertility Effects and Their Therapeutic Relevance to Steroid-Dependent Tumors

Alan Corbin, *Eugene Rosanoff, and Frederick J. Bex

*Sections of Endocrinology and *Virology, Wyeth Laboratories, Inc.,
Philadelphia, Pennsylvania 19101, U.S.A.*

The extensive developments regarding the synthesis and pharmacologic identification of luteinizing hormone (LH) releasing hormone (LHRH) have led to the generation of analogs with far superior agonistic (LH-releasing and ovulation-inducing) properties (9,10,26,27). These "super analogs," like the parent molecule, have been shown to release the gonadotropins LH and follicle-stimulating hormone (FSH), induce ovulation, and produce, in both females and males, paradoxical antifertility effects in several animal species (4–7). It has clearly been established that this trio of effects is an integral part of the reproductive pharmacologic profile of this class of peptides.

Numerous studies have demonstrated mechanisms by which these agents may produce their contradictory antireproductive effects, including partial inhibition of gonadal steroidogenesis (3,4,8,15,16). These findings have suggested the possibility that the LHRH agonists may inhibit the growth of steroid-dependent tumors (14).

This report will review the basic concepts and developments relevant to the paradoxical contraceptive effects of the LHRH agonists, the mechanisms subserving these effects, and their possible therapeutic use in the treatment of hormone-sensitive cancers.

PARADOXICAL ANTIFERTILITY EFFECTS

Female

The clearly established pregnancy-terminating effects of LHRH and agonistic analogs (3,9,22,24) are consistently associated with the ability to release LH and induce ovulation (characteristic agonist activities). In fact, the ovulation-induction (profertility) test in rats has served to identify LHRH derivatives with potential contragestational (antifertility) activity (6). The paradoxical cor-

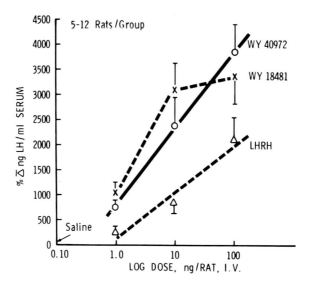

FIG. 1. Effect of LHRH agonists on serum LH levels of ovariectomized steroid blocked rats. *Triangles:* average change. (Reproduced with permission from *Int. J. Gynaecol. Obstet.,* ref. 6.)

relation between these pro- and antifertility effects are exemplified by the activities of the two LHRH agonists, Wy-18,481 (D-Ala^6-DesGly^{10}-Pro^9-LHRH ethyl-amide) and Wy-40,972 (D-Trp^6-N-MeLeu^7-DesGly^{10}-Pro^9-LHRH ethyl-amide), which are superior in potency to LHRH in stimulating release of LH (Fig. 1) and inducing ovulation (Fig. 2). Nevertheless, both compounds cause pregnancy termination when administered before implantation (days 1–7) (Fig. 3) or after implantation (days 7–12) (6,7) (Fig. 4). Additional studies in rats and rabbits, employing various modes of administration (6), reinforced the above conclusions and led to the concept that LHRH agonists may represent a novel and potent class of contraceptives. Other studies have revealed that precoital administration of the agonists to rats during the estrous cycle can delay the onset of estrus and mating, induce premature ovulation, cause ovarian and uterine regression, and lead to reduced fecundity in animals that are inseminated (1,2,22). Furthermore, such treatment inhibits the stimulatory action of human chorionic gonadotropin on the ovaries and uterus (13,23).

The mechanism by which the paradoxical antifertility effects are brought about under short-term and longer-term dosing regimens in a variety of animal models involves a down-regulatory phenomenon: administration of the agonists produces release of LH and FSH and altered patterns of prolactin secretion which, although capable of inducing ovulation under certain circumstances, result in a decrease in ovarian LH, FSH, and prolactin receptors; histologic evidence of luteolysis; interference with steroidogenesis; delayed estrogen secretion; decreased progesterone secretion; and eventual removal of uterine and/

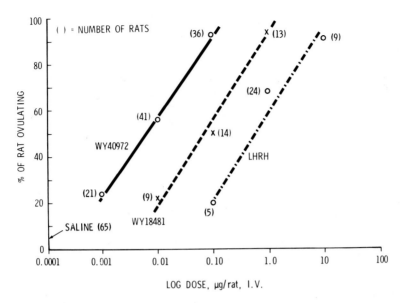

FIG. 2. Ovulation induction with LHRH agonists in pentobarbital-treated ("nembutalized") proestrous rats.

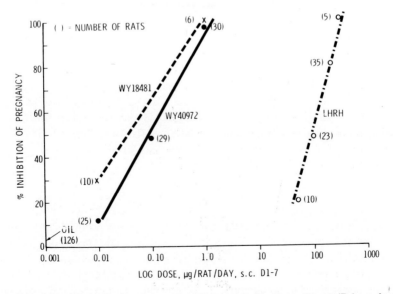

FIG. 3. Postcoital contraceptive effect of LHRH agonists in rat: treatment (R_x) on days 1–7 post coitum.

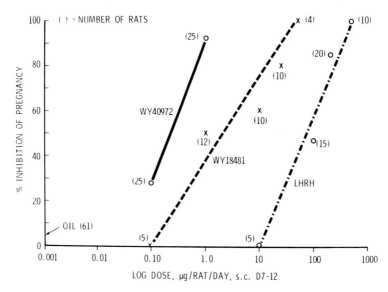

FIG. 4. Postcoital contraceptive effect of LHRH agonists in rat: Treatment (R_x) on days 7–12 post coitum.

or placental support, producing either infertile cycles or pregnancy termination (3,4,6,7,15). In immature female rats, the agonists retard pubertal development as evidenced by delayed vaginal opening and inhibition of weight gain of the ovaries and uteri (6,7). In cases of prolonged treatment, "pituitary exhaustion" ensues, resulting in reduced gonadotropin output and inhibition of ovulation. Several of these effects have been observed in the clinic in attempts to utilize the agonists to treat infertility (6,7) or, more recently, in trials specifically designed to evaluate the contraceptive potential of this class of peptides (17,21,28).

In general, in the animal models employed, the agonists eventually lead to steroid withdrawal, thereby lessening or removing support for steroid-dependent target tissues. All the suppressive effects of LHRH agonist intervention on reproductive function are reversible, since cessation of treatment leads to reactivation of pituitary responsiveness, replenishment of gonadal receptors, and restoration of normal cyclicity and breeding patterns (6,7).

Male

Administration of various LHRH agonists to male rats produces antireproductive effects analogous to those observed in female animals. Treatment with these agents results in a rapid decline in concentration of testicular LH receptors, followed by a reduction in the weights of the testes, seminal vesicles, and ventral prostate; histologic disorganization of the seminiferous tubules and spermatogonia; damage to Leydig cells; decreased spermatogenesis and testosterone production; decreased incidence of mating; and decreased capacity for fertilization (6,8,16). The severity of these effects is a function of the dose and length of administration of the agonist; the effects are reversible and the time necessary for return of full reproductive capacity after cessation of treatment is related to the intensity and duration of the treatment.

The finding that paradoxical effects of LHRH-like peptides on fertility, similar to those observed in the female, occur in the male suggests a common mechanism of action. It was originally thought that the LHRH agonists would be useful in the therapy of male reproductive dysfunction, based on the purported profertility effects (i.e., LH release, ovulation induction) of these agents. However, use of these compounds in treating retarded puberty, hypogonadotropic hypogonadism, hypospermia, and nondescended testes has met with only limited, if any, success.

ANTITUMOR EFFECTS

The data described above demonstrate that LHRH and agonists possess a reproductive pharmacologic profile predominantly contraceptive in nature, in spite of numerous and, at times, heroic attempts to stimulate human fertility with these agents in the clinic. Although, in the examples cited, decreased gonadal steroidogenesis has generally been presumed to result from effects of the agonists on pituitary gonadotropin release, a direct action on the gonad has not been ruled out. In view of the dramatic inhibitory effects on gonadal steroid-producing and gonadal steroid-dependent tissues, it was anticipated that these LHRH agonists may induce tumor regression in a manner analogous to that produced by ovariectomy or antiestrogenic drugs and, therefore, be of therapeutic value (14).

Several studies have indicated that LHRH agonists can produce regression of mammary tumors (11–13). The agonists, D-Leu[6]-DesGly[10]-Pro[9]-LHRH ethylamide (11,12,14) and D-Ser(tBU)[6]-AZGly[10]-LHRH (13,18–20) have been shown to retard the growth of mammary tumors induced by 7,12-dimethylbenz[a]anthracene (DMBA). In our laboratory, the development of tumors in 4-day-old hamsters inoculated with mouse mammary tumor cells was retarded by parenteral administration of either LHRH or Wy-18,481 for a period of 10 days. Tumor size remained depressed during the 5 days following cessation of treatment (Fig. 5). It is noteworthy that this tumor retardation occurred during suppression of the animal's own immune defense system, since these recipients had been treated with antilymphocytic serum on two occasions during the study. Thus, the peptides were capable of attenuating tumor growth under conditions which tended to promote maximal tumor growth. The results obtained suggest that the reduction of the number of tumors and the tumor regression produced by chronic treatment with these peptides is analogous to that observed following ovariectomy or treatment with the antiestrogen tamoxifen (14,19); furthermore, withdrawal of peptide treatment can lead to a recrudescence of the tumor,

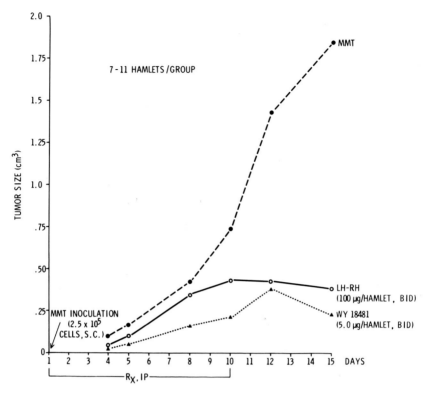

FIG. 5. Effect of LHRH or synthetic agonist on mouse mammary tumor (MMT) growth in neonatal hamsters. *Closed circles:* untreated control group.

which upon reinitiation of treatment, once again is followed by tumor regression (12). This would indicate the need for uninterrupted or long-term intermittent administration of these compounds.

It is important to note that prolactin, too, may play a role in the support of the growth of mammary tumors, through a direct effect on the tumor itself, as well as through stimulation of estrogen secretion. While treatment with the LHRH agonists reduces both blood prolactin and estradiol levels in the various animal models described, including mammary tumor-bearing animals which also show atrophy of pituitary lactotrophs (11,19), it cannot be stated conclusively that it is the reduced secretion of either or both these hormone(s) that retards the growth of the tumor. However, we assume that it is the inhibition of estradiol secretion by the LHRH agonist (i.e., "chemical castration") that is the major determinant; this assumption is based on similarities to the results derived from the ovariectomy and tamoxifen studies (11,14,19), those derived from the gonadal LH-receptor down-regulation investigations, and those suggested by pituitary LH-exhaustion studies during chronic agonist administration.

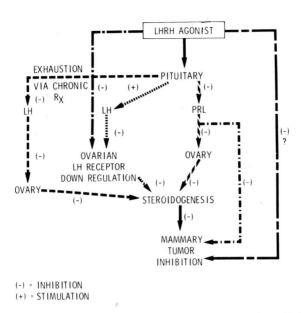

FIG. 6. Possible mechanisms of action of mammary tumor regression with LHRH agonists. R_x, treatment.

An alternative possibility is a direct action of the LHRH agonist on the tumor itself. The various means by which LHRH agonists may manifest their antitumor effects are shown schematically in Fig. 6.

These data suggest that LHRH and agonists may be valuable drugs in the treatment of gonadal steroid-dependent tumors (including, for example, prostatic hypertrophy) on their own or as therapeutic adjuncts to established procedures such as surgical extirpation, chemotherapy, radiation, and antigonadal steroid medication. However, it is likely that LHRH agonists may be of therapeutic value only in those cases of breast tumors that are estrogen-receptor positive (25). Likewise, treatment with LHRH-analogs may only be useful for those prostatic tumors that are androgen-receptor positive. Moreover, neoplasms of this general category (i.e., arising in reproductive organs) that possess receptors for additional hormones such as prolactin, progesterone, LH, and LH-like hormones (e.g., hCG), may be candidates for LHRH agonist intervention, based on the ability of such peptides to interfere with the secretion and action of these hormones, as demonstrated in studies of their antifertility effects.

CONCLUSIONS

The data reviewed indicate that LHRH and related synthetic agonists produce profound antifertility effects in both sexes in a variety of animal species. While profertility effects, such as the induction of gonadotropin release and ovulation, are also part of the pharmacologic profile of these compounds, their paradoxical antifertility effects predominate and these have been extensively evaluated for potential contraceptive use. These peptides probably produce their suppressive effects on reproduction in both males and females by a common mechanism, which ultimately results in disruption of pituitary–gonadal function, depressed steroidogenesis, and inhibition of target organs dependent on gonadal endocrine support. The utilization of these effects has been extended into the realm of cancer therapy. The ability of the LHRH-like agonists to inhibit the growth of steroid-dependent tumors (e.g., mammary cancer) is analogous to the effects produced by ovariectomy and antisteroid treatment with steroid hormone antagonists. Therefore, these peptides may represent a potentially novel pharmacotherapy for selected hormone-sensitive tumors.

REFERENCES

1. Banik, U. K., and Givner, M. L. (1975): *J. Reprod. Fertil.,* 44:87–94.
2. Beattie, C. W., and Corbin, A. (1977): *Biol. Reprod.,* 16:333–339.
3. Beattie, C. W., Corbin, A., Cole, G., Corry, S., Jones, R. C., Koch, K., and Tracy, J. (1977): *Biol. Reprod.,* 16:322–332.
4. Bex, F. J., and Corbin, A. (1979): *Endocrinology,* 105:139–145.
5. Corbin, A., and Beattie, C. W. (1975): *Endocr. Res. Commun.,* 2:445–458.
6. Corbin, A., Beattie, C. W., Jones, R., and Bex, F. J. (1979): *Int. J. Gynaecol. Obstet.,* 16:359–372.
7. Corbin, A., Beattie, C. W., Tracy, J., Jones, R., Foell, T. J., Yardley, J., and Rees, R. (1978): *Int. J. Fertil.,* 23:81–92.
8. Corbin, A., and Bex, F. J. (1980): In: *Regulation of Male Fertility, Vol. 5,* edited by G. R. Cunningham, W. B. Schill, and E. S. E. Hafez, pp. 55–63. Martinus Nijhoff, The Hague.
9. Corbin, A., Bex, F. J., Yardley, J. P., Rees, R. W., Foell, T. J., and Sarantakis, D. (1979): *Endocr. Res. Commun.,* 6:1–14.
10. Coy, D. H., and Schally, A. V. (1978): *Ann. Clin. Res.,* 10:139–144.
11. Danguy, A., Legros, N., Heuson-Stiennon, J. A., Pasteels, J. L., Atassi, G., and Heuson, J. C. (1977): *Eur. J. Cancer,* 13:1089–1094.
12. DeSombre, E. R., Johnson, E. S., and White, W. F. (1976): *Cancer Res.,* 36:3830–3833.
13. Dutta, A. S., Furr, B. J. A., Giles, M. B., Valcaccia, B., and Walpole, A. L. (1978): *Biochem. Biophys. Res. Commun.,* 81:382–390.
14. Johnson, E. S., Seely, J. H., White, W. F., and DeSombre, E. R. (1976): *Science,* 194:329–330.
15. Kledzik, G. S., Cusan, L., Auclair, C., Kelly, P. A., and Labrie, F. (1978): *Fertil. Steril.,* 30:348–353.
16. Labrie, F., Auclair, C., Cusan, L., Kelly, P. A., Pelletier, G., and Ferland, L. (1978): *Int. J. Androl. [Suppl.],* 2:303–318.
17. Lemay, A., Labrie, F., Ferland, L., and Raynaud, J. P. (1979): *Fertil. Steril.,* 31:29–34.
18. Maynard, P. V., and Nicholson, R. I. (1979): *Br. J. Cancer,* 39:274–279.
19. Nicholson, R. I., Finney, E. J., and Maynard, P. V. (1978): *J. Endocrinol.,* 79:51P–52P.
20. Nicholson, R. I., and Maynard, P. V. (1979): *Br. J. Cancer,* 39:268–273.
21. Nillius, J. S., Bergquist, C., and Wide, L. (1978): *Contraception,* 17:537–545.
22. Ripple, R. H., and Johnson, E. S. (1976): *Proc. Soc. Exp. Biol. Med.,* 152:29–32.
23. Ripple, R. H., and Johnson, E. S. (1976): *Proc. Soc. Exp. Biol. Med.,* 152:432–436.
24. Rivier, C., Rivier, J., and Vale, V. (1978): *Endocrinology,* 103:2299–2304.
25. Sarg, M. J., Jr. (1979): *J. Reprod. Med.,* 23:3–11.
26. Schally, A. V., Kastin, A. J., and Coy, D. H. (1976): *Int. J. Fertil.,* 21:1–30.
27. Vale, W., Rivier, C., and Brown, M. (1977): *Annu. Rev. Physiol.,* 39:473–527.
28. Yen, S. S. C., and Casper, R. F. (1979): *Program of the 61st Meeting of the Endocrine Society,* Anaheim, California, p. 181. (Abstr. 435).

Hormones and Cancer, edited by S. Iacobelli et al.
Raven Press, New York © 1980.

An Approach to Site-Directed Chemotherapy of Hormone-Sensitive Cancer

H. R. Lindner, F. Kohen, and A. Amsterdam

Department of Hormone Research, The Weizmann Institute of Science, Rehovot, Israel

HORMONE RECEPTORS AS TARGET SIGNALS

For many years, the oncologist's interest in the existence of hormone receptors on certain tumors has been confined to their prognostic significance in indicating whether a particular tumor is likely to respond to manipulation of the endocrine environment, be it by hormone administration or hormone deprivation. Only recently, consideration has also been given to the possibility that the presence of these specific recognition sites may be exploited to provide a homing mechanism for chemotherapeutic agents suitably linked to the homologous hormone or a cognate ligand of high affinity for the receptor.

The usefulness of cytotoxic drugs in the treatment of malignancy is severely limited, at present, by the toxicity of these agents to normal tissues, such as the rapidly proliferating cells of the bone marrow and gastrointestinal tract or the myocardium. Some attempts to impart greater selectivity of action to such drugs, for example, by coupling to lysozomotropic carriers (20) or to antibody directed to tumor antigens (4), have shown promise in model systems but still have to overcome significant obstacles before they can afford a feasible therapeutic option. As an alternative approach to a site-directed chemotherapy, the use of hormonal carriers would seem to have the advantage of ready availability compared to tumor-specific antibodies, and of greater specificity relative to general endocytosis-promoting macromolecules. On the other hand, the hormone-carrier approach is inherently limited in scope to tumors in which specific hormone receptors are expressed. In addition, it poses difficulties in view of the small number of such receptors carried even in susceptible target cells and the need for sophisticated design of hormone-drug conjugates to preserve high affinity to the receptor and ensure selective drug release within the tumor cell.

A significant proportion of neoplasms arising in hormone-target organs such as breast, ovary, uterus, prostate, melanocytes, or the lymphatic system retain, at least temporarily, their ability to bind the cognate hormone(s) with high affinity. For the purpose of this discussion, it is useful to distinguish between hormone receptors that are located within the target cell and those located on the cell surface. The receptors for steroid hormones are situated in the cytosol, and upon binding the hormone are translocated into the nucleus. By contrast, the polypeptide hormones are bound to the outer cell membrane, but as we shall see below, the bound hormone is subsequently internalized and concentrated in lysozomes which are rich in hydrolytic enzymes.

STEROID HORMONES AS DRUG CARRIERS

A number of steroid derivatives have been prepared incorporating anticancer drugs, notably of the alkylating variety, and some of these have reached the stage of clinical trial. In designing such drugs, there could conceivably be three different objectives: (a) to achieve selective concentration of the drug within the target cell due to binding of the carrier to the cytoplasmic receptor, relying on intracellular enzymes to release the active drug by cleaving a susceptible bond, and on diffusion for it to reach its ultimate site of action; (b) to cause irreversible damage to the hormone receptor by affinity labeling, thus impairing the growth potential of the tumor cell to the extent that growth is still dependent on hormonal stimulation; and (c) a more ambitious aim could be to promote the entry of an active group into the nucleus while still associated with the hormone–receptor complex, so that it will bind to an acceptor site on the chromatin, thus facilitating its attack on the genome. In each case, it would seem essential that the affinity of the hormone for its receptor be preserved in the course of derivatization. The design of nucleotropic steroid-drug conjugates [see (c)] is likely to have even more stringent structural requirements, since the ability of the cytoplasmic receptor to undergo transformation into nuclear receptor must also be preserved.

While much remains to be learned, some of the structural requirements for high affinity to steroid receptors are known from binding and competition studies, photoaffinity labeling (see ref. 10) and from work on affinity-chromatography of these receptors (see ref. 15). These studies can provide at least some guidelines as to which positions on the steroid or steroid–analog molecule are more tolerant of bulky substitution (e.g., the 7α-position of estradiol or the end of the hexane chain of hexestrol), and which modifications result essentially in complete loss of affinity for the receptor (e.g., substitution of the phenolic or the 17-hydroxyl group of estradiol), and point to the importance of the length and character of the bridge linking the hormone and drug. Obviously, the link must be such that the cytotoxic moiety is released, upon cleavage of the conjugate by intracellular enzymes, in its active form.

In the design of the first generation of steroid-nitrogen mustard conjugates these considerations have largely been ignored, and the preexisting functional groups of the hormone, which determine specificity towards the cytosol receptor, were used for derivatization. It is therefore not surprising that such compounds show only minimal affinity for the receptor. Thus, estramustine [Estracyt® (Leo 299) estradiol 3-bis(2-chloroethyl)carbamate 17β-dihydrogen phosphate] has about 10^{-5} times lower affinity than that of native estradiol (22).

The situation is reminiscent of the development of antisteroidal antisera. The most convenient way of rendering steroids antigenic was to attach them to macromolecular carriers through existing functional groups, but the antisera thus generated lacked specificity (12). Only by deliberately shifting the point of attachment to sites remote from the determinants of hormonal specificity were antisera produced with selective affinity towards particular steroid hormones (11,13). While antibody and receptor recognize different aspects of the steroid molecule, similar considerations are applicable to the design of drug-hormone conjugates likely to yield compounds with high affinity for the receptor.

Some awareness of these problems is evident in the interesting syntheses by Hamacher (8) of 2- or 4-monosubstituted estradiol mustards, which apparently retain some receptor activity (1–3%). Our own results also indicate the low affinity for receptor of steroid hormone analogs conjugated with daunomycin through positions 3 or 21 and our current efforts in this area are concentrated on derivatization at positions 7α and 6 of the steroid molecule. Often a synthetic analog of the native hormone is available with higher affinity for the homologous receptor and affords an advantageous starting point for the synthesis of drug–steroid conjugates.

PEPTIDE AND PROTEIN HORMONES AS DRUG CARRIERS

The main purpose of this chapter is to draw attention to the possibility of using a similar approach for targeting drugs to tumor cells carrying receptors for peptide and protein hormones. While these receptors are located on the outer aspect of the cell membrane, there is evidence that upon contact with the hormone the hormone–receptor complex undergoes internalization. Thus we could show by immunofluorescence and high resolution radioautographic techniques (1-3) that receptors for the glycoprotein hormone hCG (human chorionic gonadotropin) on ovarian granulosa cells are initially diffusely distributed over the cell surface (Figs. 1 and 2). After exposure for 2 hr to labeled hormone, 80% of the label was still associated with the plasmalemma, but much of it was aggregated in clusters overlying invaginations of the plasma membrane which, in turn, are related to submembranous bundles of microfilaments (1). Even at this time, about 6% of the silver grains appeared in endocytotic vesicles and 10% in lysozomes. After 8 hr, 73% of the hormone was internalized, with 50% of the radioactivity associated with lysozomes (Fig. 3). Significantly, this internalization of the hormone was accompanied by release into the medium of radioactivity that could be identified as mono- and diiodotyrosine, indicating that hydrolysis of the labeled hormone had taken place. No such hydrolysis was observed when labeled hormone was incubated with cells after prior blocking of their receptors with excess cold hormone, suggesting that the process depended on cellular uptake.

Endocytotic uptake of peptide hormones has also been documented with regard to melanocyte-stimulating hormone (MSH) (6), insulin (16,19), and epidermal growth factor (5,16). Here too, internalization occurred via formation of aggre-

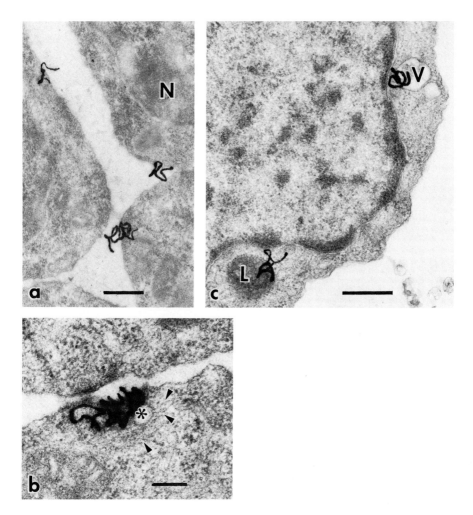

FIG. 1. Electron microscopic autoradiograms of cultured granulosa cells after 3 hr incubation with 2 IU/ml of [^{125}I]hCG. **a:** Individual silver grains as well as clustered grains are localized over cell membrane. N, nucleus; bar, 0.5 μm; ×21,900. **b:** Cluster of silver grains is evident on plasmalemma of granulosa cell. Radioactivity is associated with invagination of membrane *(asterisk).* Filamentous material appears to be associated with infolding of membrane *(arrowheads),* and this area is devoid of ribosomes. Bar, 0.2 μm; ×47,300. **c:** Part of granulosa cell. Labeling is confined to intracellular smooth vesicle (V) and lysosome-like structure (L) adjacent to plasma membrane. Bar, 0.5 μm; ×26,280. (From Amsterdam et al., ref. 3, with permission.)

gates and movement to specialized areas of the membrane identified as "coated pits" (16). Since such endocytosis was demonstrated using fluorescein or rhodamine-labeled peptides, it appears likely that the capacity of the hormone to undergo this receptor-mediated process can be preserved after bulky derivatiza-

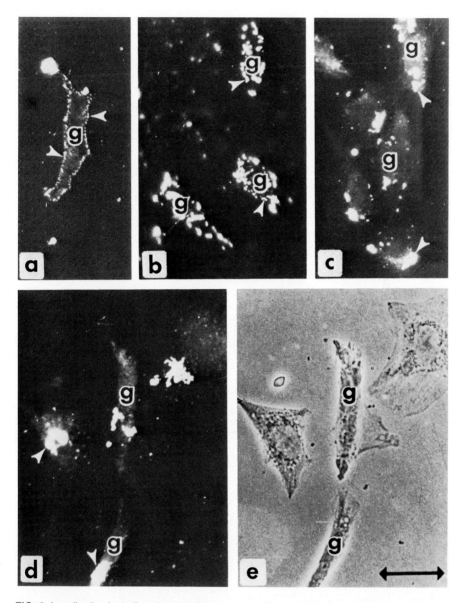

FIG. 2. Localization by indirect immunofluorescence of receptor-bound hCG in cultured granulosa cells. Calibration = 30 μm. **a:** Cells were incubated with 200 IU/ml of the hormone for 5 min and then fixed with formaldehyde. Tiny specks of fluorescence *(arrowheads)* are visible at the entire circumference of an elongated granulosa cell (g). **b:** Cells were incubated for 120 min with the hormone and fixed with formaldehyde. Clusters of fluorescence are visible *(arrowheads)* over 3 granulosa cells (g). The clusters seem to be larger than those obtained after 5 min incubation with the hormone. **c:** Cells were incubated for 90 min with the hormone and subsequently with anti-hCG without prior fixation of the cell. Large clusters are seen at the circumference of several granulosa cells (g). **d:** Treatment was as described in **c**, but the cells are incubated for an additional 1 hr after removing of excess antibodies. Note large clusters and caps *(arrowheads)* over granulosa cells (g). **e:** The same field as in **d** through phase contrast optics indicating the integrity of the cells. (From Amstedam et al., ref. 2, with permission.)

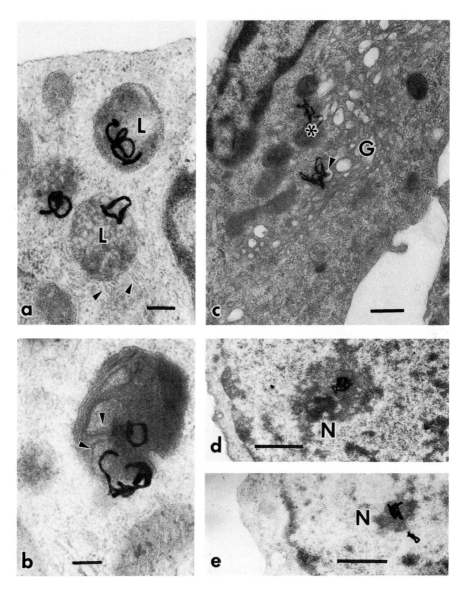

FIG. 3. Electron microscopic autoradiograms of cultured granulosa cells after 3 hr of incubation with 2 IU/ml of [125I]hCG followed by 5 hr of incubation with 20 IU/ml of unlabeled hormone. **a:** Part of granulosa cell. Silver grains are localized over lysozome-like structures (L). Note that filamentous material appears to be associated with lower lysozome *(arrowheads)*. Bar, 0.2 μm; ×35,520. **b:** Same as in **a.** Note that membrane fragments *(arrowheads)* are visible within lysozome. Bar, 0.2 μm; ×37,590. **c:** Part of granulosa cell showing Golgi complex (G). Silver grains are visible on smooth membrane vesicle *(arrowhead)*, which seems to be part of Golgi complex. Another cluster of silver grains is seen in close proximity to electron-dense granules *(astrisk)*. Bar, 0.5 μm; ×17,360. **d:** Silver grains over heterochromatin area of granulosa cell nucleus (N). Bar, 1 μm; ×13,250. **e:** Part of another granulosa cell showing labeling in a similar position to **d.** Bar, 1 μm; ×13,620. (From Amsterdam et al., ref. 3, with permission.)

tion, provided the site and method of substitution are appropriately selected.

These observations suggest that it may be possible to use peptides and protein hormone conjugates of cytotoxic drugs to achieve selected concentration of such drugs in cells carrying the appropriate receptor. Thus far, a single attempt in this direction has been reported: Varga et al. (21) prepared a β-MSH-daunomycin conjugate and showed that it was toxic at 1.4 μM to Cloudman S-91 melanoma cells but not to 3T3 fibroblasts, though the latter were sensitive to free daunomycin. The conjugate was not fully characterized chemically, but is believed to involve substitution at Asp[1], Lys[6], and Lys[17] with a molar ratio of daunomycin to β-MSH of 2.2. The mode of preparation of the conjugate should yield a saturated carbon-nitrogen bond not obviously susceptible to cleavage by known cellular enzymes. There was no clear evidence that the conjugate was significantly more potent than the free drug, per residue of alkaloid, on cultured melanoma cells, but it did exhibit selectivity with regard to cell type. Unfortunately, there has been no published follow-up to date of this brief but promising report.

In addition to MSH-receptors, human melanoma cells frequently possess receptors for estradiol, glucocorticoids (18), and nerve growth factor (NGF) (7). Thus, six of seven human melanoma cell lines were reported to carry NGF receptors (7). Some of our current efforts are directed towards preparing conjugates of NGF with cytotoxic drugs of established activity against melanoma cells. However, a recent report (17) suggests that at least some human melanoma lines secrete NGF. If so, this secretion may block the attachment of exogenous modified NGF and thus frustrate this approach.

Similar drug conjugates are being synthesized, using prolactin and glycoprotein hormones such as hCG as carriers. There is no precise information concerning the domain of these hormones involved in interaction with the homologous receptor, so that the synthetic approach has still to be largely empirical, using derivatization of either the intact hormone or individual subunits of the glycoprotein hormones. The conjugates will be assayed for ability to bind to receptor preparations, to undergo internalization, for susceptibility to cleavage by lysozomal enzymes, and ultimately for their ability, relative to the free drug, to kill selectively tumor cells carrying the relevant receptors *in vitro* and *in vivo* (see Table 1). These tests have not yet progressed to a state permitting definitive statements regarding the relative merit of individual preparations.

A recent intriguing publication by Oeltmann and Heath (14) reports a selective toxic effect on rat R2C Leydig cells of a hybrid molecule composed of the A-subunit of the seed toxin protein ricin and linked by a disulfide bond to the β-subunit of hCG. Mouse L-cells, which lack LH receptor, failed to respond to this hybrid. The results are interpreted as indicating that the β-subunit of hCG, by attachment to the LH receptor, permitted the penetration of the cell membrane by the A-subunit of ricin, upon reduction of the disulfide band. This work, primarily directed at the elucidation of the mode of hormone action, points to the degree of sophistication possible, and perhaps needed, in the design of effective site-directed chemotherapeutic agents.

TABLE 1. *Desired properties of drug–hormone conjugate for site-directed chemotherapy of hormone-sensitive cancer*

1. Retention of affinity for homologous hormone receptor.
2. Ability to undergo endocytosis (peptide hormone conjugates).
3. Susceptibility to cleavage by lysosomal or other intercellular enzymes with release of active drug—unless conjugate itself is cytostatic.
4. Cytotoxic potency on receptor-carrying cells equal to or greater than that of free drug: lower toxicity than free drug for cells devoid of receptors.
5. Appropriate solubility and pharmacodynamic properties.

DISCUSSION

One may ask whether it will be prudent to use tropic hormones as drug carriers when treating malignancies whose growth they may stimulate. However, it is possible that the hormone will help push the tumor cell into a stage of the cell cycle, such as the S phase, in which it is most susceptible to the cytotoxic action of a given "payload" drug, thus achieving a synergistic action. Again, in many cases the receptor for the hormonal carrier chosen will not be uniquely confined to the tumor cells, but this would be no serious drawback provided the receptor is not present on the normal tissues most sensitive to the toxic side effects of the drug.

Many questions remain to be answered before it can be asserted that the approach outlined above to a site-directed chemotherapy for a restricted class of malignancies is really feasible. Optimization of the design of drug-hormone conjugates for this purpose involves a multitude of variables. The task of exploring these adequately may well be beyond the resources of the individual research laboratory, and certainly requires the collaboration of the chemist, the endocrinologist, and the oncologist. Meanwhile it is humbling to remember that thus far few important drugs have been created by rational design, while many more arose by serendipity. At the same time, such episodes as the recent success in controlling choriocarcinoma should remind us, as pointed out by Hertz (9), that improved treatment of specific forms of malignancy need not await a basic understanding of all cancer. The suffering caused by current cancer therapy often approaches that caused by the disease itself (see Postscript). The ready availability of specific recognition sites on some common tumors derived from hormone target tissues seems to offer opportunities that have not yet been fully exploited.

ACKNOWLEDGMENTS

We are grateful to Mrs. B. Gaier and Mrs. S. Lichter for technical assistance; to Mrs. M. Kopelowitz for typing the manuscript; to the Developmental Therapeutics Program, Chemotherapy, NCI (Dr. J. D. Douros) for the generous gift of daunomycin and adriamycin; and to the Rockefeller Foundation and the Council for Research and Development, Ministry of Commerce, Government of Israel, for generous financial support. H.R.L. is the Adlai E. Stevenson III

Professor of Endocrinology and Reproductive Biology, and A. A. is the incumbent of the Gestetner Career Development Chair at the Weizmann Institute.

POSTSCRIPT

The following poem tries to summarize the advances in the treatment of cancer since the Stone Ages. It takes the form of a dialogue between a witch doctor and a scientifically trained oncologist. For obvious reasons, the author wishes to remain anonymous. While unduly pessimistic, the poem emphasizes that there is no cause for complacency and that there is a definite need for new therapeutic approaches.

THE DREAD MAHOGUS
A Parable of Medical Progress

The Witch Doctor speaks:

We treat the dread mahogus
  With draughts of molten lead,
And strap the luckless victim
  Down on a stony bed.

We dance around his body
  And yell into his ear;
We turn his love to hatred
  And change his hope to fear.

He must eat the loathsome piss-ant
  And drink the bitter gall,
And if he lives to tell of it
  He wasn't sick at all.

The Modern Oncologist speaks:

We treat the dread mahogus
  By scientific rule:
We analyse the serum
  And scrutinize the stool.

Put electrodes on the patient
  And probes within his veins,
We tie his arms to pulleys
  And stretch his legs with cranes.

We pleasantly relieve him
  Of any need to eat:
His nutriments are furnished
  By needles in his feet.

We tell him and his family
  "We'll do our very best,"
Though we've proved it's always fatal
  By biometric test.

(With kind permission of the Editors of *Lancet.*)

REFERENCES

1. Amsterdam, A., Kohen, F., Nimrod, A., and Lindner, H. R. (1979): In: *Ovarian Follicular and Corpus Luteum Function,* edited by C. P. Channing, J. Marsh, and W. A. Sadler, pp. 69–75. Plenum Press, New York.
2. Amsterdam, A., Nimrod, A., Kohen, F., and Lindner, H. R. (1979): In: *Molecular Mechanisms of Biological Recognition,* edited by M. Balaban, pp. 419–428. Elsevier/North-Holland, Amsterdam.
3. Amsterdam, A., Nimrod, A., Lamprecht, S. A., Burstein, Y., and Lindner, H. R. (1979): *Am. J. Physiol.,* 236:E129–E138.
4. Bernstein, A., Hurwitz, E., Maron, R., Arnon, R., Sela, M., and Wilchek, M. (1978): *J. Natl. Cancer Inst.,* 60:379–384.
5. Carpenter, G., and Cohen, S. (1976): *J. Cell Biol.,* 71:159–171.
6. DiPasquale, A., Varga, J. M., Moellmann, G., and McGuire, J. (1978): *J. Anal. Biochem.,* 84:37–48.
7. Fabricant, R. F., De Larco, J. E., and Todaro, C. J. (1977): *Proc. Natl. Acad. Sci. USA,* 74:565–569.
8. Hamacher, H. (1978): *Cancer Treat. Rep.,* 62:1259.
9. Hertz, R. (1978): *Choriocarcinoma and Related Gestational Trophoblastic Tumors in Women.* Raven Press, New York.
10. Katzenellenbogen, J. A. (1978): *Cancer Treat. Rep.,* 62:1243–1250.
11. Kohen, F., Bauminger, S., and Lindner, H. R. (1975): In: *Steroid Immunoassay,* edited by E. H. D. Cameron, S. G. Hillier, and K. Griffiths, pp. 11–31. Alpha Omega, Cardiff.
12. Lieberman, S., Erlanger, B. F., Beiser, S. M., and Agata, F. J. (1959): In: *Recent Prog. Horm. Res.,* 15:165–200.
13. Niswender, G. D., Nett, T. M., Meyer, D. L., and Hagerman, D. D. (1975): In: *Steroid Immunoassay,* edited by E. H. D. Cameron, S. G. Hillier, and K. Griffiths, pp. 61–66. Alpha Omega, Cardiff.
14. Oeltmann, T. N. and Heath, E. C. (1979): *J. Biol. Chem.,* 254:1028–1032.
15. Richard-Foy, H., and Redeuilh, G. (1979): In: *Research on Steroids, Vol. 8,* edited by A. Klopper, L. Lerner, H. J. van der Molen, and F. Sciarra, pp. 159–165. Academic Press, London.
16. Schlessinger, J., Schechter, Y., Willingham, M. C., and Pastan, I. (1978): *Proc. Natl. Acad. Sci. USA,* 75:2659–2663.
17. Sherwin, S. A., Sliski, A. H., and Todaro, G. J. (1979): *Proc. Natl. Acad. Sci. USA,* 76:1288–1292.
18. Stanberry, L. R., and Lindsey, W. F. (1979): In: *Endocrine Society Program and Abstracts, 61st Annual Meeting,* Anaheim, California, p. 151.
19. Terris, S., and Steiner, D. F. (1975): *J. Biol. Chem.,* 250:8389–8398.
20. Trouet, A., Depres-de Campeneere, D., and de Duve, C. (1972): *Nature (New Biol.),* 239:110–112.
21. Varga, J. M., Asato, N., Lande, S., and Lerner, A. B. (1977): *Nature,* 267:56–58.
22. Wittliff, J. L., Weidner, N., Park, D. C., Everson, R. B., and Hall, T. C. (1978): *Cancer Treat. Rep.,* 62:1260–1263.

Subject Index

A

4-Acetoxyandrostene-3,17-dione,
   508, 509
  breast cancer treatment with,
   510–512
  estrogen inhibition by, 510,
   512–513
Acid phosphatase, prostatic tumor
   level of, 364
Actin
  testosterone-induced changes in,
   32, 33
  viral effects on, 37
Actinomycin D, glucocorticoid
   response to, 99, 106
Acute lymphoblastic leukemia, 373
  CEM cell line from, 91, 95, 96
  glucocorticoid receptors in, 373,
   376–378, 391–393, 398
    therapy response and, 371,
    373–376, 378, 379, 395–398,
    399
  null-cell, 392–393
  remissions in, 89–90, 94, 373–375
  steroid-resistant, 90
  steroid treatment of, 91–93, 94
  T-cell, 392–393
Adenocarcinoma, endometrial
  antiestrogen effects on, 443, 444,
   445–448, 452
  estradiol effect on, 482–484
  estrone production and, 478–483
  hormone replacement therapy
   and, 496–497, 499
  nuclear aneuploidy in, 495
  progestogen effect on, 444–448,
   450–452
  radiosurgical management of,
   448–449

risk factors for, 500–501
  steroid excretion in, 474
  steroid receptors in, 495–496
  tumor-host factors in, 452–454
Adenomatous hyperplasia,
   endometrial, 490–492, 497
Adenosine monophosphate, cyclic
  in cell death, 287
  generation of, 287
  growth control by, 288, 290–292
  insulin action via, 214
  mutants of, 287–290
  protein kinase response to, 290
  in tumor regression, 275–277
Adenosine triphosphate
  glucocorticoids inhibition of, 99,
   100, 136, 137
  metabolic effects related to,
   138–142
Adenyl cyclase mutants, 287–288
Adrenalectomy, estrogen
   suppression by, 507
Adrenocortical hormone deficiency,
   125
Adrenocorticotropic hormone
   (ACTH)
  prostatic response to, 185, 186
  prostaglandins influence on, 515
  vasopressin stimulation of, 165
Alanine-preferring transport system,
   122–123
Alkaline phosphodiesterase I,
   hormonal stimulation of,
   114–121
Amanitin, glucocorticoid response
   to, 99
Aminoisobutyric acid,
   glucocorticoid role in
   synthesis of, 99, 100